SPA

The Official Guide to Spa Therapy at Levels 2 & 3

Joan Scott & Andrea Harrison

Elemis Ltd

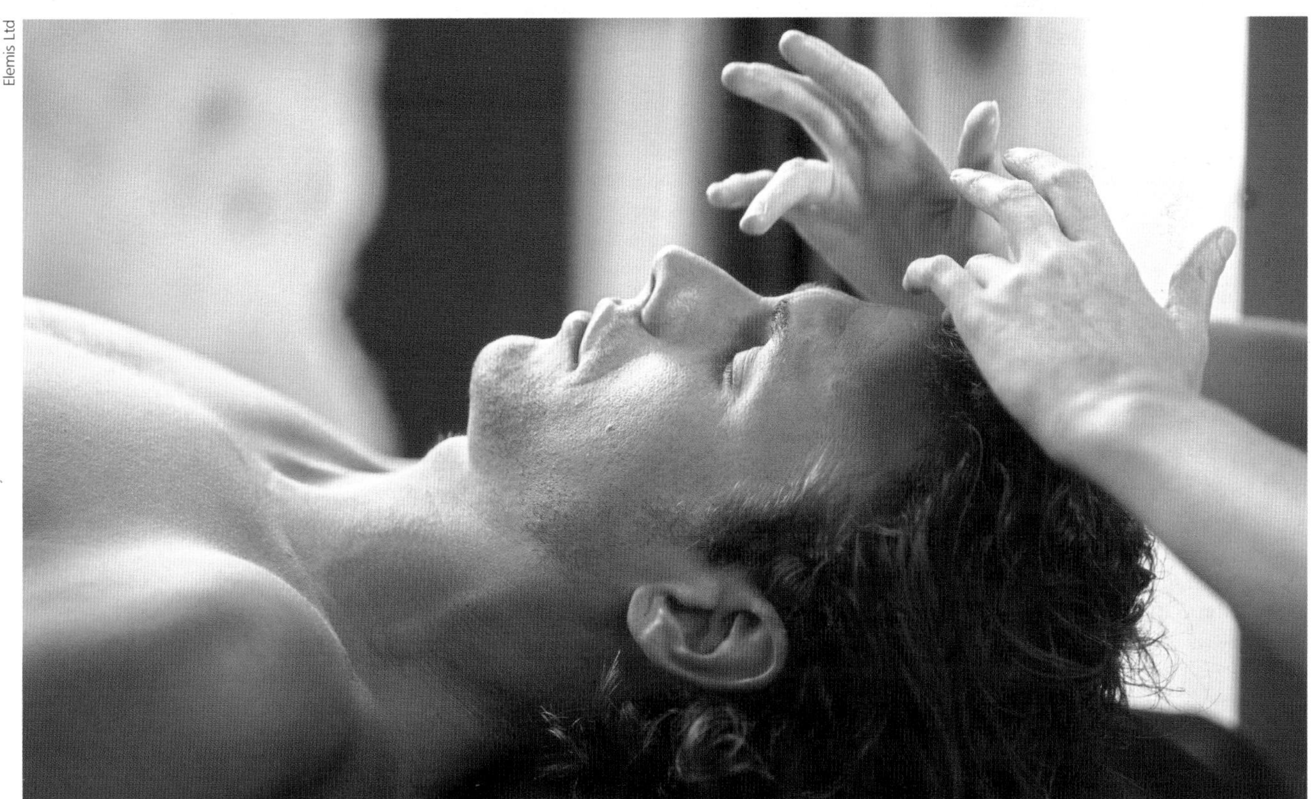

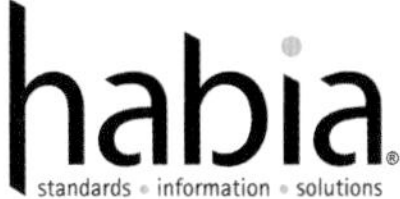
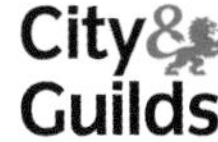
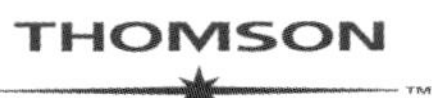

Australia • Canada • Mexico • Singapore • Spain • United Kingdom • United States

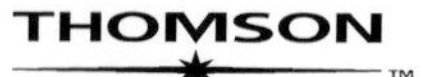

Spa: The Official Guide to Spa Therapy at Levels 2 & 3
Joan Scott and Andrea Harrison

Publishing Director John Yates	Commissioning Editor Melody Dawes	Editorial Assistant Tom Rennie
Production Editor Sonia Pati	Manufacturing Manager Helen Mason	Development Editor Lizzie Catford
Typesetter Integra	Production Controller Maeve Healy	Senior Marketing Executive Natasha Giraudel
Cover Design Harris Cook Turner	Text Design Design Deluxe, Bath, UK	Printer Canale, Italy

For more information, contact Thomson Learning, High Holborn House, 50–51 Bedford Row, London WCIR 4LR or visit us on the World Wide Web at: http://www.thomsonlearning.co.uk

ISBN-13: 978–1–84480–312–5
ISBN-10: 1–84480–312–0

This edition published 2006 by Thomson Learning.

British Library Cataloguing-in-Publication Data
A catalogue record for this book is available from the British Library

SPA

The Official Guide to Spa Therapy at Levels 2 & 3

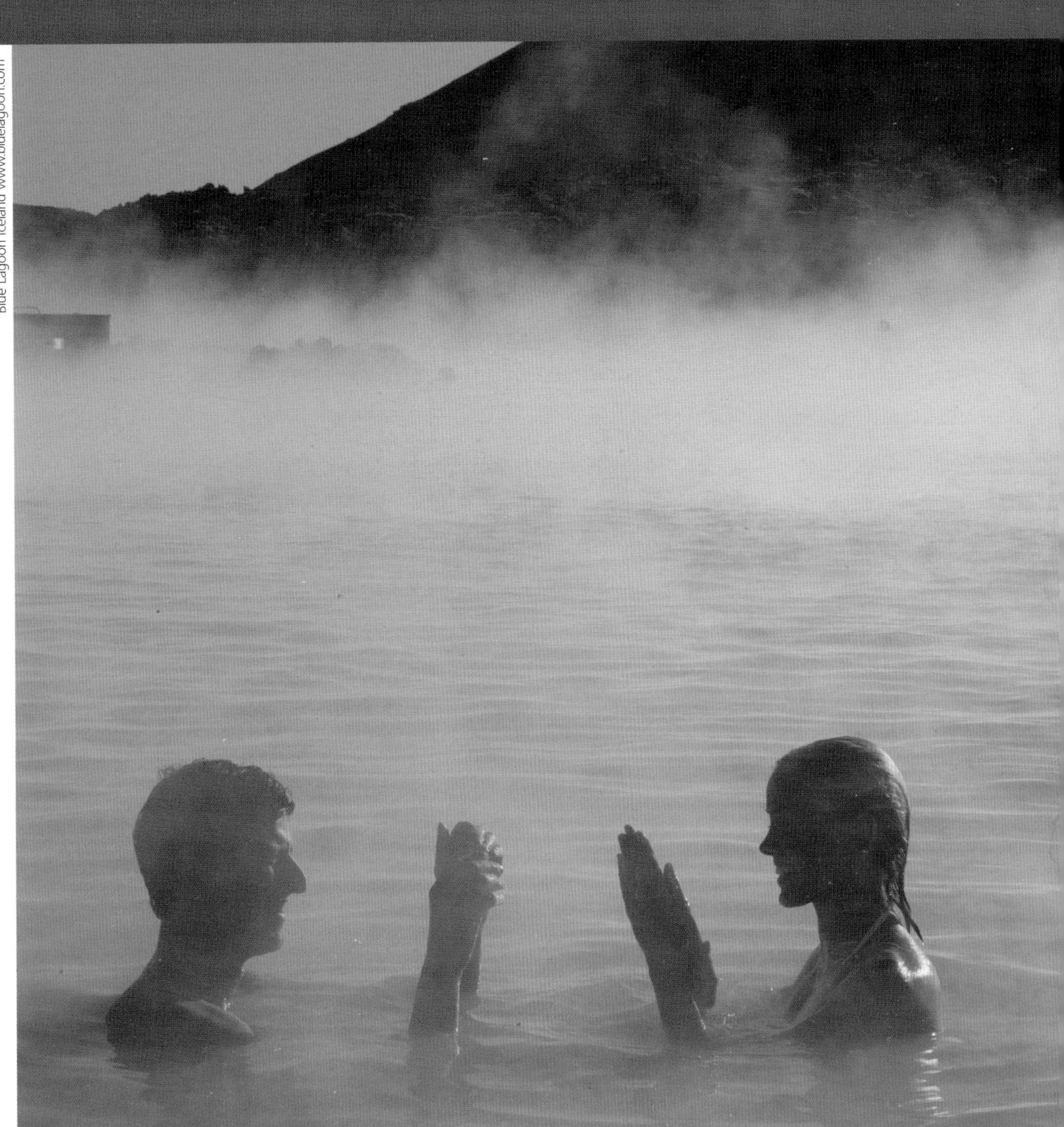

Blue Lagoon Iceland www.bluelagoon.com

HABIA SERIES – RELATED TITLES

HAIRDRESSING

Student textbooks

Begin Hairdressing: The Official Guide to Level 1 1e *Martin Green*
Hairdressing – The Foundations: The Official Guide to Level 2 5e *Leo Palladino and Martin Green*
Professional Hairdressing: The Official Guide to Level 3 4e *Leo Palladino and Martin Green*
The Official Guide to the City & Guilds Certificate in Salon Services 1e *John Armstrong with Anita Crosland, Martin Green and Lorraine Nordmann*
The Colour Book: The Official Guide to Colour for NVQ Levels 2 & 3 1e *Tracey Lloyd with Christine McMillan-Bodell*
eXtensions: The Official Guide to Hair Extensions 1e *Theresa Bullock*
Salon Management *Martin Green*
Men's Hairdressing: Traditional and Modern Barbering 2e *Maurice Lister*
African-Caribbean Hairdressing 2e *Sandra Gittens*
The World of Hair Colour 1e *John Gray*

Professional Hairdressing titles

Trevor Sorbie: The Bridal Hair Book 1e *Trevor Sorbie and Jacki Wadeson*
The Art of Dressing Long Hair 1e *Guy Kremer and Jacki Wadeson*
Patrick Cameron: Dressing Long Hair 1e *Patrick Cameron and Jacki Wadeson*
Patrick Cameron: Dressing Long Hair 2 1e *Patrick Cameron and Jacki Wadeson*
Bridal Hair 1e *Pat Dixon and Jacki Wadeson*
Professional Men's Hairdressing: The art of cutting and styling 1e *Guy Kremer and Jacki Wadeson*
Essensuals, the Next Generation Toni and Guy: Step by Step 1e *Sacha Mascolo, Christian Mascolo and Stuart Wesson*
Mahogany Hairdressing: Steps to Cutting, Colouring and Finishing Hair 1e *Martin Gannon and Richard Thompson*
Mahogany Hairdressing: Advanced Looks 1e *Martin Gannon and Richard Thompson*
The Total Look: The Style Guide for Hair and Make-Up Professionals 1e *Ian Mistlin*
Trevor Sorbie: Visions in Hair 1e *Trevor Sorbie, Kris Sorbie and Jacki Wadeson*
The Art of Hair Colouring 1e *David Adams and Jacki Wadeson*

BEAUTY THERAPY

Beauty Basics: The Official Guide to Level 1 1e *Lorraine Nordmann*
Beauty Therapy – The Foundations: The Official Guide to Level 2 3e *Lorraine Nordmann*
Professional Beauty Therapy – The Official Guide to Level 3 2e *Lorraine Nordmann*
The Official Guide to the City & Guilds Certificate in Salon Services 1e *John Armstrong with Anita Crosland, Martin Green and Lorraine Nordmann*
The Complete Guide to Make-Up 1e *Suzanne Le Quesne*
The Complete Make-Up Artist 2e *Penny Delamar*
The Encyclopedia of Nails 1e *Jacqui Jefford and Anne Swain*
The Art of Nails: A Comprehensive Style Guide to Nail Treatments and Nail Art 1e *Jacqui Jefford*
Nail Artistry 1e *Jacqui Jefford*
The Complete Nail Technician 2e *Marian Newman*
Manicure, Pedicure and Advanced Nail Techniques 1e *Elaine Almond*
The Official Guide to Body Massage 2e *Adele O'Keefe*
An Holistic Guide Massage 1e *Tina Parsons*
Indian Head Massage 2e *Muriel Burnham-Airey and Adele O'Keefe*
Aromatherapy for the Beauty Therapist 1e *Valerie Worwood*
An Holistic Guide to Reflexology 1e *Tina Parsons*
An Holistic Guide to Anatomy and Physiology 1e *Tina Parsons*
The Essential Guide to Holistic and Complementary Therapy 1e *Helen Beckmann and Suzanne Le Quesne*
The Spa Book 1e *Jane Cebbin-Bailey, Dr John Harcup, and John Harrington*
Nutrition: A Practical Approach 1e *Suzanne Le Quesne*
Hands on Sports Therapy 1e *Keith Ward*
The Encyclopedia of Hair Removal *Gill Morris and Janice Brown*

contents

PART SEVEN

about the authors

JOAN SCOTT has over twenty years' experience in the health and beauty business. Her many and varied roles include: beauty therapist, massage therapist, physiotherapy assistant, salon owner, lecturer, external examiner/verifier and curriculum manager. She is currently Director of Adult Learning at South Trafford College. Joan was co-author of the *Lecturer's Resource Packs for Beauty Therapy level 2 and 3*, and is Chair of Habia's UK Beauty Forum. She has a passion for the spa and wellness sector, and combines a wealth of knowledge with both an industry and an education perspective.

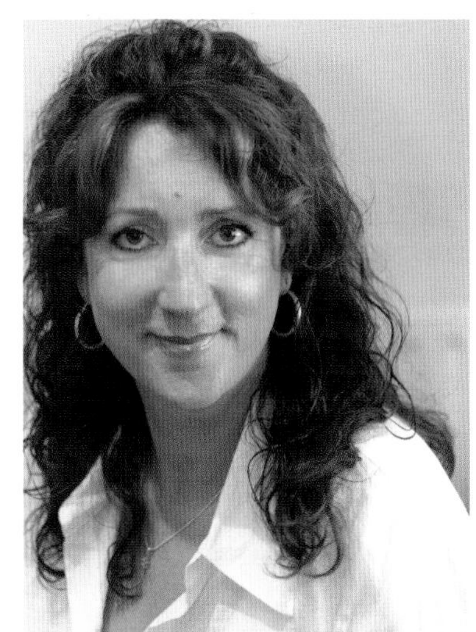

ANDREA HARRISON is currently Section Manager (Hair, Beauty and Holistic Therapy) at South Trafford College. She has extensive knowledge of the beauty business and has worked for a number of organisations as a practising therapist and manager, including working in the UK, on cruise ships and overseas. Andrea was co-author of the *Lecturer's Resource Packs for Beauty Therapy level 2 and 3*. She has combined her passions for the spa industry and travel with her experience in education.

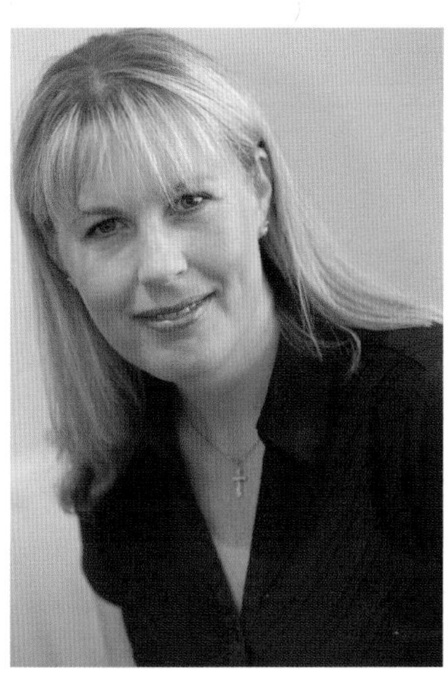

dedication

This book is dedicated to both our families for their love, support and constant encouragement.

acknowledgements

We would like to acknowledge the help of many people, without whose support this book would never have been completed. A special thank you to Melody Dawes at Thomson Learning, for her patience, humour and never-ending faith in us.

Thank you to the following for your support and help in compiling this book, and in many cases for providing images, quotes, spa profiles and treatment information:

Aghadoe Heights, Ireland
Agua, Sanderson, London
Aimia Hotel, Majorca
Ananda – in the Himalayas, India
Angela Derks
April and Daisy Harrison
Arlene Finch
Aromatherapy Associates
Assawan Spa, Burj-al-Arab, Dubai
Banyon Tree Spas
Bath House Spa
Better Living Institute, Evian les Bains, France
BISA
Bliss Spa, London
Blue Lagoon, Iceland
Brian Hunter
Bruce Hancock
Calmia Spa, London
Canyon Ranch, USA
Caracalla Spa, Le Royal Meridien Hotel, Dubai
Catherine Everest (CE) Products
Celtic Manor, Wales
Champneys Health Resorts
Chi, The Spa at Shangri-La, Bangkok
Chiva-Som International Health Resorts
Christine Meier
Clare Dickens
Clinique La Prairie, Switzerland
Colin Farndon
Colin Hall
Comfort Zone
Como Shambala, Bangkok
Corporate Edge
Cowshed Spa, Edinburgh
C-Side, Cowley Manor Hotel
Daintree Eco-lodge, Australia
Dale Sauna
Danubius Hotel Group
David Pike
Delphi Spa, Ireland
Dermalogica
De-tox box/High tech health
Devarana Spa, Bangkok
Dianne Dalgleish
Elemis Day Spa, London
Elemis

Emlyn Brown
Emma Whitelaw
Escape Photography
Eve Oxberrry
E'Spa
Exclusive Spas of Australia
EZ-Book
Finders International Ltd
Fiona Caldwell
Gemma Stewart
Geraldine Howard
Givenchy Spa, One & Only Royal Mirage, Dubai
Golden Door, California, USA
Hairdressing and Beauty Industry Authority (HABIA)
Haslauer/Kurland
Helen Norman
ISPA
Jane Crebbin-Bailey
Janice Brown, House of Famuir/HoF
Jean Sharpe
Jeff and Carol Fleming
Jez Cooper
John Brennan
Juerg Schuepbach
Kate Hudspith
Kerry Symons
Ki Day Spa, Cheshire
KLAFS
Kurumba Spa, Maldives
La Costa, California, USA
La Jolla Spa MD, California, USA
LaStone, London
Lisa Mushrow
Lissadell Towels
Lucy Clarke
Luxury Spa Finder magazine
Lynne Walker-McNees
Mandara Spas
Mandarin Oriental Hotels
Marcia Kilgore
Mardavall Hotel and Spa, Majorca
Marianne Sinar
Mike Wallace
Natalie Dzebissova
Noella Gabrielle
Nongnapat Chaiyawan
ONE Spa, Edinburgh
Oriental Spa, Bangkok
Oxypower Products
Pevonia
Phytomer
Ragdale Hall
Ritz-Carlton Hotel Grand Lakes, Orlando, USA
Rocco Forte Hotels
Royal Parc Evian, France
Samas, Kenmare Park Hotel, Ireland
Sandy Lane, Barbados
Sequoia Spa, The Grove
Serenity Spa, Seaham Hall.
Sinead Murray
Six Senses Spa, Evason Hua Hin, Thailand
Sobat Ali Din
Soneva Fushi, Maldives
Soneva Gili, Maldives
South Trafford College
Spa Business Association
Spa Capsule
Spa de Vinothérapie Caudalie, France
St Davids Hotel and Spa, Cardiff
Stobo Castle
Sughra Bibi
Susie Ellis
Susie Santiago
Termi di Saturnia Spa, Italy
Thalassa Spa, Cyprus
The Refinery, London
The Spa at Aghadoe Heights, Ireland
The Spa, Hilton Hua Hin, Thailand
The Spa, Hilton Phuket, Thailand
The Willow Stream Spa, Fairmont Hotel, Dubai
The Willow Stream Spa, Fairmont Empress, Canada
thisworks
Torrey Pines Spa & Lodge, California, USA
Tracey Corcoran
Trish Ridgway
Urban Retreat, Harrods
Victoria-Jungfrau, Switzerland
Vida Wellness Spa, Fairmont Chateau, Whistler

Contact details for many of these companies can be found in the spa directory in Part 7: Seek.

Every effort has been made to trace all of the copyright holders, but if we have inadvertently overlooked any, the publishers would be pleased to make the necessary arrangements at the first opportunity.

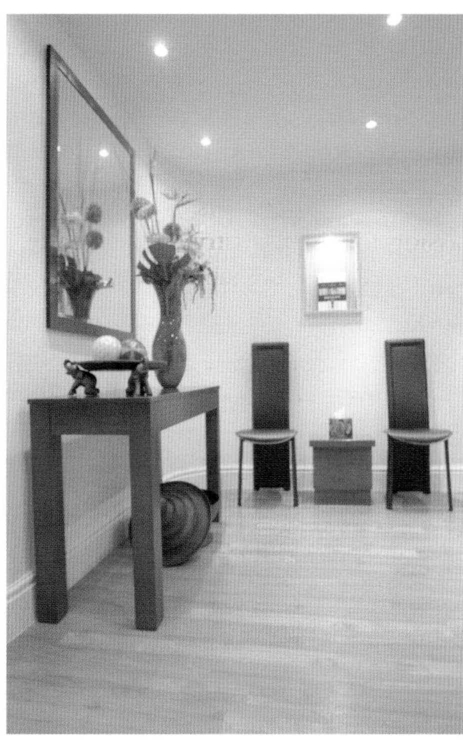

Thank you to Ki day Spa, Altrincham, Cheshire for kindly allowing the use of their establishment for the photoshoot.

foreword

Spa: The Official Guide to Spa Therapy at Levels 2 & 3 is a truly inspirational book. It is written by two experienced therapists, Joan Scott and Andrea Harrison, who combine a passion for the industry with a wealth of educational knowledge. It is also the first spa book available that relates directly to the Habia Level 3 Spa Occupational Standards.

Joan has worked in a variety of roles in her impressive career as both an educator and practitioner. Habia has had the privilege of working with Joan for many years; her input has been invaluable and the acumen she brings to her role as Chair of Habia's UK Beauty Forum is a gift to the industry.

Andrea has a vast knowledge of the spa industry. She has worked all over the world as a therapist and is also an experienced educator who has developed courses in spa therapy.

The authors have worked together for many years and their experience and strengths complement each other.

Their aim was to create a text which displayed the opportunities the spa industry has to offer and for anyone studying spa therapy to see what a fantastic sector it is, with unlimited opportunities for career progression and travel. The result is a wonderfully visual and appealing book which will entice and inspire students, lecturers, industry professionals and clients alike.

Spa: The Official Guide to Spa Therapy at Levels 2 & 3 is a pleasure to read and is a reflection of Joan and Andrea's hard work, dedication, knowledge and love for the spa industry.

Alan Goldsbro, CEO Habia

introduction

The spa sector has developed dramatically over the past couple of years. There are more opportunities than ever before to study and progress in the industry, and for individuals to have a rewarding and inspiring career in 'spa therapy'.

WHAT IS AN NVQ/SVQ QUALIFICATION?

A National Vocational Qualification (NVQ)/Scottish Vocational Qualification (SVQ) is a nationally recognized qualification that has been developed by the industry-led body to meet the needs of employers. All NVQs have a similar structure and design. NVQs/SVQs are based around the essential skills needed for a job role and are 'competence based'. This means that the person has the required level of skill and knowledge to perform the job effectively in the occupational area.

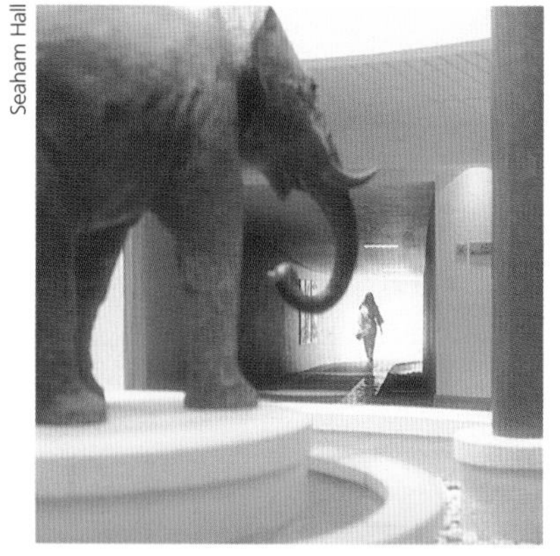
Seaham Hall

NVQ/SVQ STRUCTURE

All NVQs/SVQs have a similar structure and are made up of a number of units. Each unit can be achieved individually and a certificate of unit accreditation can be issued. Each NVQ has a number of units, some of which are:

- **Mandatory (compulsory)** – all these units need to be achieved to complete the full NVQ/SVQ award.
- **Optional (not all compulsory)** – a selection of these needs to be achieved; there is a choice of which ones.

With the Spa Therapy's NVQ Level 3 you need to achieve **6** mandatory units, plus **2** optional units.

Once all units have been completed the full NVQ qualification can be awarded.

Unit

The qualification is made up of a number of units. A unit is usually a defined task or skill, e.g. **Unit BT29** Provide specialist spa treatments.

A unit is the smallest part of a qualification that can be accredited/awarded separately.

Element

A unit is divided into 'elements'. These describe in detail the skill and knowledge parts of the unit, e.g. 'consult with and prepare the client for treatment'.

Example of a unit

Unit	Elements
Unit BT29 Provide specialist spa treatments	1. Consult with and prepare the client for treatment 2. Provide body wrapping treatments 3. Provide dry flotation treatments 4. Provide hydrotherapy treatments 5. Monitor water, temperature and spa treatments and environment 6. Provide aftercare advice

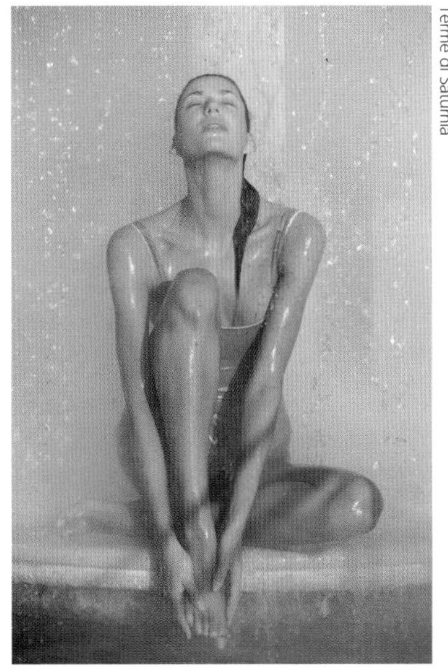

Terme di Saturnia

Performance criteria

Each 'element' has a list of 'performance criteria'. These are the necessary actions you need to perform to be competent and pass the assessment.

Range

You need to demonstrate that you can perform a skill in a 'range' of different conditions. This proves 'competence' in a wide range of situations and ensures you are prepared for the variety of clients you will meet in the industry, e.g. in Unit BT29 the range of 'treatment products' include algae, milk products, salt and aromatherapy oils.

Knowledge and understanding

Every unit has associated 'knowledge and understanding' topics. These topics need to be learned and assessed to ensure not only that you can perform a skill well, but also that you understand what you are doing and why. In addition, you will learn how to transfer your knowledge to a wide variety of situations so that you are fully prepared for working in the spa industry.

Portfolio

This is a file that contains all your evidence of assessments (projects, tests, case studies, etc.). This file needs to be very neat and professional, with a cross-referencing system that allows your assessor, internal verifier and external verifier to find easily the evidence for each unit. Some assessments are used for more than one unit, so cross-referencing is essential.

To fully achieve a unit, your portfolio should show evidence that you have achieved:

- all 'performance criteria'
- all the 'range' statements
- all the 'knowledge and understanding' topics.

SPA THERAPY NVQ/SVQ LEVEL 3

You will need to achieve the 6 mandatory units, plus 2 optional units.

Mandatory units *(all units need to be achieved)*	
G1	Ensure your own actions reduce risks to health and safety
G6	Promote additional products or services to clients
G11	Contribute to the financial effectiveness of the business
BT17	Provide head and body massage treatments
BT28	Set up, monitor and shut down water, temperature and spa facilities
BT29	Provide specialist spa treatments

Optional units *(2 units need to be achieved)*	
G12	Check how successful your business idea will be
G13	Check what law and other regulations will affect your business
BT16	Epilate the hair follicle using diathermy, galvanic and blend techniques
BT18	Improve body condition using electrotherapy
BT19	Improve face and skin condition using electrotherapy
BT20	Provide Indian head massage treatment
BT21	Provide massage using pre-blended aromatherapy oils
BT30	Provide UV tanning treatments
BT31	Provide self-tanning treatments
BT36	Improve the appearance of the skin using micro-dermabrasion

about the book

This book has been written to inspire, inform and educate those individuals entering the spa sector. It has been developed as a 'show case', featuring photographs, signature treatments, staff profiles and quotes from the best in the business! The book is based around the NVQ/SVQ levels 2 and 3 spa therapy qualifications, but includes additional areas to enhance your knowledge of the industry. The book is divided into seven parts:

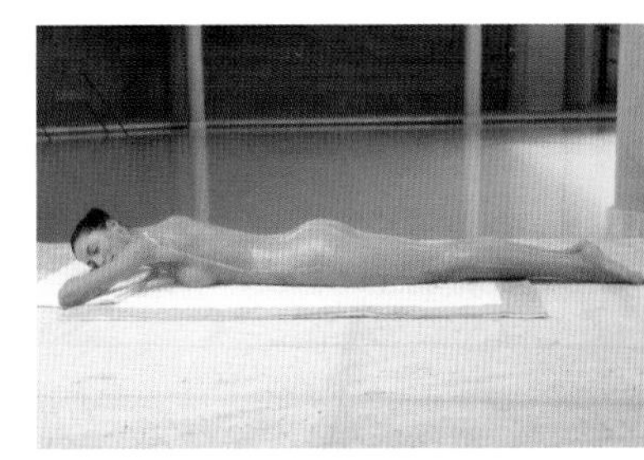
Image courtesy of Terme de Saturnia

1 **Spirit**
History and development of spa therapy

2 **Substance**
The spa sector/industry, financial effectiveness, promotion of spa services and Health and Safety

3 **System**
Anatomy and physiology

4 **Sensation**
Heat and chill treatments

5 **Splash**
Water treatments, testing and monitoring

6 **Soothe**
Body massage, Indian head massage, pre-blended massage, envelopments/exfoliation, consultation and spa etiquette

7 **Seek**
Directory of spa contacts and glossary

FEATURES WITHIN CHAPTERS

Common features appear within each chapter. An explanation for each is provided in the pages overleaf.

Health and Safety

In addition to a dedicated health and safety chapter (chapter 5), Health and Safety boxes are provided in each chapter.

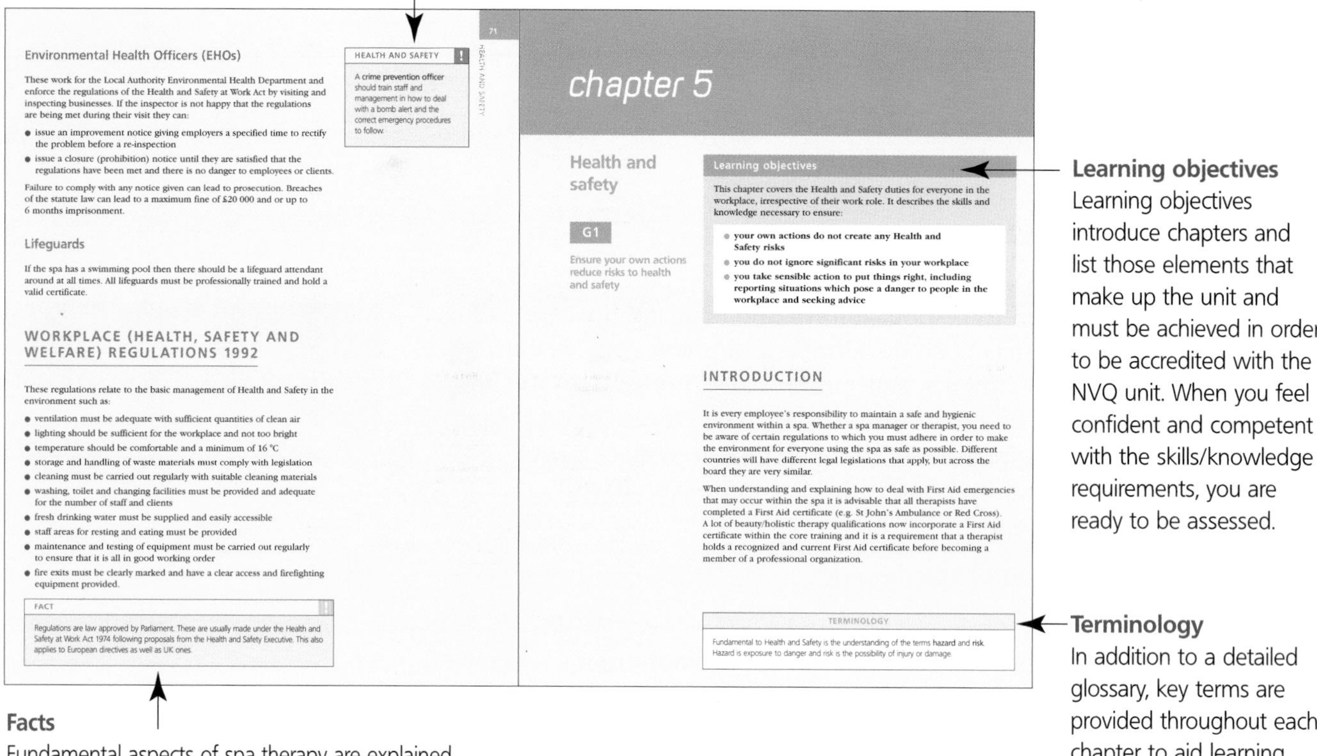

Environmental Health Officers (EHOs)

These work for the Local Authority Environmental Health Department and enforce the regulations of the Health and Safety at Work Act by visiting and inspecting businesses. If the inspector is not happy that the regulations are being met during their visit they can:

- issue an improvement notice giving employers a specified time to rectify the problem before a re-inspection
- issue a closure (prohibition) notice until they are satisfied that the regulations have been met and there is no danger to employees or clients.

Failure to comply with any notice given can lead to prosecution. Breaches of the statute law can lead to a maximum fine of £20 000 and or up to 6 months imprisonment.

Lifeguards

If the spa has a swimming pool then there should be a lifeguard attendant around at all times. All lifeguards must be professionally trained and hold a valid certificate.

WORKPLACE (HEALTH, SAFETY AND WELFARE) REGULATIONS 1992

These regulations relate to the basic management of Health and Safety in the environment such as:

- ventilation must be adequate with sufficient quantities of clean air
- lighting should be sufficient for the workplace and not too bright
- temperature should be comfortable and a minimum of 16 °C
- storage and handling of waste materials must comply with legislation
- cleaning must be carried out regularly with suitable cleaning materials
- washing, toilet and changing facilities must be provided and adequate for the number of staff and clients
- fresh drinking water must be supplied and easily accessible
- staff areas for resting and eating must be provided
- maintenance and testing of equipment must be carried out regularly to ensure that it is all in good working order
- fire exits must be clearly marked and have a clear access and firefighting equipment provided.

FACT

Regulations are law approved by Parliament. These are usually made under the Health and Safety at Work Act 1974 following proposals from the Health and Safety Executive. This also applies to European directives as well as UK ones.

HEALTH AND SAFETY

A crime prevention officer should train staff and management in how to deal with a bomb alert and the correct emergency procedures to follow.

71 HEALTH AND SAFETY

chapter 5

Health and safety

G1

Ensure your own actions reduce risks to health and safety

Learning objectives

This chapter covers the Health and Safety duties for everyone in the workplace, irrespective of their work role. It describes the skills and knowledge necessary to ensure:

- your own actions do not create any Health and Safety risks
- you do not ignore significant risks in your workplace
- you take sensible action to put things right, including reporting situations which pose a danger to people in the workplace and seeking advice

INTRODUCTION

It is every employee's responsibility to maintain a safe and hygienic environment within a spa. Whether a spa manager or therapist, you need to be aware of certain regulations to which you must adhere in order to make the environment for everyone using the spa as safe as possible. Different countries will have different legal legislations that apply, but across the board they are very similar.

When understanding and explaining how to deal with First Aid emergencies that may occur within the spa it is advisable that all therapists have completed a First Aid certificate (e.g. St John's Ambulance or Red Cross). A lot of beauty/holistic therapy qualifications now incorporate a First Aid certificate within the core training and it is a requirement that a therapist holds a recognized and current First Aid certificate before becoming a member of a professional organization.

TERMINOLOGY

Fundamental to Health and Safety is the understanding of the terms hazard and risk. Hazard is exposure to danger and risk is the possibility of injury or damage.

Learning objectives

Learning objectives introduce chapters and list those elements that make up the unit and must be achieved in order to be accredited with the NVQ unit. When you feel confident and competent with the skills/knowledge requirements, you are ready to be assessed.

Terminology

In addition to a detailed glossary, key terms are provided throughout each chapter to aid learning.

Facts

Fundamental aspects of spa therapy are explained using fact boxes to help you master the required underpinning knowledge.

Signature treatments

Real signature treatments from spas around the world are included in each chapter to inspire and demonstrate how treatments are combined to provide a unique experience.

Spa tip

The authors' experience is shared through spa tips, which provide suggestions to improve your skills and knowledge for each unit.

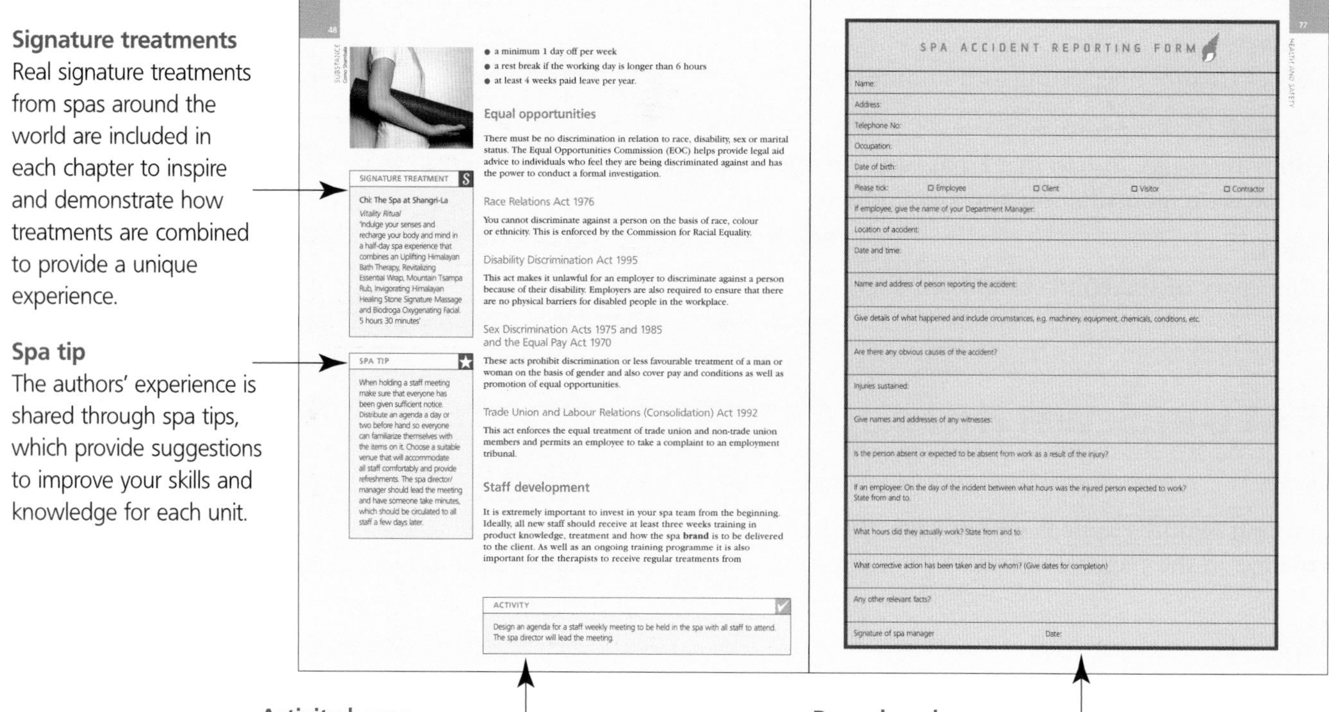

48 SUBSTANCE

SIGNATURE TREATMENT

Chi: The Spa at Shangri-La

Vitality Ritual

'Indulge your senses and recharge your body and mind in a half-day spa experience that combines an Uplifting Himalayan Bath Therapy, Revitalizing Essential Wrap, Mountain Tsampa Rub, Invigorating Himalayan Healing Stone Signature Massage and Biodroga Oxygenating Facial. 5 hours 30 minutes'

SPA TIP

When holding a staff meeting make sure that everyone has been given sufficient notice. Distribute an agenda a day or two before hand so everyone can familiarize themselves with the items on it. Choose a suitable venue that will accommodate all staff comfortably and provide refreshments. The spa director/manager should lead the meeting and have someone take minutes, which should be circulated to all staff a few days later.

- a minimum 1 day off per week
- a rest break if the working day is longer than 6 hours
- at least 4 weeks paid leave per year.

Equal opportunities

There must be no discrimination in relation to race, disability, sex or marital status. The Equal Opportunities Commission (EOC) helps provide legal aid advice to individuals who feel they are being discriminated against and has the power to conduct a formal investigation.

Race Relations Act 1976

You cannot discriminate against a person on the basis of race, colour or ethnicity. This is enforced by the Commission for Racial Equality.

Disability Discrimination Act 1995

This act makes it unlawful for an employer to discriminate against a person because of their disability. Employers are also required to ensure that there are no physical barriers for disabled people in the workplace.

Sex Discrimination Acts 1975 and 1985 and the Equal Pay Act 1970

These acts prohibit discrimination or less favourable treatment of a man or woman on the basis of gender and also cover pay and conditions as well as promotion of equal opportunities.

Trade Union and Labour Relations (Consolidation) Act 1992

This act enforces the equal treatment of trade union and non-trade union members and permits an employee to take a complaint to an employment tribunal.

Staff development

It is extremely important to invest in your spa team from the beginning. Ideally, all new staff should receive at least three weeks training in product knowledge, treatment and how the spa **brand** is to be delivered to the client. As well as an ongoing training programme it is also important for the therapists to receive regular treatments from

ACTIVITY

Design an agenda for a staff weekly meeting to be held in the spa with all staff to attend. The spa director will lead the meeting.

77 HEALTH AND SAFETY

SPA ACCIDENT REPORTING FORM

Name:

Address:

Telephone No:

Occupation:

Date of birth:

Please tick: ☐ Employee ☐ Client ☐ Visitor ☐ Contractor

If employee, give the name of your Department Manager:

Location of accident:

Date and time:

Name and address of person reporting the accident:

Give details of what happened and include circumstances, e.g. machinery, equipment, chemicals, conditions, etc.

Are there any obvious causes of the accident?

Injuries sustained:

Give names and addresses of any witnesses:

Is the person absent or expected to be absent from work as a result of the injury?

If an employee: On the day of the incident between what hours was the injured person expected to work? State from and to:

What hours did they actually work? State from and to:

What corrective action has been taken and by whom? (Give dates for completion)

Any other relevant facts?

Signature of spa manager Date:

Activity boxes

Where relevant, useful learning activities are provided within the chapter to assist learning and understanding.

Record cards

Client treatment record cards illustrate the information that you need to gain from the client and assess during the consultation in order to establish client suitability and the treatment aim.

Assessment of knowledge and understanding
Review questions are provided at the end of each chapter to assess knowledge and understanding.

Linked treatments
These lists allow you to combine treatments easily, creating fantastic spa packages and increase income from the spa.

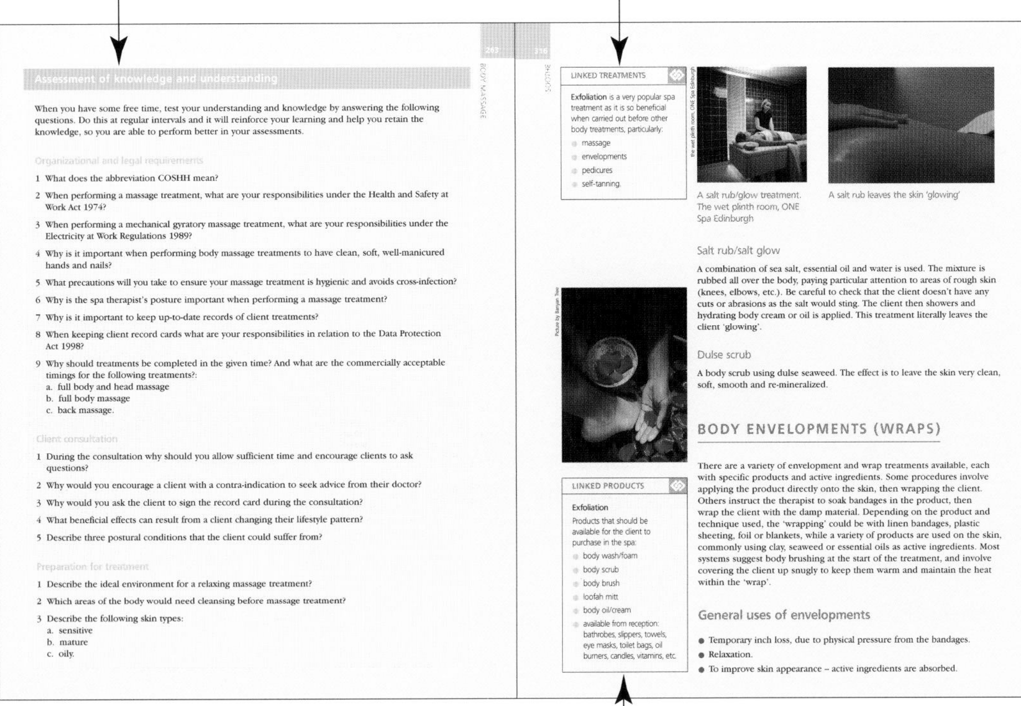

247 BODY MASSAGE

Assessment of knowledge and understanding

When you have some free time, test your understanding and knowledge by answering the following questions. Do this at regular intervals and it will reinforce your learning and help you retain the knowledge, so you are able to perform better in your assessments.

Organizational and legal requirements

1 What does the abbreviation COSHH mean?
2 When performing a massage treatment, what are your responsibilities under the Health and Safety at Work Act 1974?
3 When performing a mechanical gyratory massage treatment, what are your responsibilities under the Electricity at Work Regulations 1989?
4 Why is it important when performing body massage treatments to have clean, soft, well-manicured hands and nails?
5 What precautions will you take to ensure your massage treatment is hygienic and avoids cross-infection?
6 Why is the spa therapist's posture important when performing a massage treatment?
7 Why is it important to keep up-to-date records of client treatments?
8 When keeping client record cards what are your responsibilities in relation to the Data Protection Act 1998?
9 Why should treatments be completed in the given time? And what are the commercially acceptable timings for the following treatments?:
a. full body and head massage
b. full body massage
c. back massage.

Client consultation

1 During the consultation why should you allow sufficient time and encourage clients to ask questions?
2 Why would you encourage a client with a contra-indication to seek advice from their doctor?
3 Why would you ask the client to sign the record card during the consultation?
4 What beneficial effects can result from a client changing their lifestyle pattern?
5 Describe three postural conditions that the client could suffer from?

Preparation for treatment

1 Describe the ideal environment for a relaxing massage treatment?
2 Which areas of the body would need cleansing before massage treatment?
3 Describe the following skin types:
a. sensitive
b. mature
c. oily.

216 ENGLISH

LINKED TREATMENTS

Exfoliation is a very popular spa treatment as it is so beneficial when carried out before other body treatments, particularly:
- massage
- envelopments
- pedicures
- self-tanning.

A salt rub/glow treatment. The wet plinth room, ONE Spa Edinburgh

A salt rub leaves the skin 'glowing'

Salt rub/salt glow

A combination of sea salt, essential oil and water is used. The mixture is rubbed all over the body, paying particular attention to areas of rough skin (knees, elbows, etc.). Be careful to check that the client doesn't have any cuts or abrasions as the salt would sting. The client then showers and hydrating body cream or oil is applied. This treatment literally leaves the client 'glowing'.

Dulse scrub

A body scrub using dulse seaweed. The effect is to leave the skin very clean, soft, smooth and re-mineralized.

BODY ENVELOPMENTS (WRAPS)

There are a variety of envelopment and wrap treatments available, each with specific products and active ingredients. Some procedures involve applying the product directly onto the skin, then wrapping the client. Others instruct the therapist to soak bandages in the product, then wrap the client with the damp material. Depending on the product and technique used, the 'wrapping' could be with linen bandages, plastic sheeting, foil or blankets, while a variety of products are used on the skin, commonly using clay, seaweed or essential oils as active ingredients. Most systems suggest body brushing at the start of the treatment, and involve covering the client up snugly to keep them warm and maintain the heat within the 'wrap'.

LINKED PRODUCTS

Exfoliation
Products that should be available for the client to purchase in the spa:
- body wash/foam
- body scrub
- body brush
- loofah mitt
- body oil/cream
- available from reception: bathrobes, slippers, towels, eye masks, toilet bags, oil burners, candles, vitamins, etc.

General uses of envelopments

- Temporary inch loss, due to physical pressure from the bandages.
- Relaxation.
- To improve skin appearance – active ingredients are absorbed.

Equipment list
To assist you when preparing for each practical treatment an essential equipment list is provided.

Linked products
Key retail opportunities are highlighted by these lists of spa products that can be linked to treatments, creating fantastic spa packages that benefit the client whilst increasing business/income.

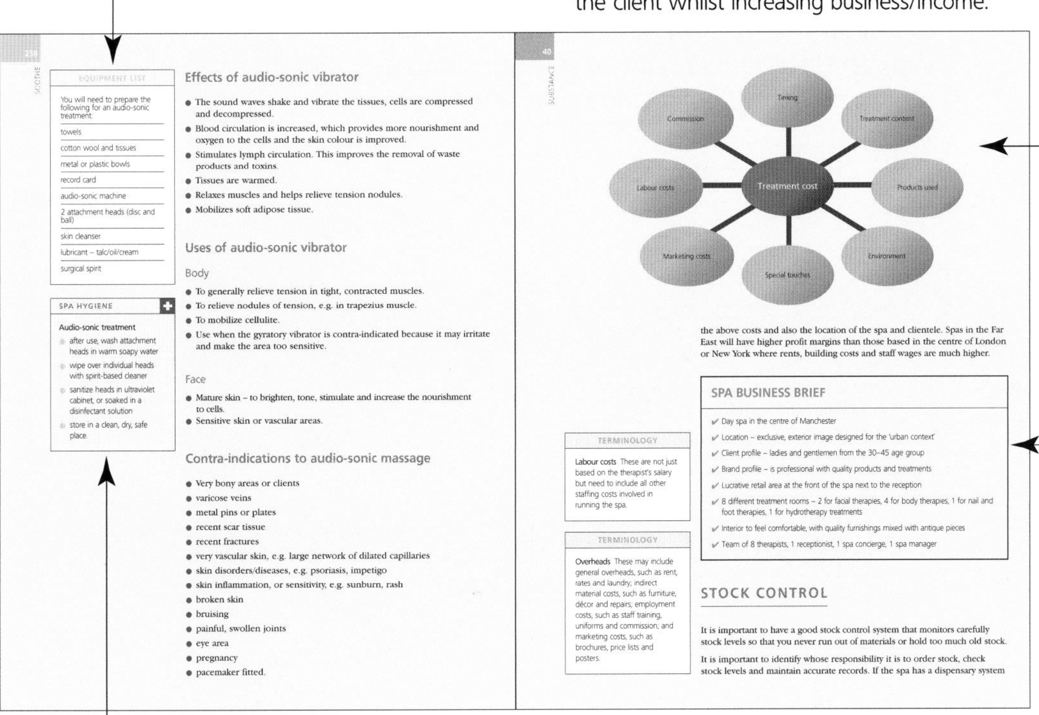

EQUIPMENT LIST

You will need to prepare the following for an audio-sonic treatment:
- towels
- cotton wool and tissues
- metal or plastic bowls
- record card
- audio-sonic machine
- 2 attachment heads (disc and ball)
- skin cleanser
- lubricant – talc/oil/cream
- surgical spirit

SPA HYGIENE

Audio-sonic treatment
- after use, wash attachment heads in warm soapy water
- wipe over individual heads with spirit-based cleaner
- sanitize heads in ultraviolet cabinet, or soaked in a disinfectant solution
- store in a clean, dry, safe place.

Effects of audio-sonic vibrator

- The sound waves shake and vibrate the tissues, cells are compressed and decompressed.
- Blood circulation is increased, which provides more nourishment and oxygen to the cells and the skin colour is improved.
- Stimulates lymph circulation. This improves the removal of waste products and toxins.
- Tissues are warmed.
- Relaxes muscles and helps relieve tension nodules.
- Mobilizes soft adipose tissue.

Uses of audio-sonic vibrator

Body
- To generally relieve tension in tight, contracted muscles.
- To relieve nodules of tension, e.g. in trapezius muscle.
- To mobilize cellulite.
- Use when the gyratory vibrator is contra-indicated because it may irritate and make the area too sensitive.

Face
- Mature skin – to brighten, tone, stimulate and increase the nourishment to cells.
- Sensitive skin or vascular areas.

Contra-indications to audio-sonic massage

- Very bony areas or clients
- varicose veins
- metal pins or plates
- recent scar tissue
- recent fractures
- very vascular skin, e.g. large network of dilated capillaries
- skin disorders/diseases, e.g. psoriasis, impetigo
- skin inflammation, or sensitivity, e.g. sunburn, rash
- broken skin
- bruising
- painful, swollen joints
- eye area
- pregnancy
- pacemaker fitted.

40

the above costs and also the location of the spa and clientele. Spas in the Far East will have higher profit margins than those based in the centre of London or New York where rents, building costs and staff wages are much higher.

SPA BUSINESS BRIEF

- ✓ Day spa in the centre of Manchester
- ✓ Location – exclusive, exterior image designed for the 'urban context'
- ✓ Client profile – ladies and gentlemen from the 30–45 age group
- ✓ Brand profile – is professional with quality products and treatments
- ✓ Lucrative retail area at the front of the spa next to the reception
- ✓ 8 different treatment rooms – 2 for facial therapies, 4 for body therapies, 1 for nail and foot therapies, 1 for hydrotherapy treatments
- ✓ Interior to feel comfortable, with quality furnishings mixed with antique pieces
- ✓ Team of 8 therapists, 1 receptionist, 1 spa concierge, 1 spa manager

TERMINOLOGY

Labour costs These are not just based on the therapist's salary but need to include all other staffing costs involved in running the spa.

TERMINOLOGY

Overheads These may include general overheads, such as rent, rates and laundry; indirect material costs, such as furniture, décor and repairs; employment costs, such as staff training, uniforms and commission; and marketing costs, such as brochures, price lists and posters.

STOCK CONTROL

It is important to have a good stock control system that monitors carefully stock levels so that you never run out of materials or hold too much old stock.

It is important to identify whose responsibility it is to order stock, check stock levels and maintain accurate records. If the spa has a dispensary system

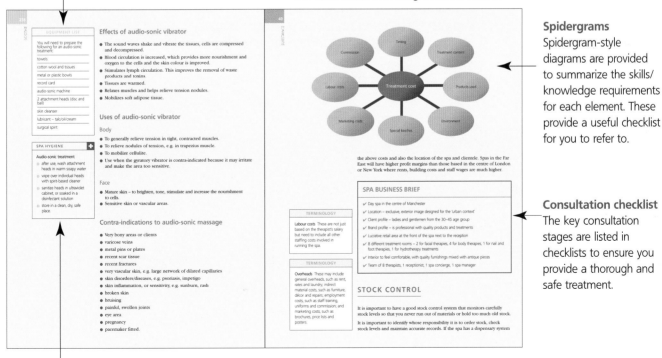

Spidergrams
Spidergram-style diagrams are provided to summarize the skills/ knowledge requirements for each element. These provide a useful checklist for you to refer to.

Consultation checklist
The key consultation stages are listed in checklists to ensure you provide a thorough and safe treatment.

Hygiene
Key hygiene tips for each treatment ensure you provide safe and professional spa therapy.

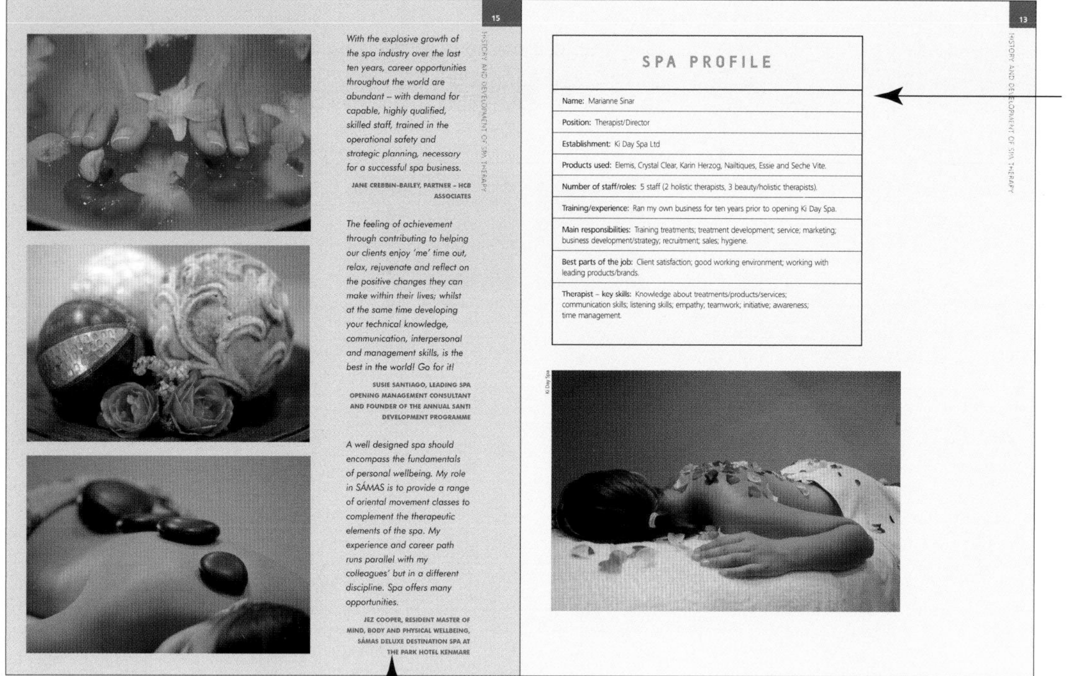

15

HISTORY AND DEVELOPMENT OF SPA THERAPY

With the explosive growth of the spa industry over the last ten years, career opportunities throughout the world are abundant – with demand for capable, highly qualified, skilled staff, trained in the operational safety and strategic planning, necessary for a successful spa business.

JANE CREBBIN-BAILEY, PARTNER – HCB ASSOCIATES

The feeling of achievement through contributing to helping our clients enjoy 'me' time out, relax, rejuvenate and reflect on the positive changes they can make within their lives; whilst at the same time developing your technical knowledge, communication, interpersonal and management skills, is the best in the world! Go for it!

SUSIE SANTIAGO, LEADING SPA OPENING MANAGEMENT CONSULTANT AND FOUNDER OF THE ANNUAL SANTI DEVELOPMENT PROGRAMME

A well designed spa should encompass the fundamentals of personal wellbeing. My role in SÁMAS is to provide a range of oriental movement classes to complement the therapeutic elements of the spa. My experience and career path runs parallel with my colleagues' but in a different discipline. Spa offers many opportunities.

JEZ COOPER, RESIDENT MASTER OF MIND, BODY AND PHYSICAL WELLBEING, SÁMAS DELUXE DESTINATION SPA AT THE PARK HOTEL KENMARE

13

HISTORY AND DEVELOPMENT OF SPA THERAPY

SPA PROFILE

Name: Marianne Sinar

Position: Therapist/Director

Establishment: Ki Day Spa Ltd

Products used: Elemis, Crystal Clear, Karin Herzog, Nailtiques, Essie and Seche Vite.

Number of staff/roles: 5 staff (2 holistic therapists, 3 beauty/holistic therapists).

Training/experience: Ran my own business for ten years prior to opening Ki Day Spa.

Main responsibilities: Training treatments; treatment development; service; marketing; business development/strategy; recruitment; sales; hygiene.

Best parts of the job: Client satisfaction; good working environment; working with leading products/brands.

Therapist – key skills: Knowledge about treatments/products/services; communication skills; listening skills; empathy; teamwork; initiative; awareness; time management.

Ki Day Spa

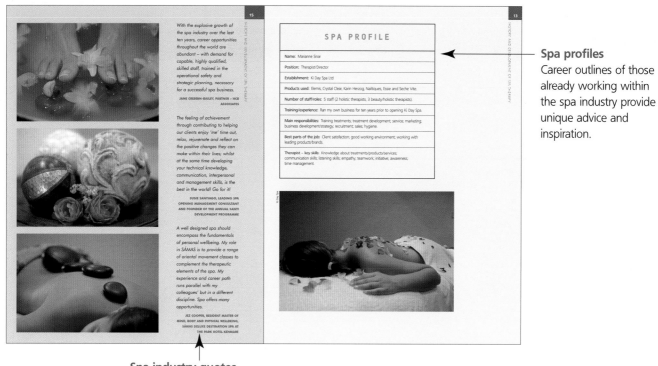

Spa profiles
Career outlines of those already working within the spa industry provide unique advice and inspiration.

Spa industry quotes
Inspiring quotes from key figures within the spa industry around the world provide inspiration and encouragement for those entering the spa sector.

A **spa directory** can be found at the end of the book, containing contact details such as UK/international spas, industry bodies, product/equipment suppliers, recruitment, etc. A **glossary** is also provided as a handy reference for spa words, technical terms and spa treatments.

NVQ/SVQ mapping grid

Chapters	1	2	3	4	5	6	7	8	9	10	11	12	13	14	15
Beauty therapy NVQ/SVQ Level 2															
BT15 Assist with spa treatments (optional unit)					x		x		x	x				x	x
Spa therapy NVQ/SVQ Level 3															
G1 Health/safety					x										
G6 Promote products/services				x											
G11 Financial effectiveness			x												
BT17 Head/body massage					x	x					x		x		x
BT28 Water, temperature and spa facilities					x		x	x	x	x				x	x
BT29 Spa treatments					x	x	x	x	x					x	x
BT20 Indian head massage (optional unit)					x	x					x	x			x
BT21 Massage with pre-blended oils (optional unit)					x	x						x			x
ITEC Level 3 Diploma in spa treatments															
History/concept	x														
Atmosphere/ambience		x													x
Exfoliation					x	x								x	x
Steam and sauna					x	x	x								x
Body masks/wraps					x	x								x	x
Seawater/seaweed					x	x								x	x
Water treatment					x	x	x	x	x	x					x
Hydrotherapy					x	x			x						x

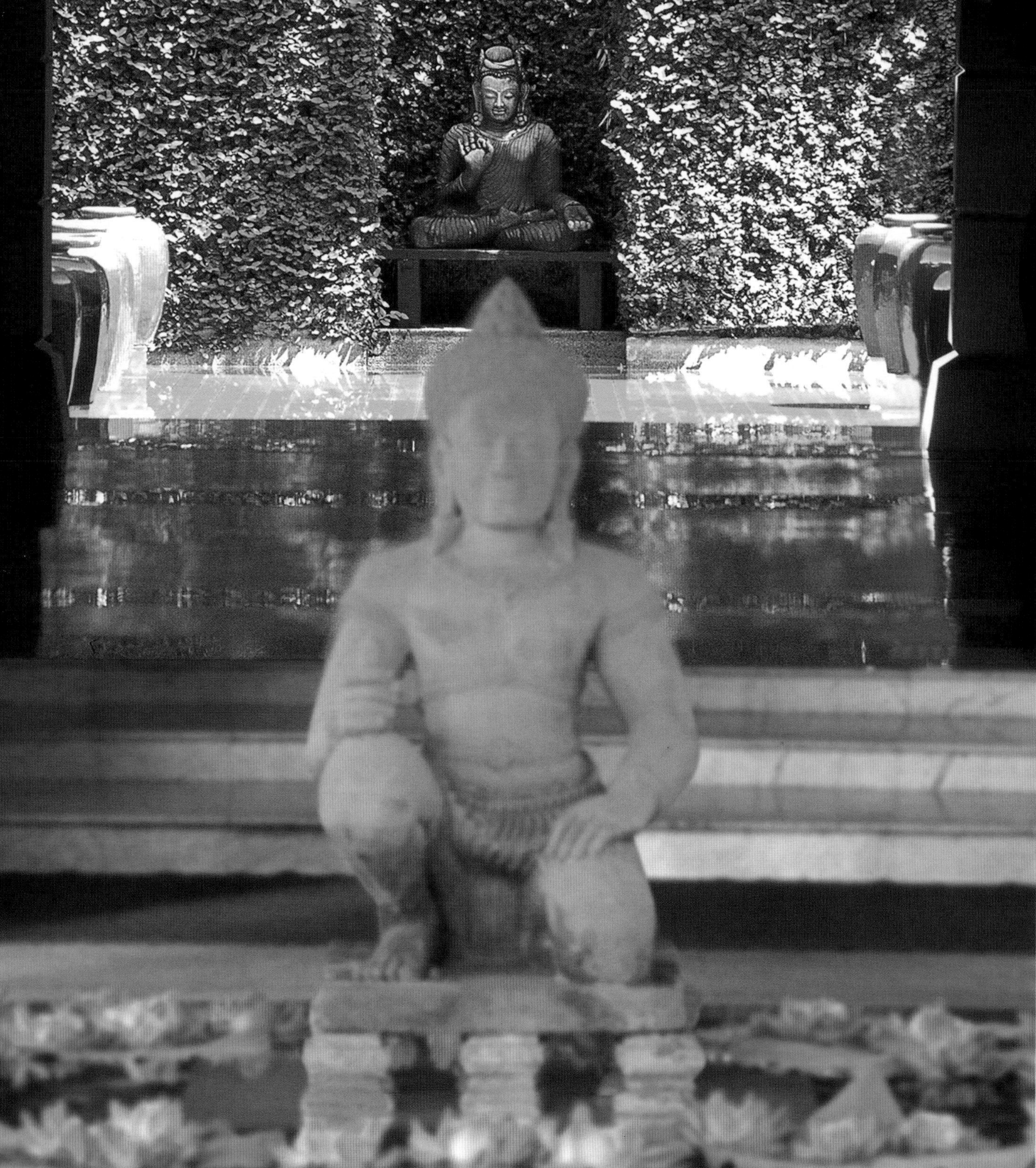
Image courtesy of Chiva-Som

Joining the spa industry? It couldn't be a ***better time*** *due to the fact globally there is an* ***incredible realization*** *that* ***spa*** *is no longer only about pampering but also a therapeutic process constantly developing. Bridging the gap between spa and other health modalities is a* ***strong focus,*** *and one which will most definitely enhance the industry at a universal level.*

BRUCE HANCOCK, DIRECTOR HEALTH AND WELLNESS, CHIVA-SOM INTERNATIONAL HEALTH RESORT

1 SPIRIT

It's such an exciting time to be joining the spa industry because it is expanding rapidly and there are lots of new improvements in treatment design. Basic treatment concepts are being developed so that the client's whole experience at a spa is becoming a better and more enjoyable journey from start to finish.

GERALDINE HOWARD, PRESIDENT, AROMATHERAPY ASSOCIATES

The spa industry has been expanding at quite a pace for some years now and is showing no signs of slowing. With new spas still opening every week and countless skincare and equipment brands keen to claim their share of this vibrant market, managers are realizing that it is no longer enough just to have a spa; they also need to offer a high level of service and a real point of difference to set them apart from others in the market.

EVE OXBERRY, EDITOR, *PROFESSIONAL SPA* MAGAZINE

chapter 1

History and development of spa therapy

Learning objectives

This chapter covers the background information you need to put the industry into perspective. It describes the skills and knowledge necessary to enable you to:

- **understand the history of spas and spa treatments**
- **recognize how the spa industry is supported and promoted**
- **identify different types of spas**
- **recognize worldwide spa opportunities**

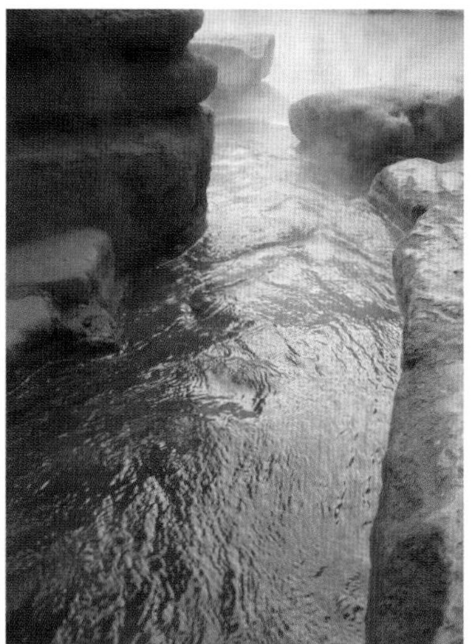

HISTORY OF SPAS AND SPA TREATMENTS

The history of spa therapy and the many associated treatments can be traced back thousands of years. In most spas, the emphasis is on water in some form, either from an artificial source or using mineral water from natural sources such as a spring, lake or sea. In other spas the focus is on therapeutic ingredients unique to them, such as mud, or the environment or the health-giving properties of grapes.

Research has found many aspects to spa history. Detailed below are some of the main developments with approximate dates:

5000 BC A form of acupressure was practised in China. It is thought to have originated in India and then travelled to China where the Chinese developed their own system.

5000 BC Ayurvedic medicine practised in India. This is accepted as the forerunner of many of the other healing systems, including

TERMINOLOGY

Spa is thought to be derived from the Latin phrase '*Solus per aqua*' which means 'health from water'.

Spa is only used in English-speaking countries. Across Europe there are a variety of names used for water related health resorts. In Germany **kurort** may be used and means 'place of cure', and **bad** is often used as part of a geographic location. **Les Bains** is the French name for spa, whereas in Italy they use **terme** and in Spain **baños**.

TERMINOLOGY

Balneotherapy a water therapy treatment using sea or mineral water, or thermal spring water.

Health spa usually the name given to a place where the main interest is health and people attend for therapeutic purposes.

TERMINOLOGY

Ayurveda is a complete philosophy that aims to create a balance between the mind and body. It encompasses every aspect of health, from nutrition and lifestyle to treatments and meditation. It is referred to as the 'mother of medicine' and is one of the oldest forms of medicine.

those developed in China, Tibet and Greece. Water was used as a treatment for a variety of diseases in early Indian medicine.

3000 BC Water therapy and herbal treatments were developed by the Egyptians.

500 BC The Greeks believed that the physical properties of water made it powerful, and that it had unique healing properties. In Greece cold water bathing was practised, with therapeutic benefits for soldiers and warriors.

380 BC Hippocrates, a famous physician and the 'father of medicine', believed hot and cold bathing was beneficial for healing. He developed the 'rule of opposites', whereby 'cold affusions recall the heat'. Hippocrates also used massage for treatment of injuries and disease. He found it to be more beneficial when rubbing towards the heart (the circulatory system was not understood then).

300 BC Water treatments were introduced to the Roman Empire by the ancient Greeks.

Buddha statue, southern Thailand

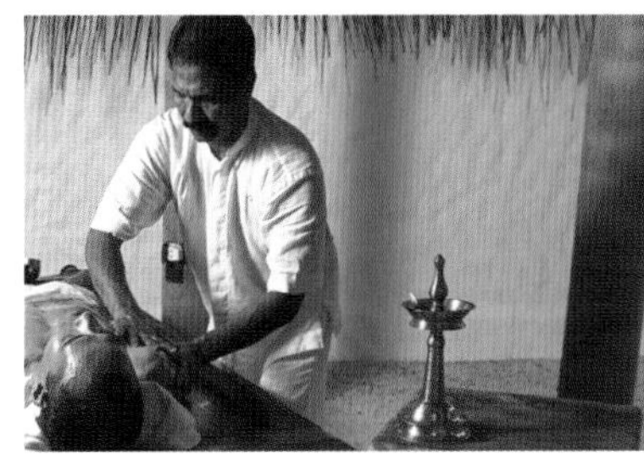

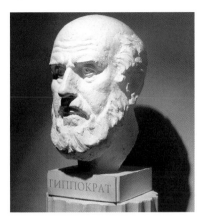

Ayurvedic treatment

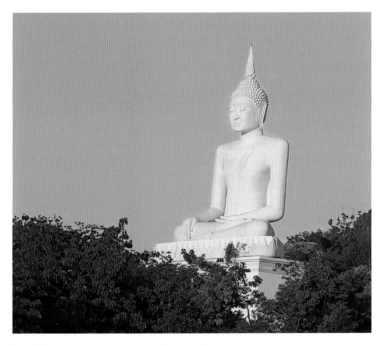

Hippocrates

TERMINOLOGY

Shirodhara is a deeply relaxing Ayurvedic treatment where warm oil is slowly poured over the centre of the forehead (or 'third eye').

FACT

Many of the soldiers and warriors instructed by Hippocrates kept fit and healthy by swimming in icy cold rivers or seas daily.

TERMINOLOGY

Thalassotherapy aims to balance the body by using seawater and marine by-products.

Algotherapy uses algae or marine products to relax and detoxify the body.

FACT

Roman gladiators were oiled and massaged until their skin was glowing red and supple before commencing battle.

FACT

The Romans associated personal hygiene with health and the bathing ritual became the focus for their social life. Advanced facilities were built, including *caldariums* (hot baths), *tepidariums* (warm baths) and *frigidariums* (cold plunge pools).

FACT

A **brine bath** uses water that is saturated with salt, similar to seawater.

A **Celtic Roman bath** combines hot and cold baths, showers and pools with heat and steam rooms.

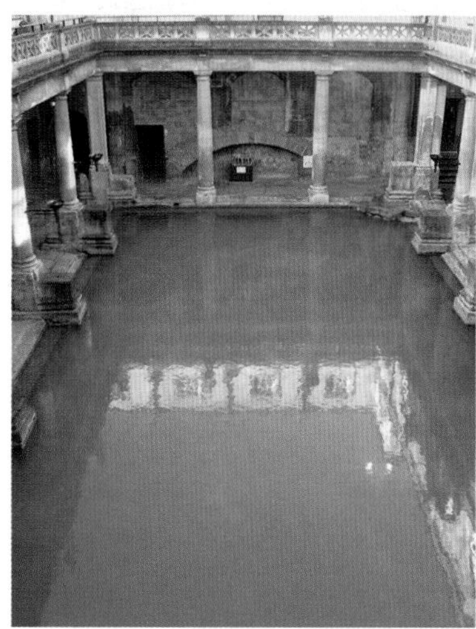

Main Roman bathing pool at Bath, England

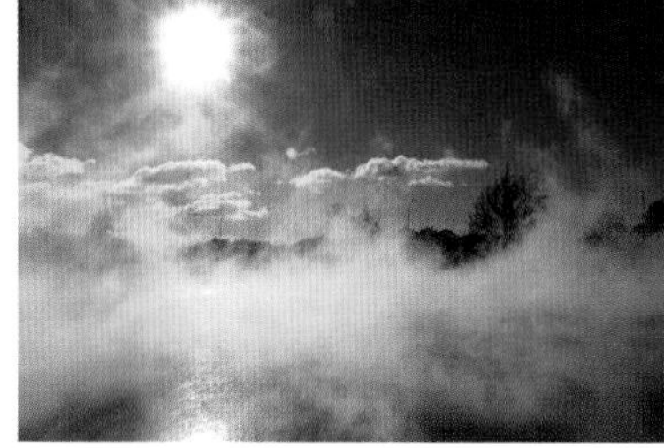

Thermal pool

100 BC Buddhism arrived in Thailand, and alongside came the development of massage and healing systems.

23 AD Antonius Musa used Hippocrates' 'rule of opposites' (e.g. cold baths) and cured the Emperor Augustus of his diseased liver.

37 AD Celsus, a doctor working in Rome, advised patients with swollen legs to bathe in a cold bath up to their neck.

50 AD Romans in England in the first century lived in towns where the waters were considered to contain special minerals and salts for healthy living, e.g. Harrogate, Buxton, Bath, Leamington, etc.

76 AD In Bath, England, a spa (Aqua Sulis) was built by the Romans.

80 AD The Romans used a spring in Belgium called Sulus Par Aqua. This is thought to be the origin of the word 'spa'. They also developed an advanced system of massage.

180 AD Galen, a doctor during the Roman era, discovered arteries were filled with blood and not air. He treated injuries and diseases with massage, varying the direction of massage. Public baths were more commonplace by this time. Galen used baths and affusions, often alternating hot and cold temperatures.

211 AD A thermal spring was discovered in Baden-Baden, Germany, by the Romans.

600 AD Shiatsu developed in Japan when Buddhism was introduced to the country. Delegations from China brought back skills in medicine, and the Japanese developed their own characteristics for shiatsu.

800 AD Turkish baths were developed in the Ottoman Empire.

1100 AD An Italian woman doctor, Trotula of Salesno, advised those preoccupied with slimming and beauty to bathe in the sea and use applications made of herbs. Her remedy involved spreading a mixture of cow dung and medicinal herbs all over the body followed by either long periods of time in a small room sweating profusely or, alternatively, hot sand baths.

1200 AD Britons discovered Turkish baths during the Crusades. This may have led to the development of 'sweat houses' in London.

1326 AD Spa, Belgium: the Sulus Par Aqua (see previously 80 AD) spring was re-discovered. Local ironmaster Collin le Loup was said to be cured by the waters from the local spring.

1350 AD Warm springs were developed in Europe, including one at Buda. Carlsbad, discovered by Emperor Charles IV, became a famous spa. Around this time the douche or shower was developed in Italy.

1360 AD In England, hot springs gained a bad reputation because of the nudity and spread of disease. The perceived immoral behaviour of bathers led to them being made to cover up while bathing.

1500 AD Bathing increased in popularity as a medical treatment during the Renaissance period in Europe.

1540 AD Baths and springs were closed in England by Henry VIII because of their links with Rome.

1551 AD William Slingsby discovered a spring at Harrogate with waters similar to the spring at Spa, Belgium. Timothy Bright named this spring the 'English Spa', and it was also referred to as the 'English spaw fountain'.

1571 AD English Catholics travelled to Spa in Belgium to 'take the water' and meet up with Catholics from all over Europe. Fears of a plot to overthrow the Protestant monarchy in England led to an Act of Parliament to limit travel to Spa in Belgium. To counter this threat, bathing in England was popularized by Elizabeth I.'Taking the waters' became popular again. Baden in Germany became the most famous spa in Europe.

1580 AD Italian spas flourished, including Abano, Padua, Montecatini and Lucca. French spas developed more slowly and included Vichy.

1631 AD Research into the chemical content of spa water claimed that English spas were as health-giving and effective as the popular European ones.

1663 AD Popularity of spas was increased by Charles II visiting spas at Bath, Epsom and Tunbridge. Samuel Pepys (diarist) commented at the time about Bath that 'methinks it cannot be clean to go so many bodies in the same water'. Each spa was unique, and was thought to have specific properties that could heal certain illnesses.

1690 AD Cold water treatment was developed as a therapy for mental illnesses.

1750 AD The therapeutic benefits of the sea and bathing were becoming increasingly accepted. Cold water was said to stimulate circulation, promote sleep and help heal burns and scalds.

1780 AD In an attempt to cure his madness, George III 'takes the waters' at Weymouth, on the southern coast of England.

1810 AD A revival in massage. Peter Henry Ling of Sweden (1776–1839) made the most dramatic contribution to massage and exercise. His influence spread to Europe and America. He understood the necessity for a knowledge of anatomy and physiology before applying massage and exercise. He emphasized that only normal conditions should be treated and the abnormal be left to the doctor. He founded the Swedish system of massage.

1826 AD At the High Rock Spring in Saratoga (New York), a European-style spa was opened.

1829 AD Grafenberg, Germany, the first hydrotherapy spa was established, encompassing diet, exercise, bathing, fresh air and health treatments. The 'Priessnitz cure' was a type of cold water cure developed to include cold wraps, cold baths plus fresh air,

TERMINOLOGY

A **douche** is a shower. The Scottish douche is a very stimulating treatment. With the client standing, the spa therapist applies a high-pressure hose of alternating warm and cold water to simulate massage movements.

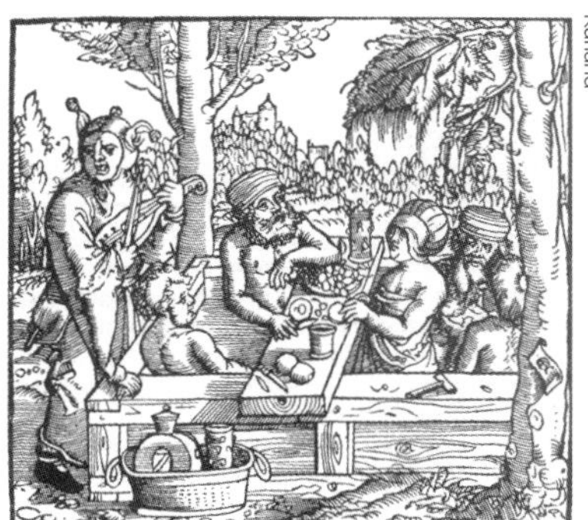

Kurland

Spa in Belgium

TERMINOLOGY

A **Vichy shower** is sometimes called an affusion shower. It is a horizontal shower with varying pressures and temperatures suspended over a wet table so that the entire body is covered with a gentle warm stream of water.

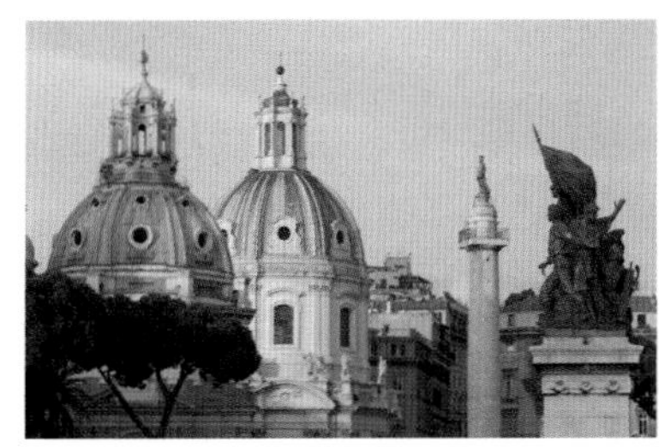

1580, Italian spas flourished

FACT

Many famous individuals extolled the benefits of taking the **'cold water cure'** at Malvern, including Charles Darwin, Alfred, Lord Tennyson and Florence Nightingale.

FACT

A **sitz bath** stimulates the immune system. It is a chair-like bath. The feet soak in alternate hot and cold water, while the hips and lower body are immersed in herbal hot water.

nutrition and exercise. Douches and 'sitz' baths (hip bath) were used to help heal within the pelvic areas.

1848 More than 30 'water cure' centres opened across the eastern coast of America. These differed from European spas as they were less demanding on the individual and did not encompass diet and exercise. They were seen as more sociable when compared to a health cure for illness and ailments.

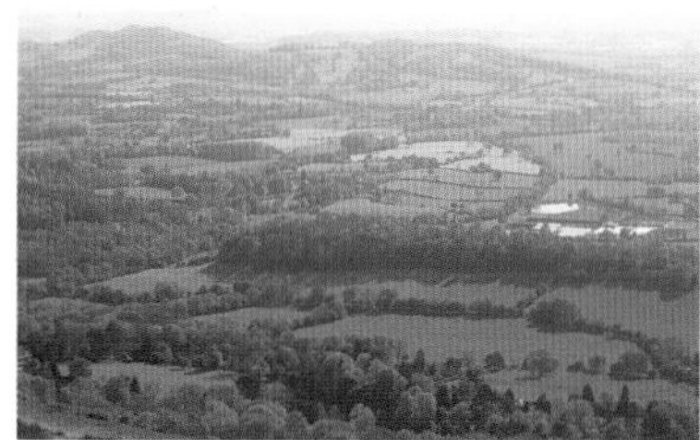

Malvern, England

1849 AD Malvern in the West Midlands had been a small spa for over a hundred years, but now became the main centre in England for treating the sick through hydrotherapy. Malvern was linked with a spa in Yorkshire called Ben Rhydding. Other spas administering the 'water cure' across the country included Manchester, Epsom, Tunbridge Wells, Bath, Matlock, Grasmere, Cheltenham and Ramsgate.

FACT

The **Swiss shower** is a cascading vertical body spray shower. Multiple sprays create a gentle or vigorous rain shower from the ankles to the shoulders from above.

1851 AD In New York the American Hydropathic Institute opened, later succeeded by the New York Hydropathic School. The 'water cure' was popular in America until the late 1850s. The end of the Civil War changed many of the spa centres. Some closed and those that survived had less of a focus on water. 'Hot springs' flourished in areas such as Arkansas, Florida and West Virginia.

FACT

Saratoga springs in New York was one of the most famous and a great influence on the **spa culture** of America.

1861 AD Vienna, Austria: a clinic and the Institute of Hydrotherapy was opened by Dr W. Winternitz.

1876 AD Dr John Kellog was a student of Dr Winternitz in Vienna, and for 46 years practised at the Battle Creek sanatorium in America. His brother invented the breakfast cereal for patients at the sanatorium.

TERMINOLOGY

Mud treatments are often referrred to as **Pelotherapy**.

1867 AD Thalassotherapy was defined and developed by Dr La Bonardhière. It involved healing the body through sea air and treatments including seawater, algae, mud and sand.

1870 AD Dr Mezger of Holland (1839–1901) helped to establish massage as a reputable means of treatment in the field of rehabilitation and medicine.

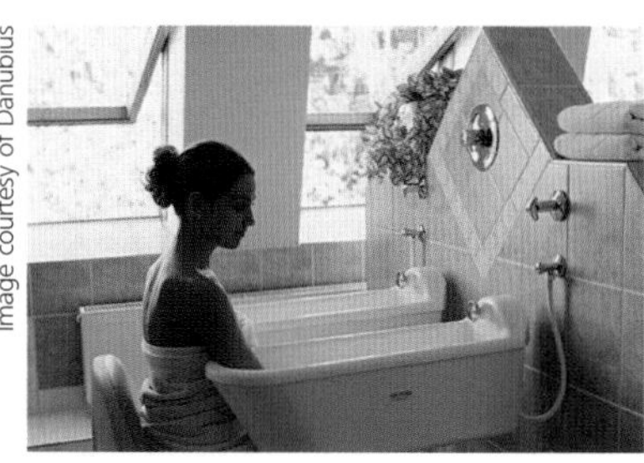

Image courtesy of Danubius

A Kneipp bath

FACT

Seawater cures became more popular in France and Sweden because their seawater was rich in minerals and trace elements, with the Dead Sea's salt concentration being ten times stronger than the Mediterranean Sea's.

FACT

Kneipp body wraps are relaxing, detoxifying and can also improve the immune system. Additives such as clay, salt and dried herbs are often used. The **Kneipp bath** was developed to use herbal or mineral baths of differing temperatures.

1880 AD Bad Worishofen, Germany: the poor benefited from the hydrotherapy treatments of Father Sebastian Kneipp, who went on to publish *My Water Cure* in 1892. The '**Kneipp cure**' was a combination of treatments encompassing plant therapy and lifestyle changes.

1894 AD A group of women joined together to form the Society of Trained Masseuses to raise the standards and reputation of massage. Rules and regulations were developed for training. Exams were set and the society flourished. It was licensed by the Board of Trade in 1900 and called the Incorporated Society of Trained Masseuses.

1895 AD The term '**naturopathy**' was developed by Dr J. Scheel to encompass natural medical cures, including water. Massage, herbs, wholefood, air and water were recommended in favour of medication and surgery. A year later the American School of Naturopathy was founded in New York.

1900 AD '**Climatotherapy**' was developed, using the healing powers of the climate combined with the mineral rich seawater treatments.

1917 AD Eight spa towns grouped together to establish the British Spas Federation (BSF).

1918 AD Individuals wounded in the First World War were treated in spas at Bath, Buxton, Cheltenham and Harrogate. The conditions treated were varied, such as shell shock, war wounds, and muscle and joint injuries.

1920 AD The Society of Trained Masseuses amalgamated with the Institute of Massage and Remedial Exercise. A royal charter was granted and it became known as the Chartered Society of Massage and Medical Gymnastics. The title was changed again in 1943 to the Chartered Society of Physiotherapy. It became state registered in 1964. Exercise in water became an acceptable and recognized part of rehabilitation programmes.

1925 AD Establishment of an institute for shiatsu by Tokujiro Namikoshi, adapting the traditional Japanese massage techniques.

1925 AD Champneys Cure resort was opened in Tring, Hertforshire, by the naturopath Stanley Leif.

1939 AD Spas treat soldiers wounded in the Second World War. Because of the cost of the war, there was no money to re-invest in British spas and inevitably they became run-down and fell into disrepair. European spas, meanwhile, continued to flourish and maintain their role as vital for health and wellbeing.

1990 AD The London Thrombosis Research Institute developed a cold water treatment involving 'head out of water immersion'. The results proved that cold water treatment helped thin the blood

TERMINOLOGY

Naturopathy encompasses natural substances and the power of nature to heal the body.

TERMINOLOGY

Climatotherapy uses the forces of nature, including air, light, wind, sun, humidity and location.

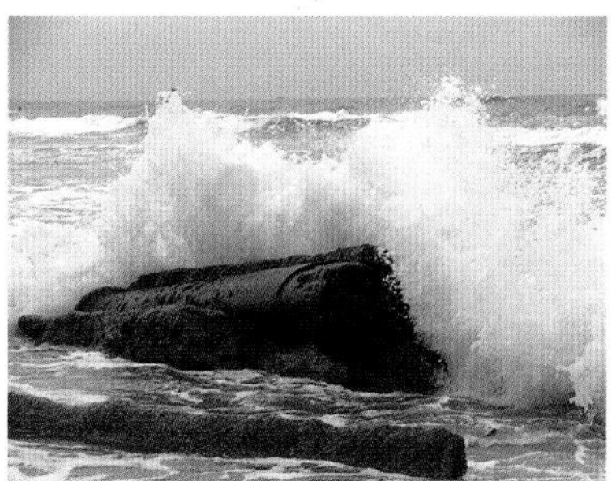

Climatotherapy includes mineral rich seawater treatments

FACT

Paraffin wax and fango mud can be combined in a **Parafango** treatment to heat, exfoliate and detoxify the body.

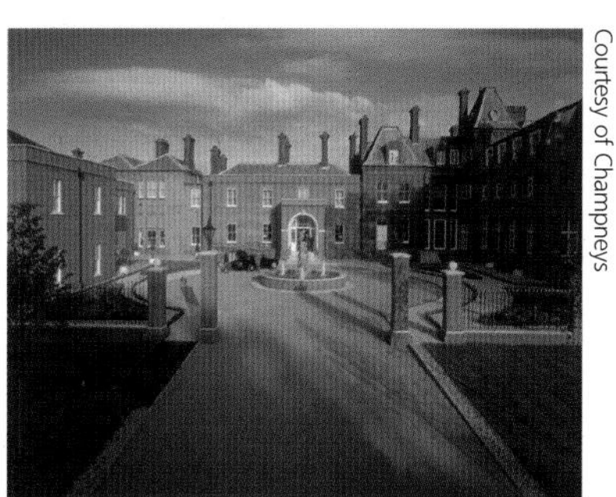

Courtesy of Champneys

Champneys, Tring, England

International Spa Association

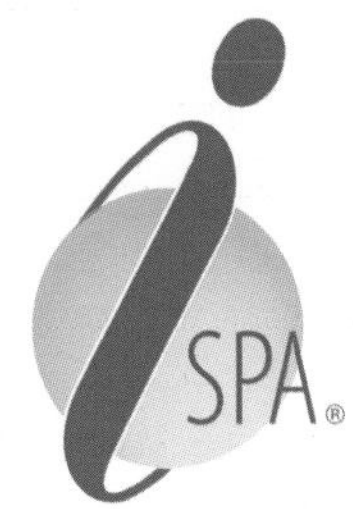

ISPA logo

Courtesy of Chiva-Som

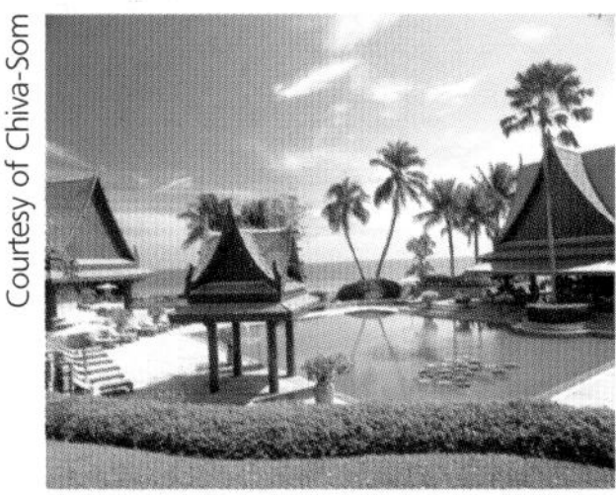

Chiva-Som, Thailand

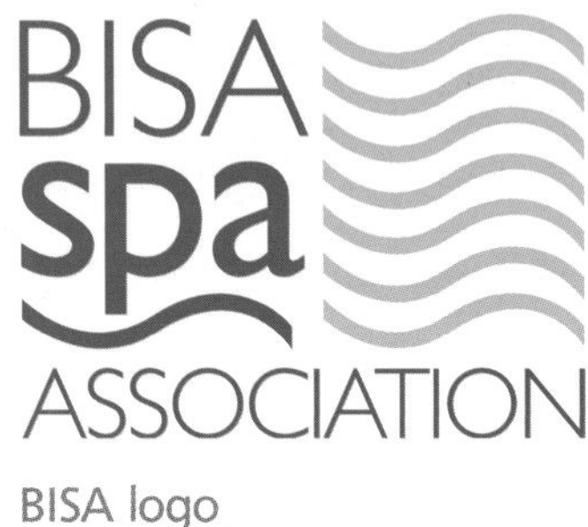

BISA logo

spa business association

SBA logo

Oriental Spa, Bangkok

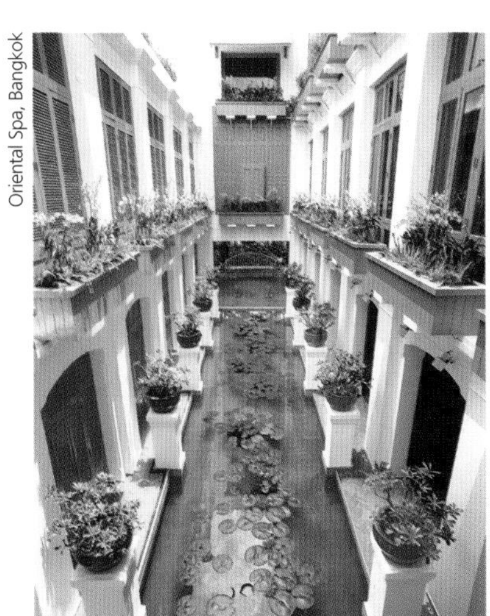

Spa therapy is a booming industry

and block the clotting mechanism. These results endorsed the claims made by many people over centuries that 'cold water cures' definitely worked and were not simply 'myth or legend'.

1991 AD International Spa Association (ISPA) was established in America.

1993 AD First spa on board a cruise liner was opened on the Queen Elizabeth 2 by Steiner Leisure Group.

1993 AD Destination and retreat spas established, such as Chiva-Som in Thailand.

1995 AD The European Spa Association (ESPA) was established.

1998 AD The British International Spa Association (BISA) was founded to establish minimum standards and quality of service to the spa industry.

2000 AD Spa therapy qualifications were developed.

2001 AD Hydrotherapy became an acceptable treatment worldwide and used in hospitals and medical centres by physiotherapists to treat a wide range of conditions.

2004 AD The British Spas Federation (BSF) became the representative body for the spa industry in the United Kingdom and Ireland and changed its name to the Spa Business Association (SpaBA).

Today A spa revolution. The 'spa business' has seen enormous growth, both within the United Kingdom and internationally. This expansion has resulted in the development of national standards and qualifications in '**spa therapy**' as a more relevant, specialized qualification for individuals wanting to work in the spa industry.

SUPPORTING AND PROMOTING THE SPA INDUSTRY

There are numerous organizations around the world supporting the spa industry and promoting the services and benefits of the sector. These are too diverse to mention individually, but the main developments are:

- The British Spas Foundation (BSF), formed in 1917, changed its name in 2004 to the Spa Business Association (SpaBA). This is a large organization representing everyone supplying, investing, employed or studying in the spa industry in the United Kingdom or Ireland and aims to 'provide one strong voice for everyone in this dynamic and vibrant industry'. SpaBA works to influence government, media, investors, legislative bodies and consumers.
- The International Spa Association (ISPA) was founded in America in 1991. The organization is recognized as the leading professional organization and voice of the spa industry. Membership comprises approximately 2000 health and wellness facilities and providers from nearly 70 countries. ISPA works to advance the professionalism of the spa industry by providing invaluable educational and networking opportunities to promote the value of the

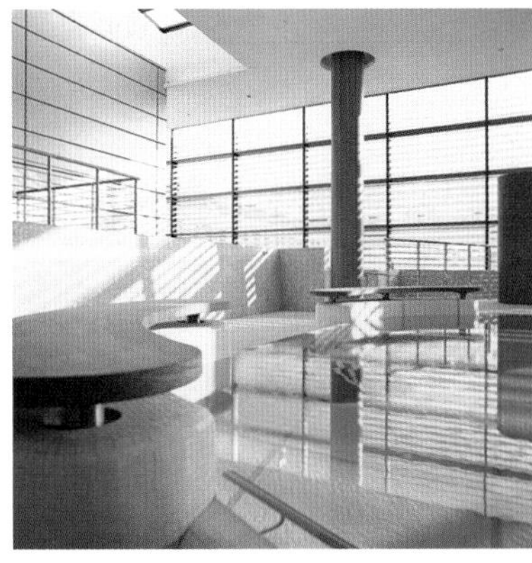
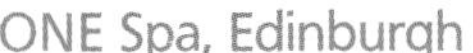

ONE Spa, Edinburgh

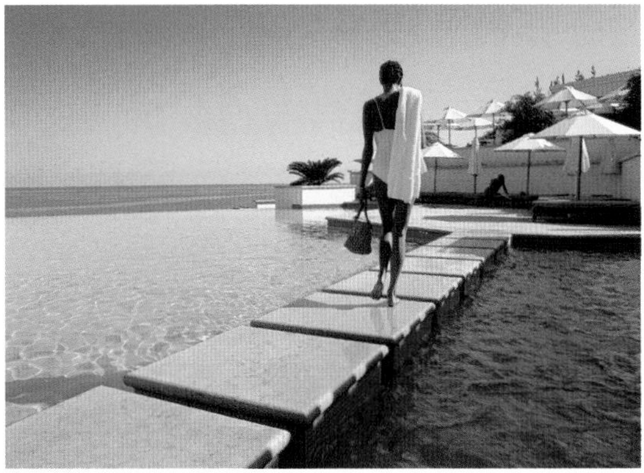

Thalassa Spa, Anassa, Cyprus

spa experience to society and to be the authoritative voice of the spa industry.

- In 1995 the European Spa Association (ESPA) was formed to promote spas and encourage a collaborative approach to training, standards setting, research and educating health and medical practitioners. This brought together the German Spa Association (DBV) and the British Spas Federation (BSF).

In addition to professional organizations, there are many other activities that promote the spa industry:

- **Publications**: there are an increasing number of glossy, aspirational 'coffee-table' books being published that feature spas. Magazines ranging from lifestyle editions to specialist trade publications all promote the services and benefits of spas.
- **Websites**: thousands of websites are available to satisfy the appetite of the public for spa knowledge and many of these can be found in the spa directory in this book.
- **Travel companies**: an increasing number of companies are specializing in 'spa tourism' and offer bespoke packages tailored to the individual's every need.
- **Hotels**: many hotel groups are promoting 'spa packages' as they see this revenue stream as essential to their expansion plans. Some organizations are going further and developing their own quality benchmarks and criteria. The Leading Hotels organization, for example, launched a global spa certification programme in recognition of the growth and popularity of the spa experience, especially in conjunction with a hotel visit. A panel of spa experts will ensure that certification means compliance with testing standards that define and distinguish a world-class spa.

FACT

Leading Hotels has become recognized as the world's largest brand of luxury hotels, encompassing more than 420 hotels in over 80 countries.

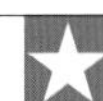

SPA TIP

Professional Spa is a high-quality publication that showcases world-class spas and treatments, as well as providing valuable information and contacts for spa professionals.

SPA TIP

Conde Nast Traveller is a fantastic, highly regarded magazine that features spas regularly and holds an annual 'Readers' Spa Awards'.

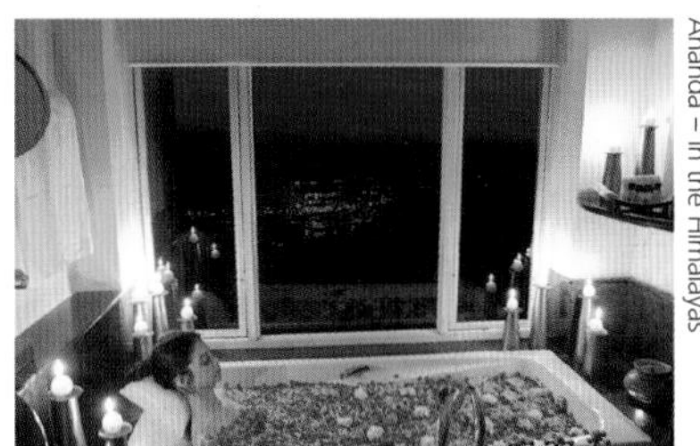

Ananda – in the Himalayas

A flower bath treatment at Ananda – in the Himalayas

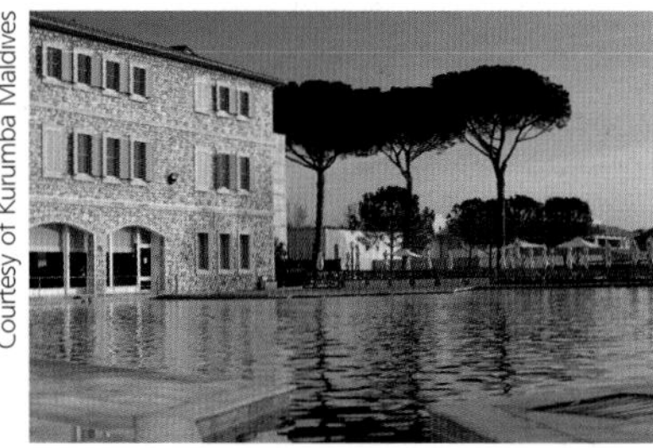

Courtesy of Kurumba Maldives

TERMINOLOGY

Glocal a word used in the spa sector to describe the combination of global influences with local culture and traditions.

World-wide opportunities

The spa business is booming and a huge variety of spas exist in different parts of the world. Spas tailored to the uniqueness of their locations include 'vineyard spas' and 'ski spas', and spa developments are springing up in countries as diverse as Cyprus, France, Greece, India, Italy, Mauritius, the Maldives, New Zealand and Switzerland. Each type of spa is aimed at a particular segment of the market and, depending on the location, they can all thrive and be successful.

The increasing popularity and media coverage of spas has made clients very well educated and informed as to the range of treatments on offer, which in turn has made them more demanding. They are prepared to spend time and money on visiting spas as they see this as an investment in their health. This investment on the part of the client leads then to high expectations of the spa experience and only the full service will meet their needs. Increasingly, clients want a full range of water and thermal experiences, combined with a variety of treatments, plus healthy eating, relaxation and fitness activities.

As individuals take more responsibility for their own health, they turn to spas to provide a full spectrum of activities, from acupressure to Zen gardens. Many clients work hard to live a longer, healthier life and want to preserve their youthfulness. Increasingly, medi spas and wellness centres are becoming popular, where medical practitioners and health therapists work together to develop new treatments for anti-ageing and improved health. There could not be a more exciting time for you to train and work in the spa industry – the opportunities open to you are fantastic – join now!

FACT

Iceland has more spas per capita than any other country, including the famous 'Blue Lagoon', which is a milky blue lake of silica-rich water.

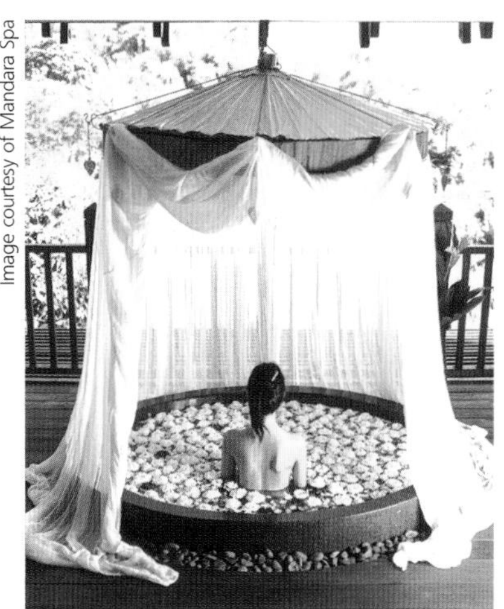

Image courtesy of Mandara Spa

A Mandara Spa treatment

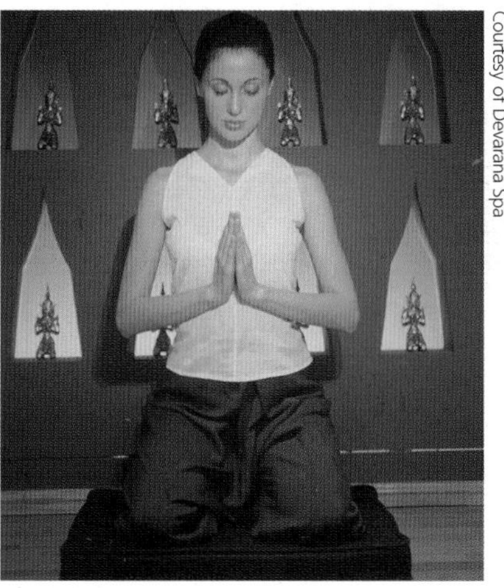

Courtesy of Devarana Spa

People have growing expectations of what spas should provide

SPA PROFILE

Name: Marianne Sinar

Position: Therapist/Director

Establishment: Ki Day Spa Ltd

Products used: Elemis, Crystal Clear, Karin Herzog, Nailtiques, Essie and Seche Vite.

Number of staff/roles: 5 staff (2 holistic therapists, 3 beauty/holistic therapists).

Training/experience: Ran my own business for ten years prior to opening Ki Day Spa.

Main responsibilities: Training treatments; treatment development; service; marketing; business development/strategy; recruitment; sales; hygiene.

Best parts of the job: Client satisfaction; good working environment; working with leading products/brands.

Therapist – key skills: Knowledge about treatments/products/services; communication skills; listening skills; empathy; teamwork; initiative; awareness; time management.

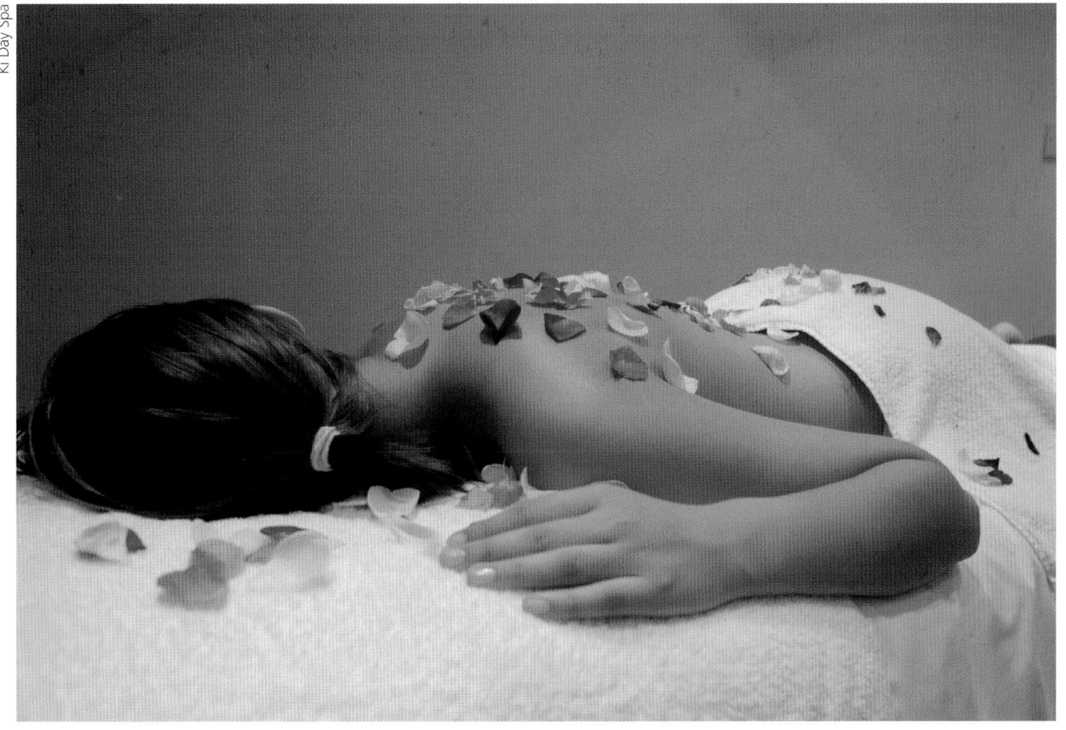
Ki Day Spa

Assessment of knowledge and understanding

When you have some free time, test your understanding and knowledge by answering the following questions. Do this at regular intervals and it will reinforce your learning and help you retain the knowledge, so you are able to perform better in your assessments.

1 What does the latin phrase '*Solus per aqua*' mean?

2 From what date was Ayurvedic medicine practised in India?

3 Who was referred to as the 'father of medicine'? And what was his 'rule of opposites'?

4 In which country is the town of Spa?

5 What is:
   a. a caldarium?
   b. a tepidarium?
   c. a frigidarium?

6 What is the name of the famous German spa where a thermal spring was discovered by the Romans?

7 Why did hot springs in England gain a bad reputation in 1360?

8 In 1551, which spa did Timothy Bright name the 'English Spa'?

9 Which diarist said 'methinks it cannot be clean to go so many bodies in the same water'?

10 Who said 'The sea washes away all the evils of mankind'?

11 Which English king attempted to cure his madness by bathing at Weymouth?

12 Who founded the Swedish system of massage?

13 What is the 'Priessnitz cure'?

14 What is a 'sitz' bath?

15 Which English spa became the main centre for treating the sick by hydrotherapy in the mid-nineteenth century?

16 For the patients of which American sanatorium was Kellog's breakfast cereal invented?

17 What is a 'Kneipp bath'?

18 What is 'climatotherapy'?

19 In which year was the British Spas Federation (BSF) established?

20 In what year did the Chartered Society of Physiotherapists become state registered?

21 What year did Champneys Cure resort open?

22 Which association was established in America in 1991?

23 What is the aim of the Spa Business Association (SpaBA)?

24 In which country is the 'Blue Lagoon' spa?

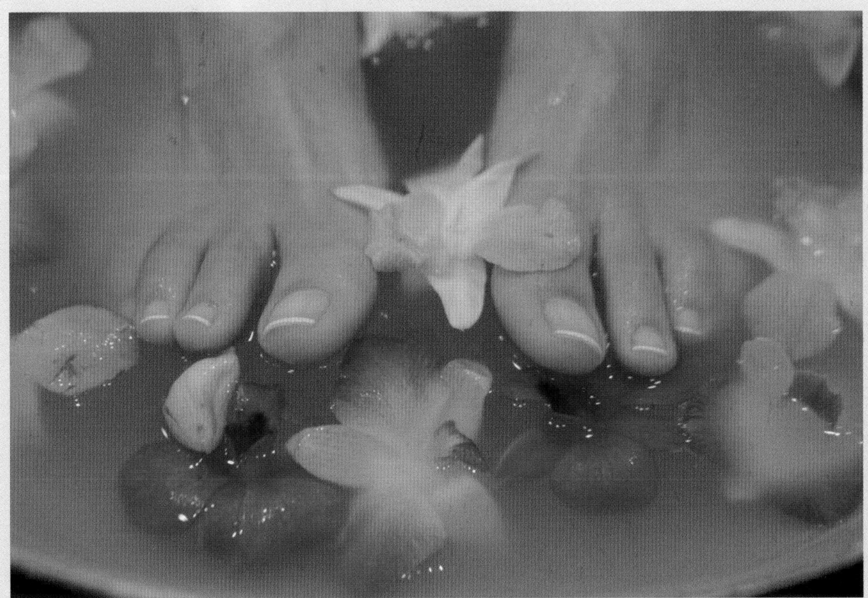

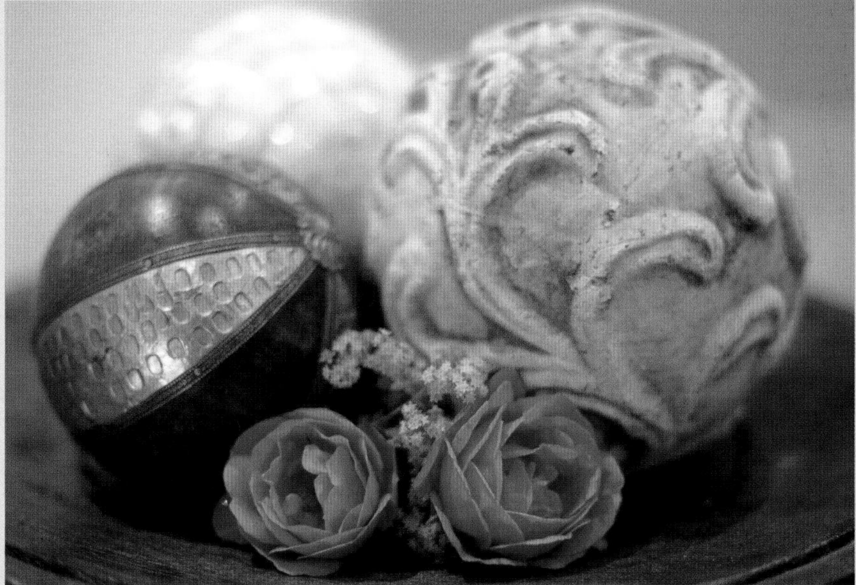

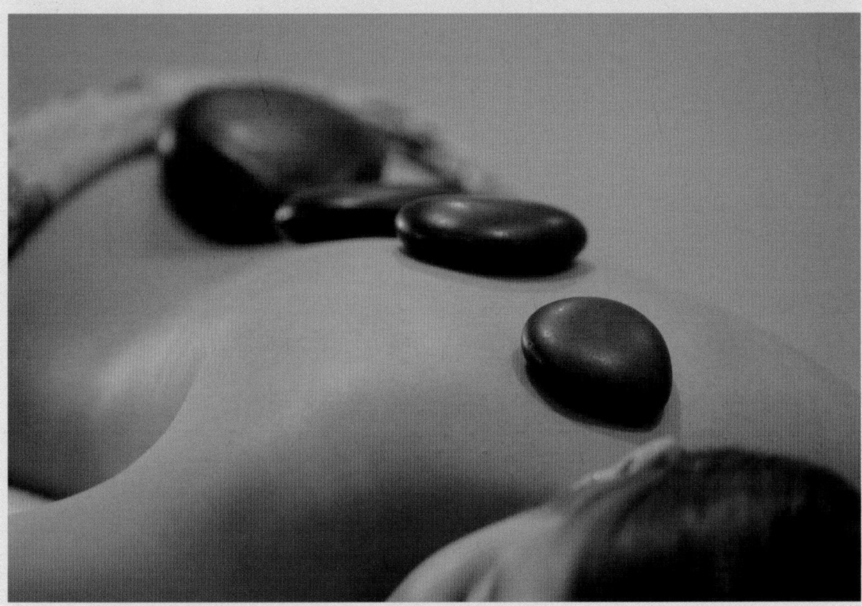

With the explosive growth of the spa industry over the last ten years, career opportunities throughout the world are abundant – with demand for capable, highly qualified, skilled staff, trained in the operational safety and strategic planning, necessary for a successful spa business.

JANE CREBBIN-BAILEY, PARTNER – HCB ASSOCIATES

The feeling of achievement through contributing to helping our clients enjoy 'me' time out, relax, rejuvenate and reflect on the positive changes they can make within their lives; whilst at the same time developing your technical knowledge, communication, interpersonal and management skills, is the best in the world! Go for it!

SUSIE SANTIAGO, LEADING SPA OPENING MANAGEMENT CONSULTANT AND FOUNDER OF THE ANNUAL SANTI DEVELOPMENT PROGRAMME

A well designed spa should encompass the fundamentals of personal wellbeing. My role in SÁMAS is to provide a range of oriental movement classes to complement the therapeutic elements of the spa. My experience and career path runs parallel with my colleagues' but in a different discipline. Spa offers many opportunities.

JEZ COOPER, RESIDENT MASTER OF MIND, BODY AND PHYSICAL WELLBEING, SÁMAS DELUXE DESTINATION SPA AT THE PARK HOTEL KENMARE

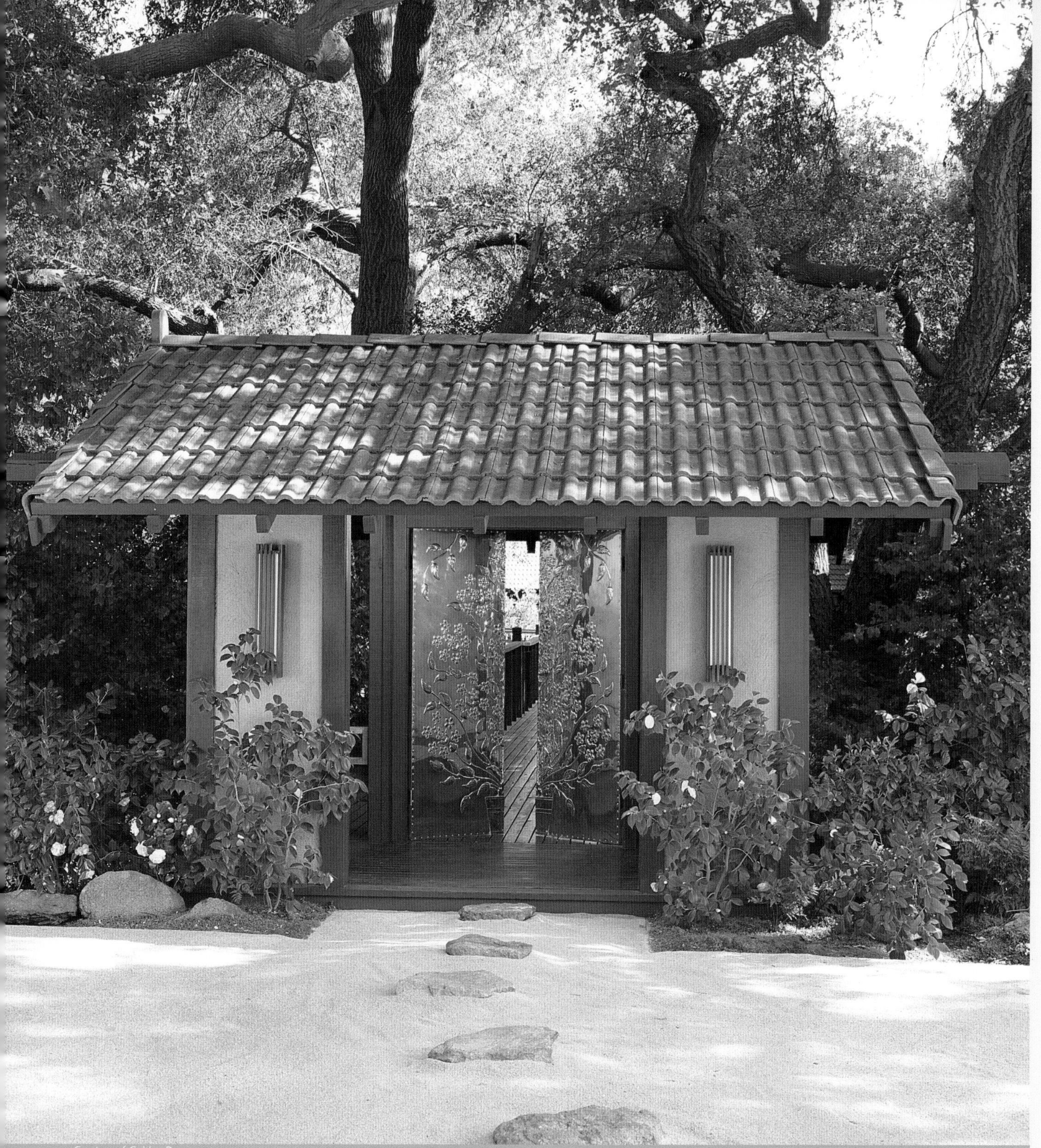

Courtesy of Golden Door

The continuing growth of awareness amongst the general population of the body/mind connection makes this an exciting time to be involved in the spa movement. The need to replenish and create balance by incorporating various types of bodywork into wellness regimes, in conjunction with exercise programmes, is seen more and more as a necessity rather than a luxury.

DIANA TURK, MASSAGE SUPERVISOR, GOLDEN DOOR

2 SUBSTANCE

It is a very exciting time to be part of the spa industry. Spas are now mainstream as consumers are demanding the nurturing and healing environment offered during the spa experience. Spas have gained respectability as the emphasis for spa-goers is increasingly that of self-preservation, stress relief and relaxation. People are busier than ever before and want to reward themselves for working so hard. Everyone deserves a 'time out' to recharge their batteries.

LYNNE WALKER MCNEES, ISPA PRESIDENT

In today's world, where the pace of life seems to only increase, we need to be reminded how to slow down, take a deep breath and think about what we are doing. Increasingly, spas are becoming holistic centres that consider your whole being and help you to get in touch with your natural healing potential and show you how it can be utilized. Gone are the days when a spa retreat was an indulgence enjoyed by the wealthy; instead, it is something that many of us are seeking in order to maintain the balance to achieve and maintain good health.

SUGHRA BIBI, CORPORATE TRAINING MANAGER, SIX SENSES SPAS

chapter 2

The spa sector, market and industry

Learning objectives

This chapter covers the background information you need to recognize different types of spa. It describes the skills and knowledge necessary to enable you to:

- **identify the seven ISPA spa types**
- **recognize other spa types**
- **understand where the spa industry is heading**
- **understand the key spa roles**

INTRODUCTION

As the number of spa visitors is rapidly increasing, the clients' demands for services offered at a spa are becoming more specialized and with a greater emphasis on lifestyle programmes. There are many types of spa offering a variety of services to meet clients' needs, varying from day spas to luxury resort spas where every need is catered for. The International Spa Association (ISPA) has categorized them into seven types to help consumers choose their preferred type of spa experience:

- Destination spa.
- Day spa.
- Resort/hotel spa.
- Medi spa.
- Cruise ship spa.
- Spa town.
- Mineral spring spa.

Destination spa

This type of spa provides guests with a whole lifestyle programme as well as a vast range of therapies. The guests are all here to experience the spa and achieve personal goals, e.g. lose weight, de-stress, eat healthily or just to take a break from their hectic lifestyles and have some personal space.

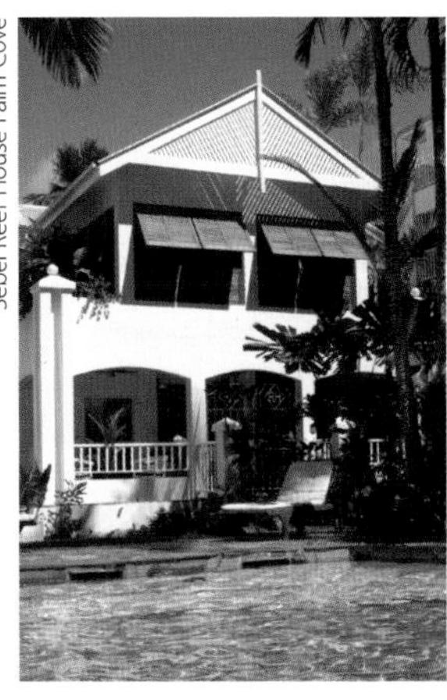
Exclusive Spas Australia. Image Collection – Copyright, Sebel Reef House Palm Cove

Spa exterior

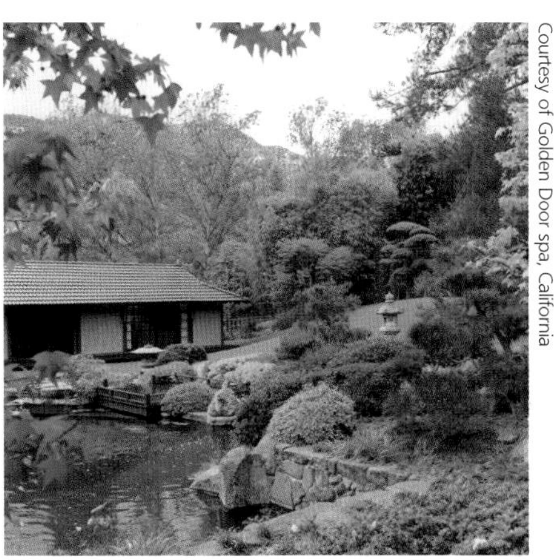
Courtesy of Golden Door spa, California

Koi pond

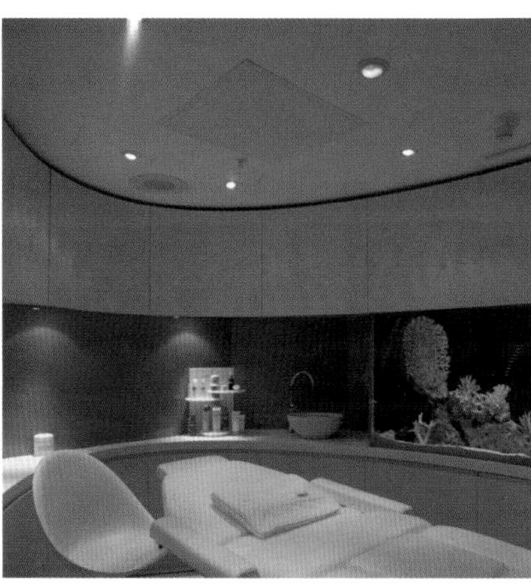
Urban Retreat at Harrods

Crème de la mer treatment room

The main facilities should include:

- On-site accommodation
- Healthy food – spa cuisine
- Physical fitness programmes which include outdoor activities
- A variety of spa treatments – these may vary depending on the style of the spa
- Relaxation areas
- Tailor-made packages aimed at different client requests
- Spectacular location/surroundings
- Spa facilities – swimming pool, hydrotherapy baths, etc.
- Medical supervision
- Educational programmes – talks, lectures, workshops
- Professional, qualified staff
- Gym/fitness facilities

FACT

The Golden Door in California has regularly received awards for the best US destination spa and the world's best destination spa.

Day spa

A lot of beauty salons have changed their names to join the trend of the 'day spa' but some are just a salon offering basic spa services. Day spas are targeting the busy professional client who wants to access spa services on a day-use basis.

The main facilities should include:

- A clean, calm, relaxing, nurturing environment
- Changing facilities with lockers for storing personal belongings and outdoor wear
- Spa robes and slippers
- Private treatment rooms for each client, which include shower facilities
- Professional, qualified therapists
- Body and face treatments, including some form of hydrotherapy/water-based therapies
- Half and full day spa treatment programmes
- Relaxation area
- Optional facilities include: hair services, manicures and pedicures, spa cuisine/health food and fitness facilities: personal trainer, yoga/pilates/meditation classes

SPA TIP

A **Couples Day Suite** is a treatment room containing his and hers couches, showers, relaxation area, outdoor spa pool (if the climate allows), music system, etc.

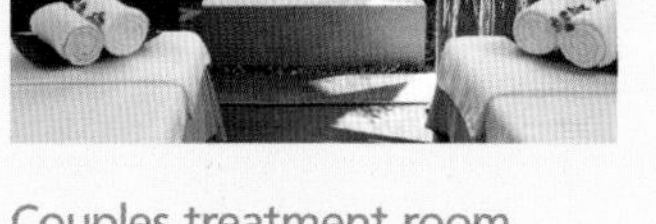
Courtesy of Mandara Spa

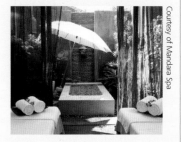

Couples treatment room

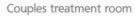

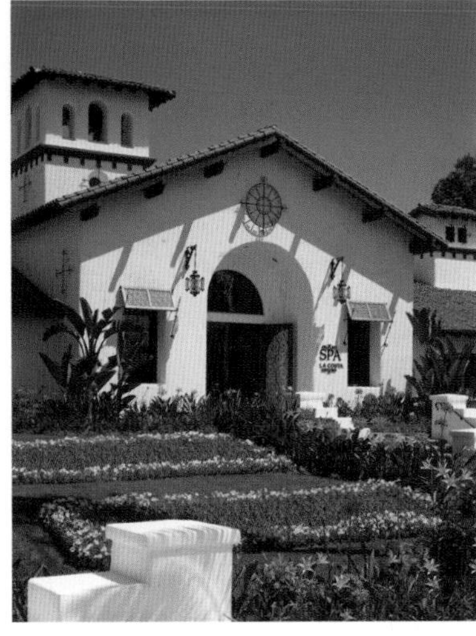

Spa entrance, La Costa Resort & Spa, California

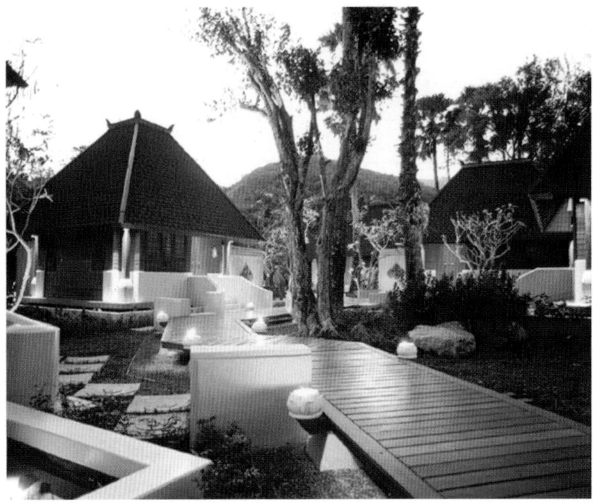

Spa entrance, Hilton, Phuket

SPA TIP

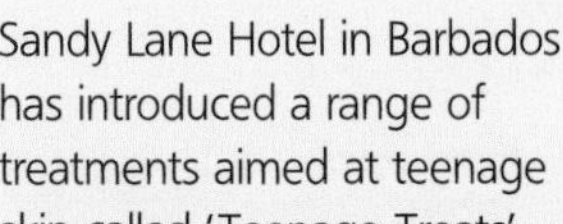

Sandy Lane Hotel in Barbados has introduced a range of treatments aimed at teenage skin called 'Teenage Treats'.

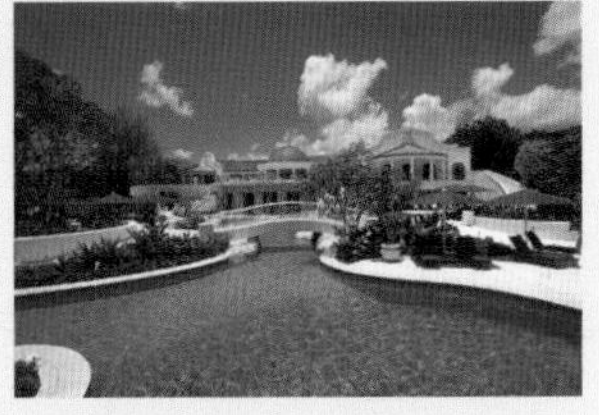

Image courtesy of Sandy Lane, Barbados

View to the spa, Sandy Lane Spa, Barbados

Resort/hotel spa

Located within a hotel or resort, the resort/hotel spa may be owned by the hotel or a franchise provision and will provide professional spa services to guests, which may include outside guests who pay a daily rate to use the facilities. They may also be situated adjacent to the hotel if not directly inside the building.

The main facilities should include:

- Changing facilities with lockers for storing personal belongings and outdoor wear
- Spa robes and slippers
- Private treatment rooms for each client, which include shower facilities
- Professional, qualified therapists
- Body and face treatments, including massage
- Half and full day spa treatment programmes
- Relaxation area
- Swimming pool/gym/fitness facilities, which may also include tennis courts, golf course
- Spa cuisine, but also the option of finer foods, desserts and alcohol for clients not following specific weight-loss programmes and who are looking more for luxuries
- Optional facilities include: hair salon services, manicures and pedicures, some form of hydrotherapy/water-based therapies and a hydrotherapy suite (sauna, steam, thermidarium, rasul, etc.)

Medi spa

The medi spa integrates traditional spa services with aesthetic services. As cosmetic surgery is on the increase, this environment allows for clients to receive spa treatments recommended by the doctors to increase their recovery after surgery and still experience the benefits of spa therapy.

Clinique La Prairie, Montreux

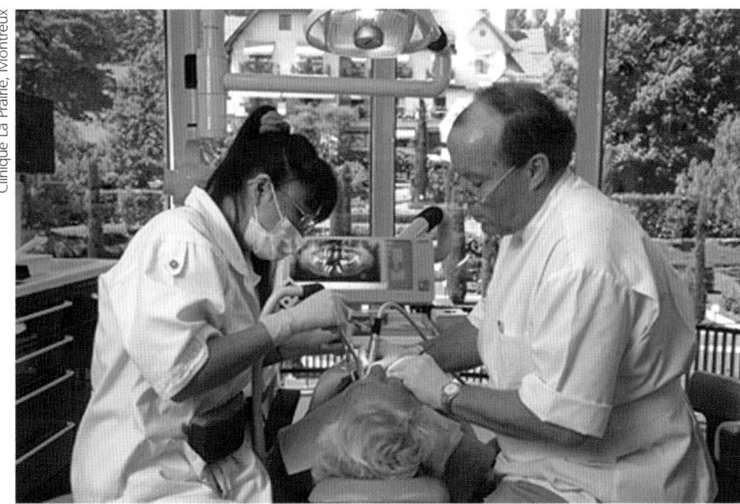

Medical treatment, Clinique La Prairie, Switzerland

SPA TIP

La Jolla Spa MD in California has created its own Spa MD skin therapy product line to support their commitment to skin therapy and the correction of sun damage and fine lines.

The main facilities should include:

- Changing facilities with lockers for storing personal belongings and outdoor wear
- Private treatment rooms for each client, which include shower facilities
- Relaxation and waiting areas
- Body and facial spa services, including massage
- Spa cuisine
- Hydrotherapy pool
- Weight-loss programmes
- Qualified professional therapists and double board-certified surgeons
- Medical procedures, which may include acupuncture, botox, laser therapy, liposculpture, plastic surgery, laser hair removal

Cruise ship spa

An increasingly popular form of vacation and one of the fastest growing industries, a spa aboard a cruise ship provides a full range of facial and body treatments, fitness facilities and exercise programmes and has similar facilities to a hotel/resort spa. Most cruise ships are now like floating hotels!

FACT

Steiner Leisure Group has nearly 200 spas on board cruise ships around the world.

The main facilities should include:

- Private treatment rooms
- A full range of body and facial therapies
- Gym and fitness facilities
- Relaxation area
- Hair salon services including manicures and pedicures
- Optional facilities include: some form of hydrotherapy/water-based therapies, a hydrotherapy suite (sauna, steam, rasul, etc.), personal training sessions

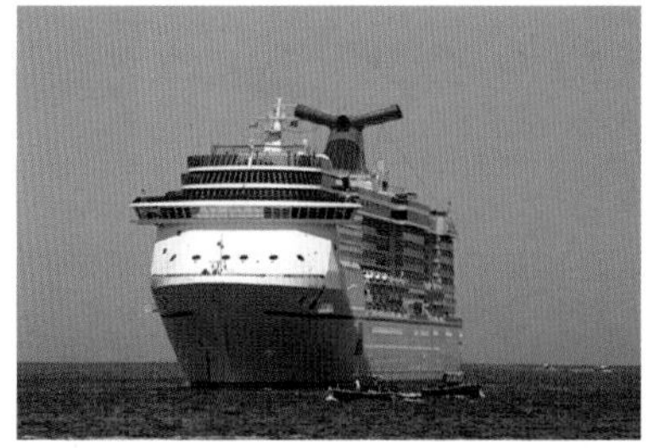

Cruise ship at sea

SPA TIP 

Chiva-Som in Thailand was one of the first destination spas to open in the Far East and has been voted one of the top destination spas in the world for many years, leading to a surge in spa development in that part of the world.

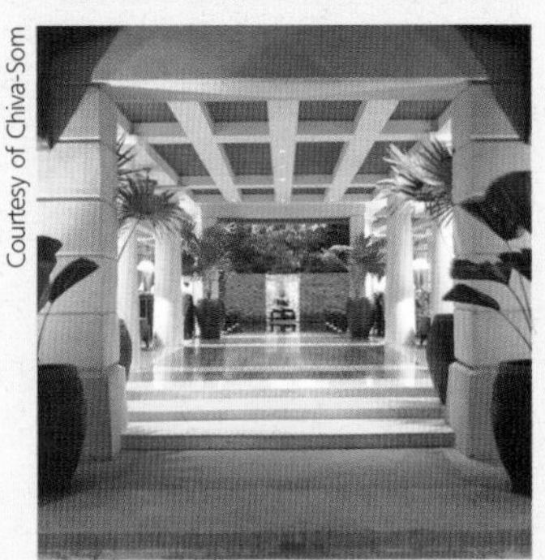
Courtesy of Chiva-Som

Entrance to Chiva-Som

FACT !

One of the oldest spa towns in Europe is Baden-Baden in Germany.

Spa town

These were the only source of spa treatments for centuries and are now undergoing a resurgence in popularity. Built on a natural thermal mineral water source that is used both for bathing and incorporated into a variety of hydrotherapy treatments.

A traditional spa town would include:

- Natural mineral/thermal/seawater source
- A vast range of hydrotherapy treatments and bathing facilities
- Historical buildings
- Cultural activities
- An outdoor, healthy environment with parks, etc., for walking in and relaxing

Mineral spring spa

This may be a stand-alone spa facility or be combined with a destination spa or medi spa. Usually there is a naturally occurring source of thermal or mineral water, or in some cases seawater. Mud treatments may also feature at these spas.

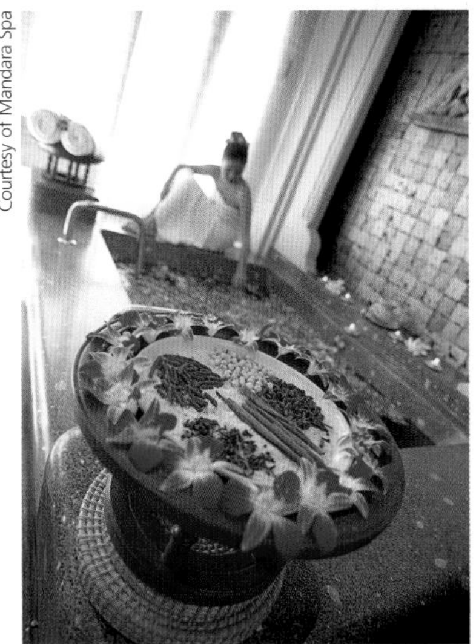
Courtesy of Mandara Spa

Plunge pool

Other spa types

In addition to the seven ISPA categories of spa, several other types can be identified:

Club spa

A club spa is part of the health club industry, whose main purpose is fitness but whose clients wish to access spa facilities on a day-use basis. Ideally the spa area should be situated away from the fitness facilities – which can be very noisy – in a more peaceful and quiet location.

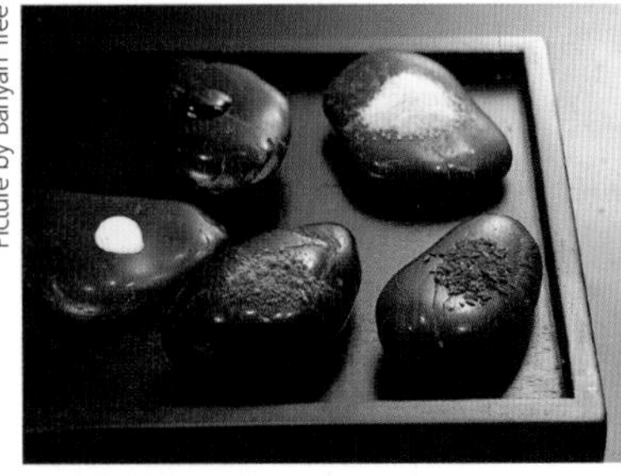
Picture by Banyan Tree

Herbs and spices, Banyan Tree

Tropical/Asian experience

Spas offering a tropical/Asian experience employ local treatments which have been carried out for centuries as traditional healing systems and since adapted into treatments to suit a modern clientele. The core of the treatments is tapping into natural resources from the region, e.g. herbs, spices, local plants and being aware of the environment, something which is incorporated into the design of a spa with an ecological approach. The spa experience also includes nurturing the client, an approach which has long been part of the culture, and creating a serene, stress-busting retreat.

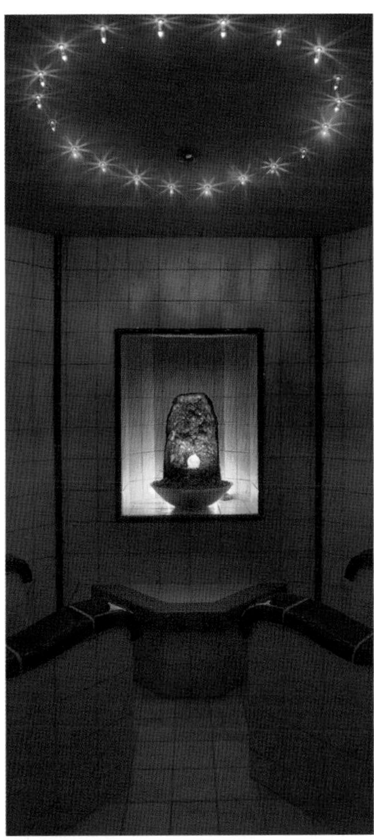

Precious stone chamber, Aghadoe Heights, Ireland

Treatments you may experience at this type of spa are:

- Thai massage
- Balinese massage
- Coconut scrubs
- Balinese boreh
- Lulur
- Indian head massage
- Shirodhara
- Essential oil massage
- Floral bath
- Herbal heat packs

Spiritual spa

As life becomes more frantic, people are looking for a space to re-energize themselves and cleanse the mind, body and soul. More and more spas are adopting a more spiritual feel in the services and treatments they offer, adapting eastern philosophies and beliefs along with the traditional holistic therapies that are an important part of this type of spa.

Treatments you may experience are:

- Yoga
- Meditation
- Shirodhara
- Four-hand massage
- Medicated oil massage
- Self healing
- Reiki
- Honey seed scrub

Elegant spas

Luxurious elegance, reflecting the spa treatments and the service each guest receives, distinguishes these spas from the rest. It is the detail that is applied every day, from the way that the towels are folded and the flowers are placed around the spa to the music played, everything the client experiences in the spa blends into this desirable environment.

Treatments you may experience are:

- Hydrotherapy massage
- Blitz showers
- Algae wraps
- Age-management facials
- Hot stone massage
- Body toning treatments
- Manual lymphatic drainage massage
- Mud mask
- Anti jet lag therapy massage
- Flotation

ACTIVITY

Write a short paragraph on a spa of your choice describing the types of treatments and particular experiences a client would receive when visiting.

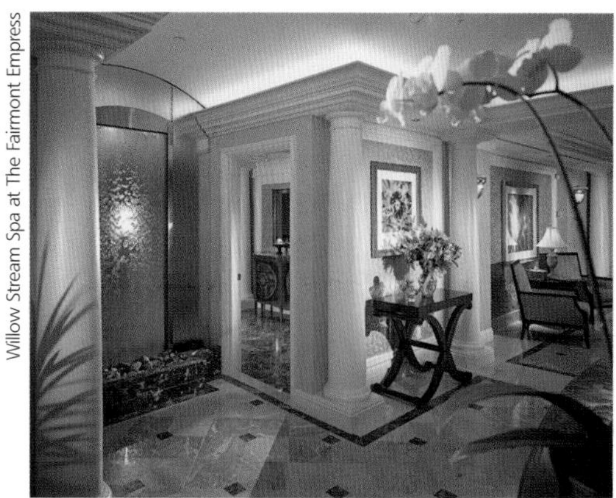

Willow Stream Spa at The Fairmont Empress

Reception, Willow Stream Spa at The Fairmont Empress

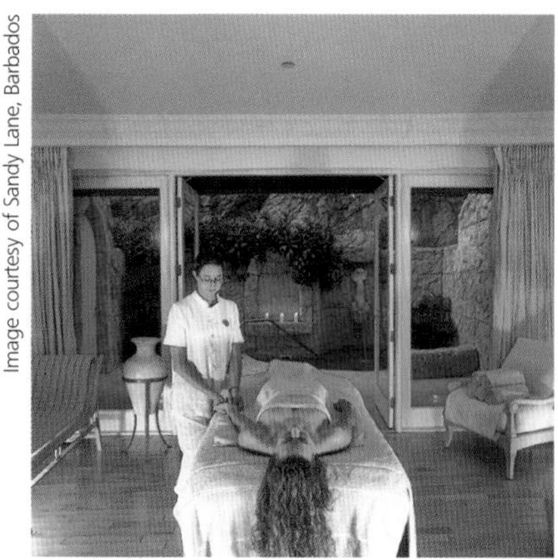

Image courtesy of Sandy Lane, Barbados

Treatment room with private garden and pool, Sandy Lane Spa, Barbados

THERAPEUTIC EUROPEAN SPAS AND THE FUTURE

Traditionally European spas were mainly medical centres for the treatment of diseases such as arthritis, rheumatism and some respiratory and circulatory disorders. Treatments were based around a natural resource such as thermal water, mud, mineral drinking water, salt and even natural gas.

This spa concept tended to follow the same structure: treatments, such as physiotherapy, electrotherapy, hydrotherapy, packs, balneotherapy (i.e., treatments involving thermal water) and rehabilitation massage, were controlled and prescribed by doctors. Guests would visit the spa for two- or three-week stays, many subsidized by state health insurance systems. The range of problems encountered would vary from guests merely wanting to relax and have a break from the stresses of life to those with more serious problems connected to disorders of the locomotor system.

The past ten years has seen a dramatic change in this traditional spa concept in Europe. There have been two major influences. Firstly, the withdrawal of support from state insurance companies and, secondly, as people started to travel and have different 'spa experiences', higher customer expectations.

The result has been a huge swing to **wellness** and the building of extensive aqua facilities in many spas in Europe. This new direction in the spa concept has in many cases taken precedence to the extent that the medical aspect has become almost neglected.

An excellent example of this European shift to wellness is the Danubius Hotel Group. A Danubius health spa contains six key elements:

1. natural resources – 'the centerpiece of our spas'
2. medical excellence and supervision
3. therapeutic treatments
4. wellbeing and relaxation treatments

5 fitness and beauty

6 healthy spa cuisine.

Their treatments are based on their natural resources. Every Danubius health spa is closely supervised by experienced doctors, expert in the field of spa medicine. Their therapeutic services include: physiotherapy, medical massage, electrotherapy, hydrotherapy, packing and balneotherapy.

As people become more travelled and 'spa-experienced', spas will have to compete to attract a share of the market. This will require more imagination with respect to treatments and concepts (in particular using the earth's natural resources) and competitive pricing. Spas are currently a luxury product. This will change in the future, opening the possibility of more 'affordable' treatments and spa experiences.

FACT

Spa cruises are being developed that encompass the total spa experience – treatments, activities and cuisine. In addition, many of the port visits include spa activities, such as visits to yoga centres, temples, thermal springs, hiking, etc.

SPAS OF THE FUTURE

These will be influenced by today's culture and the current social climate and the industry is already beginning to embrace what the customer of today is looking for in a spa experience.

Workspace spas

Our working environments will adapt to teach the concept of wellbeing and give the space to create and work as people demand. Employees and employers are already meeting these demands with the introduction of on-site massage and yoga/pilates sessions being offered in offices.

Airport spas

Once confined to first class passengers only, the latest developments are now available to all travellers. More and more people are flying long distance or travelling everyday for work purposes and airport spas provide all the basic treatments plus treatments designed specifically for jet lag and weary travellers.

Medi spas

This type of spa will be on the increase as the retirement age of the population rises and more people look for ways to maintain their youth whilst incorporating relaxation and wellbeing.

Spa living/communities

As more people search for a whole new way of living that incorporates the holistic approach of wellbeing, communities will start to be built around spas (as in the Roman times), which will become the focus of activities.

SPA EXPERIENCES AND SIGNATURE PACKAGES

A **signature treatment** is a treatment unique to the spa that has been devised to 'showcase' the best the spa can offer. When developing your signature treatment, you want to create an experience that sets you apart from other spas and that is not on offer elsewhere. A lot of time and thought should go into the development stages, and the piloting and testing out of practical skills. It may take many months of research and development before the package is ready to be included in the spa menu. A signature treatment or package can last an hour, three hours, a whole day or even a week in some cases.

When creating your signature treatment you should consider:

- The concept of the spa
- The spa environment
- The clientele/guests
- The demand for different types of treatments
- The products used in the spa
- The resources and equipment
- The skills of the staff
- The geographical location and culture
- The entire 'spa journey'

SPA ROLES

Spa director

Is responsible for the day to day management of the entire operation of the spa. The spa director's job responsibilities include:

Responsibilities	*Qualifications/skills*
• Maintain and preserve the spa's vision	• Ability to understand financial statements and manage a spa operating budget
• Prepare and analyse financial budgets and report the spas financial performance	• Excellent customer service and communication skills
• Hire, train and manage the spa staff	• A confident team player
• Plan special spa events, spa nights and spa promotions	• Enthusiastic about their profession and self-motivated
• Demonstrate high standards of service and interpersonal skills	• Good computer skills
• Build spa teams, mentor and motivate staff	• Manage their time efficiently with the ability to meet deadlines

SIGNATURE TREATMENT S

COMO Shambhala

'The Metropolitan Bath: This cleansing treatment works to gently exfoliate and soften your skin. After dry brushing the body, COMO Shambhala's specially prepared Invigorate Salt Scrub (infused with essential oils, macadamia oil and oat bran) is applied to the body. After a rinse in a revitalizing bath, this treatment concludes with a relaxing COMO Shambhala Massage. Healthy Juice from Glow. 120 min'

- Hold regular staff meetings
- Establish performance and revenue goals for all spa departments
- Order and maintain spa supplies and equipment
- Research competitor spas
- Be active and visible within the spa
- Mediate in any disputes

- Some experience of working as a spa therapist

Spa manager

Is directly responsible to the spa director. Some spas only employ a spa manager rather than a spa director and it really depends on the size of the spa. A large spa with over 50 staff ideally needs both roles.

The spa manager's job responsibilities include:

Responsibilities	*Qualifications/skills*
• Liaise between management, staff and clients • Conduct spa tours and be visible within the spa • Mentor and motivate staff • Hold regular staff appraisals • Mediate in any disputes • Maintain and monitor the inventory of all spa products • Supervise daily spa tasks – check appearance of treatment rooms and communal areas • Arrange monthly front desk schedules for all spa staff • Meet monthly sales plans • Make sure that all displays are presented fresh, clean and eye catching • Monitor client satisfaction • Create staff incentive programmes	• Same as for a spa director

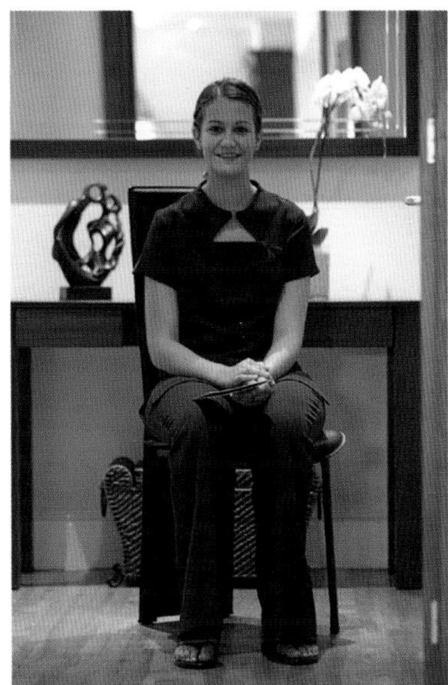

Spa therapist

Spa therapist

Depending on the size of the spa, you may be employed to do only body therapies or specialize as an aesthetician that carries out all the facial treatments, waxing, manicures, etc. Always check the job description first.

Job responsibilities of a spa therapist:

Responsibilities	*Qualifications/skills*
• To maintain client comfort at all times • Provide treatments and services • Be on time for appointments • Set up and maintain high standards throughout the day in the treatment room – making sure everything is neat and that it is well stocked • Demonstrate respect, sensitivity and concern for guests' needs • Promote spa treatments to clients • Participate in staff training • Maintain high levels of health and safety at all times • Maintain your own spa schedules and work hours	• Recognized certificates in massage therapies/beauty therapy/holistic therapies • At least two years' experience within your field • Preferably a member of a professional association • Recognized first aid qualification

Spa consultant

With the boom of interest in the spa market and tough competition developing, a spa consultant has become necessary in order to clarify exactly what is to be achieved, research the proposal and manage the event at all stages of development.

Some of the job responsibilities of a spa consultant are:

Responsibilities
• Plan the spa concept, prepare the design brief and the schedule for the work to be completed • Develop spa services, treatment menus, signature treatments and spa packages • Select product lines

- Develop service protocols, procedures, spa rituals and wellness programs
- Analyse data to price spa treatments and develop menu costs

It is also essential to have research and computer skills along with a wide range of experiences within the spa industry.

Spa product trainer

This is a dual role delivering product and treatment training to therapists and maintaining promotion work for spas who are established with the treatment line. This type of work often requires the trainer to travel extensively.

The responsibilities of a spa product trainer include:

Responsibilities

- Good presentation skills
- Time management
- Mapping lesson plans and schedules
- Understanding customer needs
- Good communication skills
- Awareness of the spa industry as a whole, particularly direct competition
- Personal presentation to a high standard
- A passion for the spa industry

SPA PROFILE

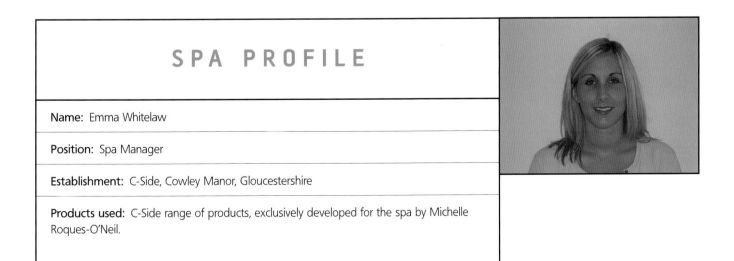

Name: Emma Whitelaw

Position: Spa Manager

Establishment: C-Side, Cowley Manor, Gloucestershire

Products used: C-Side range of products, exclusively developed for the spa by Michelle Roques-O'Neil.

Number of staff/roles: 16 in total, including spa therapists, gym leader, receptionists.

Training: Gloucester College of Arts and Technology; Santi Spa Management programme.

Main responsibilities: 'Every aspect of ensuring C-Side provides an outstanding level of customer care. Staff selection and recruitment, treatment development and training is a huge part of my role; we have a very detailed and comprehensive training programme for all our staff.'

Best parts of the job: 'Helping my team to develop, watching them grow into their role. Especially rewarding is seeing how their communication skills and confidence develop. I still find time to do some treatments; it's important to me that I retain a high level of practical skill so I'm able to train all the staff to a very high standard. It's also great seeing guests enjoying themselves and loving what we offer at C-Side. I love being part of a world-class spa, meeting a variety of guests, many who return time after time.'

Secrets of a successful spa therapist: 'Motivation: they need to know what their goals are. Within a spa environment a therapist needs to focus totally on customer care and exceeding the guests expectations. A spa therapist must have a passion for the job.'

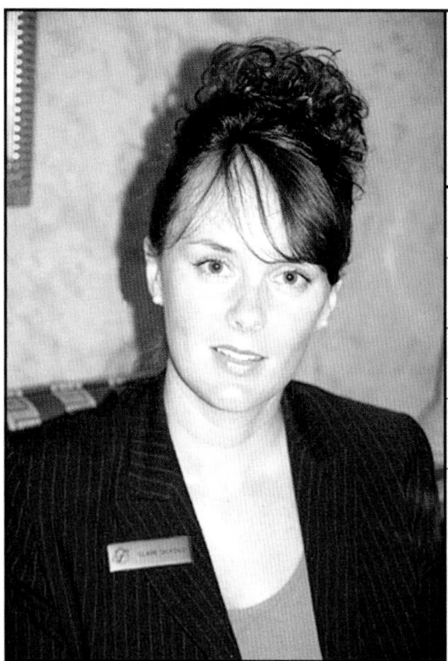

SPA PROFILE

Name: Clare Dickens

Position: Spa Director

Establishment: Willow Stream, the spa at The Fairmont, Dubai, UAE

Products used: Phytomer, Aromatherapy Associates, Willow Stream.

Number of staff/roles: 4 experienced coordinators to run the reception; 4 male and 3 female therapists (to increase to 10 in total); 4 lifeguards (to increase to 6 in order to provide swimming lessons); 4 spa attendants responsible for maintaining the public areas; 3 personal trainers; plus an assistant spa manager and a floor supervisor to be recruited.

Training: Trained as a therapist at Farnborough College of Technology in 1992/3 and awarded IIHHT/IHBC diplomas. Additional courses in RSA aerobics, Sports Massage and Sports Therapy Diploma.

Trained as reflexologist with IFR in 1994.

City and Guilds 7306 teaching certificate in adult education 1997.

Regular attendance at spa seminars and conferences.

Main responsibilities: Spa operations, including monthly profit and loss statements, annual budget, recruitment, research for new brands and treatments, team training, promotion and marketing plan, submissions to spa/beauty magazines, treatment and membership tariffs, monitor competitors, implement corporate standards, ensure thorough team communication, motivation/incentives plans.

Best parts of the job: Daily variety, from creative photo shoots and marketing plans to analysing charts and figures; guest contact – meeting new people/building relationships with regular members; working with and learning about different cultures; industry constantly developing – implementing changes and improvements.

Secrets of a successful spa therapist: Knowledge, empathy and active listening skills combined with 'natural talent'. I believe that you can teach anyone the skills necessary to perform a treatment, but there is a special quality a therapist requires to provide a guest with a true 'experience'. Plus an understanding of both business and guest requirements, providing retail advice to the guest in order to support the treatment at home and therefore receive the results desired without feeling the discomfort of a heavy sell, in balance with the need for retailing to grow business levels.

Assessment of knowledge and understanding

When you have some free time, test your understanding and knowledge by answering the following questions. Do this at regular intervals and it will reinforce your learning and help you retain the knowledge, so you are able to perform better in your assessments.

1 What type of facilities would you expect at the following spas?:
   a. destination
   b. day
   c. medi

2 Give five examples of treatments you may experience on a tropical/Asian spa.

3 Describe three treatments which adopt a more spiritual/holistic feel in their practice.

4 Give six main responsibilities of a spa director.

5 List three qualities that you would look for in a spa manager.

6 Who is the spa manager responsible to?

7 List four responsibilities a therapist would have in a spa.

8 Briefly describe the role of a spa consultant.

9 Give five responsibilities of a spa product trainer.

chapter 3

Financial effectiveness

G11

Contribute to the financial effectiveness of the business

Learning objectives

This chapter describes how to contribute to the financial effectiveness of the business, check how successful your business idea will be and check what law and other regulations will affect your business.

It describes the skills and knowledge necessary to enable you to:

- **contribute to the effective use and monitoring of resources**
- **meet productivity and development targets**
- **explain your business idea**
- **make sure there is a market for the business**
- **decide if your business will be a success**
- **make sure that the business is set up and will trade legally**
- **meets the current regulations for health and safety**

When providing spa therapy services it is important to use the skills you have learnt in the two following core units:

G1 Ensure your actions reduce risks to health and safety

G6 Promote additional products or services to clients

INTRODUCTION

The long-term success of a spa relies on how efficiently it is managed in relation to staff, resources, stock control and meeting both product delivery and financial targets. However 'holistic' the spa may be it will need to make a profit to survive in this highly competitive market.

It is also imperative to have a well structured business plan that identifies clearly the aims and objectives of the business. Before the business plan is written you will need to conduct market research for your idea – does it meet the client's needs and what is the competition like from local businesses and the spa industry?

SPA TIP 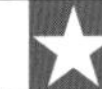

When starting a spa business you must consider your market thoroughly before any financial investment is taken – see chapter 4 for more details.

PLANNING

Whether you are starting a new business, taking over an existing one or managing a spa it is important to have a business plan which addresses your chosen:

- spa concept
- outcomes/goals
- customer profile
- targeted part of the spa market
- competitors
- brand
- business team.

Ideally a business plan should only be 1–2 pages in length, with clear objectives set according to the **SMART** principles:

- **Specific** – relate to your overall outcome/goals
- **Measurable** – appropriate to achieving your objectives and plan
- **Achievable** – realistic objectives, which can be accomplished
- **Relevant** – relate to the spa concept, brand and team
- **Timed** – a date and time limit must be given to the project.

Most companies also have a mission statement, which is a simple statement giving an overall philosophy as to what the business is about and what it is hoped to achieve.

FACT

The Mandarin Oriental's **mission statement** is: 'Our mission is to completely delight and satisfy our guests. We are committed to making a difference every day: continually getting better to keep us the best.'

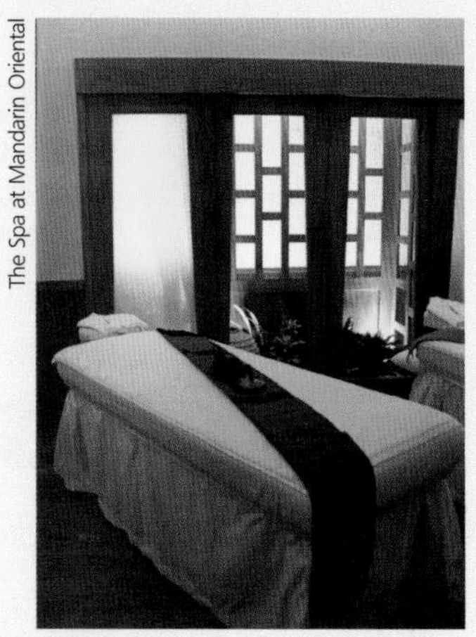
The Spa at Mandarin Oriental

Treatment room, Mandarin Oriental

BUSINESS TYPES

If you are setting up your own spa business it is important to decide what type type of business organization it will be and who will run it.

Sole trader

A one-man business, where you are your own boss and do not have to take anyone else into account when making decisions.

Advantages

All profits are your own. You decide the financial arrangements. Easy to set up if you are using your own capital. You can make all the decisions on the concept and design of the business.

Disadvantages

Responsibility for all debts. Long hours at work can be occurred. May be constricted by how much capital you have.

Partnerships

Two or more joint owners. You put capital into the business and share the work and profits. An agreement should be drawn up stating the requirements of the partnership.

Advantages

More capital available. Shared responsibility. Financial status remains confidential.

Disadvantages

Shared profits. Responsibility for all debts. A partnership would break up on death, retirement or bankruptcy unless stated in a contract agreement.

Private limited company

Any number of people can be involved with a board of directors. An agreement has to be formed between all members involved on the running of the business, which must be sent to the Registrar of Companies. If they are happy with the business then they will issue the company with permission to trade, i.e. a Certificate of Incorporation.

Advantages

More capital to invest. Limited liability. Directors continue with the business whoever dies or retires.

Disadvantages

Expensive to set up. Carefully audited accounts have to be kept and inspected.

Franchising

This gives you the opportunity to operate someone else's business as your own. A franchiser is the person/company who owns the rights to the franchise. A franchisee is the person who operates the franchise.

Advantages

Complete business concept. Support and training is given. Having the backing of a known large company.

Disadvantages

Profits have to be shared.

BYELAWS AND LEGISLATION RELATING TO RUNNING A BUSINESS

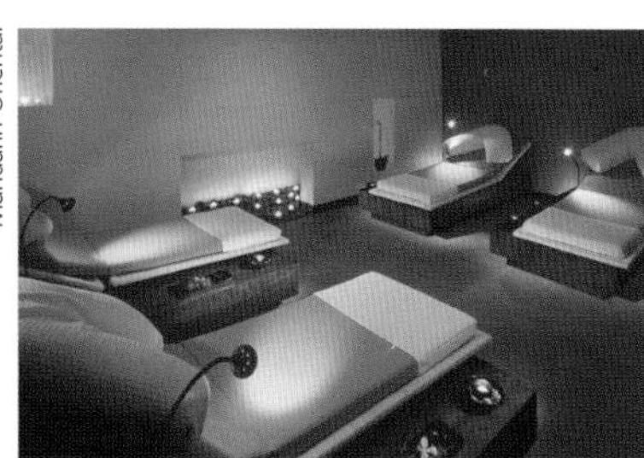
Courtesy of the Spa at Mandarin Oriental

You need to be aware of all the current legal requirements relating to health and safety and the byelaws that apply to all businesses. These are identified in chapters 4 and 5.

INSURANCES

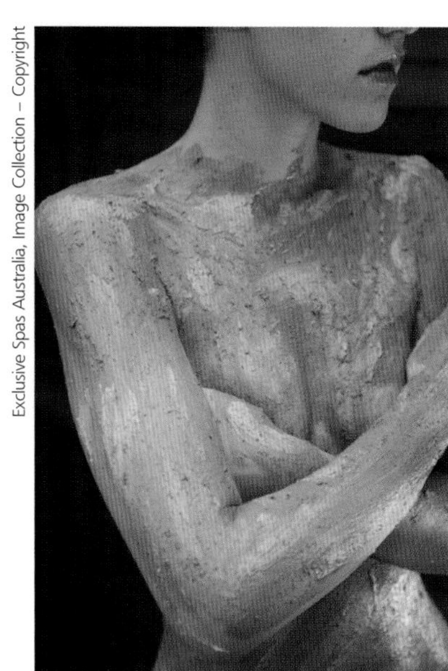
Exclusive Spas Australia, Image Collection – Copyright

It is fundamental when you undertake a business to have insurances to protect against any misfortune that may occur. An insurance document is a legal contract between the insured party and the company from whom you are buying. It requires you to disclose any information that may affect the insurance policy and any changes that occur against the risk insured. Failure to do so may affect any claims made.

The following classes of insurance are essential when setting up a business:

- Property insurance – to include buildings, contents, equipment, etc., against fire, theft, damage, etc.
- Income provision – particularly for small businesses in case of illness, etc.
- Liability insurance – this covers the business if an injury or illness occurs to a client whilst on your premises and is classified as follows:
  - public liability any damage to a member of the public whilst on your premises
  - product liability injury occurred to a client from products used or sold by the business
  - employer's liability every employer with employees must take out this insurance to protect the employees. Both employers and employees have a 'duty of care'.

RAISING CAPITAL FOR THE BUSINESS

> **FACT**
>
> Professional organizations and associations specialize in liability insurances for therapists, which are important to have if you are working freelance.

There are various financial avenues you may wish to take in order to raise money and they must be looked at very carefully. You need to have a clear idea as to how much money you wish to borrow, the level of repayments you can afford and what commitments you are tied to in the contract. Most finance sources will ask to see your business plan and a cash flow forecast for the first few years of business (always keep it realistic!).

Banks

Usually the main source of finance for small businesses as they are able to offer professional advice and have had plenty of experience. If a loan is agreed then you will need to open up a business account with them into which your income is paid and from which bills, etc., are paid. Usual customer contracts and conditions will apply.

Building societies

These work in exactly the same way as banks and most now have the same facilities as a bank.

Private investors

You may be able to borrow money from family or a friend. This may be a cheaper and easier way to finance the business but does have some pitfalls, such as family feuds and fall-outs and the people in question may decide they want a say in the running of the business. If you choose this route then it is advisable to first have a legal document drawn up.

Finance houses

If a bank or building society will not lend you the money then you may wish to take a loan from one of the many finance houses in the market. Beware that borrowing money this way may lead to high interest rates and repayments and you may be asked to put up some security against the loan. Always read the small print on the contract to make sure there are no other forfeits.

SPA TIP 

Your local council will be able to give advice on any local schemes available to help small business. Once of the most popular in assisting young enterprises has been the **Prince's Trust**, which provides grants to people between the ages of 18 and 30 who wish to start their own business.

TAXATION

Income tax is the most common form of direct taxation and can be paid to the state in four different ways.

PAYE (Pay As You Earn) from employee's wages

Devised by the Inland Revenue to deduct tax directly from the employee's wages. Each employee is given a code from the Inland Revenue that shows how much allowance they are entitled to before starting to pay tax.

ACTIVITY 

Visit your local bank and ask for an information pack on starting up a new business.

National Insurance contributions

These payments cover national health, state pension and unemployment. The employer has to collect these from the employee and pay contributions

> **FACT**
>
> HM Customs and Revenue (HMCR) requires a quarterly VAT return and has the right to examine your business records at any time.

to the Inland Revenue based on the employee's earnings. The classifications are as follows:

- Class 1 relates to the amount you earn (both employee and employer pay this).
- Class 2/4 flat rate contributions for the self-employed.
- Class 3 voluntary to help you qualify for benefit (if you do not work).

If you are self-employed you will need an accountant to deal with the tax office but your can pay your National Insurance contributions by either buying a stamp from the Post Office or making payments monthly or yearly direct to the Social Security Office.

Value added tax (VAT)

This tax is collected on all business transactions – goods and services – and is a tax on turnover and not profit. The Chancellor of the Exchequer can alter the rate of VAT. The main rate of VAT at the moment is 17.5 per cent, which is added to the supply of goods and services (food, medicine, books, etc., are exempt). To register for VAT you should apply to your local HMCR office, who will issue you with an identity number. You must keep accurate records of all tax paid on purchases and received from sales. These records must be retained for a minimum of six years.

Corporation tax on the profits from a limited company

The spa owner is required to pay income tax on their own salary as well as on any profit they draw out of the company.

ACCOUNTS

Depending on the size of your business you may have a finance department that deals with all financial transactions, or for a small business you may wish to do your own accounts and employ an accountant to help with the end-of-year finance sheets which you must present to your tax office.

You are required by law to make a true return of your income each year, including profits. The tax office requires that the accounts supplied are a true reflection of the business. For sole traders and partnerships you will need to supply a trading account and a profit and loss account along with a concluding balance sheet.

> **FACT**
>
> The Spa Business Association is pressing for the VAT on spa treatments to be reduced in line with treatments provided by medical practitioners, osteopaths, dentists, occupational therapists, etc.

> **TERMINOLOGY**
>
> A **balance sheet** shows what the business has earned, spent, has as assets in the bank, who owes you money and what investments you may have made, such as new equipment, etc.

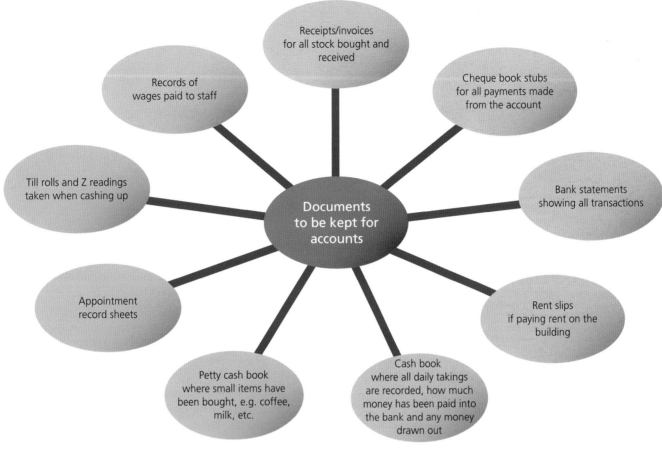

Documents to be kept for accounts:

- Receipts/invoices for all stock bought and received
- Cheque book stubs for all payments made from the account
- Bank statements showing all transactions
- Rent slips if paying rent on the building
- Cash book where all daily takings are recorded, how much money has been paid into the bank and any money drawn out
- Petty cash book where small items have been bought, e.g. coffee, milk, etc.
- Appointment record sheets
- Till rolls and Z readings taken when cashing up
- Records of wages paid to staff

BUDGETING AND CASH FLOW FORECASTS

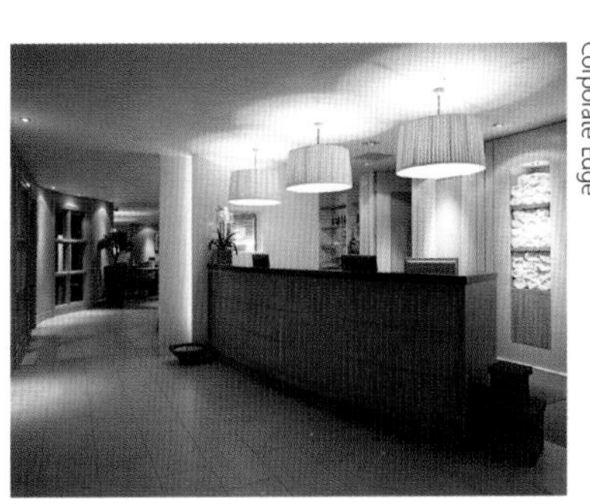

Corporate Edge

Spa reception, Calcot Manor

To be a profitable spa it is important to have a strict budget to control all overheads, consumables, staffing and income. This budget may be set monthly, quarterly or yearly depending on how finances are managed. The budget may be an estimate if it is a new business or if it is an existing business it is advisable to base the budget on previous years' costs and incomes. Budgets need to be slightly flexible in case of an increase in treatment demand and more consumables and staffing costs being required, as long as it can be balanced by the increase in income.

COSTING TREATMENTS

Most new businesses have a problem when ascertaining what is the right price to charge for a treatment. The price has to cover all associated costs along with a profit margin.

Treatment content and timing should also be reflected in the price to ensure that it offers value for money for the client whilst making a healthy profit for the spa. A profit margin can range from 20 to 80 per cent, depending on all

SPA TIP 

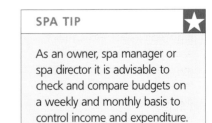

As an owner, spa manager or spa director it is advisable to check and compare budgets on a weekly and monthly basis to control income and expenditure.

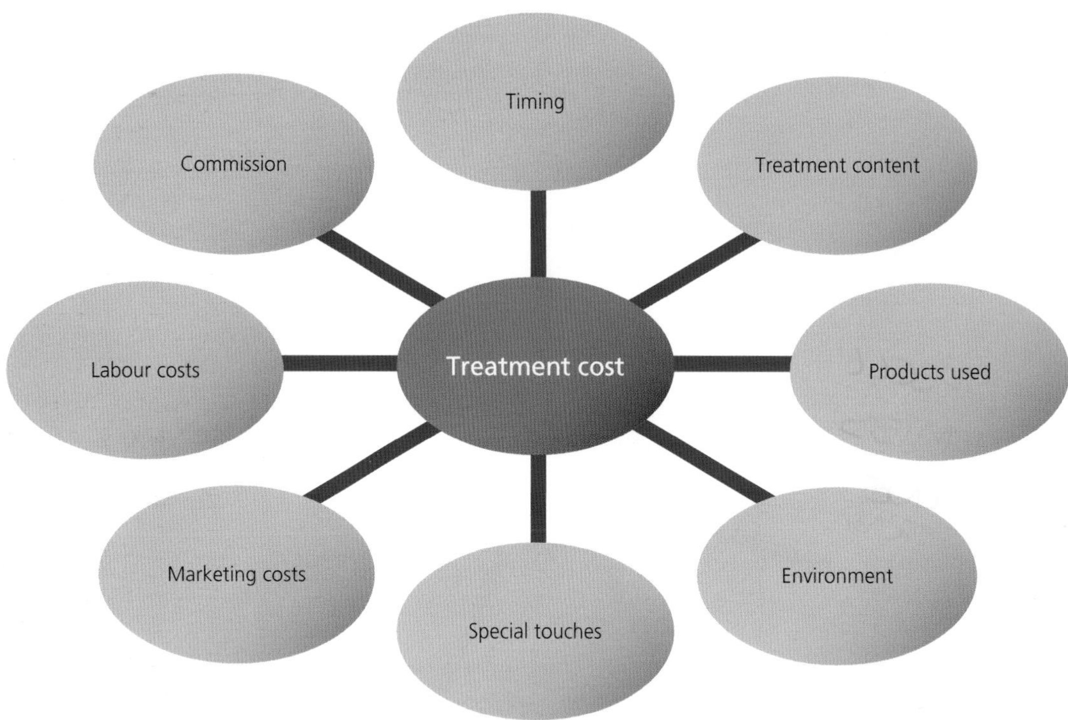

the above costs and also the location of the spa and clientele. Spas in the Far East will have higher profit margins than those based in the centre of London or New York where rents, building costs and staff wages are much higher.

SPA BUSINESS BRIEF

- ✔ Day spa in the centre of Manchester
- ✔ Location – exclusive, exterior image designed for the 'urban context'
- ✔ Client profile – ladies and gentlemen from the 30–45 age group
- ✔ Brand profile – is professional with quality products and treatments
- ✔ Lucrative retail area at the front of the spa next to the reception
- ✔ 8 different treatment rooms – 2 for facial therapies, 4 for body therapies, 1 for nail and foot therapies, 1 for hydrotherapy treatments
- ✔ Interior to feel comfortable, with quality furnishings mixed with antique pieces
- ✔ Team of 8 therapists, 1 receptionist, 1 spa concierge, 1 spa manager

TERMINOLOGY

Labour costs These are not just based on the therapist's salary but need to include all other staffing costs involved in running the spa.

TERMINOLOGY

Overheads These may include general overheads, such as rent, rates and laundry; indirect material costs, such as furniture, décor and repairs; employment costs, such as staff training, uniforms and commission; and marketing costs, such as brochures, price lists and posters.

STOCK CONTROL

It is important to have a good stock control system that monitors carefully stock levels so that you never run out of materials or hold too much old stock.

It is important to identify whose responsibility it is to order stock, check stock levels and maintain accurate records. If the spa has a dispensary system

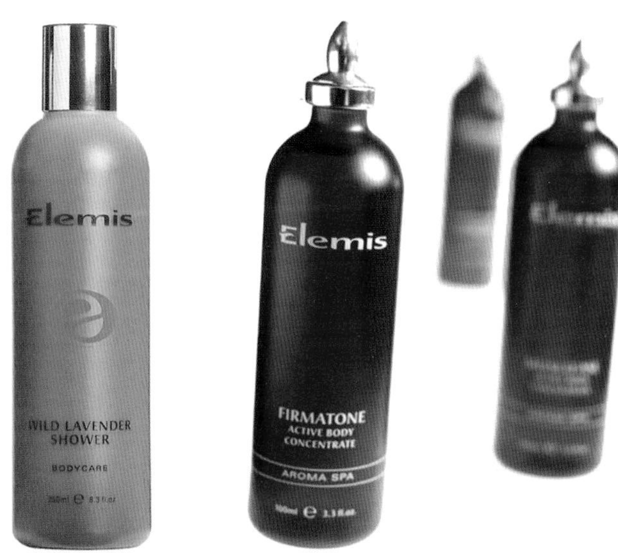
Elemis
WILD LAVENDER SHOWER
BODYCARE
Elemis
FIRMATONE
ACTIVE BODY CONCENTRATE
AROMA SPA

Elemis Ltd

Spa products

SPA TIP

Wholesalers are ideal when buying stock in bulk to keep costs low on items such as tissues, bedroll, cotton wool, towels, oil, etc.

SPA TIP

As there are so many **product companies** vying for business, make sure you are receiving a good price on the product, that deliveries are frequent and on time and that you receive rewards for loyal custom, including staff training and updates on the latest products and promotions.

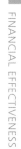

then it may be included into their job role to receive and unpack stock as it arrives and store it in the appropriate areas. Ideally, the spa manager should maintain stock records so as to see which products are used a lot or are selling well and which are the most popular treatments. All this information will build up over time and give a good idea as to which stock to hold more of and which to keep at the basic level. Every spa will identify different roles that hold this responsibility and it may be down to the spa therapist to maintain stock levels in their treatment room.

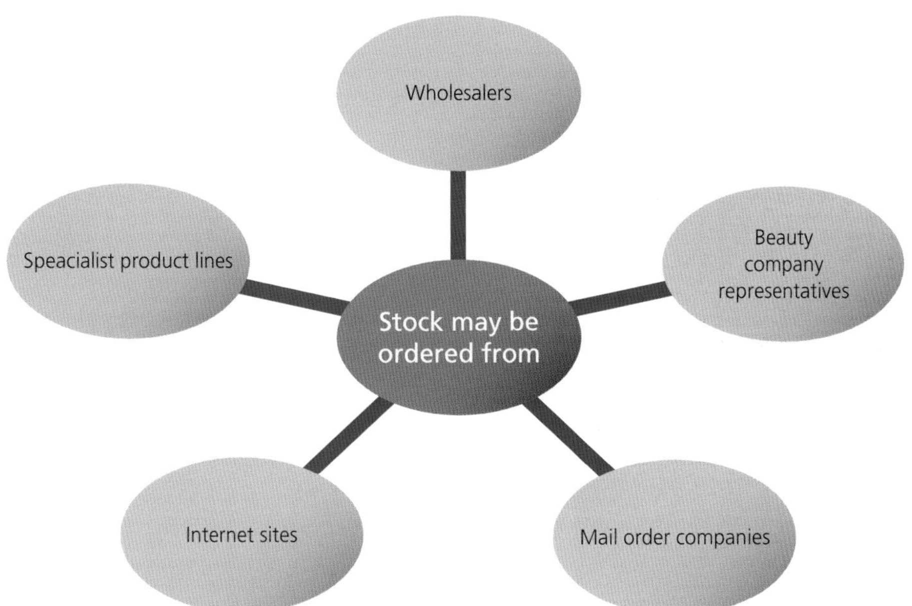
Wholesalers
Speacialist product lines
Beauty company representatives
Stock may be ordered from
Internet sites
Mail order companies

Monitoring stock levels

Stock levels can be monitored manually but it is now more common to use a computerized system. Stock should be divided into two areas: consumables (such as tissues, bedrolls and products used within a treatment) and retail

FACT 

Some software can analyse retail sales per staff and which product range they sell the most of. They can also produce purchase orders, match deliveries to orders and monitor stocktakes.

SPA TIP 

A lot of companies have a set-up price for ordering your first stock line, which could be around £2000. You must look into this if you are opening a small business.

SPA TIP

It is important that your retail area is eye-catching and has a good choice of products to enhance visual appeal as this is often a way of drawing the client in for a sale.

items that are sold to the client. This is easier if there is a shop within the spa where all products are sold.

Stock levels

It is important to maintain accurate stock records to get a clear indication as to which products are the most popular and which move slower. When purchasing retail stock concentrate on two or three brands that offer a good choice. It is important not to over buy stock or hold too many products, as you could be left with money tied up in stock that is not selling.

The important things to remember when ordering stock are:

- Order stock on a regular basis so that you do not run out and have to cancel treatments – large spas may have special deals with companies whose products they are using and may hold higher levels of stock than would a small day spa.
- Aim for minimum 'safe' stock levels for each line of retail products.
- Check on delivery times and add a safety margin when placing an order.
- Continually re-assess order levels as some products may be moving quicker than others.
- At busier times of the year, such as Christmas, more stock will need to be ordered the month before.
- For seasonal products such as sun creams (unless working in a hot country), order more of in the summer months and keep levels at a minimum the rest of the year.
- Check regularly with company representatives on the special offers and promotions they run to entice clients, such as gift boxes and free products with specific treatments.

Handling stock

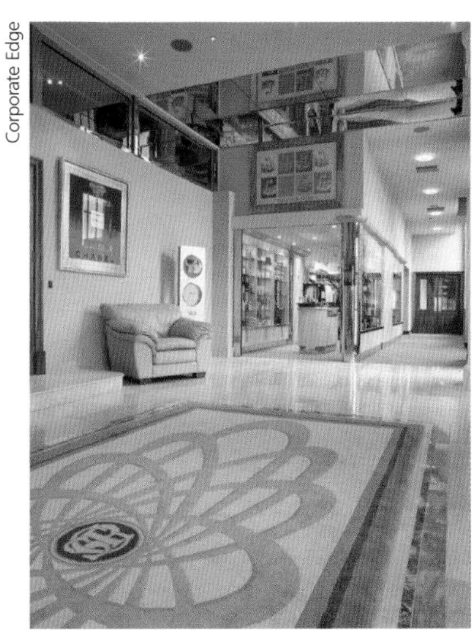

Corporate Edge

Retail area at Stoke Park

It is important to inspect the stock thoroughly when it arrives to check for any damage, such as dents in packages, scratches, dirty or out of date products. Check also that all the stock requested has arrived by matching the original order with the delivery note. Mistakes can be made in warehouses, etc., when distributing a large order. If you are returning damaged goods then telephone the company first with your complaint, then pack the goods and send them back to the sender with any relevant paperwork.

Stock rotation

Always place new stock at the back of the shelf and move older items to the front so that you are not left with out of date products. Always keep your stock cupboard and shelves clean, tidy and organized so that you can see the products clearly. Always place heavier items on lower shelves.

Spa works	REP: Sarah Brown
TEL: 470392	

		Min	Max	Mar	Apr	May	Jun
Coral							
Cleanser	500 ml	10	20	5/15	10/10	12/8	9
	200 ml	20	30	22/8	20/10	19/11	20
Toner	500 ml	10	20	10/10	11/9	9/11	10
	200 ml	20	30	20/10	20/10	21/9	19
Moisture	250 ml	5	10	5/5	6/4	5/5	4
Cream	50 ml	15	25	12/13	16/9	15/10	11
Height	250 ml	5	10	5/5	8/2	5/5	6
Cream	50 ml	15	25	14/11	16/9	14/11	10

Manual stock recording system

If you use a computerized stock control system then it is easy for the products to be bar-coded. As they are sold, the computer reads the code number and automatically adjusts the stock levels.

If a computerized system is not used then you will have to employ a manual stock-recording system. This recording system needs to show:

- product range
- description of product and size
- how many items are left in stock
- minimum and maximum stock levels of each item
- new stock that has just arrived.

Usually at the end of a financial year all stock held within the spa would be counted and records kept. This will show how much capital you are holding in stock.

Stock security

This is always a problem in spas and salons. Regular stock checks should identify if there is a problem with stock disappearing quicker than is normally expected. An ideal preventative measure is to install security cameras in all areas holding a large amount of stock, such as the reception, shop and dispensary area. Dummy stock can be purchased from most retail companies to display in open areas around the spa and in treatment rooms with the main retail stock locked safely away.

SPA TIP

If regular mistakes are occurring with orders then contact the supplier or inform their representative that you are not happy with the service you are receiving.

SPA TIP 

If the packaging changes on the products you are selling then ask the company to take the old ones back and replace with the new design.

HEALTH AND SAFETY

When lifting any boxes in the spa do not struggle if they are too heavy – get someone to help. When you have to lift, always keep a straight back, stand feet apart and bend from the knees, keeping your head up and elbows close to your body to give extra support.

HEALTH AND SAFETY

Any hazardous chemical substances should be stored in a metal cupboard inside the stock room and marked clearly as containing a hazardous substance. Water testing chemicals should be stored this way.

HEALTH AND SAFETY 

Management should regularly brief staff on issues regarding stock and how theft is dealt with.

SPA TIP

Look into leasing rather than buying, especially if the piece of equipment is very expensive. This used to be done a lot in beauty salons with sun beds and tanning booths as the lessor will also cover any repairs and breakages that occur.

HEALTH AND SAFETY

A qualified electrician must test all electrical equipment every 12 months in compliance with the Electricity at Work Regulations 1989.

HEALTH AND SAFETY

Always make sure that staff are correctly trained in the use of equipment and know how to clean it.

PURCHASING TOOLS AND EQUIPMENT

As well as holding retail stock and salon products, a lot of a spa's capital is tied up in equipment that over the years will be subject to a lot of wear and tear. As with all purchases it is important to source the best deals when buying equipment. Try different manufacturers as prices will differ and the more equipment you buy from one supplier the better deal you will get. More specialized equipment such as flotation tanks, hydro baths, wet tables, etc., may need to be purchased from specialist suppliers, but if purchasing say

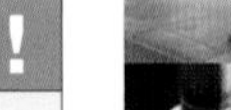

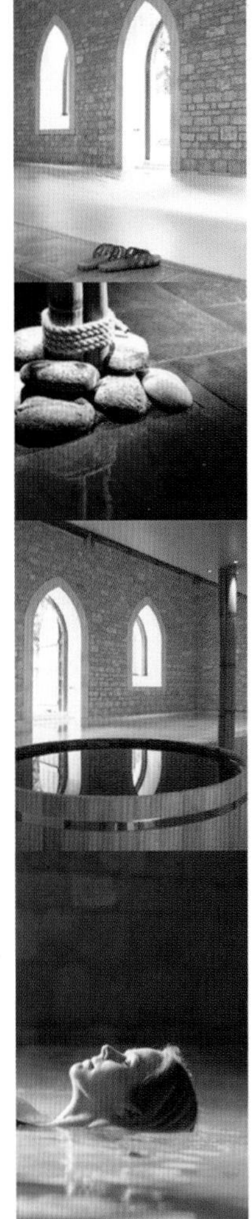

NEW PARK MANOR

is opening BATH HOUSE SPA

A sensational new spa in the heart of the New Forest, boasting a 16 metre swimming pool, hydro pool, sauna and steam rooms, gymnasium, six treatment rooms and a unique relaxation terrace with exceptional views of the parkland and forest.

Exciting opportunities are available for:

HEAD THERAPIST
BEAUTY THERAPISTS
HOLISTIC THERAPISTS

Full and Part time positions available.

We offer a competitive salary and benefits package with an opportunity for further development within the group.

Duties will include:

- Hosting duties
- Delivering treatments to an exceptional standard
- Involvement in day to day running of the spa

Main requirements:

- Exceptional client care
- Excellent communication and organisation skills
- NVQ level 3 or equivalent professional qualification "

Please apply in writing to
Madeleine Petzer, Human Resources Manager
New Park Manor Hotel
Lyndhurst Rd, Brockenhurst, SO42 7QH
or e-mail: madeleine.petzer@newparkmanorhotel.co.uk

Sample job advert

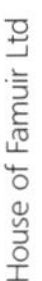
House of Famuir Ltd

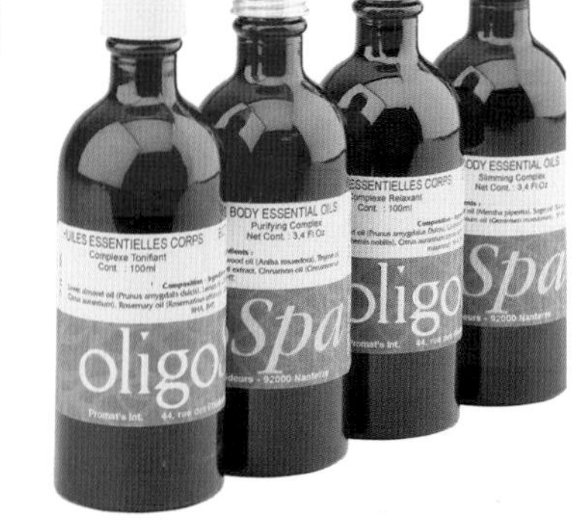

Treatment products

12 massage couches, 25 chairs and 12 trolleys then it may be best to give one company the business to get the best deal. As with retail stock, at the end of each financial year all equipment must be recorded as it is counted as capital.

SPA TIP

Hold regular team meetings and involve staff in decision making, such as how to present the treatment rooms, fold towels, what herb teas to serve to clients, etc. If staff are involved they will feel valued.

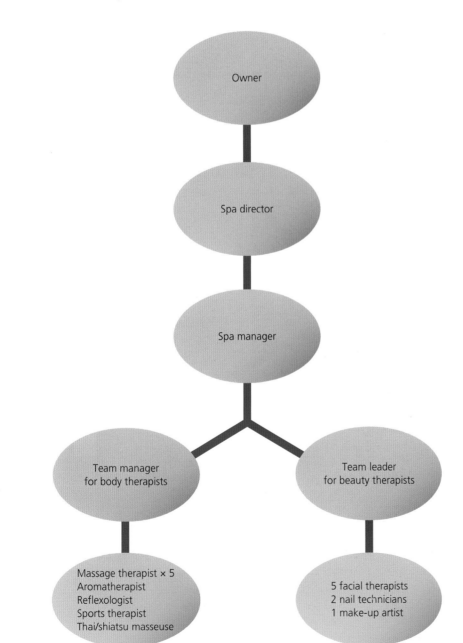

HUMAN RESOURCES

One of the most difficult and exciting parts of setting up a spa business is developing the spa team. Staff are the most important asset of the business and should share your philosophy or know what your spa ethos and vision are. Staff should be nurtured as they provide the main source of income for the spa through 'the treatments to the client'. A good therapist who is motivated, praised and paid well will stay with the business for a long time, which is something that regular clients like to see, a familiar face.

Employment contracts

When a new employee is hired they should be given a thorough induction before any training begins. The spa director may do this themselves or in a large establishment a member of staff from the personnel section may carry it out. During this induction the member of staff should be given a job description, detailing their job role and responsibilities, and be told about the establishment's grievance and disciplinary procedures.

Employment contracts should be issued to an employee within the first month of them starting work and should be signed by the member of staff. The employee and the human resources department or spa owner then both hold a copy. The contract should state:

- the rate of pay and payment details
- hours to be worked
- how many paid and unpaid holidays are allowed
- sick pay details
- maternity leave details
- any schemes such as pension or healthcare that they can pay into.

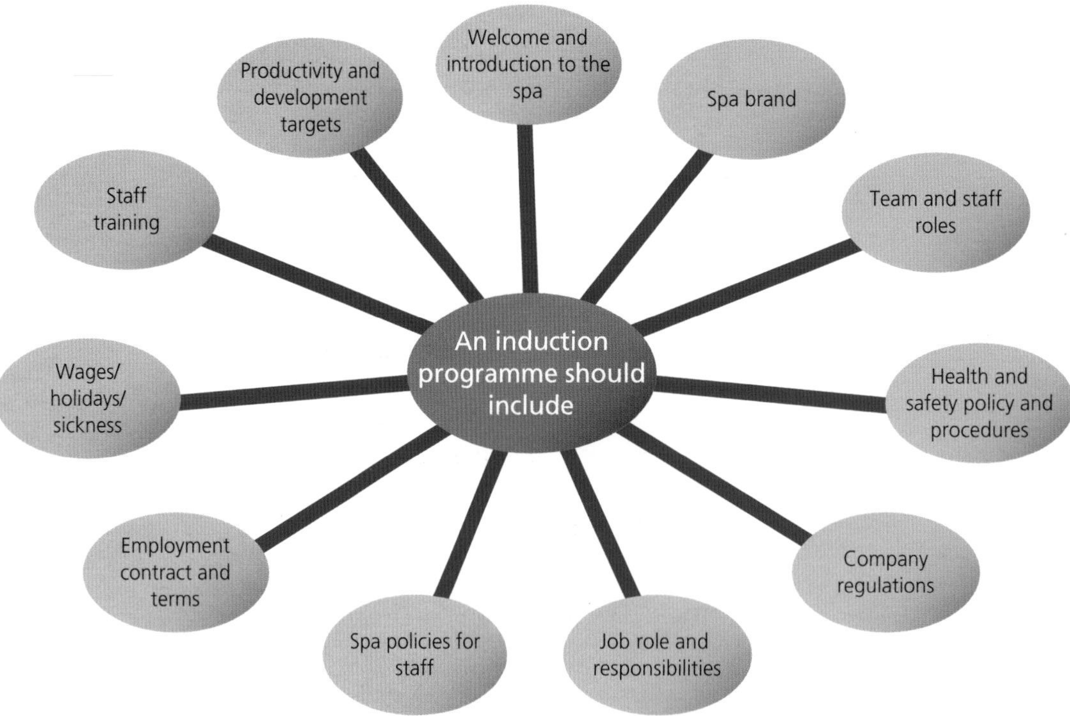

FACT

All employees should receive a wage slip when they get paid which states their gross monthly or weekly salary (depending when they are to be paid). It should itemize any commission or bonuses paid and all deductions made, and what they were for.

SPA JOB DESCRIPTION

Job Description: Spa Manager

Responsible to: Spa Director

Job purpose: To manage and develop a team of therapists providing Western and Oriental therapies. To maintain a high standard of customer service and client care and to mentor and motivate your team. To provide administrative support ensuring the effective and efficient day-to-day running of the spa.

Major responsibilities:

- to manage a team of therapists within the spa
- to develop services and treatments in line with the spa brand
- to promote services to existing clientele and assist in developing a new client base
- to provide treatments if required at busy times
- to achieve designated performance targets for the team
- to participate in staff training and professional development
- to undertake administrative and marketing activities
- to manage the provision of resources and stock levels
- to maintain professional standards and hygienic practices within the spa
- to undertake other duties that may be reasonably required by the Spa Director

Grievance procedure

If you have a grievance relating to your employment then you have a right to express it. If you feel that you are being treated unfairly then you should try to resolve the issue informally in discussion with your manager. Sometimes a more formal means of appeal is required and it is important to familiarize yourself with the spa's grievance and appeals procedures. The aim of all grievance procedures is to ensure all problems are thoroughly investigated and resolved as soon as possible.

Employment legislation

Working Time Directive 1998

This protects employees from being required to work more than 48 hours a week. It also contains provisions regarding shift work, night work, rest breaks and minimum holiday entitlement.

The provisions include:

- a maximum 48 hour working week
- night shifts must be a maximum of 8 hours work in 24 hours

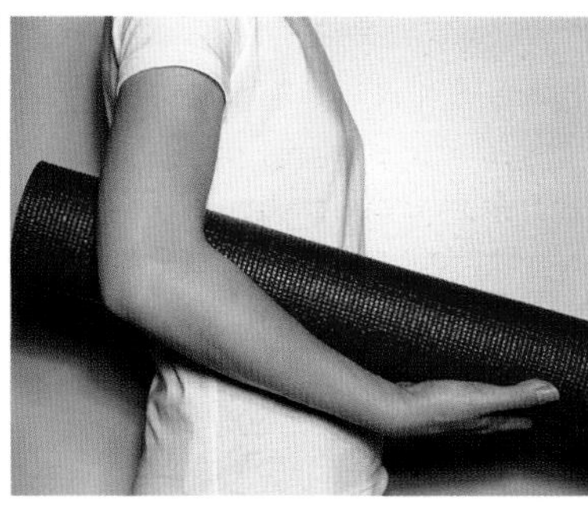
SUBSTANCE
Como Shambala

- a minimum 1 day off per week
- a rest break if the working day is longer than 6 hours
- at least 4 weeks paid leave per year.

Equal opportunities

There must be no discrimination in relation to race, disability, sex or marital status. The Equal Opportunities Commission (EOC) helps provide legal aid advice to individuals who feel they are being discriminated against and has the power to conduct a formal investigation.

Race Relations Act 1976

You cannot discriminate against a person on the basis of race, colour or ethnicity. This is enforced by the Commission for Racial Equality.

Disability Discrimination Act 1995

This act makes it unlawful for an employer to discriminate against a person because of their disability. Employers are also required to ensure that there are no physical barriers for disabled people in the workplace.

Sex Discrimination Acts 1975 and 1985 and the Equal Pay Act 1970

These acts prohibit discrimination or less favourable treatment of a man or woman on the basis of gender and also cover pay and conditions as well as promotion of equal opportunities.

Trade Union and Labour Relations (Consolidation) Act 1992

This act enforces the equal treatment of trade union and non-trade union members and permits an employee to take a complaint to an employment tribunal.

Staff development

It is extremely important to invest in your spa team from the beginning. Ideally, all new staff should receive at least three weeks training in product knowledge, treatment and how the spa **brand** is to be delivered to the client. As well as an ongoing training programme it is also important for the therapists to receive regular treatments from

SIGNATURE TREATMENT 

Chi: The Spa at Shangri-La

Vitality Ritual
'Indulge your senses and recharge your body and mind in a half-day spa experience that combines an Uplifting Himalayan Bath Therapy, Revitalizing Essential Wrap, Mountain Tsampa Rub, Invigorating Himalayan Healing Stone Signature Massage and Biodroga Oxygenating Facial. 5 hours 30 minutes'

SPA TIP

When holding a staff meeting make sure that everyone has been given sufficient notice. Distribute an agenda a day or two before hand so everyone can familiarize themselves with the items on it. Choose a suitable venue that will accommodate all staff comfortably and provide refreshments. The spa director/ manager should lead the meeting and have someone take minutes, which should be circulated to all staff a few days later.

ACTIVITY 

Design an agenda for a staff weekly meeting to be held in the spa with all staff to attend. The spa director will lead the meeting.

Canyon Ranch

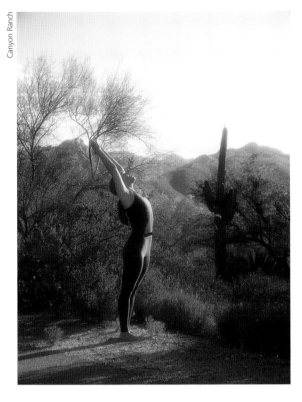

SPA TIP

Some spas have been known to arrange beach yoga and meditation sessions with staff to develop a team spirit.

ACTIVITY

Design a two-day induction programme for a new spa therapist.

each other as you can always learn new techniques this way and it is also important to experience the 'spa journey' from the client's perspective.

The setting, agreeing and recording of individual staff targets is a key part of staff development and is covered in chapter 4.

Staff appraisals

To enable staff to contribute successfully to the delivery of spa services and also to achieve their full potential it is essential for them to understand the purpose of their role and to possess the necessary knowledge and skills. This can be done informally, but a more formal appraisal allows you to identify how well they are doing, review their job role if necessary and identify any development needs they may have.

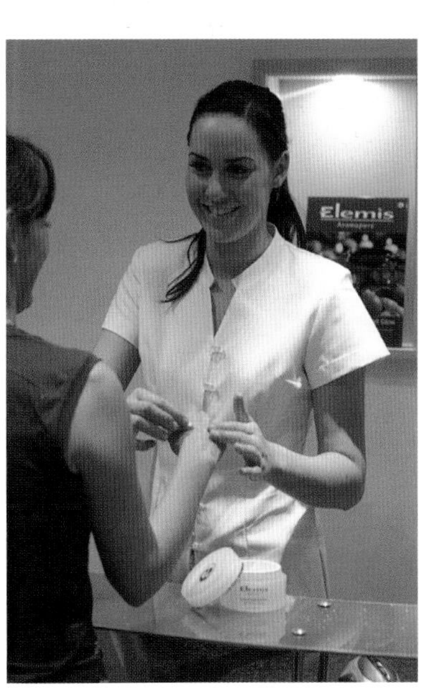

An appraisal form should contain the following information:

- staff name, job role, date of the review and the person carrying out the appraisal
- any changes/responsibilities in their role
- identify strengths and weaknesses, such as meeting targets, etc.
- whether staff training objectives from the last appraisal were met
- any training and development requirements for their job role
- how their development targets would fit into the spa's business plan and targets for the year
- agreed objectives for continuing professional development and a target date for review.

SPA PROFILE

Name: Tracy Corcoran

Position: Director

Establishment: Ki Day Spa Ltd

Products used: Elemis, Crystal Clear, Karin Herzog, Nailtiques, Essie and Seche Vite.

Number of staff/roles: 5 staff (2 holistic therapists, 3 beauty/holistic therapists).

Training/experience: Worked for Marks & Spencer in commercial management for 12 years prior to opening Ki Day Spa.

Main responsibilities: Operations; training retailing/service; reception; marketing; business development/strategy; recruitment; sales; finance; hygiene.

Best parts of the job: Client satisfaction; good working environment; working with leading products/brands.

Secrets of a successful spa therapist:
Director – key skills: Leadership; communication; listening; teamwork; negotiation; problem solving; influencing; marketing awareness; initiative; awareness; delegation; organization and planning; time management.

KEY/CORE SKILLS OPPORTUNITIES

To be an excellent spa therapist you must be able to communicate well, both orally and in writing. To be able to succeed and progress in the spa industry, it is also essential that you have an ability to work with numbers and information technology (IT). Increasingly, employers are looking for spa therapists with these 'key' skills when they recruit staff. NVQ/SVQ unit **G11** provides you with an opportunity to develop evidence for the following:

KEY SKILLS	CORE SKILLS
Communication Level 1; C1.3	Communication Access 3; Task 2
Communication Level 2; C2.2	Communication Intermediate 1; Task 1
Communication Level 3; C3.1a	Communication Intermediate 2; Task 3
Application of number Level 1; N1.1, N1.2	Numeracy Access 3; Task 4
Working with others Level 3; WO3.1, WO3.2, WO3.3	Working with others Intermediate 2; Tasks 1, 2, 3 and 4
Improving own learning and performance Level 3; LP3.1, LP3.2, LP3.3	(no parallel unit in core skills)

Assessment of knowledge and understanding

When you have some free time, test your understanding and knowledge by answering the following questions. Do this at regular intervals and it will reinforce your learning and help you retain the knowledge, so you are able to perform better in your assessments.

1 What is the importance of having a business plan?
2 What is a mission statement?
3 What are the advantages and disadvantages of being:
   a. a sole trader?
   b. a franchisee?
4 Why does a spa business need to have insurance?
5 Give three financial avenues you may explore to raise capital for your business.
6 What is VAT and how is it paid?
7 What type of documents must a business produce for an accountant at the end of the tax year?
8 What do you need to take into consideration when costing a treatment?
9 How and where can you order stock?
10 How can a spa manager monitor stock levels?
11 Why is it important to rotate stock?
12 How must you lift boxes in a stock room?
13 Where would you store water-testing chemicals?
14 When should stock be returned?
15 How often should electrical equipment be tested and by whom?
16 What should be included in a staff induction programme?
17 List four examples of effective teamwork.
18 What information should an employment contract contain?
19 If you had a grievance at work, to whom and how would you report this?
20 What is meant by equal opportunities at work?
21 Why is it important for staff in the spa to receive regular professional development?
22 Give six signs of good communication behaviour.
23 Why is it necessary to conduct staff appraisals?
24 If you were a spa manager, what action would you take if a member of staff did not meet their individual targets?

chapter 4

Promotion of spa services and products

G6

Promote additional products or services to clients

Learning objectives

This chapter discusses ways to promote products and services to clients. It describes the skills and knowledge necessary to enable you to:

- **identify additional products or services that are available**
- **inform clients about additional products or services**
- **gain clients' commitment to additional products or services**

When providing spa therapies it is important to use the skills you have learnt in the following core units:

G1 Ensure your own actions reduce risks to health and safety

G11 Contribute to the financial effectiveness of the business

INTRODUCTION

In today's competitive spa market a therapist has to be able to do so much more than just give a good treatment. They need to look at the client as a whole and offer advice and recommendations on everything from treatment products, nutrition and alternative treatments to changes in lifestyle to promote wellbeing to the client. A good spa therapist will inspire loyalty from the client and help to establish a reputation and set standards that will allow the business to grow.

SPA IMAGE

The treatment services and products used in your spa should reflect who and what your philosophies are. It is important that this statement is reflected in everything you do, from the name of the spa, the menu of treatments, the design of the spa and marketing pictures, to the products and how many ranges are used and the training of therapists and management.

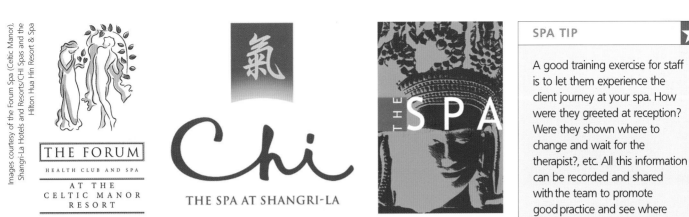

Images courtesy of the Forum Spa (Celtic Manor), Shangri-La Hotels and Resorts/CHI Spas and the Hilton Hua Hin Resort & Spa

THE FORUM
HEALTH CLUB AND SPA
AT THE
CELTIC MANOR
RESORT

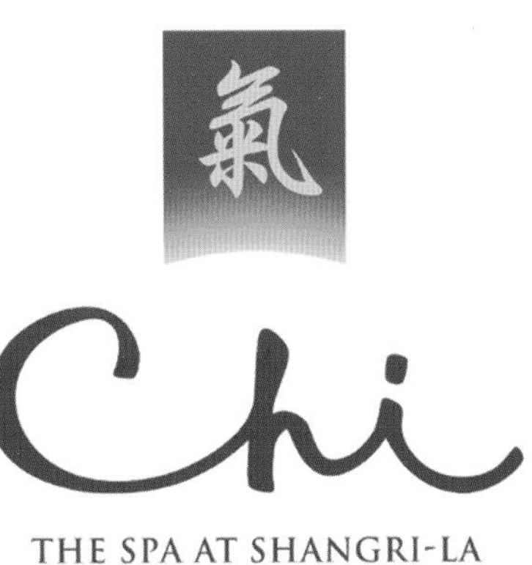
Chi
THE SPA AT SHANGRI-LA

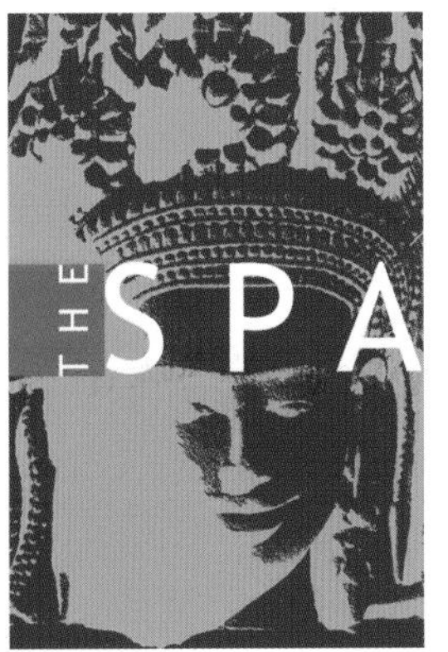
THE SPA

Spa logos

> **SPA TIP**
>
> A good training exercise for staff is to let them experience the client journey at your spa. How were they greeted at reception? Were they shown where to change and wait for the therapist?, etc. All this information can be recorded and shared with the team to promote good practice and see where improvements can be made.

Selecting product ranges for the spa

Clients like a selection of products and treatments to choose from when they visit a spa and the range should reflect what your spa stands for. There is a wide range of spa products available to enable spas to create treatments that reflect their brand. Companies such as Elemis, Espa, Phytomer, Pevonia, Thalgo, and Finders have created their own signature treatments that reflect their product brands and philosophies and can be adopted by the spa. But some spas mix well-known brand treatments along with their own product range, which are designed specifically so that their own signature treatments can be designed around them. Ideally, 3–4 product ranges are sufficient as too many can be confusing for the client.

You may decide to use client surveys or focus groups to find out what the consumer would like to see at your spa and the type of treatments and services they would like to use. There are a lot of factors to consider – don't just choose a range because you like it!

Phytomer

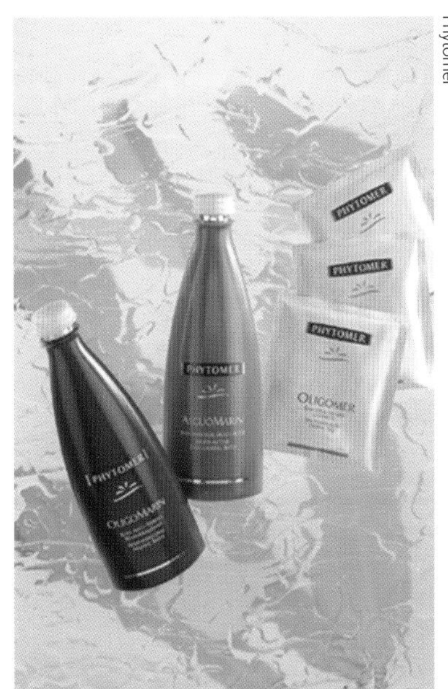
PHYTOMER
OLIGOMER
PHYTOMER
OLIGOMARIN

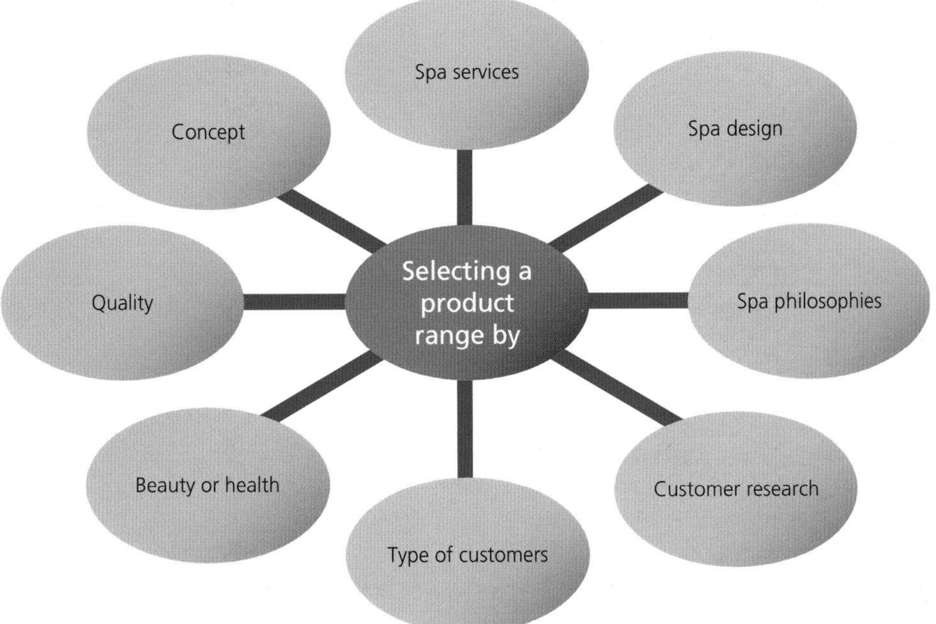
Selecting a product range by
Spa services
Concept
Spa design
Quality
Spa philosophies
Beauty or health
Customer research
Type of customers

> **SPA TIP** 
>
> If you specialize in **thalassotherapy treatments** then you can use product lines such as Thalgo, Finders or Phytomer, which use natural minerals and seaweed in their range. If your spa is based around natural/organic treatments then you can use Aveda or Elemis, or create your own range of organic products.

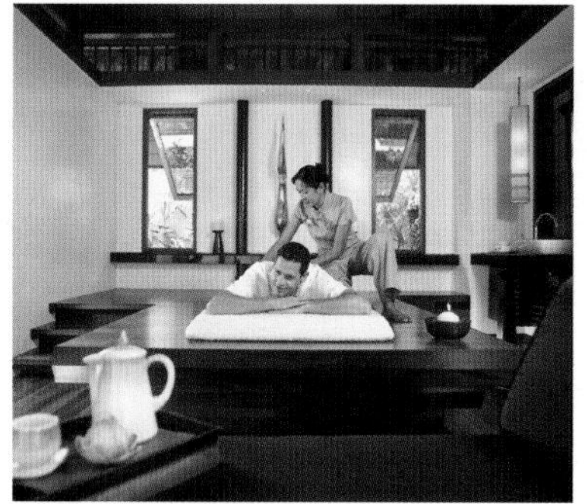

Thai massage, Hilton, Phuket

SPA TIP 

Any new treatments introduced should be tried and tested by all the staff before being presented to customers, as staff feedback can be a valuable source of research.

FACT

Receptionist is one of the most important roles in the spa as they are usually the first person the customer meets and can make a great impression. It is important that the receptionist has sampled all the treatments on offer and gained product knowledge as they should be able to talk freely and recommend from all the services offered on the spa menu.

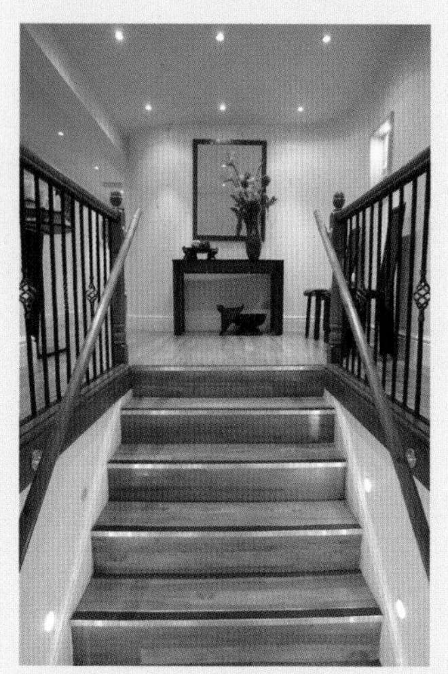

Spa reception area, Ki Day Spa

Staff training in products and treatments

In order for products and treatments to be successful in a spa all staff need to be trained thoroughly in all ranges before being allowed to work on clients. Ideally training should last a minimum of a month and will depend on the range of products and treatments offered at the spa. The larger product companies tend to do most of the training at their own centres, but some may send a trainer out to the spa depending on staff numbers.

It is important that the therapist is trained in all aspects of the spa to include:

- product knowledge
- treatments
- spa concept and philosophies
- how to present treatment rooms and treatments, e.g. placement of towels and flowers on the couch
- small details, e.g. how is water served to the client, music
- appearance of the therapist, e.g. uniform style, hair, shoes – flip flops or none!

Training of staff should be continuous in order to increase motivation, professionalism, confidence and promote the high standards expected.

Once accounts have been set up with product companies they then should regularly send a representative to keep you updated on the products and treatments, answer any queries that you may have and help with any promotional activities that you would like to offer. It is beneficial for the product company to provide a good service to you as your spa is a marketing tool for their brand, as well as your being a valued customer.

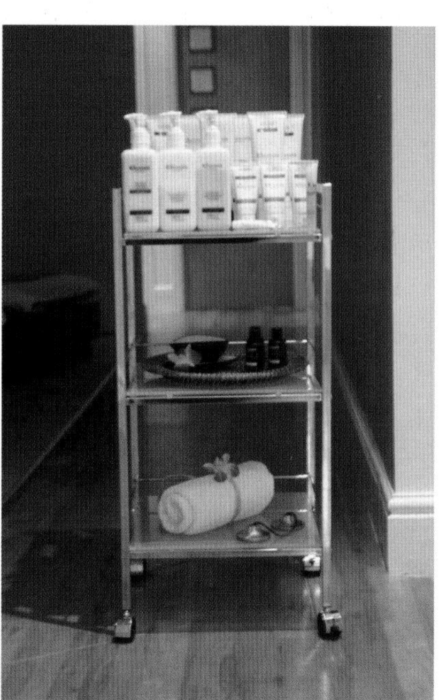

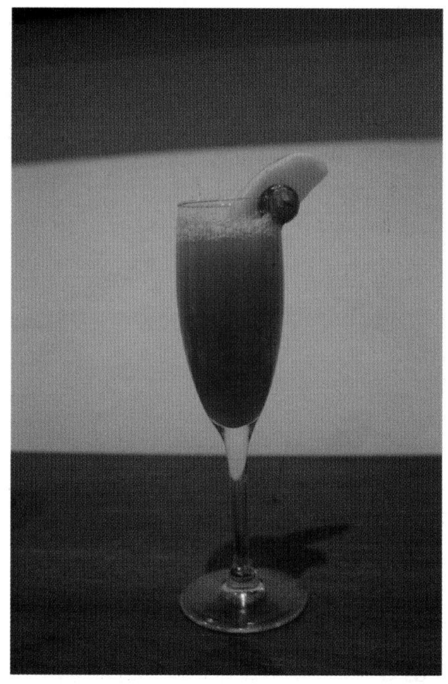

Attention to detail is vital

FACTORS WHICH AFFECT CLIENT SALES

There are several issues to consider as to why the customer has chosen your spa and services from this expanding market and it is important to analyse this first as it may affect both how much money the client spends and return business.

- Advertising – did the client read about the spa in a magazine article, on the internet or in a newspaper advert?
- Is this their first spa visit or are they regular customers in the spa market?
- Have they come on recommendation from a friend?
- Is this an indulgence treatment for them or an escape from work/family life?
- Is their visit for weight loss, beauty or complementary/preventative treatment?

All of these details should be covered as part of the consultation and will give you an idea as to how serious they are about their treatments and their intention to continue a maintenance programme at home.

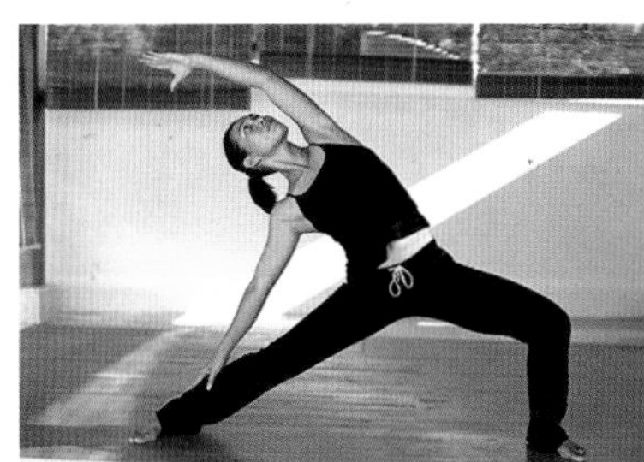
Courtesy of Kurumba Spa, Maldives

Client in yoga position

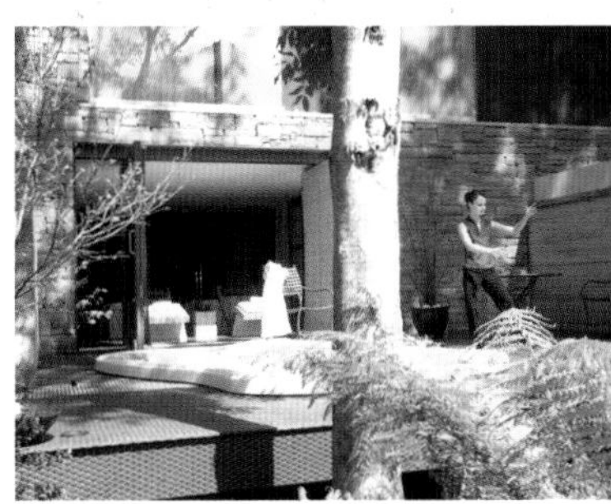
Courtesy of Sàmas

Client doing t'ai chi

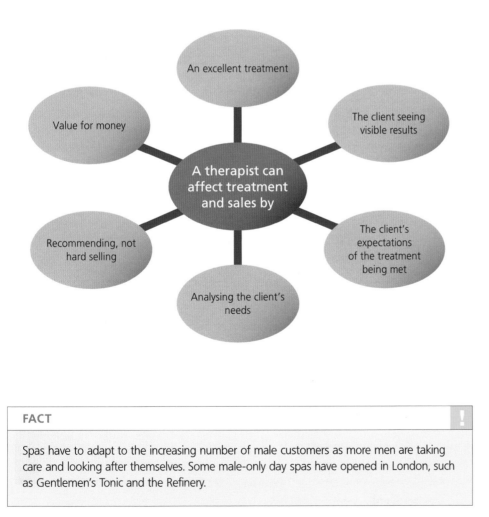

FACT

Spas have to adapt to the increasing number of male customers as more men are taking care and looking after themselves. Some male-only day spas have opened in London, such as Gentlemen's Tonic and the Refinery.

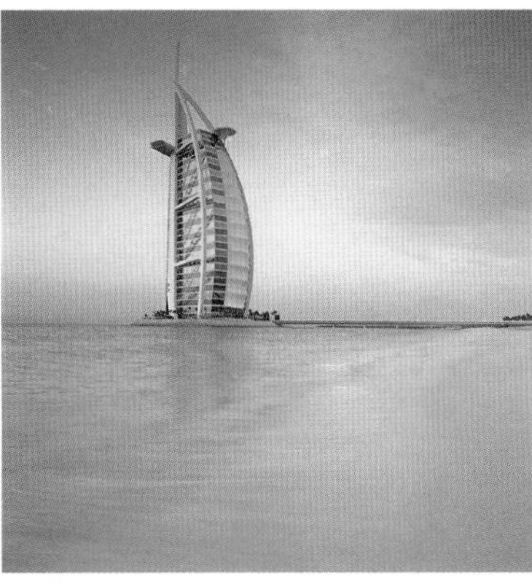

Burj-al-Arab, Dubai

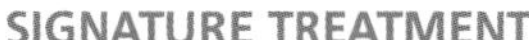

SIGNATURE TREATMENT S

From Burj-al-Arab, Dubai:

'Assawan Around the World Massage: An exclusive treatment created for our Assawan guests to experience a wonderful combination of Shiatsu, Thai, Swedish and Balinese massages, a full 90 minutes of pure indulgence for the body and mind.'

TECHNIQUES IN SELLING AND RECOMMENDING PRODUCTS

Most therapists find selling products difficult and this has always been a complaint from managers in the spa/beauty industry to colleges and training establishments when they employ their students. Most therapists learn their selling techniques and skills through experience in the industry and it can take time to build their confidence. The secret to retailing products is the training of staff, so that they know the product ranges thoroughly and believe in the treatments and products used.

Retailing products can be very profitable for the spa owner and also for the therapist as most spas work on a commission basis. It is also an important part of the client service and staff should be trained in the skills of recommending further services and treatments to the customer. Training of staff should include:

- Sharing personal experiences – have they ever felt pushed into buying something, how did they feel afterwards and did they go back? Therapists who regularly hit targets should share tips and techniques that they think may help.
- Role-play – get staff to work in teams, either following scripts or allowing them to try and sell products to each other. Get feedback on how they felt and where strength and weaknesses have been identified. Always offer positive solutions to motivate staff.
- Staff should be encouraged to use the products and (as mentioned previously) try all the treatments. Products could be offered for them to purchase at cost price or as bonuses/incentives on meeting targets. Most product companies also offer product incentives for staff to encourage retail sales.

Products can be sold at the following points in a treatment:

- Consultation – identify what the client wants from the treatment, do they have regular treatments, is there room in their lifestyle for a homecare routine (simple or complex), how soon do they want to see results. At this point you could up-sell from the basic treatment the client has booked to a more elaborate service.

Phytomer

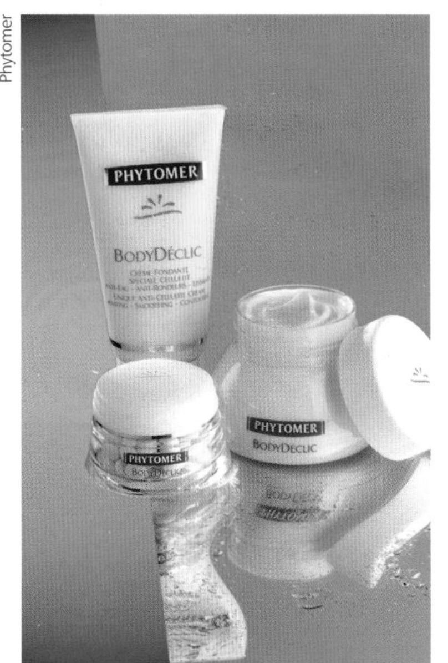

Body products

SIGNATURE TREATMENT S

From The Spa, Hilton Hotel, Phuket:

'Princess for the Day (under 12 years)
Floral Foot bath * Kids Massage * Floral Bath * Shampoo & Blow Dry * Hair Braiding * Princess Nail Art * Cookies * Fruit Juice'

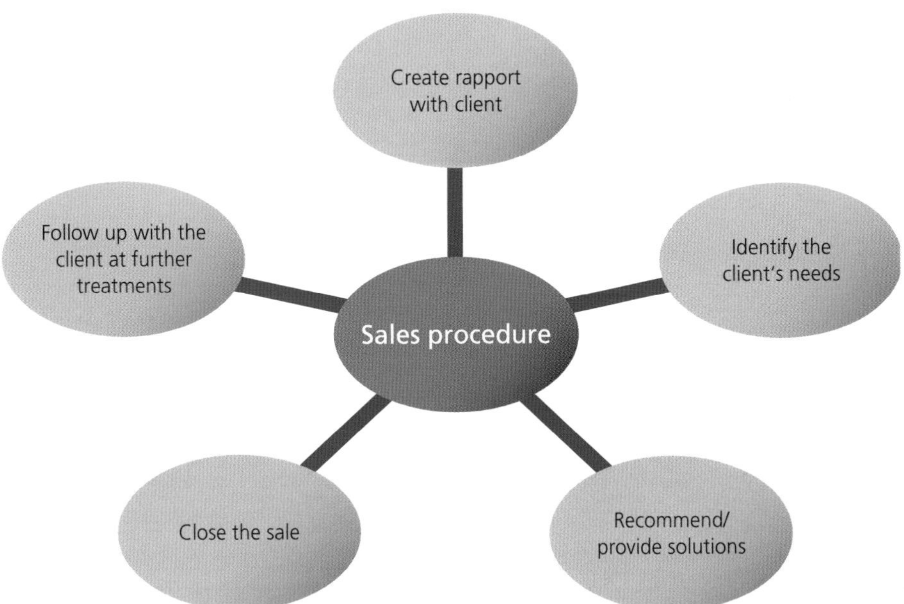
Create rapport with client
Identify the client's needs
Recommend/ provide solutions
Close the sale
Follow up with the client at further treatments
Sales procedure

ACTIVITY 

Write down all the different tools available in the spa to assist in treatment and retail sales. How would you use these effectively?

- Treatment – explain the treatment to the client and the benefits they will receive from the products being used and then leave the client to relax throughout the treatment. Do not sell to the client during the treatment as it comes across as pushy and may spoil the treatment.
- Close of the treatment – write down on a prescription card the products/treatments you recommend for the client and the benefits they will see from regular homecare/treatments. If the client asks to be shown the products (keep it simple if they do not normally use a lot of products at home), always explain how they should be used. If you believe in the treatments and products this will come across to the client.
- Close the sale – listen to the client. If they are sending out signals that they do not want to buy anything then give them a leaflet or sample as they may come back later. If the client has been impressed with the treatment and sees visible results then they will follow your recommendations.

Retail displays

Displaying products in the spa can be a good advertising tool to catch the customer's eye. Displays should be very simple, eye catching and may incorporate a display stand, show cards or posters/adverts produced to market the company. Some spas may have a street-front window where displays can be used to attract customers to the treatments and products on offer.

If products are being displayed in the treatment room then ideally dummy products should be used as these are easily replaced if the stock becomes

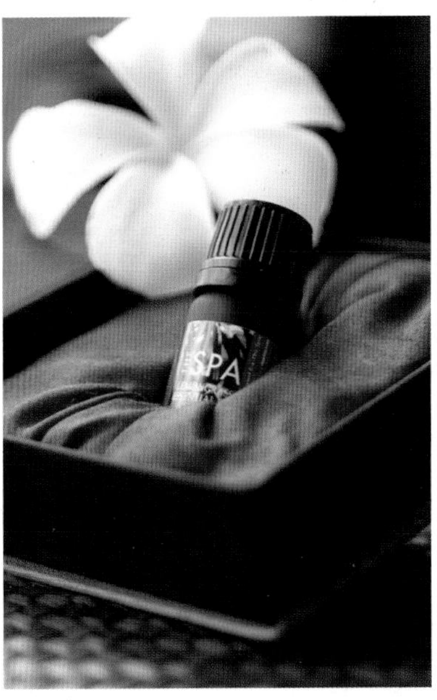
SPA
Spa product, Hilton, Phuket

SPA TIP 

Always replace stock from the back so that old stock is sold first.

SPA TIP 

If creating a display always look at it from a distance and from different angles in order to see how it can best attract the customer's eye and to judge its overall visual appeal.

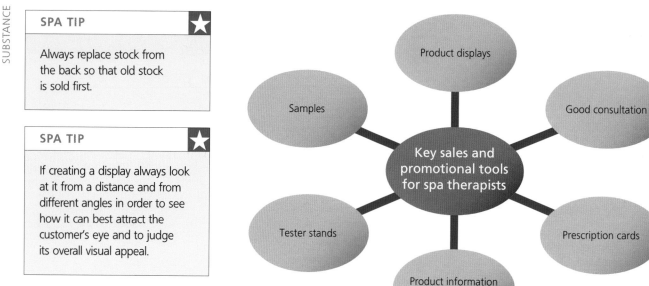

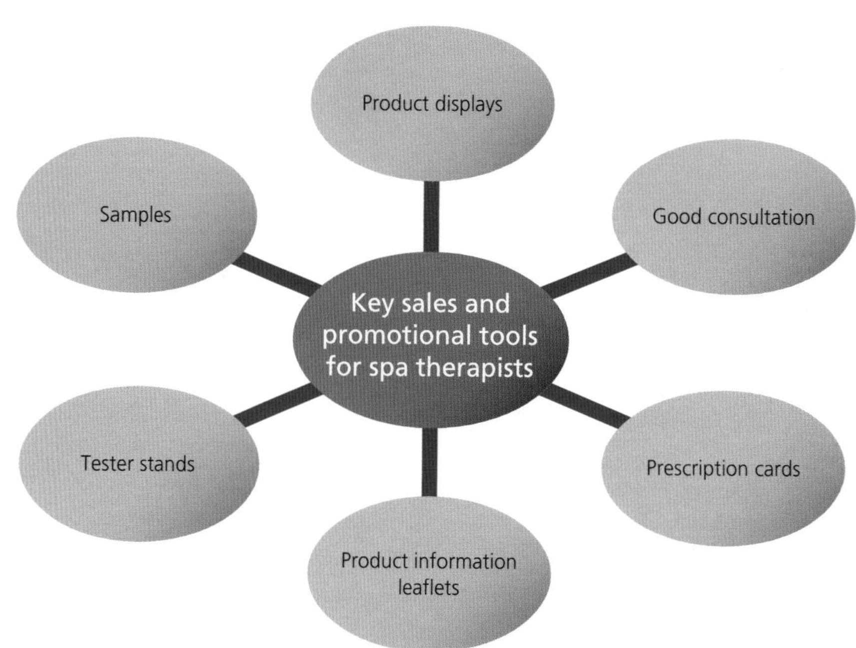
Key sales and promotional tools for spa therapists
Product displays
Good consultation
Prescription cards
Product information leaflets
Tester stands
Samples

damaged or if a client is tempted to steal them. All display stock should be kept clean, dust free and rotated regularly so that products do not spoil. Most product companies provide marketing material to promote new product lines or special promotion lines. This should be changed regularly so that it does not look dated and to entice the customer with new product lines as they are introduced. In larger spas a dresser may be used to create eye-catching displays and present promotional material within the spa so that it reflects the overall look of the brand.

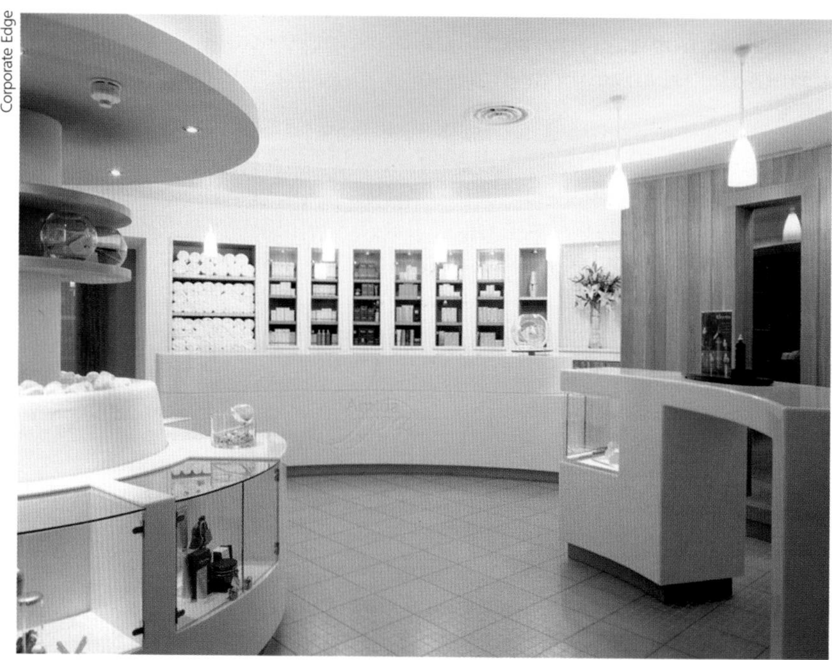

Corporate Edge

Products on display in a reception area, Stoke Park

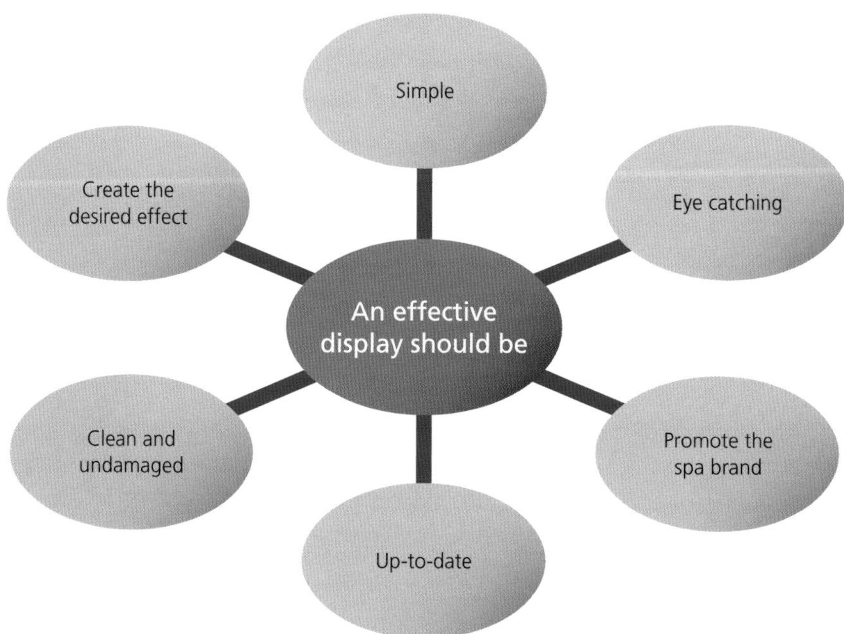

Retail sales within a spa

It is not just the therapist who can promote products and treatments; all staff should be given incentives to work as a team in promoting the brand. The receptionist is in an ideal position to close a sale and encourage repeat business to the customer. Most spas have a retail area within the reception where clients can purchase the products that have been used during the treatment and recommended by the therapist.

Tester stands can be positioned around the reception for the client to try the products in a relaxed environment without being ushered out of a treatment room as the next client is due. The more relaxed and comfortable the client feels the greater the chance of them purchasing products.

A shop incorporated within the spa/health club is very popular for selling a wide range of products to the customer. Not only can it sell the range of treatment products but also other consumables that the customer may require, such as perfume, make-up, hair products, dressing gowns, towels, books, handbags, small gifts, etc. As there is a good profit margin on retail products this can be a very good source of revenue for the business.

SPA TIP 

Some spas, such as the Ajune Day Spa in New York, have taken away the pressure of retailing from the therapist by introducing a **spa concierge** who takes care of the client at the end of their treatments. They recommend products used by the therapist and introduce new products that the customer has not tried before.

IMPORTANCE OF SETTING TARGETS

An important part of the business is setting targets for the spa and the staff. Staff targets can form the basis of the commission that they are paid on the sale of services and products. A lot of spas are trying to move away from a hard sell approach from therapists but it is integral to the revenue of the

FACT

Management motivation of staff is very important for creating a happy team and keeping good staff.

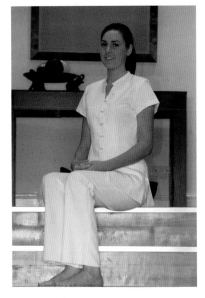

Spa therapist

Spa therapist's targets

Staff role or name	*Weekly target £*	*Daily target £*	*Day 1*	*Day 2*	*Day 3*	*Day 4*	*Day 5*
Massage therapist	£1500	£300	£				
Beauty therapist							

spa and can motivate and encourage friendly competition between staff. If therapists are employed on a salary only basis with no incentive to retail further treatments and products, it is all too-easy for them to just carry out a treatment and for the client leave without the possibility of maybe seeing them again!

Set weekly targets for the spa team and break these down into individual weekly targets. Weekly targets are often broken down further into daily targets. These targets should take into account whether the therapist is full-time or part-time, and set accordingly. The targets should be displayed for staff to see – ideally in a staff room – as this encourages staff to be aware of the revenue of the business.

The targets for the spa team could be broken down further if you knew how many clients were booked in for a particular day and divided the daily target by that number so as to find out how much is needed per client. Increase the rate of commission paid once the therapist has met their target and exceeded it, e.g. 10 per cent on weekly target and 20 per cent on anything above that target.

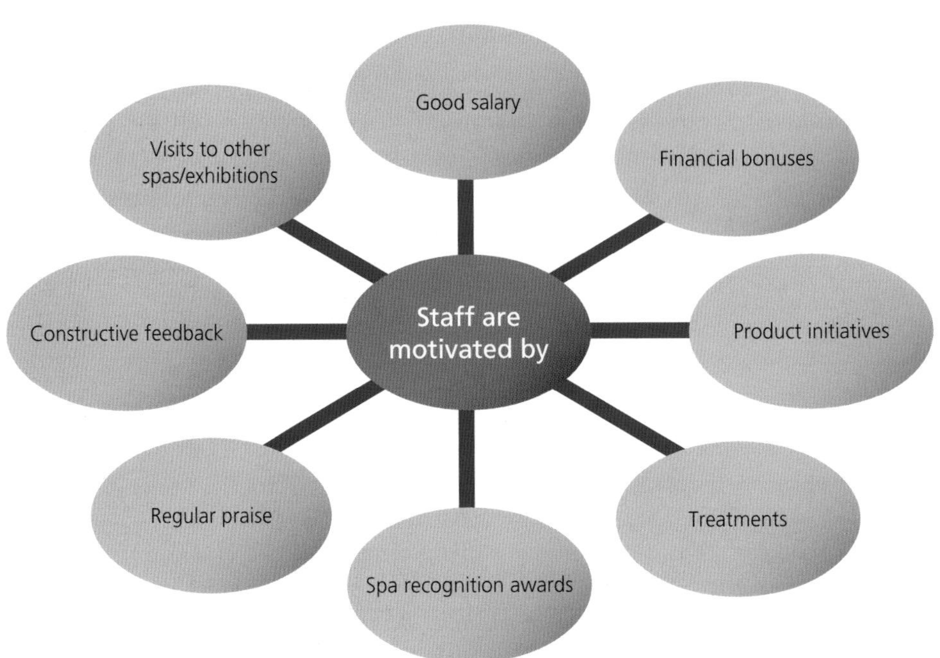

ADDITIONAL TREATMENTS 2006

BODY TREATMENTS

Body Exfoliation (a) (sd) (14) — £36.00 (25 mins)
A complete treatment to eliminate dead skin cells and leave the body soft and hydrated.

Massage by hand — £58.00 (55 mins)
Full body Swedish massage, to ease tension and sooth tired muscles.

Back Massage (14) — £36.00 (25 mins)
Using essential oils to relax tired muscles.

Paraffin Wax Full body with essential oils (P) — £58.00 (55 mins)
A very relaxing and hydrating treatment for the whole body to nourish and soften the skin.

Paraffin wax for back, neck and shoulders (14) — £32.00 (40 mins)
Localised deep heat treatment to alleviate tension and relax muscles.

Aromazone (E) — £34.00 (25 mins)
A lymphatic leg and thigh treatment to boost circulation and minimise fluid retention.

Stobo Castle Luxury Mud Wrap* — £58.00 (55 mins)
A mud envelopment to nourish, rejuvenate as well as detoxify. This 100% organic mud offers natural healing with a multitude of bio-minerals. This treatment also includes a scalp massage.

Finders Dead Sea Inch Wrap* (P) (E) (T) (L) — £75.00 (1 hr 50 mins)
The Dead Sea Inch Wrap treatment will detoxify the body, emulsify fat, reduce cellulite and improve skin tone. This is the perfect choice for those wanting to enhance the effects of a diet or detoxification programme as there is an added benefit of inch loss. This treatment is also excellent for those suffering from eczema & psoriasis.

Finders Dead Sea Algimud I Area (P) (L) (T) — £50.00 (55 mins)
The purifying and detoxifying Algimud body mask is applied to problem areas. Local circulation and cell metabolism are increased. This treatment is ideal for stretch marks, cellulite and skin that has lost its elasticity.

* Includes a Body Exfoliation

TREATMENTS LINE: 01721 760344 9am - 5.30pm
spa@stobocastle.co.uk 9

Part of a treatment price list, Stobo Castle Health Spa, Scotland

TREATMENT PRICE LISTS/BROCHURES

How you present your treatments can increase sales and should always reflect the brand of the spa. Your brand statement should be reflected through the design of the marketing material used to promote the spa and its treatments – visual stimulants are important to clients.

A treatment menu should be comprehensive but not too long and 'waffly' as clients will switch off from reading it. List treatments under headings so that it is easy for the client to locate the type of treatment they want, e.g. spa signature treatments, body therapy, water therapy, facial therapy, additional experiences, etc. Give a brief description of the treatment and how long it will last and cost. Some spas provide treatments in packages, which include use of spa facilities and lifestyle programmes of meditation, yoga, t'ai chi, etc.

WEBSITES

Is your website a good advertisement for your business? So many websites are not used effectively to promote the spa and the services offered and this could be a missed opportunity. More and more people are booking their

SPA TIP 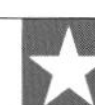

Hold regular team meetings and appraisals to discuss what motivates staff and give incentives accordingly.

ACTIVITY 

Write down a list of what motivates you and your colleagues.

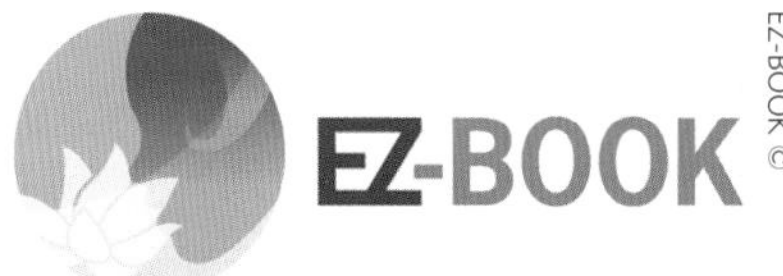

Spa software

Image courtesy of EZ-BOOK ©

SPA TIP 

Willowstream Spas produced unique marketing artwork by creating photographs of landscapes using bodies to convey their connection to the land.

SPA TIP 

Invest in creating a good website as over the next few years it may become your major source for business.

SPA TIP 

E-tail retailing through your website.

Image courtesy of the Forum Spa (Celtic Manor)

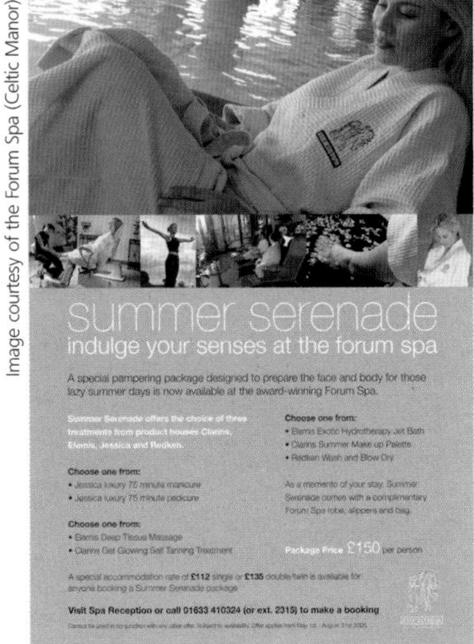

Sample of a spa promotion

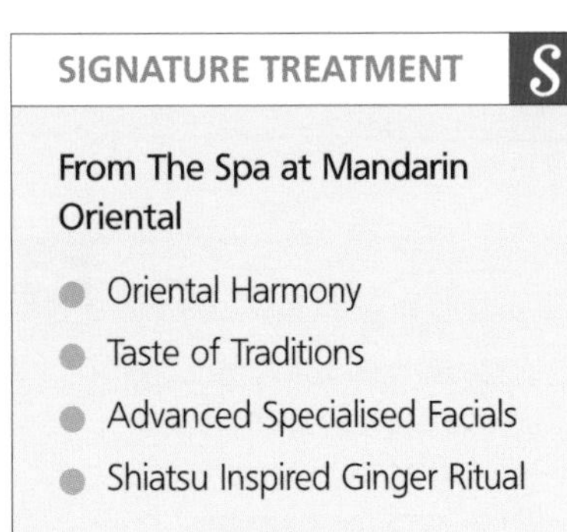

SIGNATURE TREATMENT S

From The Spa at Mandarin Oriental

- Oriental Harmony
- Taste of Traditions
- Advanced Specialised Facials
- Shiatsu Inspired Ginger Ritual

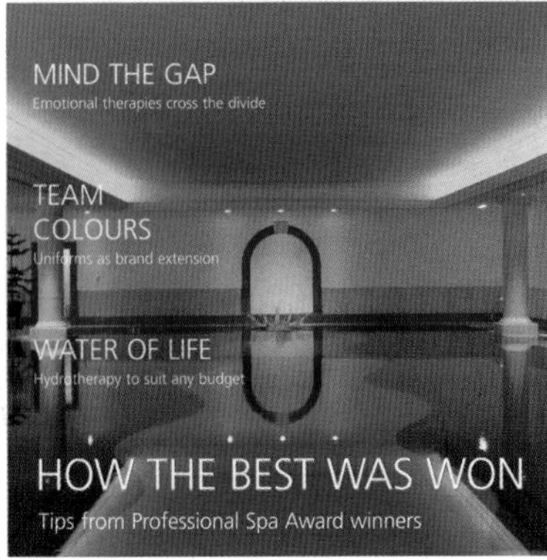

Professional Spa magazine

holidays and trips over the internet and the first impressions they receive are gleaned from images on a computer screen!

Your website should be visually appealing and promote your best assets. Include pictures of staff looking relaxed and happy and of treatments being carried out, and include testimonials from satisfied customers. A price list should be incorporated with brief descriptions of the treatments as this will entice customers sat at their workdesks feeling stressed and in urgent need of some 'pampering'.

PROMOTIONS IN THE SPA

If you need to entice new customers into the spa or encourage back old clients who have not visited for a while, a promotional evening or a product offer is a good way of stimulating client interest. Most large product companies run regular special offers where clients purchase a product or have a treatment and receive a complimentary gift of other products to try. These usually offer good value to the customer and at the same time introduce new products into their homecare routine. Marketing material is usually provided before the promotion is due to start and can be displayed in order to catch the client's attention.

Promotion events or demonstrations are a popular marketing venture to stimulate interest in new products or a new treatment whilst making it more of a social event for the clients. The event could include:

- A brief talk from a spa expert on a new treatment, lifestyle tips such as the benefits of a more holistic approach to wellbeing, a theme such as specialist Far Eastern treatments, healthy eating or 'living a stress-free life'.
- Launch of a new beauty/spa product – which could include gift bags containing small trial sizes and product information.
- An open evening for clients to browse around the spa whilst drinking a glass of 'bubbly' and observe staff carrying out different treatments available on the menu – with a discount on all treatments booked and paid for that evening.
- Make sure that staff are available to answer customer questions and give personal treatment advice.
- Provide drinks and nibbles, such as healthy snacks or, if following a theme, bite-size taster food from that country/region.
- Always give clients a 'goody bag' as most people like to take something away – put in a treatment menu, product information, samples or trial sizes (try to get some to cover all the product ranges offered in the spa), newsletter if you have one, and something personal like an affirmation card or crystal or marble stone!
- Invite a magazine such as *Professional Spa* or *Vogue* to cover the event for their publication.

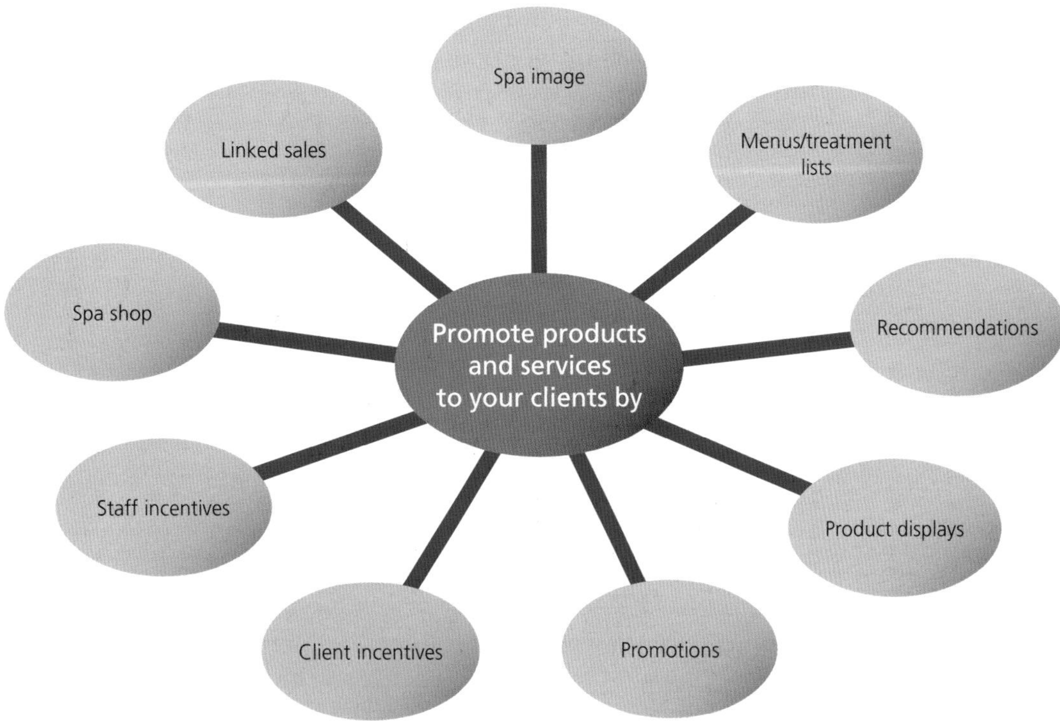

LINKED PRODUCTS

A client may only visit the spa monthly so it is important that you recommend products for them to use at home to continue the effects of your treatments. Clients are beginning to expect an in-depth consultation, followed by a type of 'prescription' that gives details of the products that will suit their individual requirements. It is the spa therapist's responsibility to make sure that the client knows that the products on offer in the spa are the same as those used in the treatments and that continued use will prolong the effectiveness of the treatment. Otherwise

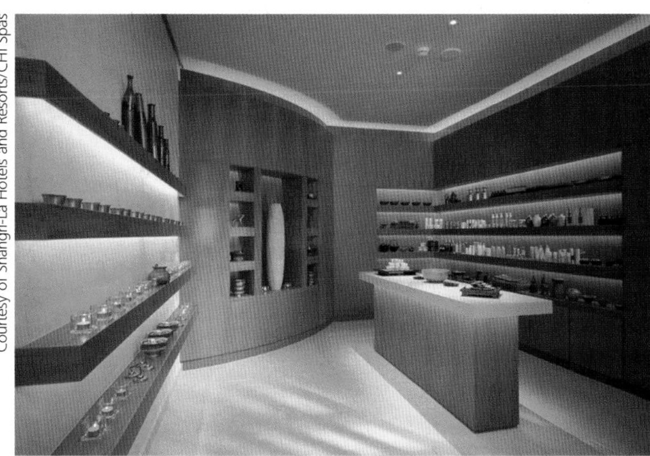
Courtesy of Shangri-La Hotels and Resorts/CHI Spas

Retail area at Chi Spa, Shangri-La

SPA TIP 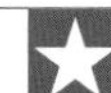

Make sure you maximize on retail opportunities by making sure the following items are available to purchase in the spa:

- body wash/foam
- body scrub
- body brush
- loofah mitt
- body oil/cream
- also available to purchase – bath robes, slippers, towels, eye masks, toilet bags, oil burners, candles, vitamins, etc.

SIGNATURE TREATMENT S

From Serenity Spa, Seaham Hall:

'Time to Share (for couples)

* Rasul * Indian Head Massage * Serenity Wellbeing Massage * Serenity Face Treat

Girls Together

* Serenity Wellbeing Massage * Serentiy Face Treat * Serenity Manicure * Make-up lesson

Mum and Bump

* Nurturing Massage for Mother to Be * Serenity Face Treat * Serenity Pedicure

Yummy Mummy

* Serentiy Face Treat and Cosmequanique * Aroma Stone Therapy * Serentiy Manicure'

clients make quick 'knee-jerk' purchases in places such as supermarkets and chemists and products may be wasted as they are not as effective or do not suit their skin. If clients invest in retail products at the spa they can recreate the 'spa experience' at home – this is something that should be highlighted and encouraged.

LEGISLATION AND CONSUMER RIGHTS

There are certain legal duties that apply to any person who purchases products or services from you. As with health and safety legislation, it is imperative that the spa follows this legislation to protect the customer.

Data Protection Act 1998

This act covers any personal information obtained from the client during a consultation. All consultation cards and clients' personal details should be kept in a secure area and only viewed when consent is gained from that person. This also applies to personal information kept on employees.

Consumer Protection Act 1987

The client is protected against products or services that are sold and are found not to be safe. It is the supplier's responsibility to make sure that all consumables meet the approved standards and clear directions are given on their correct use. If the business is found at fault then they may face legal action.

Trade Descriptions Act 1968 and 1972

These acts protect the consumer from being sold goods or services using misleading information or false descriptions. The retailer must not:

- give false descriptions of services, e.g. claiming that the client's wrinkles will disappear after one treatment
- make misleading comparisons on prices
- give false information about the effect of a product.

All products must be clearly labelled, contain accurate information about the product and be in a good condition – no damaged boxes or half-empty bottles!

Sales and Supply of Goods Act 1994

All goods sold must be of a good standard, not damaged, free from any defects and meet the description supplied. If goods are faulty and do not meet the description then this act entitles the customer to receive a refund.

Consumer Protection (Distance Selling) Regulations 2000

If you sell goods or services to consumers by any of the following:

- the internet
- digital television
- mail order, including catalogue shopping
- phone
- fax

then you must give consumers clear information, including details of the goods or services offered, delivery arrangements and payment, the supplier's details and the consumer's cancellation rights before they buy. The consumer has seven working days in which they may cancel their purchase.

SIGNATURE TREATMENT S

Bliss Spa, London

'The triple oxygen treatment: Our most-popular all-around complexion reviver includes intensive cleansing, exfoliating, a fruit acid wash, a pre-extraction oxygen wrap, the necessary extractions, a calming oxygen and milk mask, hydrating enzyme pack, and vitaminized oxygen spray. Fantastic for all skin types. Forget O2, this capital O is for "glow". 85 min'

Prices Act 1974

All retail products must be clearly marked with the price so that the client can see what they are going to be charged before they make a purchase.

Disability Discrimination Act 1995

This act gives people with a disability rights in access to services, goods and facilities. It is the spa's responsibility to make sure that these clients are not discriminated against because of their disability.

Since 2004 service providers have to consider making permanent physical adjustments to their premises if there are physical barriers prohibiting disabled people from using them.

SPA PROFILE

Name: Kerry Symons

Position: Spa Manager

Establishment: Champneys Henlow

Products used: Champneys, Clarins, Babor, Elemis, Tisserand, Orly, Nailtiques.

Number of staff/roles: Approximately 115 staff in total in the treatment department. Around 100 of those are therapists ranging from spa assistants to premier therapists. Behind the scenes staff include schedulers and stock assistants.

Training/experience: Trained at Henlow Grange College in 1990 and gained IHBC and City and Guilds. After initial training, trained in several product companies, completed my Assessors Award. I worked my way up working in various different roles in the department – Specialized Therapist, Senior Therapist, Scheduler, Assistant Manager to where I am today – Spa Manager.

Main responsibilities: The overall running of the treatment/spa department; staff appraisals, training and development; standards and procedures; client care; interviews and recruitment; budgets.

Best parts of the job: Seeing staff progress and enjoying their job. Being busy, one day is never really the same as another. Seeing the spa industry grow. Receiving feedback from the clients.

Secrets of a successful spa therapist: Never be frightened to give something a go, volunteer for whatever is available to you – it gave me a lot of confidence, e.g. working at other sites, carrying out demonstrations, etc. Have respect for your employers – allow a bit of give and take, trial whatever they suggest: you never know, it could work.

Have an interest in what your clients want, not only what you want.

To be ready for hard work.

KEY/CORE SKILLS OPPORTUNITIES

To be an excellent spa therapist you must be able to communicate well, both orally and in writing. To be able to succeed and progress in the spa industry, it is also essential that you have an ability to work with numbers and information technology (IT). Increasingly, employers are looking for spa therapists with these 'key' skills when they recruit staff. NVQ/SVQ unit **G6** provides you with an opportunity to develop evidence for KEY/CORE SKILLS. Details can be obtained from the Institute of Customer Service (ICS).

Assessment of knowledge and understanding

When you have some free time, test your understanding and knowledge by answering the following questions. Do this at regular intervals and it will reinforce your learning and help you retain the knowledge, so you are able to perform better in your assessments.

1 What factors must you consider before selecting a product range for the spa?

2 Why is it important for staff to be thoroughly trained in all aspects of the spa?

3 List five benefits of the service offered by product companies to the spa.

4 How can the receptionist help in increasing retail and treatment sales?

5 How can a therapist affect treatments and sales?

6 What is the basic sales procedure used by a therapist with a client?

7 At what points in a treatment can retail products be introduced to a client?

8 Name five selling tools that a therapist can use in promoting sales.

9 Give six key points of an effective display.

10 Why is it important to set income targets for staff?

11 List six things that motivate staff in a spa environment.

12 Produce a list of the key ingredients of a good spa promotion event.

13 What does the Data Protection Act 1998 cover?

14 Which act protects the consumer from being sold goods using misleading information?

15 How does the Disability Discrimination Act 1995 affect a disabled person's rights within a spa?

chapter 5

Health and safety

G1

Ensure your own actions reduce risks to health and safety

Learning objectives

This chapter covers the Health and Safety duties for everyone in the workplace, irrespective of their work role. It describes the skills and knowledge necessary to ensure:

- **your own actions do not create any Health and Safety risks**
- **you do not ignore significant risks in your workplace**
- **you take sensible action to put things right, including reporting situations which pose a danger to people in the workplace and seeking advice**

INTRODUCTION

It is every employee's responsibility to maintain a safe and hygienic environment within a spa. Whether a spa manager or therapist, you need to be aware of certain regulations to which you must adhere in order to make the environment for everyone using the spa as safe as possible. Different countries will have different legal legislations that apply, but across the board they are very similar.

When understanding and explaining how to deal with First Aid emergencies that may occur within the spa it is advisable that all therapists have completed a First Aid certificate (e.g. St John's Ambulance or Red Cross). A lot of beauty/holistic therapy qualifications now incorporate a First Aid certificate within the core training and it is a requirement that a therapist holds a recognized and current First Aid certificate before becoming a member of a professional organization.

TERMINOLOGY

Fundamental to Health and Safety is the understanding of the terms **hazard** and **risk**. Hazard is exposure to danger and risk is the possibility of injury or damage.

HEALTH AND SAFETY AT WORK ACT 1974 (HASWA)

This is the basis of UK health and safety law, which sets out the general duties that employers have towards their employees and members of the public and that employees have to each other.

- It is the employer's responsibility to ensure that the workplace is maintained to high standards of Health and Safety for both clients and employees.
- Employers must provide adequate training and instruction to employees to maintain Health and Safety.
- This act must be displayed clearly for employees to see.
- All staff must abide by these regulations and report to management any hazards they notice that could be of potential danger to clients and employees.

HEALTH AND SAFETY !

An employer does not have to take measures to avoid or reduce risk if it is technically impossible or if the time and cost of the measure is extortionate in relation to the risk.

ACTIVITY ✓

Devise a Health and Safety policy for a day spa.

MANAGEMENT OF HEALTH AND SAFETY AT WORK REGULATIONS 1999

Employers are required to formally provide a healthy and safe working environment and to ensure that this is maintained through regular training and carrying out of risk assessments. Assessing risks and hazards in the workplace is important to the employee and the public using the spa in order to determine that sufficient precautions have been taken.

Key hazards that may occur are:

- slipping/tripping hazards – on stairs or wet floors around the spa pool
- fire/flammable materials – storing rubbish, empty boxes, not emptying full bins, candles placed too near material/towels
- chemicals – spillage/tops left off
- electrical equipment – poor wiring, trailing wires
- poor lighting in an area – could lead to trips/falls
- manual handling – employees being responsible for lifting heavy equipment.

It is usually the managers' and employers' responsibility to carry out risk assessment and to do this they should have been on a recognized risk assessment training course – usually 2 to 3 days – where they can gain a certificate, e.g. the Risk Assessment Principles and Practice Certificate awarded by the Chartered Institute of Environmental Health (CIEH).

Once a risk assessment has been carried out on the spa environment and a risk or hazard has been identified then it must be reported to the appropriate people and measures implemented to reduce the risk where possible. Always share information with employees and provide training for them if necessary. A risk assessment should be carried out on a regular basis, and specifically if any new equipment or treatments have been introduced to the spa.

SPA TIP 

Risk assessment forms should be kept in a secure and safe place where they can be easily accessed.

FACT

HSE stands for the Health and Safety Executive, whose aim is to protect the health, safety and welfare of employees, the public and anyone who may be exposed to risks at work. If you require any information relevant to Health and Safety then contact them and they will send out the appropriate leaflets.

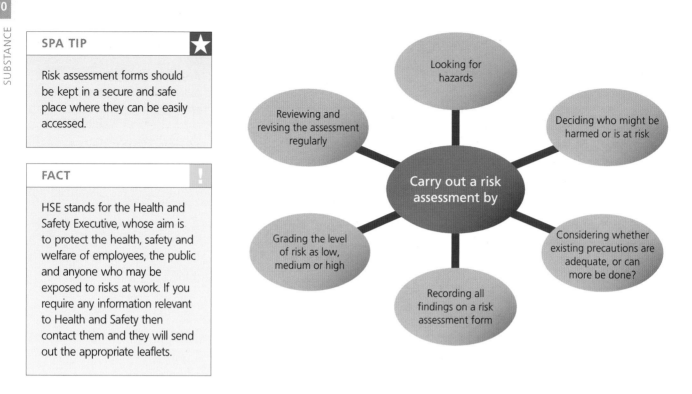

Carry out a risk assessment by
Looking for hazards
Deciding who might be harmed or is at risk
Considering whether existing precautions are adequate, or can more be done?
Recording all findings on a risk assessment form
Grading the level of risk as low, medium or high
Reviewing and revising the assessment regularly

COSHH Risk Assessment

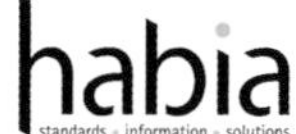

standards • information • solutions

Staff Member Responsible: Natasha Smith   Date: 1st September 2005   Review Dates: 10th January 2006

Hazard	What is the risk?	Who is at risk?	Degree of risk High/Med/Low	Action to be taken to reduce/control risk
Aerosols (List aerosols used in your salon)	These can contain flammable gases and irritant chemicals. There is a risk of fire, explosion and intoxication.	Everyone in the salon, but in particular the user of the aerosol and the client.	Low	Look for aerosols with non-flammable gases if possible. Do not expose to temperatures above 50'C. Do not pierce or burn containers. Do not inhale.
Permanent wave neutraliser (List products used in your salon)	Irritant to the skin and eyes. Moderately toxic is swallowed or inhaled.	Stylists, juniors, trainees and clients.	Medium	Store in a cool place. Reseal after use. Do not use on damaged or sensitive skin. Avoid breathing in. Never place in an unlabelled container.

EXAMPLE

 HSIP2a

A COSHH Risk Assessment form. *Health & Safety for Beauty Therapists. Author: Habia.* To order your copy contact the Habia sales team on 0845 612 3555 or visit www.habia.org to buy online.

Environmental Health Officers (EHOs)

These work for the Local Authority Environmental Health Department and enforce the regulations of the Health and Safety at Work Act by visiting and inspecting businesses. If the inspector is not happy that the regulations are being met during their visit they can:

- issue an improvement notice giving employers a specified time to rectify the problem before a re-inspection
- issue a closure (prohibition) notice until they are satisfied that the regulations have been met and there is no danger to employees or clients.

Failure to comply with any notice given can lead to prosecution. Breaches of the statute law can lead to a maximum fine of £20 000 and or up to 6 months imprisonment.

HEALTH AND SAFETY !

A **crime prevention officer** should train staff and management in how to deal with a bomb alert and the correct emergency procedures to follow.

Lifeguards

If the spa has a swimming pool then there should be a lifeguard attendant around at all times. All lifeguards must be professionally trained and hold a valid certificate.

WORKPLACE (HEALTH, SAFETY AND WELFARE) REGULATIONS 1992

These regulations relate to the basic management of Health and Safety in the environment such as:

- ventilation must be adequate with sufficient quantities of clean air
- lighting should be sufficient for the workplace and not too bright
- temperature should be comfortable and a minimum of 16 °C
- storage and handling of waste materials must comply with legislation
- cleaning must be carried out regularly with suitable cleaning materials
- washing, toilet and changing facilities must be provided and adequate for the number of staff and clients
- fresh drinking water must be supplied and easily accessible
- staff areas for resting and eating must be provided
- maintenance and testing of equipment must be carried out regularly to ensure that it is all in good working order
- fire exits must be clearly marked and have a clear access and firefighting equipment provided.

FACT !

Regulations are law approved by Parliament. These are usually made under the Health and Safety at Work Act 1974 following proposals from the Health and Safety Executive. This also applies to European directives as well as UK ones.

ACTIVITY 

Risk assessment Carry out your own risk assessment. List the potentially hazardous substances handled in spa therapy. What protective clothing should be available?

PERSONAL PROTECTIVE EQUIPMENT AT WORK REGULATIONS 1992 (PPE)

Appropriate equipment and clothing must be provided for employees where a risk or hazard in their job/duties has been identified through a risk assessment. Employees have a legal obligation to wear this equipment and are breaking regulations if they chose not to. Potentially hazardous substances used in the spa area are the chemicals used in treating spa pool water, cleaning products and the possible leakage of toxic gases bromine or ozone in the plant room.

MANUAL HANDLING OPERATIONS REGULATIONS 1992

These regulations cover all employees who have to lift and move objects during their work. To reduce the risk of injury a risk assessment must be carried out to cover all tasks that may involve moving or lifting objects. The employee has a responsibility to the employer to inform them of any physical condition they may have which might affect their ability to undertake manual handling.

The types of injury that may occur from manual handling activities are:

- back strain
- cuts
- bruises
- crushing of limbs
- scrapes
- pulled muscles.

To reduce the risk from manual handling activities, control methods must be put in place, such as:

- assess the risk
- inform the employee and provide the necessary training and instruction on how to lift and handle objects safely
- if specialist equipment is provided to lift heavy objects then it must be used
- employees must be given protective equipment to wear if this reduces the risk of injury
- all activities must be regularly reviewed through the risk assessment.

SPA TIP 

The CIEH offers a short course in the principles of manual handling, which can be offered to staff who need training.

HEALTH AND SAFETY (DISPLAY SCREEN EQUIPMENT) REGULATIONS 1992

This regulation is to support employees who regularly use a visual display unit or computer screen as a large part of their job. The regulations specify:

- acceptable levels of radiation emitted from the screen
- correct seating position and desk height
- length of time allowed at the screen and appropriate rest periods.

Employees at risk would be identified through a risk assessment and it is then the employer's responsibility to reduce that risk through the above regulations.

> **HEALTH AND SAFETY !**
>
> Some employees may require an eye test if they are suffering from headaches or eye strain due to looking at a screen for long periods. It is the employer's responsibility to pay for an eye test if this is something that has been highlighted in a risk assessment.

HEALTH AND SAFETY INFORMATION FOR EMPLOYEES REGULATIONS 1989

Employers are required to display a poster and provide information to staff regarding Health and Safety regulations.

A Health and Safety policy needs to be written for any spa employing more than five people and must be given to each employee so that they understand their own Health and Safety responsibilities. It should state:

- who has the responsibility to carry out regular Health and Safety checks
- the employee's responsibilities to maintain regulations
- who hazards should be reported to
- the correct storage of chemical substances
- fire precautions and evacuation procedure
- accident procedures and who to report to (the designated first-aider)
- emergency contact details for the manager
- how often risk assessments are carried out, and that all electrical equipment is checked and PAT tested.

> **HEALTH AND SAFETY !**
>
> All places of work should display the Health and Safety Regulations notice, ideally in a staff room where it is visible to all staff.

EMPLOYER'S LIABILITY (COMPULSORY INSURANCE) ACT 1969

All employers must have employer's liability insurance cover as it is a legal requirement. This is to cover employees against ill health and any accidents that may occur whilst at work and provide financial compensation in the event of injury.

REPORTING OF INJURIES, DISEASES AND DANGEROUS OCCURRENCES REGULATIONS 1995 (RIDDOR)

ACTIVITY 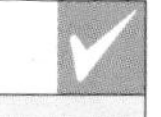

Devise an accident report form to be used in a spa.

These regulations cover the employer, employees and clients who suffer a personal injury whilst at work or visiting the premises. Employers are required to notify the local Health and Safety authority where occupational injuries or diseases have resulted in the person's absence from work for 3 or more days. If a more serious accident occurs resulting in a hospital stay or even a fatality then it must be reported immediately by telephone.

All accidents that occur within the workplace must be written in an accident book or on a report form and kept securely for a minimum of 3 years. The accident report should contain the personal details of the person who has sustained the injury or been involved in an accident, the location, date and time of the occurrence, details of what happened, treatment given, any witnesses and contact details for them, who the incident was reported to and the action taken. The manager and the person who has filled in the report must sign the document.

ELECTRICITY AT WORK REGULATIONS 1989

These regulations ensure that all electrical equipment used is maintained to a high standard and that all staff have been correctly trained in its safe use.

A qualified electrician should test all pieces of electrical equipment every 12 months. The date of the test and electrician's signature should be put on the equipment as well as on a full report, which needs to be kept safely. The report should contain:

- electrician's details
- date of the test
- serial numbers for all equipment
- when the equipment was purchased
- whether equipment was disposed of.

In addition to annual testing, a trained member of staff should regularly check all electrical equipment for safety – ideally every 3 months.

SPA TIP 

Where possible it is important that a professional electrician installs electrical equipment, particularly in a spa environment where water is being used which can be highly dangerous if it comes in to direct contact with electricity.

It is also important for the spa therapist to maintain equipment and use it safely according to the manufacturer's guidelines by storing it safely, keeping it clean, checking that wires are not frayed and plugs are not cracked, and to report any faults or concerns to the manager.

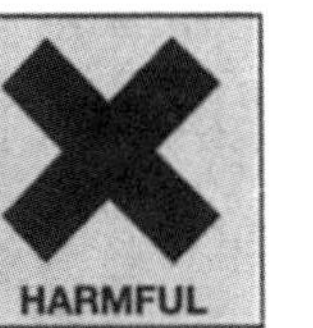

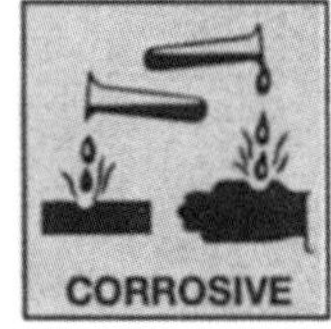

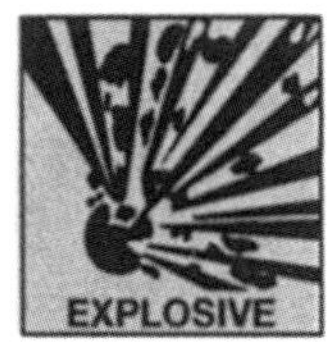

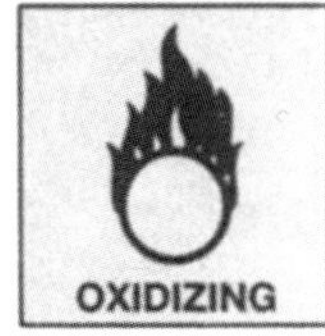

COSHH hazards symbols

CONTROL OF SUBSTANCES HAZARDOUS TO HEALTH REGULATIONS 2002 (COSHH)

These regulations require employers to assess the risks from hazardous substances used in their workplace and take the appropriate measures to minimize risk, such as:

- Substances that are hazardous to health must be clearly identified and stored in the correct place.
- Manufacturers have to provide clear guidelines on how the product should be stored and handled.
- Chemicals – such as those used in water testing and maintenance – should be stored securely in a fire-resistant room or cupboard, away from public areas.
- All staff who use hazardous materials should be trained correctly in their safe use and follow guidelines given.

Hazardous substances should be highlighted through the risk assessment and identified as a low, medium or high risk. High-risk substances should ideally be replaced with lower risk substances, and if not, stored securely.

HEALTH AND SAFETY

Hazardous substances must be stored in a cool dry place, out of direct sunlight, away from naked flames and in a well-ventilated room.

FIRE PRECAUTIONS (WORKPLACE) REGULATIONS 1997

As outlined in the Management of Health and Safety at Work Regulations 1999, a risk assessment must be carried out by the employer to identify possible fire hazards and measures taken to reduce the risk. To comply with these regulations the following must be in place:

- fire detection equipment, such as smoke alarms
- fire exits must be free from any obstruction and clearly marked
- a fire alarm system, which should be tested weekly to ensure it is fully operational
- the correct type of firefighting equipment must be available, and all staff trained in its use
- all staff should be trained in the fire evacuation procedure and be aware of their responsibilities

FACT

If working in a spa on a cruise ship you will have a responsibility to make sure that passengers are evacuated to their allocated lifeboat safely. You also must undergo training in the use of different types of firefighting equipment and be able to demonstrate how it is used.

HEALTH AND SAFETY

In the case of electrical fires the first priority is to switch off the power supply and isolate the equipment. Only then tackle with the appropriate firefighting equipment, if it is safe to do so.

HEALTH AND SAFETY !

If a person's clothes are on fire they should be smothered/rolled in a fire blanket.

HEALTH AND SAFETY !

Always contact the emergency services for even small fires as they can quickly spread.

FACT

Further leaflets on fire safety are available from the Health and Safety Executive.

- a full annual check and test of the fire alarm system by a competent service engineer
- for a large spa/hotel there must be designated fire marshals who check that all areas have been evacuated and that the building is clear.

Types of portable fire extinguisher

Colour	*Type of fire*	*Extinguisher used*
Red	Paper, wood, fabric, material	Water
Black	Electrical	Carbon dioxide (CO_2)
Cream	Flammable liquid	Foam
Blue/green	All of the above	Dry powder

CHECKLIST Do you have the correct fire precautions?

- ✔ Have we the correct extinguishers for the types of fire hazard?
- ✔ Are the extinguishers maintained and recorded?
- ✔ Are they adequately positioned and signed?
- ✔ Are there enough extinguishers for the circumstances?
- ✔ Are people trained to use the extinguishers?
- ✔ Do you hold regular fire drills?
- ✔ Would you recognize your fire alarm?
- ✔ Do you know how to raise the alarm?
- ✔ Do you know your nearest fire exit?
- ✔ Do you know your assembly point?
- ✔ Are there sufficient fire signs to direct clients to the assembly point?

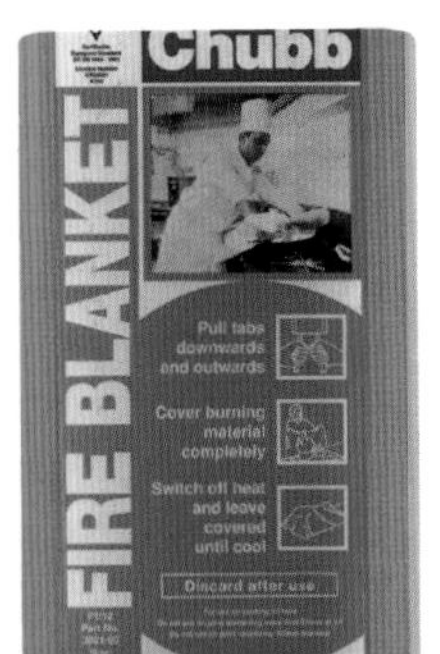

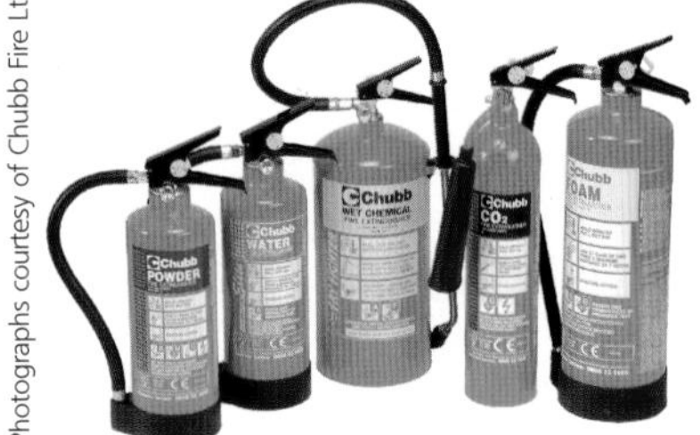

Photographs courtesy of Chubb Fire Ltd

Firefighting equipment

HEALTH AND SAFETY (FIRST AID) REGULATIONS 1981

All employers must cover the requirements of these regulations for First Aid arrangements in the workplace. Ideally, all employees should have received basic First Aid training and, depending on the size of the spa, there should be several employees skilled in the application and treatment for a person following an accident or illness. First Aid is the approved method of treatment until the casualty is placed, if necessary, into medical care. Employees need to know to whom they report an accident and where to locate a First Aid box. All accidents or illnesses that have happened on the

SPA ACCIDENT REPORTING FORM

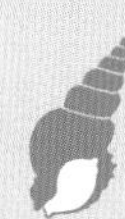

Name:

Address:

Telephone No:

Occupation:

Date of birth:

Please tick: ☐ Employee ☐ Client ☐ Visitor ☐ Contractor

If employee, give the name of your Department Manager:

Location of accident:

Date and time:

Name and address of person reporting the accident:

Give details of what happened and include circumstances, e.g. machinery, equipment, chemicals, conditions, etc.

Are there any obvious causes of the accident?

Injuries sustained:

Give names and addresses of any witnesses:

Is the person absent or expected to be absent from work as a result of the injury?

If an employee: On the day of the incident between what hours was the injured person expected to work?
State from and to.

What hours did they actually work? State from and to:

What corrective action has been taken and by whom? (Give dates for completion)

Any other relevant facts?

Signature of spa manager Date:

premises should be recorded in an accident book or report form, which should contain the following details:

- date, time and place of incident
- name and details of the person involved
- details of the injury/illness and any first aid given
- what happened to the casualty afterwards – did they go home, back to work, hospital etc.?
- the name and signature of the person who dealt with the incident.

The manager, who ideally needs to monitor any re-occurring accidents/ illnesses, should sign the accident book or report form as there may be areas of improvement needed in Health and Safety.

Contents of the First Aid box

A basic First Aid box should contain the following items:

- 10 individual sterile adhesive dressings (plasters)
- 1 triangular bandage
- 1 sterile covering for a serious wound
- 6 safety pins
- 3 medium-sized sterile unmedicated dressings
- 1 large sterile unmedicated dressing
- 1 extra large sterile unmedicated dressing
- 1 sterile eye pad.

The size of the spa and the number of employees and clients will dictate how many First Aid kits need to be available. These boxes should be regularly monitored and re-stocked as necessary. The above is only a basic guide and you may want to put some small scissors and tweezers in the box.

When carrying out a First Aid procedure the following guidelines are given:

- assess the situation
- decide on a diagnosis for the casualty
- provide immediate treatment
- if required, ring for an ambulance
- always report any accident, either in the accident book or, in more serious cases, to the police.

SIGNATURE TREATMENT S

Golden Door, California

Golden Door Signature Citrus Blend Sea Salt Scrub with Avocado: 'Inspired by our lush groves and verdant hillsides, this ambrosial treatment available exclusively at the Golden Door is fresh and fragrant with the natural essences of lemon, chamomile, and lavender plus a soothing blend of avocado, sweet almond and olive oils. Begin with a gentle sea salt exfoliation using silk mitts. A warm-water wash with our richly lathering Signature Citrus Scent bath gel is followed by Signature Citrus Shea Butter moisturizer and Golden Door Botanical Body Oil.'

SPA PROFILE

Name: Darcie DeBartelo

Position: Corporate Director of Spas for Evans Hotels

Establishment: The Spa Torrey Pines, The Lodge Torrey Pines, La Jolla, California

Products used: Torrey Pines signature line, Phytomer, Babor, Li'tya from Australia, Napa Valley grapeseed products.

Number of staff/roles: 75 part and full time staff, including massage therapists, aestheticians, nail technicians, fitness staff and locker room spa attendants.

Training/experience: 'Originally studied on a Hotel Restaurant Management Programme and started as a spa receptionist, working her way up through the business side of the spa industry.' Previous roles have been at: Claremont Resort and Spa in Berkeley, California; Assistant Spa Director at the Phoenician Centre for Wellbeing in Scottsdale, Arizona; Spa Director of the Mirbeau Inn & Spa in the Finger Lakes region of New York.

Main responsibilities: 'Creating the spa environment for guests and staff. Developing and designing treatments and products (including the Torrey Pines signature line) focusing on the integrity and therapeutic value of each service. The spa menu focuses on the real physiological and psychological benefits of a treatment rather than trendy gimmicks. I am also responsible for financial budgets, marketing and promoting the spa and developing in-house training and educational days for staff. Recently I have been in charge of creating a new spa at the Catamaran Resort Hotel on Mission Bay in San Diego which has included the development of a new product line and designing the spa menu and treatments based upon spa traditions from the French Polynesian and Asian cultures.'

Best parts of the job: 'Creating spas from the beginning and being able to develop products and treatments reflecting the spa brand. I also enjoy training and mentoring staff about the spa experience and the service that each client will receive, educating the client through treatments. In my role, everyday is different which is what makes the position so enjoyable.'

Secrets of a successful spa therapist: 'A spa therapist should be truly passionate about what they are doing. A good therapist will also educate themselves by learning from their colleagues.'

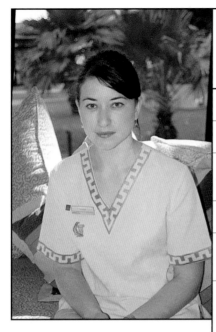

SPA PROFILE

Name: Natalie Dzebissova

Position: Spa Manager

Establishment: Caracalla Spa and Health Club, Le Royal Meridien Beach Resort & Spa, Dubai

Products used: Elemis, Decleor, O-Lys, Ionithermie

Number of staff/roles: Spa Manager, 4 therapists (female), 2 therapists (male), Spa Receptionist

Training/Experience:

Steiner School, Dubai – Therapist training

Caracalla Spa – Spa Therapist

Caracalla Spa – Head Therapist

Caravalla Spa – Spa Manager since 2002

Main responsibilities:

Day-to-day operational running of the spa.

Development of new treatments and techniques.

Recruiting and training staff.

Marketing and advertising.

Best parts of the job:

Communicating with people; staff and guests.

Meeting lots of new people within the Spa industry, it's a constantly changing industry and you need to keep up to date with developments and new treatments. Clients are increasingly well-educated and knowledgeable about the Spa concept and treatments on offer. They demand a high level of service, especially in a Spa within a 5-star hotel such as Le Royal Meridien.

I enjoy working with my team of therapists. They are the most important resource in a Spa and I love working closely with them to develop a team of individuals with excellent practical skills and exceptional customer service.

Secrets of a successful spa therapist:

Passion! You must be passionate about the whole spa business. 'Attitude' and passion cannot be developed easily if it's not there in the first place. You've got to love the job!

A sense of responsibility to the guest, everything should be about making the treatment a 5-star experience.

Expertise. The therapist's touch will reflect their emotion, you need to be calm, balanced, relaxed, focused and enjoy what you are doing.

KEY/CORE SKILLS OPPORTUNITIES

To be an excellent spa therapist you must be able to communicate well, both orally and in writing. To be able to succeed and progress in the spa industry, it is also essential that you have an ability to work with numbers and information technology (IT). Increasingly, employers are looking for spa therapists with these 'key' skills when they recruit staff. NVQ/SVQ unit **G1** provides you with an opportunity to develop evidence for KEY/CORE SKILLS. Details can be obtained from ENTO.

Assessment of knowledge and understanding

When you have some free time, test your understanding and knowledge by answering the following questions. Do this at regular intervals and it will reinforce your learning and help you retain the knowledge, so you are able to perform better in your assessments.

1 What are your responsibilities under the following legislations:
   a. Health and Safety at Work Act 1974?
   b. Workplace (Health, Safety and Welfare) Regulations 1992?
   c. Control of Substances Hazardous to Health Regulations 2002?

2 Who should give First Aid in the workplace?

3 By whom and how often should electrical equipment be tested?

4 What type of fire is a carbon dioxide extinguisher used for?

5 How should a heavy box be lifted?

6 What type of information should be contained in a spa's Health and Safety policy?

7 How would you carry out a risk assessment?

8 What does an EHO do?

9 Give three examples of personal protective equipment (PPE) that might be used by a member of staff in a spa.

10 What does the Health and Safety Executive do?

11 What does the abbreviation COSHH stand for?

12 Give five measures than can be taken to prevent a fire in a spa.

13 What information must be obtained for an accident report form?

14 Name six items found in a First Aid kit?

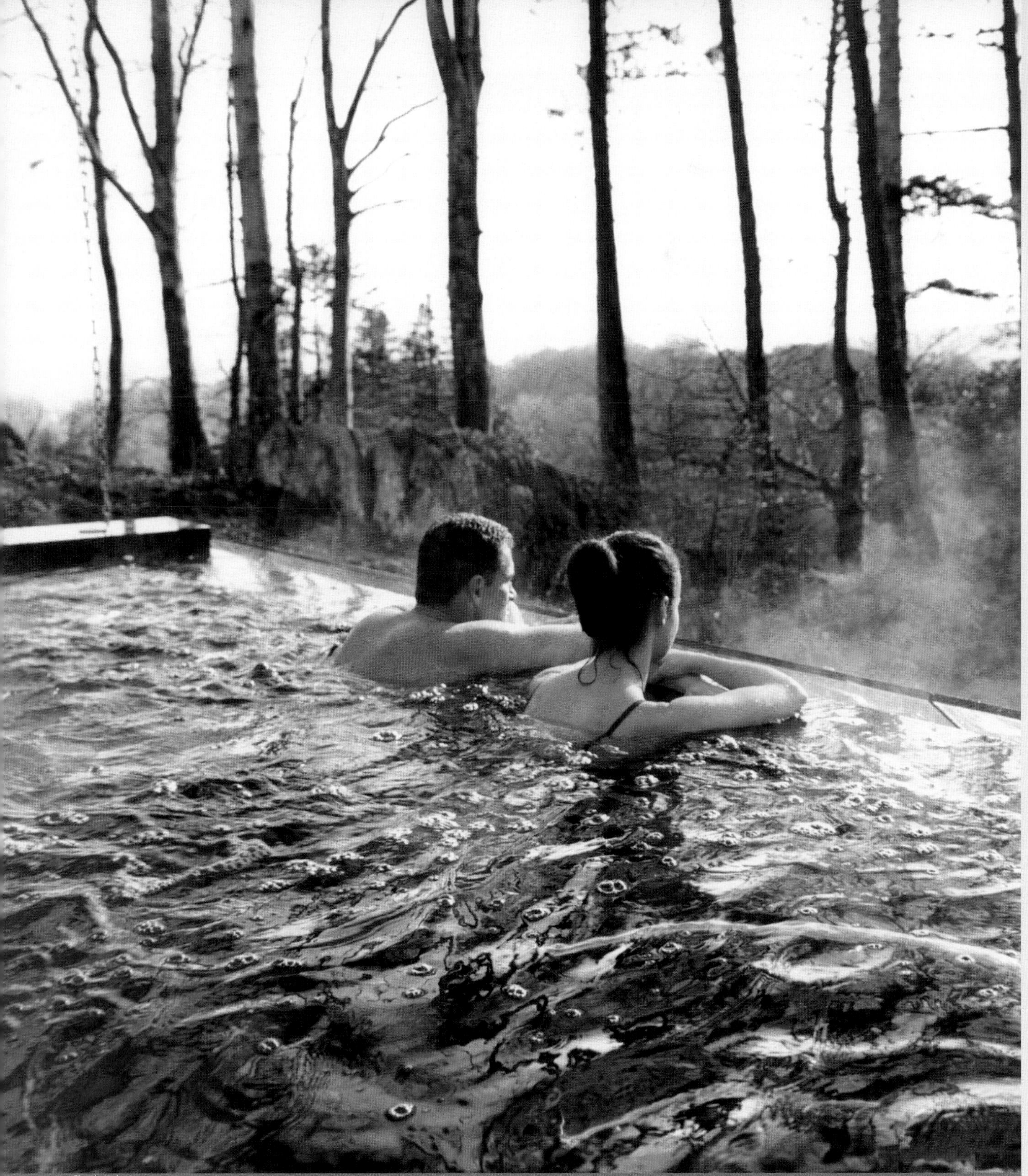

Elemis Ltd

career *in the spa industry is a* ***license to travel*** *and* ***see the world****.*
Regardless of which area a person is interested in, it offers ***wonderful opportunities*** *to those dedicated to the philosophy and ethos of true spa.*
The world is their oyster*.*

JOHN BRENNAN, GENERAL MANAGER, PARK HOTEL KENMARE AND SÁMAS DELUXE DESTINATION SPA

3 SYSTEM

I feel that there has never been such an exciting time to join the spa Industry as now. The growth, the opportunities, the challenges and the rewards in return for commitment and enthusiasm – it's never been so good!

TRISH RIDGWAY, SPA DIRECTOR, STOBO CASTLE HEALTH SPA

We are now at a time when people, through travel, are just starting to experience different cultures of 'spa'. As ideas come together and customers become more discerning, this will have a huge impact on our industry, not just in terms of business growth on an international level, but in terms of spa concepts as well. I see opportunities, in what will become an exciting, diverse industry, in imaginative new enterprises, working across borders, with a wide choice of career options.

MIKE WALLACE, SPA AND FITNESS DEVELOPMENT DIRECTOR, DANUBIUS HOTELS GROUP

chapter 6

Anatomy and physiology

Learning objectives

This chapter covers the essential knowledge a spa therapist needs to safely and effectively provide a range of spa treatments, and includes:

- **the skeletal system**
- **the muscular system**
- **the cardiovascular system**
- **the lymphatic system**
- **the digestive system**
- **the respiratory system**
- **the nervous system**
- **the urinary system**
- **the endocrine system**
- **the reproductive system**
- **cells and tissues**
- **the skin**
- **the five senses**

THE SKELETAL SYSTEM

The skeletal system is composed of bones, joints and cartilages. Its functions are to:

- support the body
- give shape to the body
- protect vital organs and tissues such as the heart, lungs, brain and spinal cord
- aid movement (bones act as levers for muscles)
- provide attachment for muscles and tendons
- store minerals, e.g. calcium
- produce blood cells in the red bone marrow.

Classification of bones

The bones of the skeleton can be classified into five types:

1 Long – these bones are strong, hollow and light, e.g. the femur bone in the thigh.

2 Short – these are strong, light and resilient, e.g. the wrist and ankle bones.
3 Irregular – these are uniquely shaped to carry out their function, e.g. the vertebrae.
4 Flat – these bones are strong and light, and protect organs and tissues, e.g. the skull.
5 Sesamoid – these are small bones that develop in certain tendons, e.g. the patella.

The skeleton

The skeleton is made up of 206 individual bones. These are divided into two parts:

1 The axial skeleton, which is central and forms the main axis of the body. It includes:
   - skull
   - vertebral column
   - sternum
   - ribs.
2 The appendicular skeleton, which supports the appendages or limbs, and attaches them to the body. It includes:
   - shoulder girdle and arms
   - pelvic girdle and legs.

TERMINOLOGY

Ossification the process of bone formation.

Osteoblast bone building cells.

Osteocyte osteoblasts that have become calcified.

Centre of ossification cluster of osteoblasts where bone tissue develops. There are three such centres in a long bone.

Anatomical terms

Superior	Above/upper
Inferior	Below/lower
Anterior/ventral	Front surface
Posterior/dorsal	Back surface
Median line	Imaginary line through the body from crown of head to feet
Medial	Towards the mid-line of the body
Lateral	Away from the mid-line of the body
Proximal	Nearest (to point of reference)
Distal	Furthest (from point of reference)
Supine	Lying face upwards
Prone	Lying face down
Plantar	Front surface/sole of foot
Dorsal	Back surface/top of foot

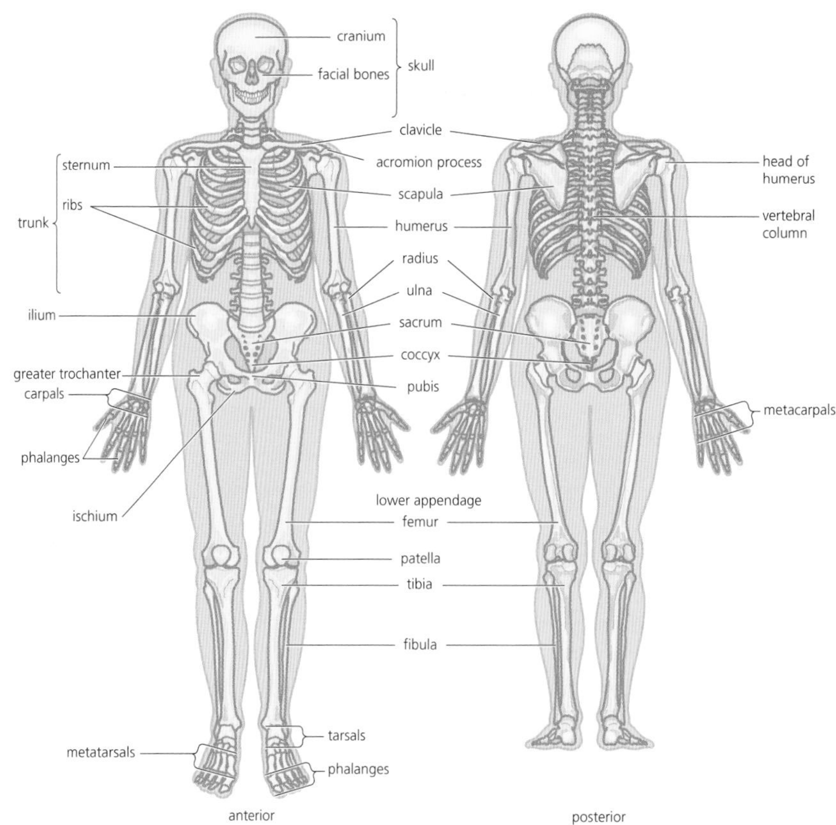

The skeleton

As a spa therapist it is important for you to be able to identify bones and bony points. This will ensure that you can massage and treat the body safely, without any causing any harm or discomfort for the client.

Bones of the head

The bones of the head are usually referred to as the skull, and can further divided into:

- bones of the cranium
- bones of the face.

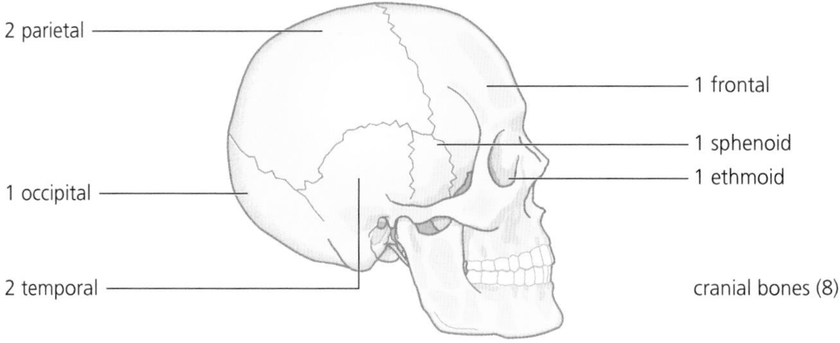

Bones of the cranium

Bones of the cranium

Name?	*How many?*	*Where?*	*What does it do?*
Frontal	1	Forehead	Forms the forehead and upper part of the eye sockets
Occipital	1	Lower back of the head	Forms lower back part of the cranium. Has a large hole called the foramen magnum; the spinal cord, nerves and blood vessels pass through it
Temporal	2	Lower sides of the head	Forms lower sides of the head, has two bony points to which muscles attach known as the mastoid process and the zygomatic process
Parietal	2	Upper sides of the head	Both are fused together to form the top of the head, i.e. the crown
Sphenoid	1	Internal base of cranium, at the back of the eye sockets	A bat-shaped bone that brings together and joins all the bones of the cranium
Ethmoid	1	Between the two eye sockets	Forms part of the nasal cavities

Bones of the trunk

The trunk is made up of the following bones:

- 1 sternum (breast bone)
- 12 ribs
- vertebral (spinal) column, which consists of 33 vertebrae:
  - 7 cervical vertebrae
  - 12 thoracic vertebrae
  - 5 lumbar vertebrae
  - 5 sacral vertebrae, fused together to form the sacrum
  - 4 coccygeal vertebrae, fused together to form the coccyx.

The individual vertebrae are separated by discs of cartilage, and held together by strong ligaments, providing strength and flexibility to the body.

ACTIVITY 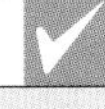

Think of a word that will remind you of the bones . . . use the word **PESTOF** to remind you of the six different bones of the cranium.

ACTIVITY 

Fill in a blank outline of the facial bones as many times as necessary until you know all the bones off by heart. Then, when you are practising your facial massage, go over the names of the bones. Get a colleague in your class or spa to ask you to name all the bones frequently; the more you practise the quicker it will embed in your long-term memory.

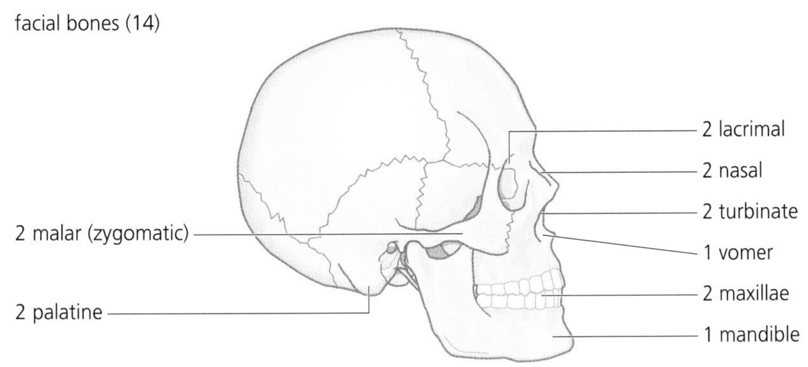

Bones of the face

Bones of the face

Name?	*How many?*	*Where?*	*What does it do?*
Mandible	1	Lower jaw	Forms the lower jaw and holds the lower teeth
Maxilla	2	Upper jaw	Fused together to form the upper jaw. Holds the upper teeth
Malar (Zygomatic)	2	Cheek	Forms the cheek bones
Lacrimal	2	Eye sockets	Forms the inner walls of the eye sockets
Nasal	2	Nose	Forms the bridge of the nose
Vomer	1	Nose	Forms the dividing bony wall of the nose
Palatine	2	Nose	Forms the floor and wall of the nose, and roof of the mouth
Turbinate	2	Nose	Forms the outer walls of the nose

SPA TIP

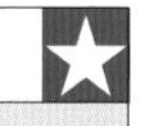

Remember which side of the forearm the ulna is on by thinking 'the little finger side goes with the little word (ulna)'. Or, the thumb **R**otates and **R** is for radius.

Bones of the shoulder girdle and arms

The shoulder girdle consist of:

- 2 clavicles (collar bones)
- 2 scapulae (shoulder blades).

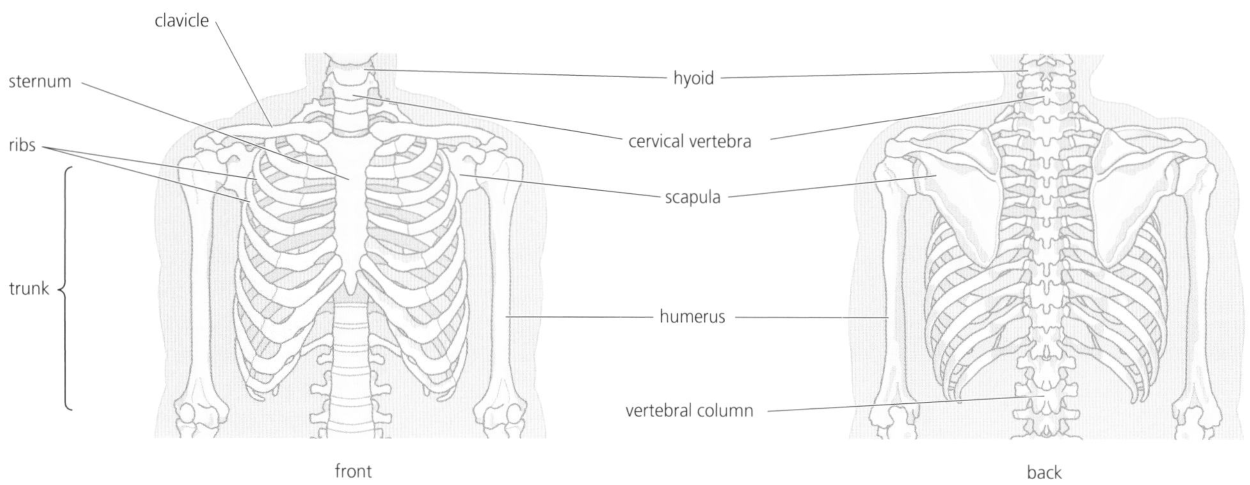

The shoulder girdle and upper arm

The bones of each arm include:

- humerus (upper arm)
- radius (forearm – thumb side)
- ulna (forearm – little finger side).

The bones of the wrist and hand consist of:

- 8 carpals (wrist)
- 5 metacarpals (hand)
- 14 phalanges (fingers).

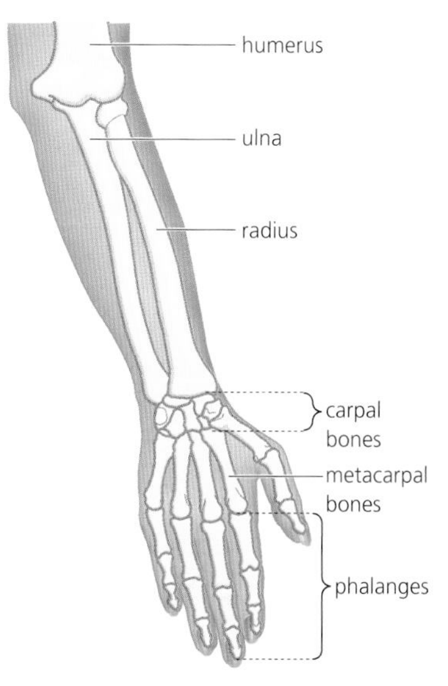

Bones of the arm

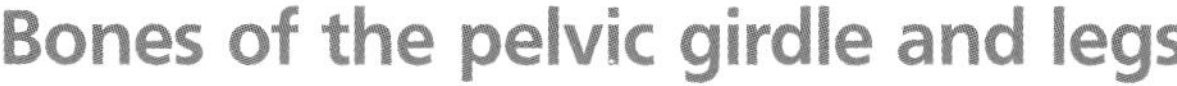

Bones of the pelvic girdle and legs

The pelvic girdle consists of 2 innominate bones, made up of 3 bones fused together:

- ilium – upper part
- ischium – posterior/back part
- pubis – anterior/front part.

The bones of each leg include:

- femur (thigh)
- patella (knee cap)

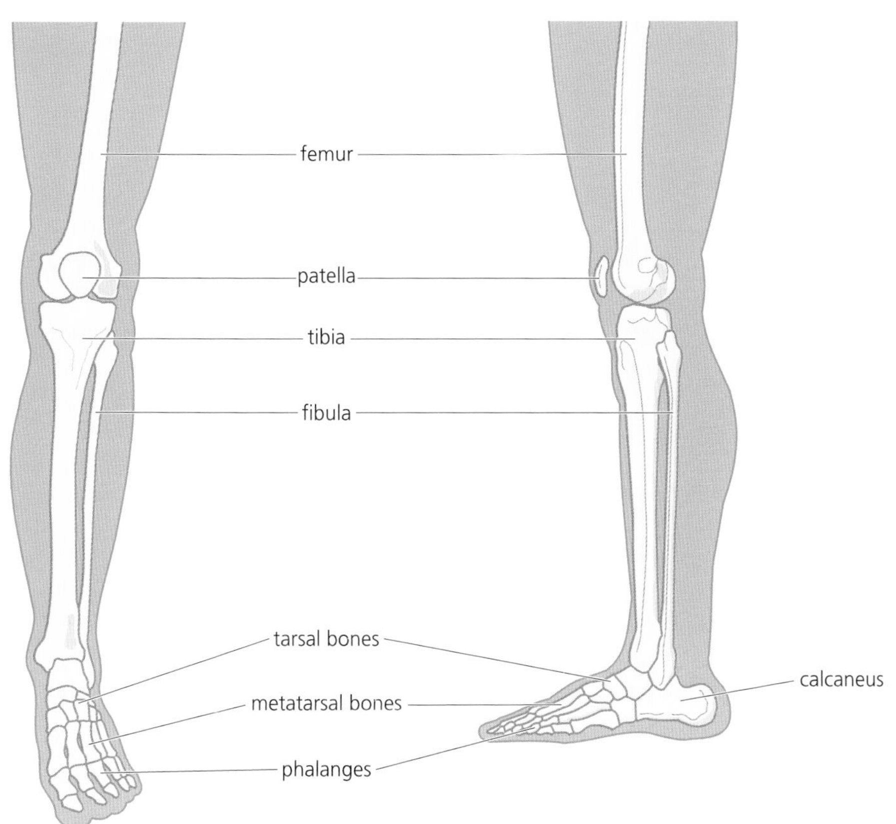

Bones of the lower leg

- tibia (foreleg – inner side)
- fibula (foreleg – outer side).

The bones of the ankle and foot consist of:

- 7 tarsals (ankle)
- 5 metatarsals (foot)
- 14 phalanges (toes).

Arches of the feet

FACT

Clients with **fallen arches** or **flat feet** find walking any distance painful, and often seek the help of a **podiatrist**.

ACTIVITY

Look at a footprint in the sand . . . you can often tell if someone has flat feet as the whole of their instep is visible, whereas it is usually sculpted out.

The bones of the feet are arranged in a series of arches. These arches are formed by the bones and joints, and are supported by strong ligaments. The arches are necessary to ensure the weight of the body is supported, and provide leverage when walking, so helping to maintain balance.

Longitudinal arches

These run along the length of the foot, and are in two parts. The medial (inner) longitudinal arch is the higher and forms what is known as the 'instep'. The lateral (outer) longitudinal arch is lower and supports the outer part of the foot.

Transverse arches

The transverse arch runs across the foot and is formed by the ankle bones and the posterior (back) part of the metatarsals.

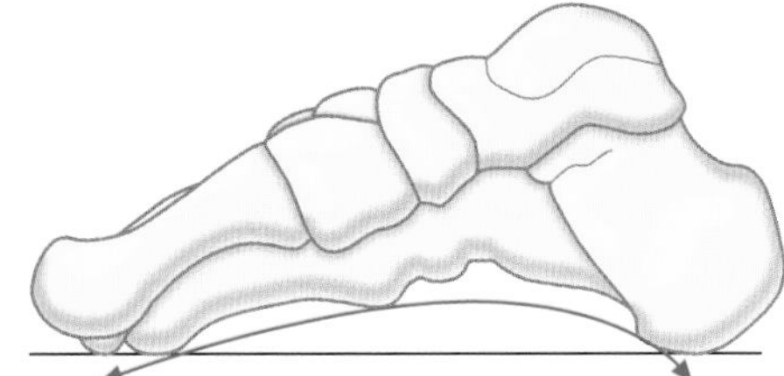
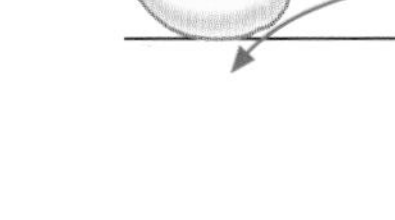
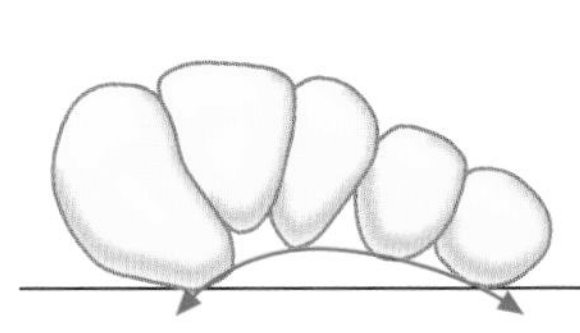

Arches of the foot

Movement terms

Flexion	Bending. Decreasing of the angle between two bones, at a joint
Extension	Straightening. Increasing of the angle between two bones, at a joint
Lateral flexion	Movement of the vertebral column when it bends sideways
Dorsi-flexion	Toes point upwards
Plantar flexion	Toes point downwards
Inversion	Sole of foot turned to face inwards

continued

Eversion	Sole of foot turned to face outwards
Abduction	Movement away from the mid-line of the body
Adduction	Movement towards the mid-line of the body
Elevation	Upward movement
Depression	Downward movement
Supination	Movement of forearm – palm turns upwards
Pronation	Movement of forearm – palm turns downwards
Rotation	Pivoting or moving of a bone on its own axis
Circumduction	Bone follows an imaginary cone-shaped path as it moves, combining flexion, extension, abduction and adduction

ACTIVITY

Copy the table of movement terms . . . blank out either the name or its explanation. Fill it in to revise . . .

Joints

Bones are static and rigid, and do not move independently. Joints are formed wherever one bone meets another. Some joints do not move at all, others have varying degrees of mobility. There are three main types of joints:

1 Fibrous – in immovable joints the bones fit very tightly together and are joined by fibrous connective tissue, e.g. the sutures of the cranium.
2 Cartilaginous – in slightly movable joints the bones are connected by discs of cartilage; usually there is no joint cavity, e.g. vertebral column.
3 Synovial – there are many freely moveable joints in the body and they are all synovial joints. They all have the following characteristics:
   - a joint cavity
   - hyaline cartilage, which covers the surfaces of the bones that articulate with each other
   - a capsule – like a sleeve that surrounds the joint. Ligaments surround the capsule to add strength and help stabilize the joint
   - synovial membrane – this lines the capsule and produces synovial fluid
   - synovial fluid – this lubricates and nourishes the joint.

There are six different types of synovial joint, and they are classified according to their structure and range of movement.

TERMINOLOGY

Tendon joins muscles to bones. If a tendon is very flat and broad it is called an aponeurosis.

Ligaments joins bone to bone. They are made of very strong fibrous tissue and are responsible for the stability of joints and the body generally.

TERMINOLOGY

Discs/menisci these are pads of fibro-cartilage which are attached to the bones and allow the joint to fit better, e.g. cartilage in the knee joint.

Bursae these are small sacs of synovial fluid that help reduce friction between a tendon and a bone. An inflammation of the sac results in bursitis.

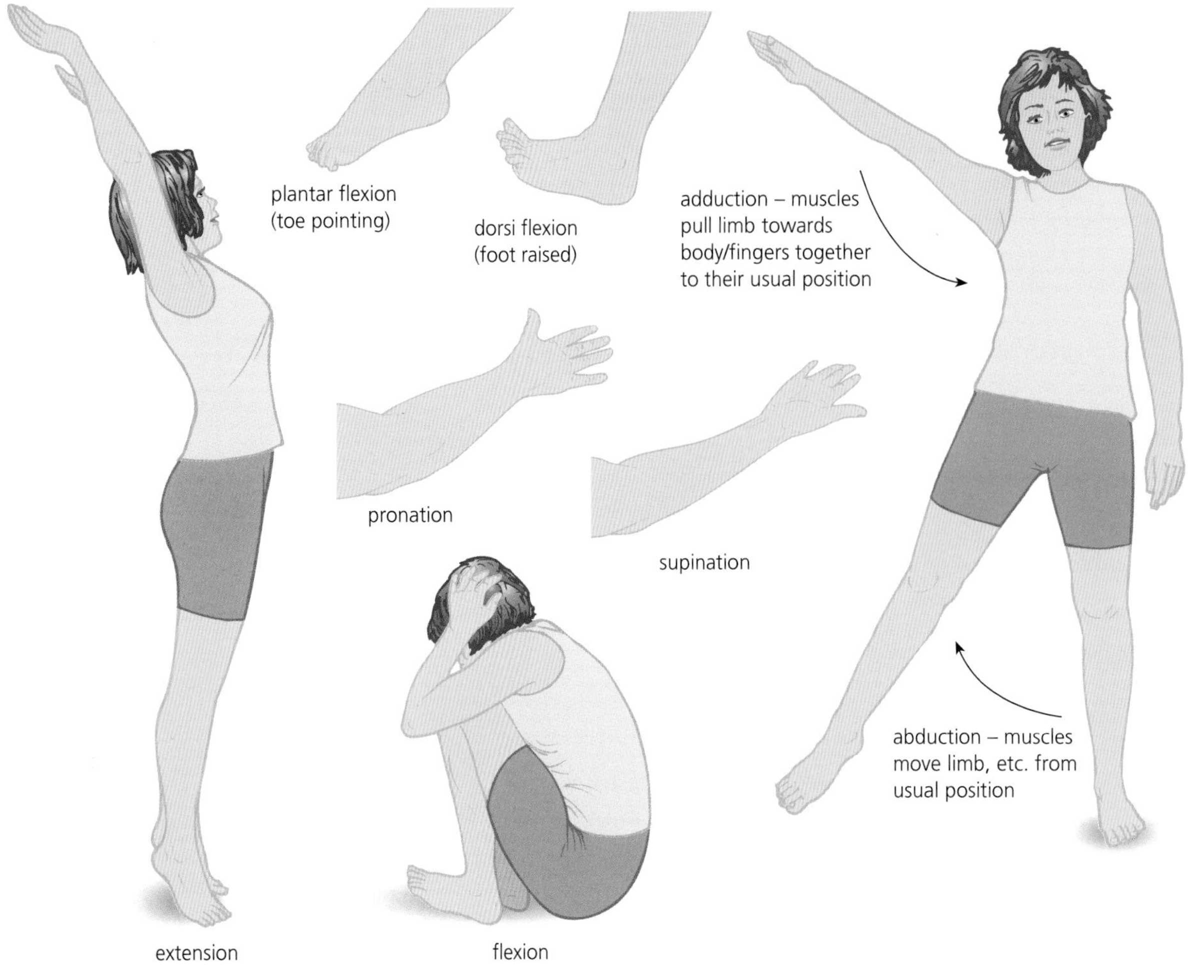

plantar flexion
(toe pointing)
dorsi flexion
(foot raised)
adduction – muscles pull limb towards body/fingers together to their usual position
pronation
supination
abduction – muscles move limb, etc. from usual position
extension
flexion

The main muscle movements

fibrous connective tissue joins bones of the cranium
cartilage pad (intervertebral disc)
fibrous connective tissue surrounds the joint

Bone connections

bone
synovial fluid
articular cartilage
sleeve-like ligament – forming joint capsule
synovial membrane

A synovial joint

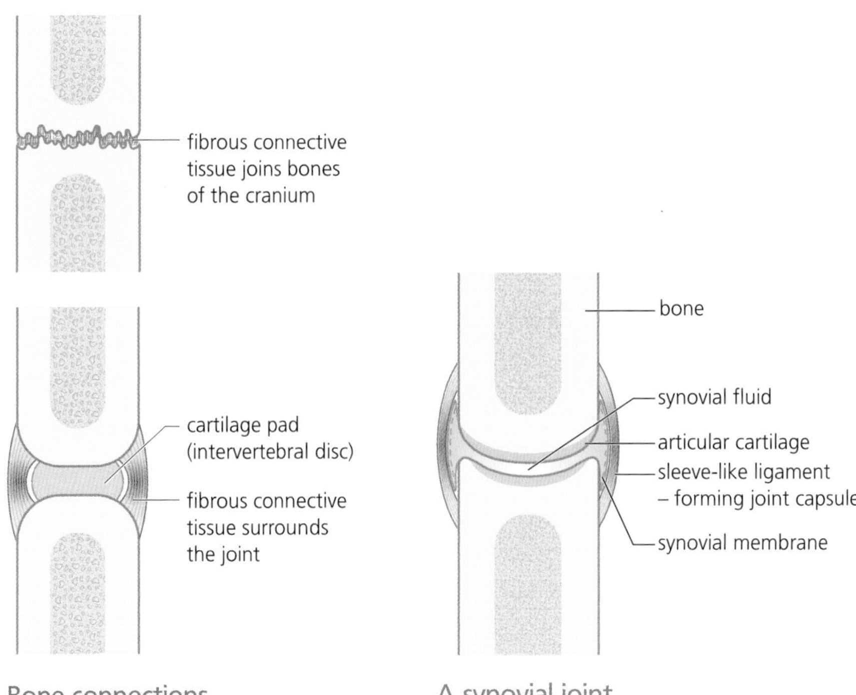

Six types of synovial joint

Type	*Range of movement*	*Example in body*
Ball and socket	Very wide. flexion/extension abduction/adduction circumduction/rotation	Shoulder joint
Plane/gliding	Short gliding movement	Intercarpal joints
Hinge	One plane only: flexion/extension	Elbow
Pivot	Rotation only	Atlas on axis (neck)
Condyloid	Two planes: flexion/extension abduction/adduction restricted circumduction	Wrist
Saddle	Two planes: flexion/extension abduction/adduction circumduction	Base of thumb

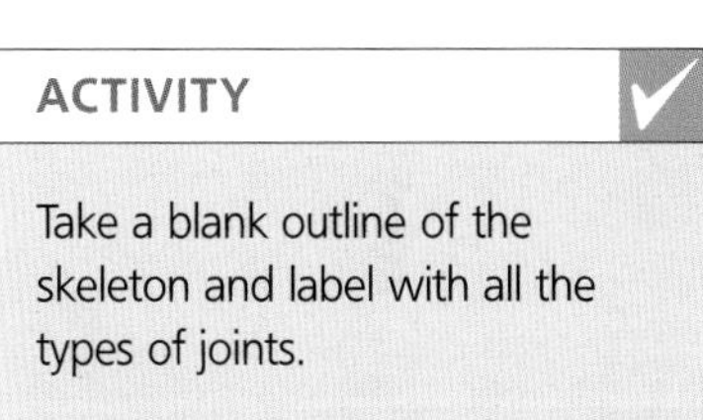

ACTIVITY

Take a blank outline of the skeleton and label with all the types of joints.

Main synovial joints of the body

Joint	*Type*	*Movement*
Hip	Ball and socket (between head of femur and pelvis)	Flexion/extension Abduction/adduction Rotation
Shoulder	Ball and socket (between head of humerus and scapula)	Flexion/extension Abduction/adduction Rotation

intracapsular ligament

socket (pelvis)

ball (head of femur)

Hip joint

shallow socket (scapula)

ball (head of humerus)

tendon of biceps muscle runs through the joint capsule

humerus

Shoulder joint

continued

Joint	*Type*	*Movement*
Knee	Hinge (between femur and tibia)	Flexion/extension
Elbow	Hinge (between humerus and ulna)	Flexion/extension
Forearm	Pivot (between radius and ulna)	Supination (palm up) Pronation (palm down)
Ankle	Hinge (between tibia/fibula and talus)	Dorsi-flexion (toes point up) Plantar flexion (toes point down)
Wrist	Condyloid (between radius/ulna and carpals)	Flexion/extension Abduction/adduction
Foot	Gliding	Inversion/eversion
Hand	Gliding	Flexion or clenching Extension or stretching
Toe	Hinge	Flexion/extension Base of toes – abduction/adduction
Finger	Hinge	Flexion/extension Base of fingers – abduction/adduction

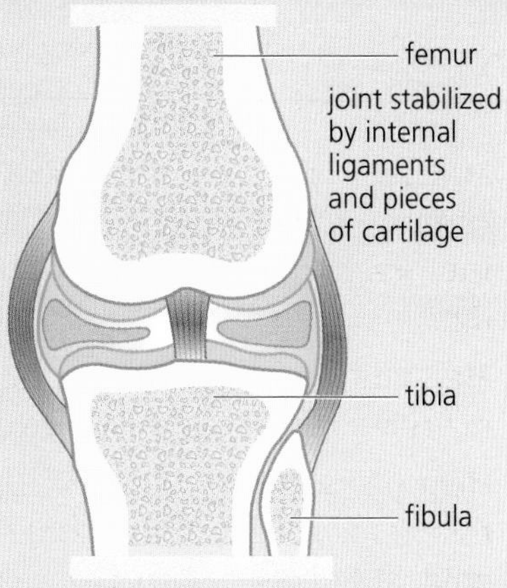

femur
joint stabilized by internal ligaments and pieces of cartilage
tibia
fibula

Knee joint

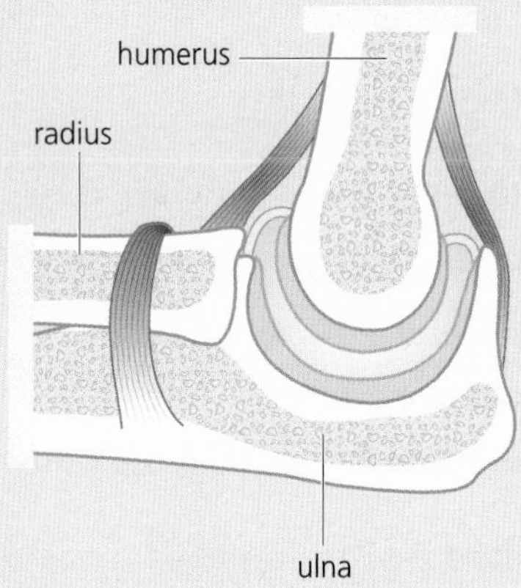

humerus
radius
ulna

Elbow joint

THE MUSCULAR SYSTEM

The skeleton is the framework of the body, but alone it cannot move. The functions of muscle tissue are as follows:

- Motion – this includes all voluntary activity and movements, from running to blinking an eyelid. It also covers involuntary actions, such as the heart beating and peristalsis (movement of food through the digestive system).
- Maintain posture – the continuous contraction of the skeletal muscles maintains the body's posture.
- Heat production – when a skeletal muscle contracts, heat is produced and this helps the body to maintain a normal body temperature. If the body is cold, shivering occurs in an effort to produce more heat. If the body is hot the muscles will relax.

Types of muscle

Within the body there are three different types of muscle:

1. skeletal muscle
2. visceral muscle
3. cardiac muscle.

Characteristics of muscles

- Extensibility – ability to stretch or extend.
- Contractability – ability to contract or shorten.
- Elasticity – ability to return to its original length after stretching.
- Excitability – ability to receive a signal (nerve stimulation) and respond.

Types of muscle

Type	*Description*	*Striated/non-striated*	*Voluntary/involuntary*
Cardiac muscle	• Only found in the heart • Fibres are short, thick and dense • Contracts rhythmically • Does not tire easily	Striated	Involuntary
Visceral	• Found in the walls of blood and lymph vessels, the stomach, the alimentary canal, the respiratory tract, etc.	Non-striated (smooth)	Involuntary
Skeletal	• Usually attached to bones • Protected by fascia, which is connective tissue • Muscles are held together in functioning groups • Allows free movement	Striated	Voluntary

Nerve and blood supply to muscles

Nerve supply	*Blood supply*
● Voluntary muscles only contract when they have a healthy nerve supply ● For a muscle to contract, it needs to be stimulated by a nerve impulse	● Muscle contraction requires energy, and this is provided by tissue respiration inside the muscle cells ● Glucose and oxygen supply the energy, and carbon dioxide and water are the waste products ● When exercising, muscles need a good blood supply to bring oxygen and glucose, and also to remove the waste products

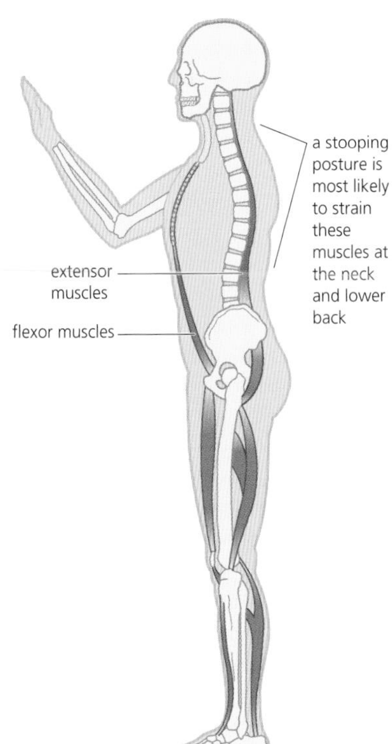
a stooping posture is most likely to strain these muscles at the neck and lower back
extensor muscles
flexor muscles

The main flexors and extensors used in posture

Muscle conditions

Muscle tone

A muscle never fully relaxes, there are always some fibres that are contracted. If there was not a certain amount of 'tautness' then postural muscles would completely relax and the body would not be held upright. This partial contraction is called **muscle tone**. Tone is essential for good posture, and helps keep the body upright and the muscles ready for action. The body can maintain an upright position only if the flexor and extensor muscles are both partially contracted; this helps stabilize the joints.

Good posture

The head is balanced on top of the spine, all vertebrae are correctly positioned, hips are level, feet square on the ground.

Poor posture

The back and neck muscles will tire quickly if the posture is poor. The internal organs can be compressed, and breathing and digestion can be affected. Poor posture needs to be corrected by education, constant effort and regular exercise.

Flaccid muscle

This is a muscle with less than normal tone. A muscle may become flaccid because of damage to the motor nerve supply. Another reason is lack of use, e.g. during an illness where the person is bedridden. If a muscle is not used, it can start to loose tone within days and become flaccid and then atrophy (waste away).

Spastic muscle

This is a muscle with a greater than normal degree of tone. Muscle 'spasm' can result from an injury or illness.

Muscle strength

This indicates how strong the muscle is. Muscles get stronger when they work against some kind of resistance, e.g. during weight training.

Muscular fatigue

If a skeletal muscle has been contracted for a long time it can become tired, and eventually does not respond at all. Fatigue means a lack of response to stimulation. It can be the result of a poor blood supply and consequent lack of oxygen. Another cause can be a build up of lactic acid and carbon dioxide, which can both accumulate in the muscle during exercise.

Muscle cramp

This is an involuntary total contraction in the muscle. It can be extremely painful as the entire muscle feels 'locked'.

Shivering

As a muscle becomes colder, the tone increases. The toned muscles start to contract spasmodically. This is an involuntary muscle action making the muscle work and therefore produce heat, helping to raise the temperature of the body.

Stiffness after muscle activity

When muscles contract, they use energy. Heat builds up and carbon dioxide, water and lactic acid are formed. After strenuous exercise lactic acid can accumulate because there is not enough oxygen available for metabolism. The muscles are affected and an aching sensation results with a 'heaviness' in the limbs. Cramp can happen if lactic acid builds up at the same time as the body is being deprived of salt and water or oxygen.

Muscle endurance

Endurance refers to the capacity of a muscle to sustain repeated contractions.

Origins and insertions of muscles

A muscle usually has a tendon at each end. The tendons join the muscle to the bones. When the muscle contracts, the fibres shorten and the ends of the muscles are pulled towards the middle. The bones that are attached to the tendons are pulled, and the result is movement at the joint. The muscle is usually attached to two bones, one attachment is referred to as the 'origin' and the other the 'insertion'. Very often the 'origin' remains fixed during the contraction to allow the movement at the 'insertion' end of the muscle.

Facial muscles

These muscles are responsible for facial expression. Many of the muscles are very small, and instead of being attached to bone their 'insertion' is often another muscle or the skin of the face.

SIGNATURE TREATMENT S

Banyan Tree Spa, Bangkok

'Rejuvenation: Two ways to experience total rejuvenation – the choice is yours. Combine a 30-minute body scrub and a 60-minute massage by choosing your preferred treatments from our menu. Alternatively, you may wish to forgo the body scrub in favour of a full 90-minute massage. Whichever you choose, our unique techniques combined with the privacy and natural environment of our spa pavilions are sure to make this luxurious treatment a wholly satisfying experience. 2 hours'

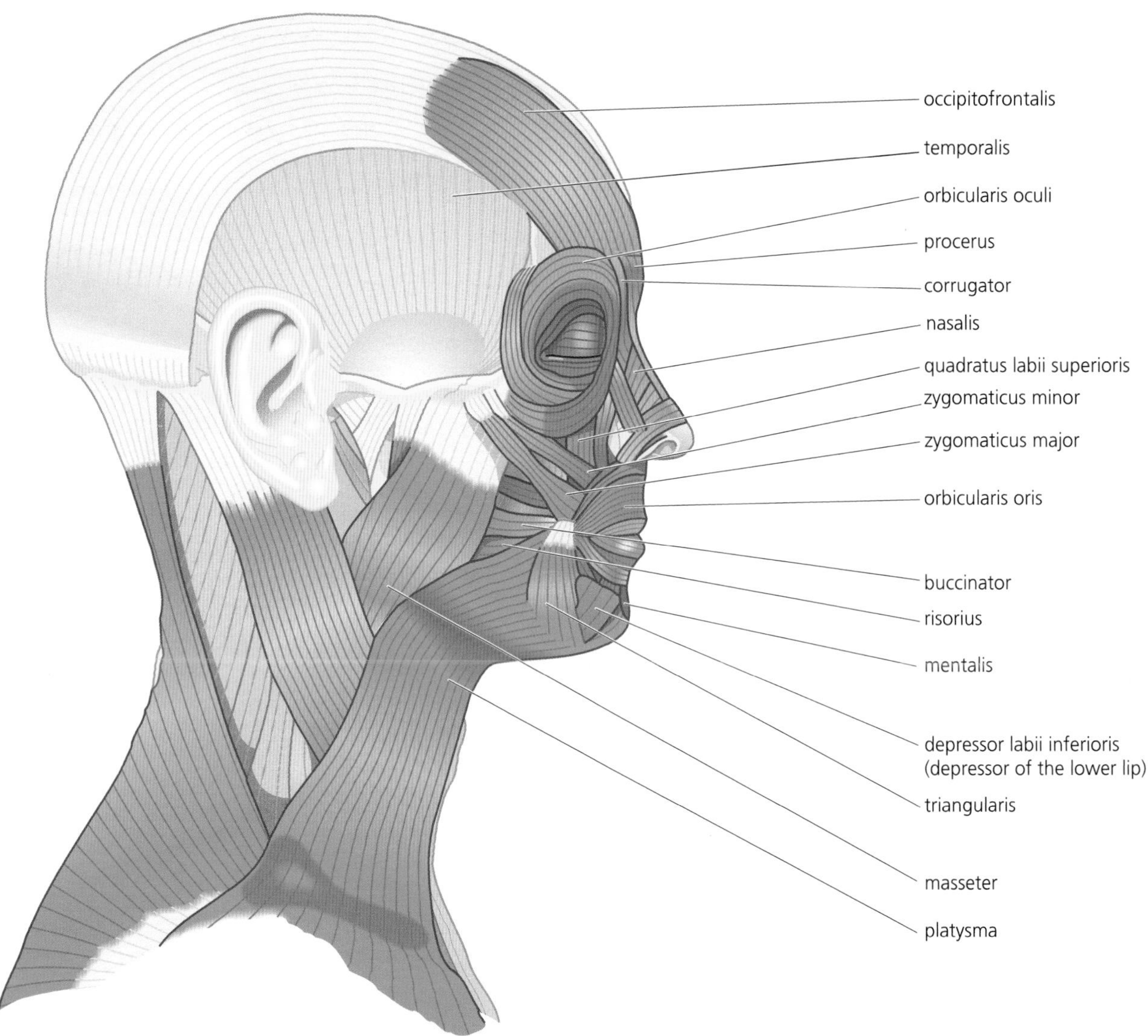

Muscles of the face

Muscles of facial expression

Name	*Where*	*Expression*	*Action*
Occipito-frontalis	Forehead	Surprise	Raises the eyebrows
Corrugator	Between the eyebrows	Frown	Pulls eyebrows together
Orbicularis oculi	Around the eye	Winking	Closes the eyelid, screws the eye up
Risorius	Extends diagonally from the corners of the mouth	Smiling	Draws the corner of the mouth outwards
Buccinator	Inside the cheek	Blowing	Compresses the cheek
Zygomaticus (major and minor)	Extends diagonally from the corners of the mouth	Smiling, laughing	Lifts the corner of the mouth upwards and outwards

continued

Procerus	Covers the bridge of the nose	Distaste	Wrinkles the skin over the bridge of the nose
Nasalis	Covers the front of the nose	Anger	Opens and closes the nasal openings
Quadratus labii superioris	Surrounds the upper lip	Distaste	Raises and draws back the upper lips and nostrils
Depressor labii	Surrounds the lower lip	Sulking	Depresses the lower lip and draws it slightly to one side
Orbicularis oris	Surrounds the mouth	Kiss, pout, pucker, doubt	Purses the lips, closes the mouth
Triangularis	Corner of lower lip, extends over chin	Sadness	Draws down the corner of the mouth
Mentalis	Chin	Doubt	Raises the lower lip, causing the chin to wrinkle
Masseter	Cheeks	Anger/aggression	Raises the jaw and clenches the teeth
Platysma	Sides of neck and chin	Fear, horror	Draws the corner of the mouth downwards and backwards

Muscles of mastication (chewing)

Name	*Where*	*Action*
Masseter	Cheek area, extends from the zygomatic bone to the mandible	Clenches the teeth, closes and raises the lower jaw
Temporalis	Extends from the temple region at the side of the head to the mandible	Raises the jaw and draws it backwards in a chewing motion

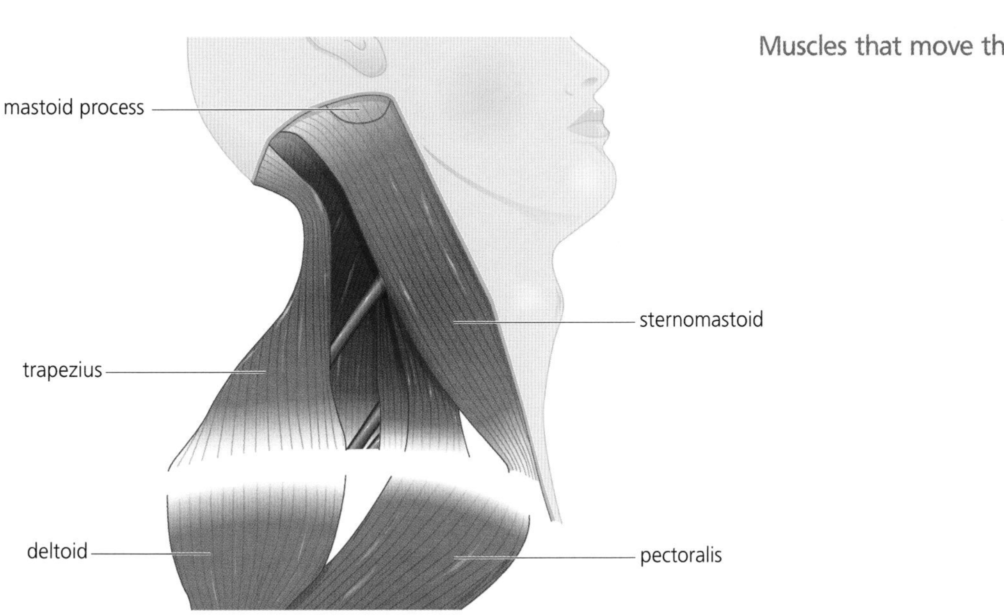

Muscles that move the head

Muscles that move the head

Muscle	*Position*	*Action*
Occipitalis	Covers the back of the head	Draws the scalp backwards
Trapezius	Triangular muscle covering the back of the neck and the upper back	Draws the head backwards, elevates and braces the shoulder, rotates scapula and allows movement at the shoulders
Sterno-cleido-mastoid	Side of the neck, from behind the ear to the sternum and clavicle	Both sides together flexes the neck, rotates and bends the head sideways

Abdominal muscles

Name	*Position*	*Action*
Rectus abdominus	Front of abdomen, runs from the pelvis to the sternum and costal cartilages of the lower ribs	Flexes the spine, compresses the abdomen, tilts the pelvis
Obliques	Internal obliques lie on either side of the rectus abdominus and the external obliques lie on top. Their fibres run in opposite directions so they form a strong network of muscle	Together they compress the abdomen and twist the trunk. One side working independently will bend the body to one side

The abdominal muscles

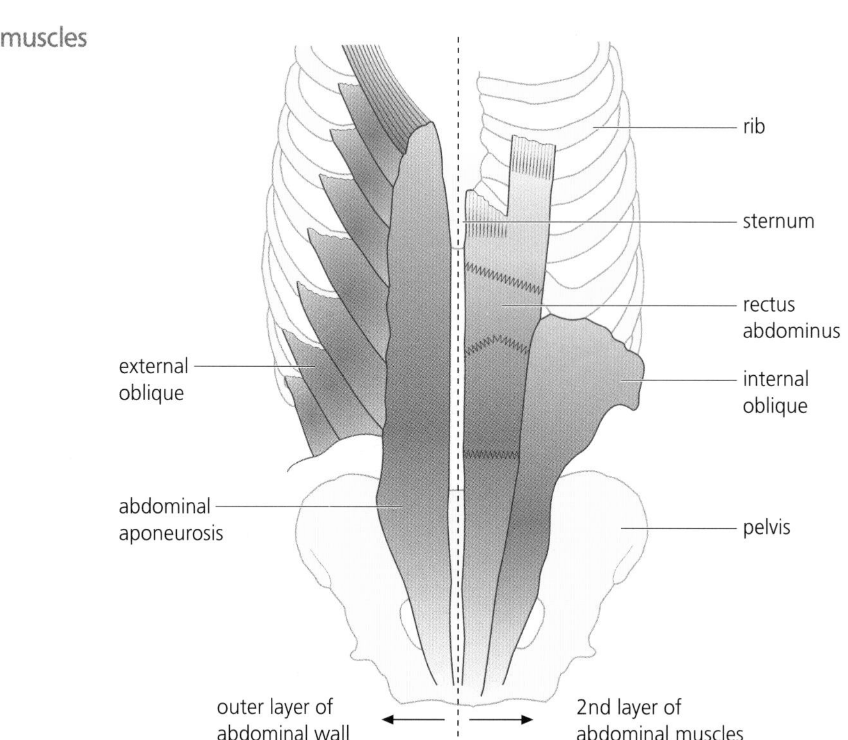

Muscles of the chest and upper arm

Name	*Position*	*Action*
Pectoralis major	Across the upper chest, from the clavicle, sternum and ribs to the top of the humerus. Forms the front wall of the axilla	Adducts the arm, draws it forwards and rotates it medially. Used in throwing and climbing
Pectoralis minor	Underneath the pectoralis major. Originates from the 3rd, 4th and 5th ribs, and it inserts into the outer corners of the scapula	Draws the shoulders downwards and forwards
Deltoid	Covers the top of the shoulder, from the clavicle and scapula to the upper part of the humerus	Abducts the arm to a horizontal position. Aids in further abduction and in drawing the arm backwards and forwards
Biceps	Covers the front of the upper arm. Its two origins are on the scapula and its insertion is on the radius	Flexes the elbow, supinates the forearm and hand.
Triceps	Only muscle at the back of the upper arm. Three origins, one on the scapula and two on the humerus. It inserts into the ulna	Extends the elbow
Brachialis	Under the biceps at the front of the humerus, from halfway down its shaft to the ulnar near the elbow joint	Flexes the elbow

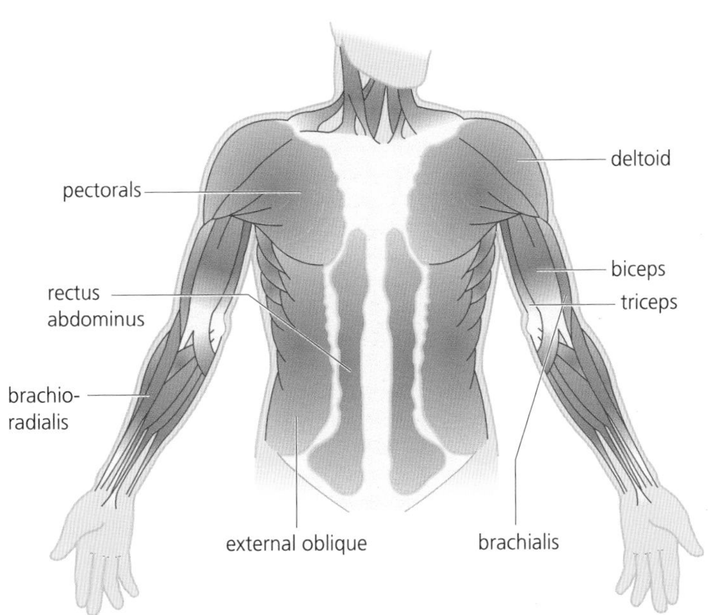

The muscles of the chest, arm and trunk

Muscles of the hand and arm

Muscle	*Position*	*Action*
Brachio-radialis	Thumb side of forearm. Its origin is on the shaft of the humerus. Its insertion is at the end of the radius bone	Flexes the elbow
Flexors	Middle of the forearm	Group of muscles that flex and bend the wrist, drawing it towards the forearm
Extensors	Little finger side of the forearm	Group of muscles which extend and straighten the wrist and hand
Thenar muscles	In the palm of the hand, below the thumb	Flexes the thumb and moves it outwards and inwards
Hypothenar muscles	In the palm of the hand, below the little finger	Flexes the little finger and moves it outwards and inwards

Muscles of the hand and arm

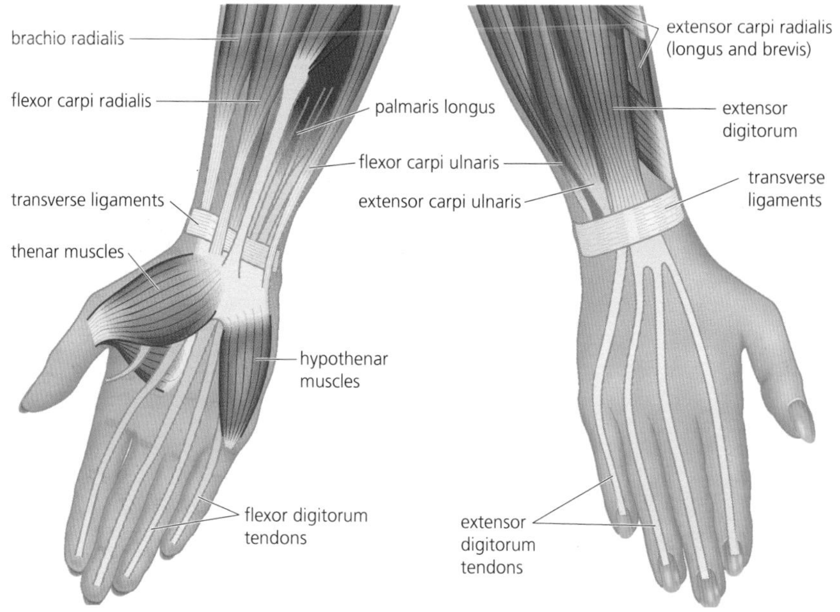

Muscles of the back

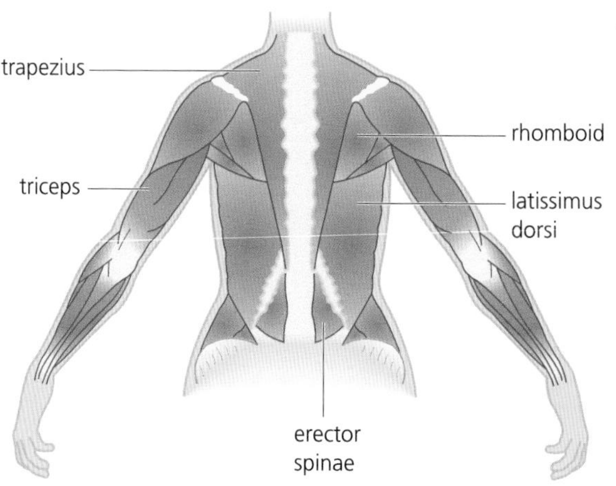

Muscles of the back (shoulder and trunk)

Muscle	*Position*	*Action*
Trapezius	Back of the neck and shoulders, its origin runs from the base of the skull down the spines of the thoracic vertebrae. It inserts into the scapula and clavicle	Moves the scapula up, down and back. Raises the clavicle, can also be used to extend the neck
Latissimus dorsi	Crosses the back, from the lumbar region, up to insert into the top of the humerus. It forms the back of the axilla	Adducts the shoulder downwards and pulls it backwards. Used in rowing and climbing
Erector-spinae	Three groups of overlapping muscles which lie either side of the spine from the neck to the pelvis	Extends spine, keeps the body in an upright position
Rhomboids	Between the shoulders, originating from the thoracic vertebrae and inserting on the scapula bone	Braces the shoulders, and rotates the scapula, moving the shoulder

Muscles used in breathing

Muscle	*Position*	*Action*
External intercostals	Connects the lower border of one of the ribs to the one below, the muscle fibres run down and forwards	Used in breathing movements to draw the ribs upwards and outwards when breathing in (inspiration)
Internal intercostals	Between the ribs, the fibres run upwards and forwards to the rib above	Draw the rib downwards and inwards when breathing out (expiration)
Diaphragm	Divides the thorax from the abdomen	Contraction of this muscle increases the volume of the thorax

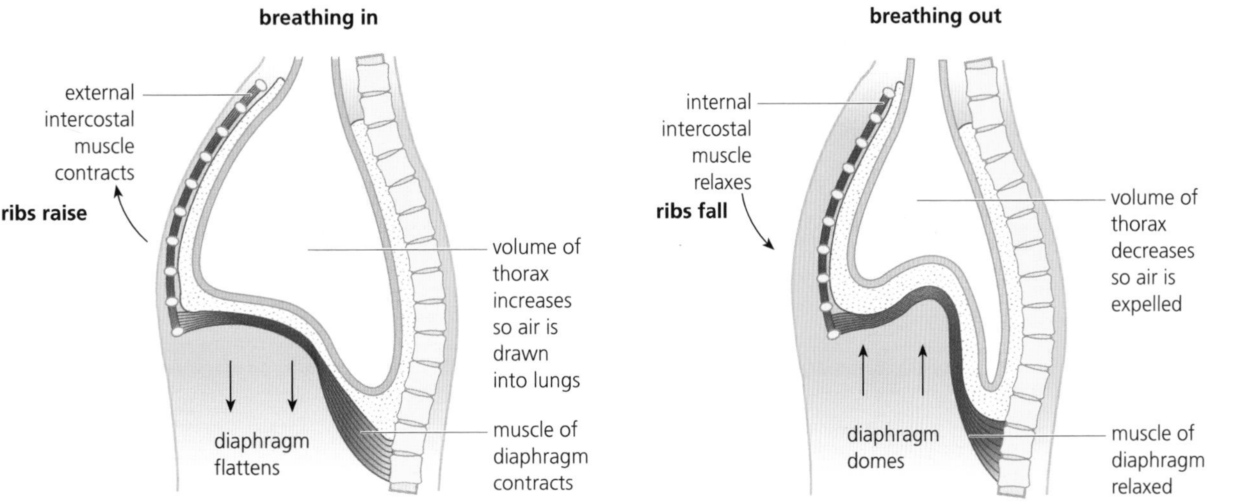

Inspiration and expiration

Muscles of the legs and buttocks

Muscle	*Position*	*Action*
Gluteals	Form the buttock, connecting the pelvis and femur. A group of three muscles: 1 gluteus maximus 2 gluteus medius 3 gluteus minimus	Extends the hip. Abducts and rotates the femur, used in walking and running. Also used to raise the body to an upright position
Hamstrings	Back of the thigh. A group of three muscles: 1 biceps femoris 2 semitendinosus 3 semimembranosus. They run from the pelvis and top of the femur to the bones on the lower leg below the knee	Flex the knee, extend the thigh. Used in walking and jumping
Gastrocnemius	Calf of the leg	Flexes the knee, plantar-flexes the foot
Soleus	Calf of the leg, below the gastrocnemius, inserts through the achilles tendon on to the heel bone	Plantar-flexes the foot. With gastrocnemius is used to push-off when walking and running
Quadriceps femoris	Front of the thigh. A group of four muscles: 1 rectus femoris 2 vastus medialis 3 vastus intermedialis 4 vastus lateralis. They run from the pelvis and top of the femur to the tibia through the patella and patellar ligament	Extend the knee, used in kicking. The rectus femoris helps to flex the hip
Sartorius	Crosses the front of the thigh from the outer front rim of the pelvis to the tibia at the inner knee	Flexes the knee and hip, abducts and rotates the femur. Used to sit cross-legged
Adductors	Inner thigh	Adducts the hip, flexs and rotates the femur
Tibialis anterior	Front of lower leg	Inverts the foot, dorsi-flexes the foot, rotates foot outwards

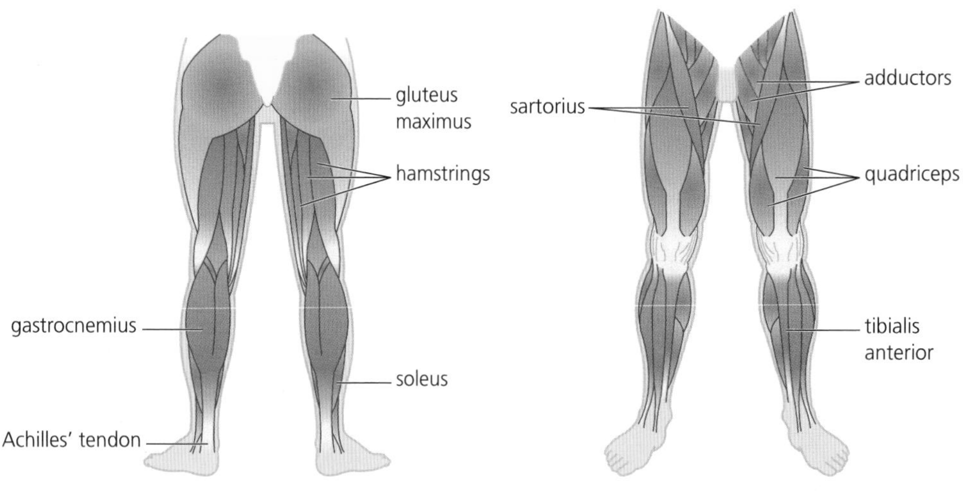

Anterior and posterior leg muscles

Muscles of the foot

All the muscles in the foot work together to move the body when walking and running. The foot is similar to the hand in that a lot of the muscles are situated in the lower leg, and their tendons run into the foot; when these are pulled they move the foot and toes.

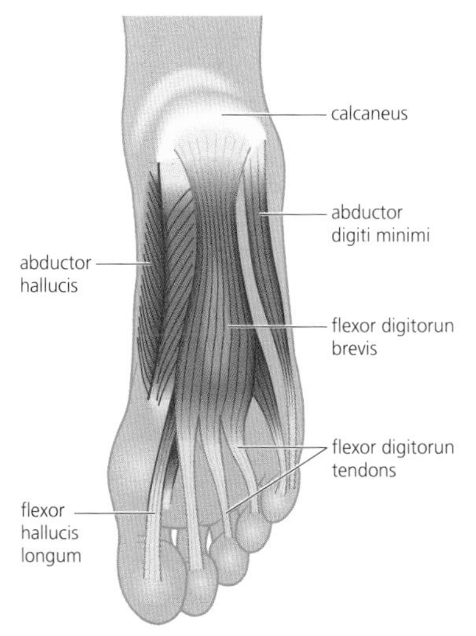

Muscles of the foot

THE CARDIOVASCULAR (CIRCULATORY) SYSTEM

Heart

The heart is a large muscular organ that pumps blood through the vessels. Its position in the body is between the lungs in the thoracic cavity.

Structure of the heart

- The pericardial sac is a loose-fitting membrane surrounding the heart.
- The wall of the heart is in three parts:
  - epicardium – the thin and transparent external layer
  - myocardium – middle layer of specialized cardiac muscle
  - endocardium – inner layer that covers the valves and associated tendons.

Blood circulation through the heart

The flow of blood around the body is a continuous circuit:

- Blood circulates from the heart, through vessels called arteries to the organs and tissues bringing oxygen and nutrients.
- Blood returns to the heart in veins. All the oxygen has been absorbed by the tissues and cells.
- The heart pumps the blood around the lungs to replace the oxygen, then it is ready to start the cycle again by pumping the oxygenated blood around the body in the arteries.

> **FACT**
>
> The heart can beat over 100 000 times a day.

> **FACT**
>
> The heart is divided into 4 chambers or cavities:
>
> - right and left **atria** – the upper 2 chambers
> - right and left **ventricles** – the lower 2 chambers.
>
> The left and right sides of the heart are kept apart by a wall called the septum. This prevents the blood from the right side of the heart contacting the arterial blood on the left side.

Stages of a heartbeat

Diastole During this phase the heart fills with blood from the veins.

Systole Strong contractions of the atria and then the ventricles force blood out of the heart through the arteries. The pulmonary artery carries blood from the right ventricle to the lungs to become re-oxygenated. The aorta carries oxygenated blood from the left ventricle around the rest of the body.

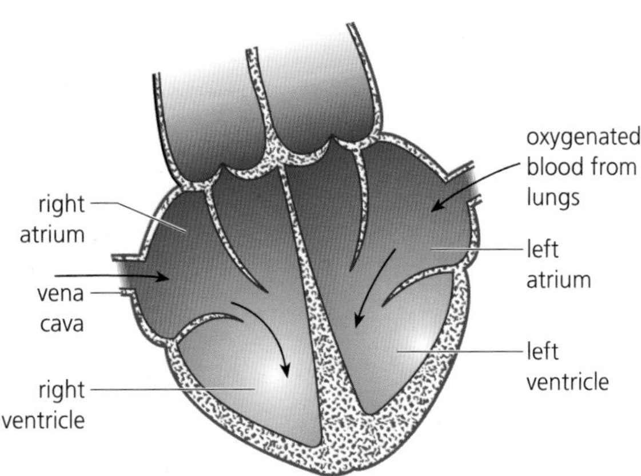

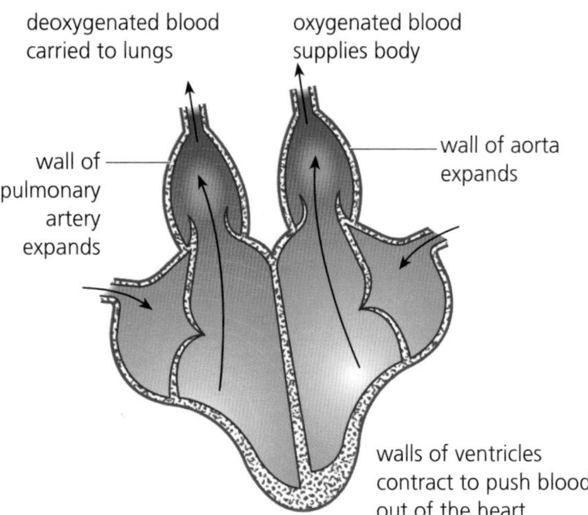

Diastole and systole

Blood

There are four main functions of blood:

1 Transport
   – oxygen is transported from the lungs to the cells of the body in the red blood cells
   – carbon dioxide is carried from the cells of the body to the lungs
   – nutrients are carried from the digestive tract to the cells of the body
   – cellular waste, such as water, lactic acid, and urea, are carried in the blood to be excreted
   – hormones are carried from the endocrine glands by the blood to target organs.
2 Defence
   – white blood cells – called leucocytes – protect the body by combating disease and fighting infection.
3 Clotting
   – special blood cells – called platelets – clot the blood when the skin is damaged. This prevents both excessive loss of blood and bacteria entering.
4 Regulation
   – blood absorbs heat from the liver and muscles and transports it around the body to maintain a constant internal temperature
   – blood helps to regulate the body's pH balance.

> **FACT**
>
> Blood consists of approximately: 55% plasma; 45% corpuscles.

> **FACT**
>
> **Blood shunting** is where blood can suddenly be diverted to wherever the body needs it most. It happens because certain arteries have direct connection with veins. When the connections open they act as 'shunts' which allow blood in the artery to have direct access to a vein. Spa treatments should not be given after a heavy meal because blood will have shunted to the intestines to aid digestion, resulting in a decreased supply to other areas of the body.

Blood vessels

Blood vessels are the channels or tubes through which blood travels. There are three types:

1 arteries
2 veins
3 capillaries.

Blood vessels

Vessel	*Direction of blood flow*	*Valves*	*Blood pressure*	*Walls*	*Function*
Artery	Carry blood away from the heart	None	High pressure	Very thick, strong, muscular and elastic	● To carry oxgenated blood from the heart to the organs, tissues and cells ● Deep location, apart from over pulse spots ● Become small vessels called arterioles which connect with capillaries
Vein	Towards the heart	Many valves at intervals to prevent backflow of blood	Low pressure	Less thick and muscular	● To carry de-oxygenated blood from the organs, tissues and cells back to the heart ● Superficial location ● Become small vessels called venules which connect with capillaries
Capillary	Between the arterioles and venules	None	Low (but higher than a vein)	Thin, single cell layer (allows diffusion of dissolved substances to and from the tissues)	● Supply the tissues and cells with nutrients ● Smallest vessels, some the size of a hair ● Unite arterioles and venules to form a fine network in the tissues

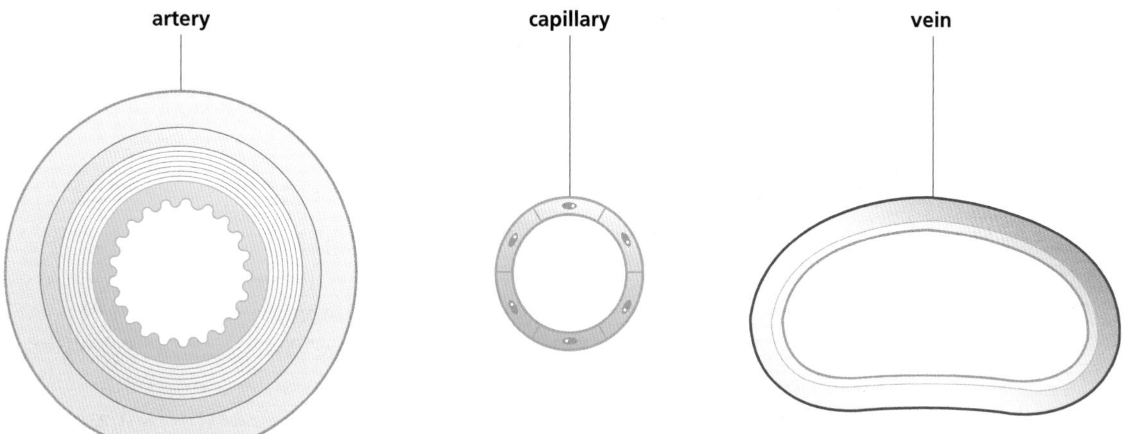

Cross-sections of blood vessels

Nervous control of blood supply

The autonomic nervous system controls most of the arteries in the body. Two sets of nerves are involved:

1 Vasoconstrictor nerves – these reduce the supply of blood to an area by narrowing the vessels. If this happens on a large scale the blood pressure will be raised.

2 Vasodilator nerves – these increase the blood supply to an area by dilating the blood vessels. During strenuous activity these nerves will allow the vessels to dilate and allow extra blood to reach the muscles.

Blood circulation around the body

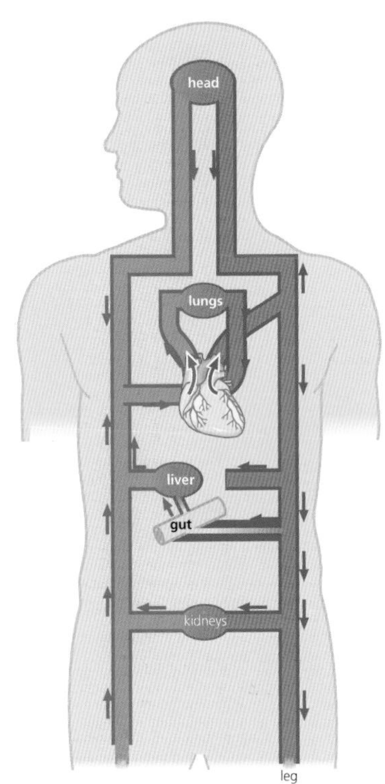

The circulatory system

Flow of blood in arteries

Blood flow in the arteries is maintained by blood pressure caused by the pumping of the heart. Blood pressure (BP) is measured in the arteries. Normal BP has a value of approximately 115 mm mercury over 70 mm mercury.

- The first value (115 mm) is the pressure reached when the heart is contracting and pushing blood around the body.
- The second value (70 mm) – is the pressure when the heart is relaxed and filling up with blood.

BP is always higher when standing than when sitting or lying down, and increases with exercise or stress and anxiety. **High blood pressure** would be in the region of 160 over 100 (referred to as **hypertension**), and long-term this can damage the heart, brain and kidneys so needs medical treatment. **Low blood pressure** would be 100 over 60, which can cause frequent fainting to occur.

Blood flow through the organs

Within each major organ there is a network of capillaries. Arterioles are the small thin arteries that feed these capillaries with fresh oxygenated blood. The arterioles can control the blood flow through an organ by constricting to reduce the flow of blood, or dilating to increase it. With exercise the blood flow is improved, enabling it to supply the muscles with extra oxygen and glucose, and to carry away waste products, such as carbon dioxide and lactic acid.

HEALTH AND SAFETY !

Heat treatments can cause dizziness and fainting as the blood is diverted to the skin to help reduce the rising body temperature. Therefore the blood pressure falls resulting in a reduced blood flow to the head and brain. Similarly this can happen when a client stands up too quickly after lying down for a treatment.

Blood flow through the skin

The body's normal temperature is 37 °C, and blood helps maintain this. When blood circulates through the internal organs and muscles it becomes warm. If the body temperature starts to rise, then blood flows near the surface of the skin to release some of the heat to the environment. The skin will appear red and feel warm (or hot) but the rise in body temperature will be stopped.

Blood vessels in the skin are organized in such a way that they can either direct blood close to the surface of the skin or pass it via shunt vessels deeper in the dermis. This helps to regulate the body temperature:

- Body temperature drops – blood flows deeper through the dermis, preventing heat being lost to the environment.
- Body temperature rises – blood flows closer to the surface of the skin to allow heat to be lost.

This process of vasodilation and vasoconstriction is controlled by the autonomic nervous system.

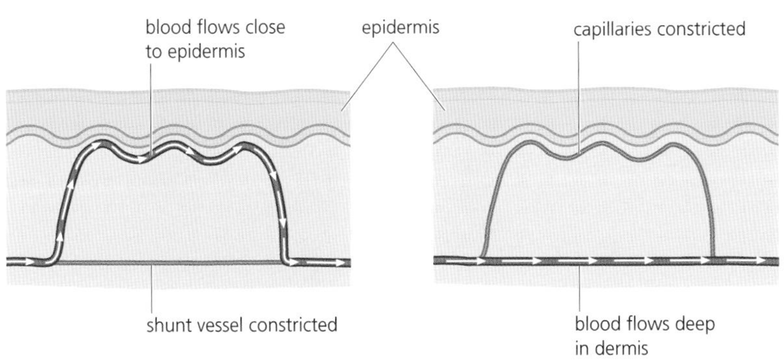

Vasoconstriction and vasodilation

TERMINOLOGY

Erythaema a reddening of the skin, caused by dilation of the blood vessels. It can result from physically increasing the blood flow, for example through massage, or because the body is hot or affected by injury or infection.

Flow of blood in veins

Blood flows slower and under less pressure in the veins. Muscle contractions help squeeze the blood along the veins, especially in areas such as the legs where the blood is travelling against gravity. Varicose veins result from problems with valves in the veins, whereby blood is allowed to flow backwards, which weakens and stretches the vein walls. The superficial leg veins are the ones most commonly involved, as they do not have as much help from muscle contractions as the deeper veins.

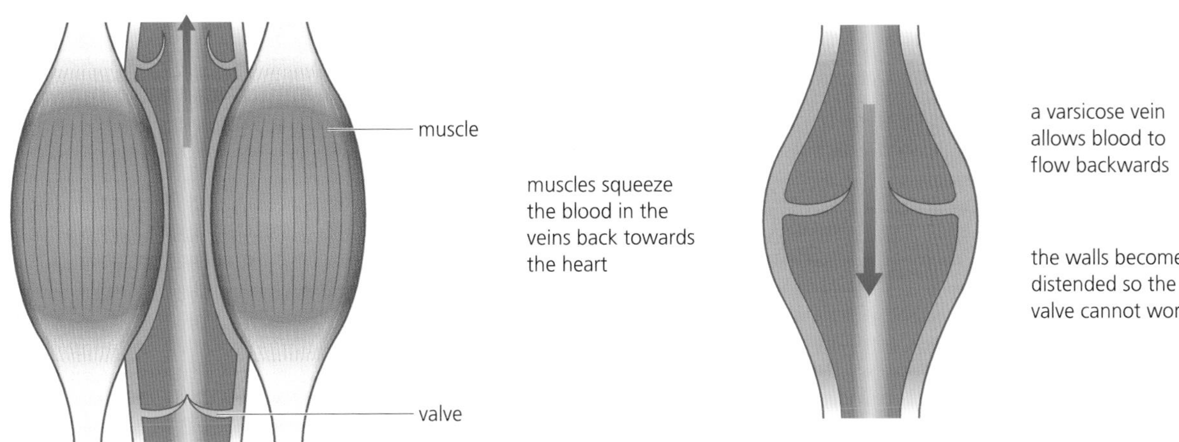

Control of blood flow by valves

Blood circulation of the head

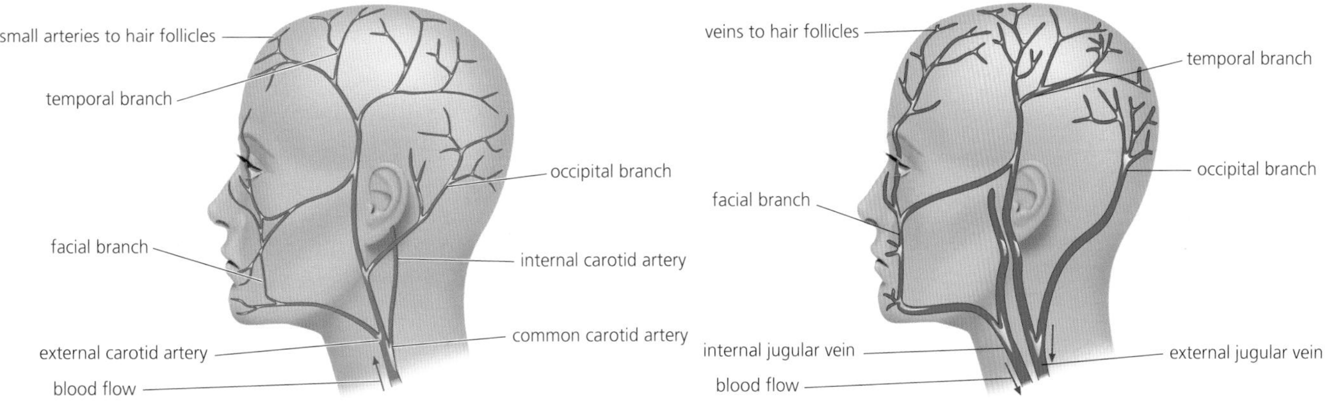

Blood supply to and from the head

Blood flow to the head

Blood circulation is under the control of the **heart**

Blood leaves the heart in large elastic tubes called **arteries**

Blood to the head arrives via the **carotid arteries**. There are two main carotid arteries, one on each side of the neck

These arteries divide into smaller arteries: the **internal cartotid artery** and the **external carotid artery**

Internal carotid artery passes the temporal bone and enters the head, taking blood to the brain

External carotid artery stays on the outside of the skull, and divides into three branches:

1 **occipital branch** – supplies scalp and back of head
2 **temporal branch** – supplies scalp, head, sides of face and skin
3 **facial branch** – supplies muscles and tissues of the face

The arteries and arterioles constantly divide until they become very tiny **blood capillaries**. Because their walls are only one cell thick they allow substances from the blood to pass through them into the **tissue fluid** which bathes and nourishes the tissues and cells of the body

Blood capillaries start to join up again, forming **venules** then larger vessels called **veins**. Veins carry blood to the heart

The main veins are the external and internal jugular veins. The **internal jugular vein**, and its main branch the **facial vein**, carry blood from the face and head. The **external jugular vein** carries blood from the scalp and has two branches: the **occipital branch** and the **temporal branch**

The jugular veins join to enter the **subclavian vein**, which lies above the clavicle

Blood returns to the heart, it is then pumped to the **lungs**, where the red blood cells **absorb fresh oxygen**, and **carbon dioxide is expelled** from the body

Blood returns again to the heart, and **starts the next journey** around the body: the circle of life.

Arteries of the arm and hand

A system of arteries supply the arm and hand. A network of veins can be seen on the inside of the wrist, with the arteries located much deeper. It is the blood that gives the nail bed its healthy pink colour, as the blood capillaries are seen beneath the nail.

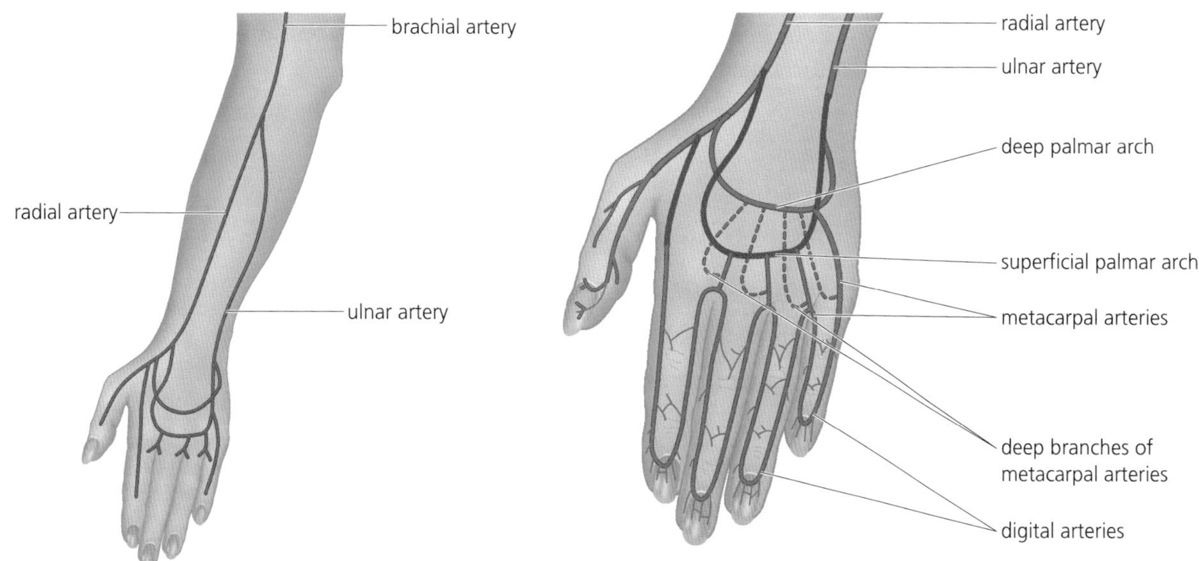

Arteries of the arm and hand

Arteries of the foot and lower leg

A system of arteries nourish the skin and nails of the feet by bringing blood to the tissue. Cold temperatures and poor circulation mean insufficient blood reaches the feet and they feel cold, while extreme circulation problems may cause chilblains.

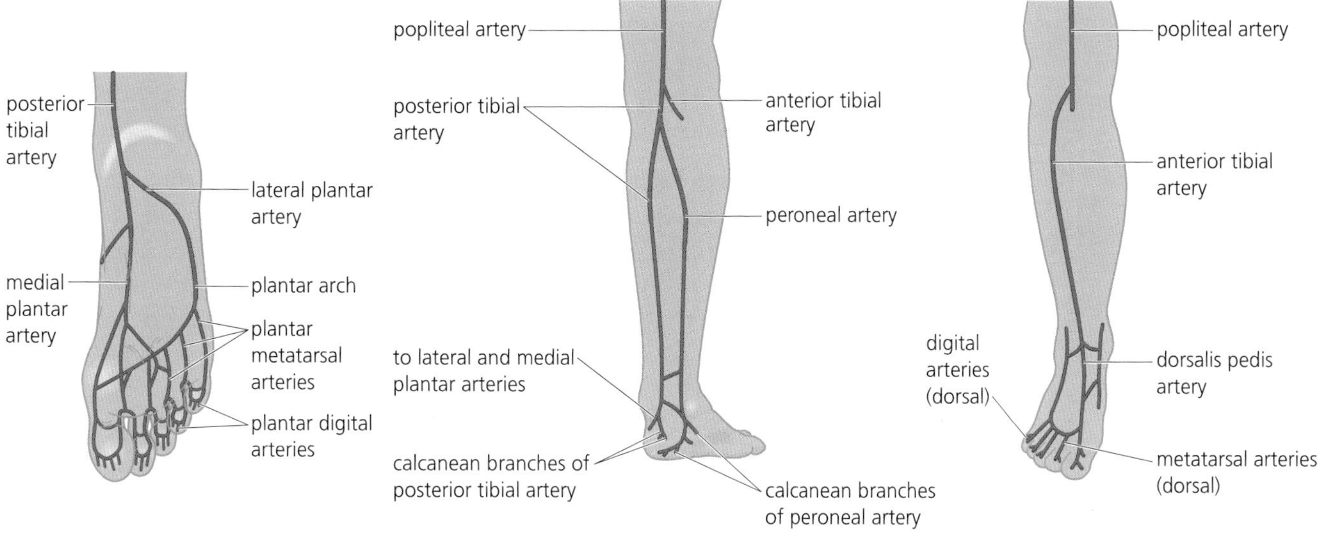

Arteries of the foot and lower leg

FACT

If you have been ill and have had **swollen glands**, these are lymph glands that have enlarged to fight the infection.

TERMINOLOGY

Oedema means 'swelling', where the tissue fluid accumulates instead of draining away and returning to the blood system. This can be caused by poor circulation or a medical condition (contra-indicated).

THE LYMPHATIC SYSTEM

The lymphatic system is very closely linked to the cardiovascular system, and connects with it. The primary function is defensive: to protect the body from disease. Functions of the lymphatic system are:

- Drains tissue fluid from the spaces between the cells.
- Tissue fluid and protein are returned to the blood circulation, via the subclavian veins.
- Lymphocytes are produced that defend the body against infection and disease.
- Lymph nodes act as a filter, removing toxins, waste products and foreign substances.
- Transports fats in a fluid called 'chyle', from the small intestine to the blood.

The main parts of the lymphatic system are:

- lymph fluid
- lymph capillaries, vessels and trunks
- lymph nodes (glands)
- lymph ducts
- lymphatic organs.

Lymph fluid

Fluid from blood passes through the walls of the tiny capillaries and enters the tissue spaces. This 'interstitial fluid' then becomes 'lymph' when it enters the lymph vessels. Lymph consists mainly of water, and certain substances found in blood plasma, such as fibrinogen.

Lymph capillaries, vessels and trunks

Lymph vessels start as blind-ended capillaries, which form a network among the tissue spaces. Their walls are very thin, which allows the tissue fluid to pass through and into the capillaries. The small capillaries join together and form larger vessels. These vessels are similar in structure to veins, but have thinner walls and a lot more valves at intervals to prevent backflow.

The lymph vessels join together to form 'lymph trunks', eventually the lymph is emptied into two main ducts – the thoracic duct and the right lymphatic duct. These ducts drain into the subclavian veins, and thereby the lymph returns to the blood system. This is a constant cycle – fluid moves into tissues, enters fine lymph vessels, is transported to the ducts, and then is returned to the bloodstream.

Lymph nodes

Lymph vessels drain into lymph nodes at various stages along the route to the two main ducts. Lymph nodes are a group of small, bean-shaped structures; they can be superficial or deep nodes. Lymph enters the node

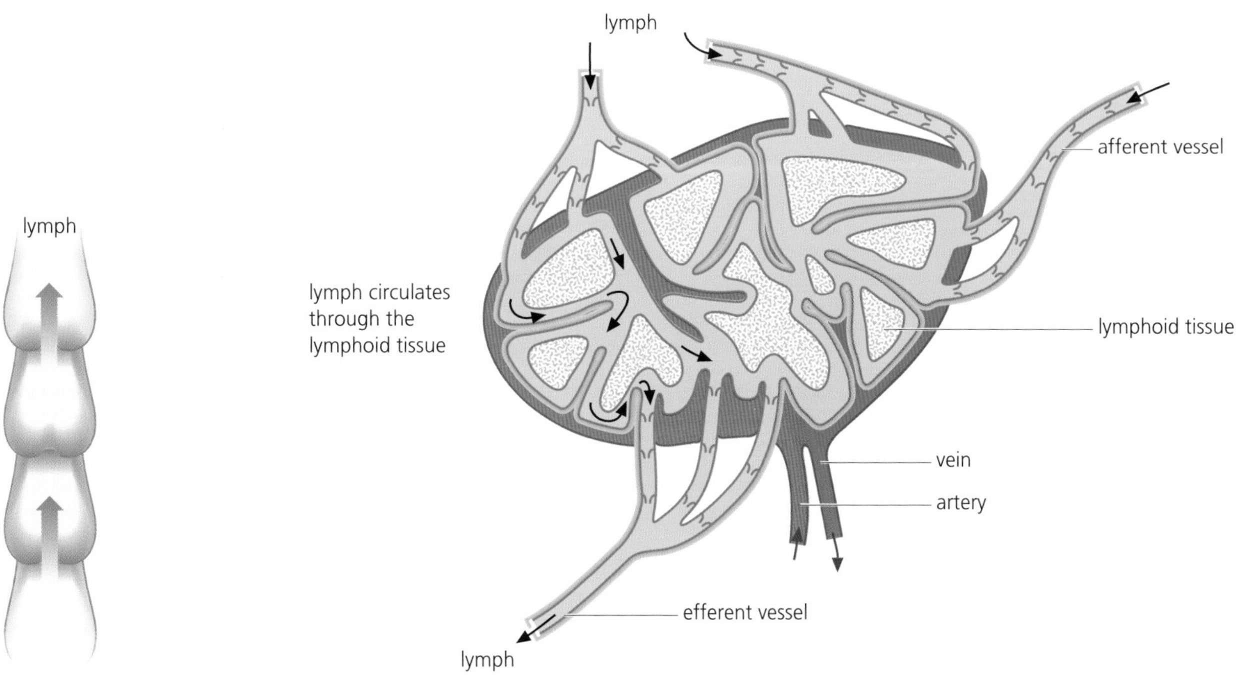

A lymph vessel and a lymph node

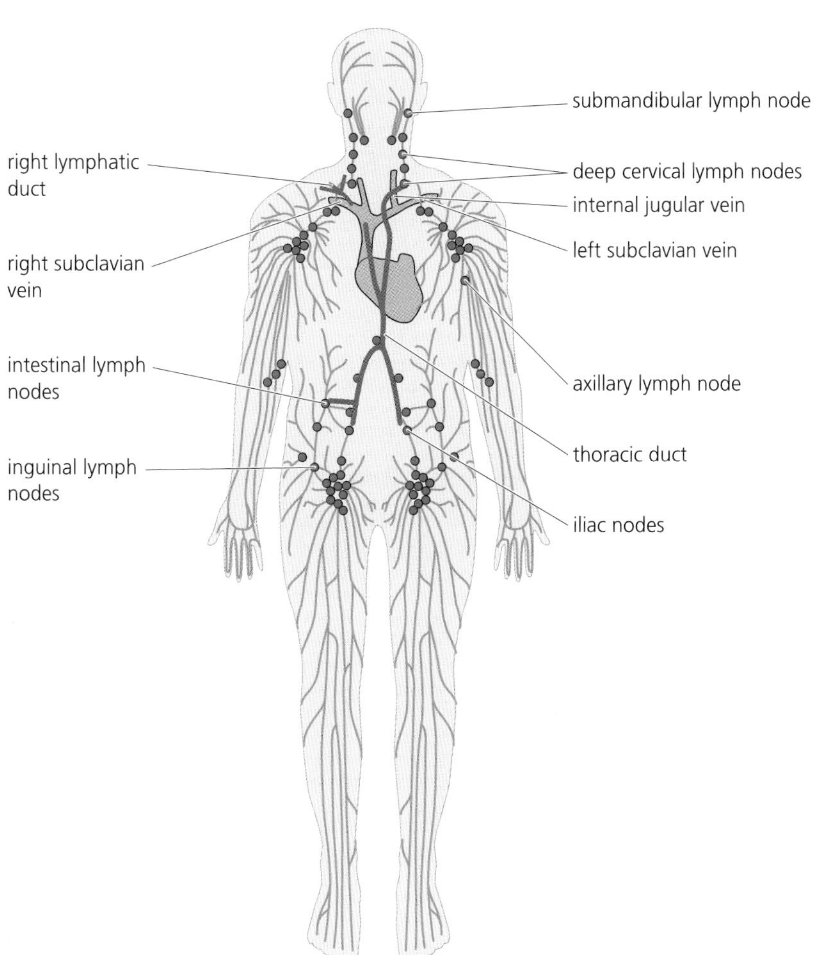

The lymphatic system

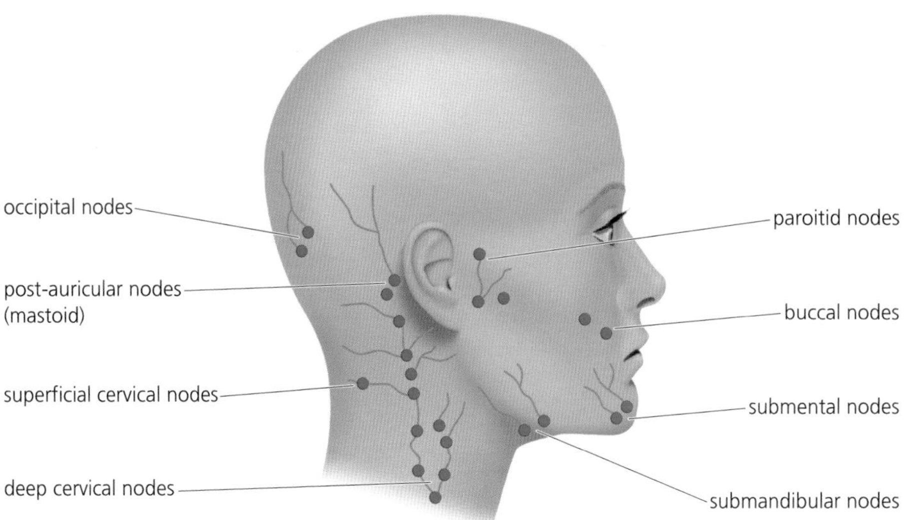

Lymph nodes of the head

through an 'afferent' vessel, it is then filtered, and leaves through an 'efferent' vessel. A main function of the nodes is to act as a filter, cleaning the lymph so that bacteria, toxins and other substances are prevented from entering the bloodstream. There are two types of white cells inside the lymph node: macrophages and lymphocytes. The macrophage cells engulf and destroy foreign substances and debris in the lymph. Lymphocytes produce antibodies to fight bacteria. They can flow into the bloodstream with the lymph. When infection is present, the lymph nodes closest to the infection can swell and become painful because the white cells are fighting to destroy the bacteria.

Lymph ducts

The lymph vessels join together to form 'lymph trunks' and eventually the lymph is emptied into two main ducts:

1 The thoracic duct – receives lymph from the left side of head and chest, left arm, and all the body below the ribs.
2 The right lymphatic duct – receives lymph from the right side of the head and the chest and right arm.

Lymphatic organs

- Tonsils – part of the body's defence against disease. Lymphocytes and antibodies produced in the tonsils fight local infection.
- Thymus gland – situated in the upper thoracic cavity, produces antibodies to fight foreign substances.
- Spleen – a large mass of lymphatic tissue, situated alongside the stomach. As well as filtering and cleaning blood, it produces antibodies which destroy foreign particles.

Swelling (oedema)

If there is a problem with the lymphatic system, then drainage will not be as effective as it should be. This can lead to swelling of the tissues. This is known as oedema. Generally, lymph flow varies from person to person. If a person is very active this can help speed up the flow, as the contractions of the muscles helps exert physical pressure on the vessels. If lymph flow in an area is slowing down, and becoming stagnant, then moving the limbs and exercising the muscles can be beneficial.

SPA TIP 

Massage can be extremely useful for lymphatic drainage. The massage strokes should be directed towards the nearest lymph gland, and can often be interspersed with 'squeezing', kneading movements. Massage physically puts pressure on the vessels, pushing the lymph in the direction of drainage.

THE DIGESTIVE SYSTEM

Digestion is the process whereby foods are gradually broken down into their basic components to provide the body with energy for growth and repair.

The digestive system is composed of:

- mouth
- pharynx
- oesophagus
- stomach
- small intestine
- large intestine
- rectum and anal canal.

The digestive system

Structure	*Description*
Mouth	Food is mechanically broken down by the teeth, and chemically broken down by the saliva (contains the digestive enzyme amylase)
Pharynx	Each mouthful of food is formed into a ball-like mass (bolus) which is pushed by the tongue to the back of the mouth. The muscles in the wall of the pharynx contract and the food is swallowed
Oesophagus	The oesophagus walls involuntarily contract and peristalsis carries the food towards the stomach
Stomach	The food enters the stomach and is thoroughly mixed with gastric juice by the churning action of the stomach's strong muscular walls. The gastric juice consists mainly of strong hydrochloric acid, protective mucus and pepsin, a digestive enzyme. When the food has been reduced to a pulp (chyme) it passes through the pyloric sphincter into the duodenum
Small intestine	The main part of digestion and absorption takes place along the length of the small intestine. Digestive juices pour into the duodenum from the pancreas and gall bladder. Furthermore, the lining of the small intestine secretes a range of digestive enzymes. Absorption of the digested nutrients into the bloodstream is helped by the heavily folded surface, with thousands of minute finger-like projections known as villi
Large intestine	Any waste products that are not of use to the body, pass through the ileocaecal valve into the large intestine to be removed. Peristalsis is the wave-like movement of the large intestine that moves the food material along the ascending, transverse and descending colon. The final part of the colon before the rectum is the sigmoid colon
Rectum and anal canal	Solid waste/faeces are stored in the rectum, until they are released through the anus

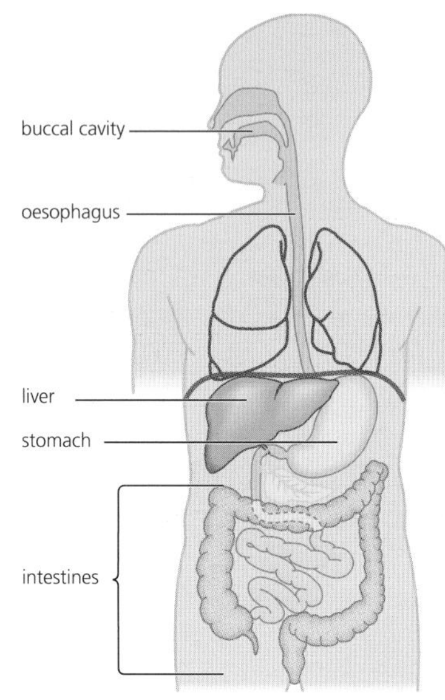

The digestive system

Four stages of digestion

1 Ingestion – food is taken in through the mouth.
2 Digestion – food is broken down by mechanical and chemical means.
3 Absorption – the tissues and cells of the body absorb the water and nutrients, to provide energy.
4 Excretion – food that is indigestible or of no use to the body is excreted (passed out).

THE RESPIRATORY SYSTEM

The function of the respiratory system:

- Ensures the oxygen transported from the lungs by the blood reaches all the cells of the body.
- Oxygen is used to provide energy for cell respiration.
- The waste product of cell respiration – carbon dioxide – is removed by being breathed out through the lungs.

The respiratory system is composed of:

- nose
- pharynx
- larynx
- trachea
- lungs
- bronchi
- bronchioles
- intercostal muscles
- diaphragm.

FACT

The small intestine is so called because of its diameter rather than its length – it measures approx 7 metres (or 23 feet)!

FACT

Between 1 and 2 litres of gastric juice is secreted daily by the glands in the stomach lining.

FACT

Respiration is the process by which energy is released from food. It involves every part of the body because it is at a cellular level that the release of energy occurs. It is one of the most important aspects of human physiology.

The respiratory system

Structure	*Description*
Nose	Air enters the nose, is warmed to body temperature, and tiny hairs (cilia) and mucous help filter the air
Pharynx (throat) Trachea (windpipe) Larynx (voice-box)	Air enters the lungs via a series of pipes. Air forced through the larynx (voice-box) causes the vocal cords to vibrate producing sound. The trachea is a flexible windpipe ringed with cartilage, air is funnelled through the trachea, which then forks to become the left and right bronchi
Lungs	The 2 lungs fill the deep thoracic cavity. The right lung consists of 3 lobes; the left lung is slightly smaller with 2 lobes and is indented to make way for the heart. The bronchioles end in air sacs called alveoli. It is here that the exchange of oxygen and carbon dioxide takes place. The pulmonary arteries enter the lungs and branch into small capillaries at the alveoli
Bronchi	The trachea divides to become 2 branches that enter the lungs; the right bronchus and the left bronchus
Brochioles	Inside the lungs the bronchi divide further, and eventually become smaller branches/tubes – bronchioles
Intercostal muscles	Muscles situated between the ribs that move the ribcage and increase and decrease lung volume during inspiration and expiration
Diaphragm	A sheet of muscle that forms the floor of the thoracic cavity. It contracts and flattens to allows the lungs to fill with air during inspiration, and during expiration it helps squeeze the air out of the lungs

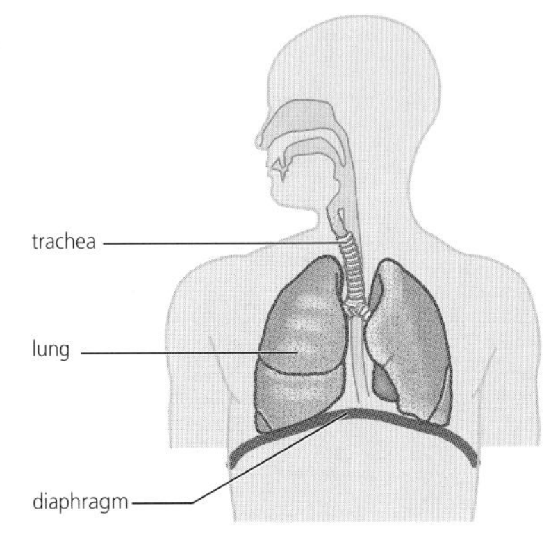

The respiratory system

THE NERVOUS SYSTEM

The nervous system enables the body to discover the world outside and monitor the world within. Without it the body could not survive. It allows the body to respond and react to changes in the environment by moving muscles and co-ordinating the actions of the various organs. The nervous system works very closely with the endocrine system, usually in a much faster way.

The nervous system is divided into two parts:

1 the central nervous system (CNS)
2 the peripheral nervous system (PNS).

FACT

The nervous system is very fragile and needs protection. The brain and spinal cord are covered by tough membranes called meninges and cushioned by being bathed in a liquid called cerebrospinal fluid.

Central nervous system

This consists of the brain and the spinal cord. The brain is housed in the skull, which protects it, and the spinal cord has the support and protection of the vertebrae.

The brain is one of the largest organs in the body, and is divided into different parts, each with a specific function.

Spinal cord

The spinal cord is a continuation of the medulla oblongata. The main function is to:

- relay nerve impulses to and from the brain and the peripheral nervous system
- help maintain the body's internal balance (homeostasis) by providing rapid responses to external or internal stimuli.

The spinal cord is made up of bundles of nerve fibres carrying messages to and from the brain. The pathways cross so that sensations from one side of the body register in the cortex of the brain on the other side.

Functions of the brain

Part	*Location*	*Function*
Brainstem ● Medulla oblongata ● Pons varolii ● Mid-brain	Continuation of the spinal cord	● A bridge connecting the spinal cord with the brain, and parts of the brain with each other ● Areas of it help control heart rate, depth/rate of breathing and reflexes such as coughing and sneezing
Cerebrum	Major part of the brain, divided into 2 hemispheres, and 4 lobes: – frontal lobe – occipital lobe – temporal lobe – parietal lobe	● Centre of thought, memory, intelligence, responsibility and reasoning ● Initiates and controls all voluntary muscular movement ● Receives sensory information, such as touch, sight, sound, smell, taste and pain
Thalamus	Situated above the mid-brain	● Main centre for sensory impulses, it interprets messages to the brain. Also involved with memory and some emotions
Hypothalamus	Situated above the pituitary gland, and is linked to it	● Controls many body activities, such as: – body temperature – thirst and hunger – sleeping/waking patterns – autonomic nervous system
Cerebellum	Located at the back of the brain, butterfly shaped with 2 lateral wings	● Motor area of the brain, maintaining posture, coordination, balance and fine movements
Ventricle	A cavity in the brain containing cerebrospinal fluid	● The fluid protects the brain, acting as a shock absorber. Also delivers nutrients and removes waste

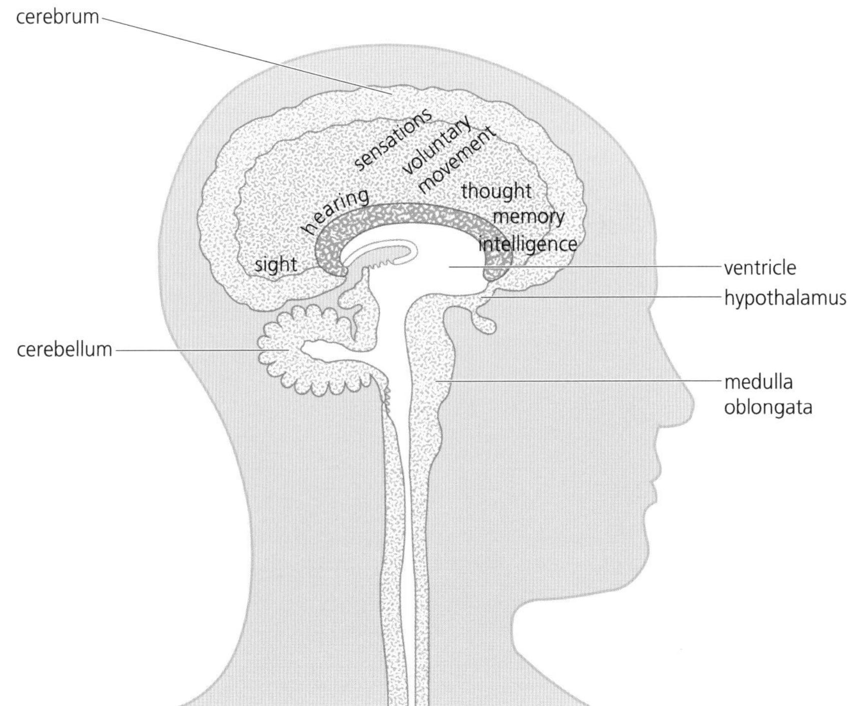

Vertical section through the brain

The peripheral nervous system

There are 12 pairs of cranial nerves originating from nuclei in the brain, 10 of which originate directly from the brainstem. Each pair is numbered, indicating the order in which they leave the brain. Some cranial nerves are sensory, others are 'mixed' meaning they have both a 'motor' and a 'sensory' function.

Nerves of the face and neck

The cranial nerves of concern to the spa therapist are:

- 5th cranial nerve – trigeminal nerve
- 7th cranial nerve – facial nerve
- 11th cranial nerve – accessory nerve.

5th cranial nerve (trigeminal nerve) This nerve conveys messages to the brain from the sensory nerves of the mouth, nose, teeth and skin. Furthermore, it also has a motor function, and helps create the chewing action when eating. This nerve has three branches:

1 opthalmic nerve – tear glands, skin on forehead and upper cheeks
2 maxillary nerve – upper jaw and mouth
3 mandibular nerve – lower jaw muscle, teeth and muscle involved with chewing.

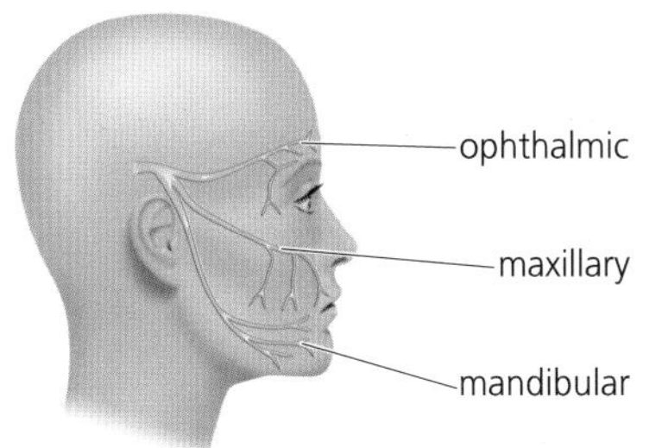

5th cranial nerve

7th cranial nerve (facial nerve) This nerve passes through the temporal bone behind the ear, and then divides. It is a 'mixed' nerve that covers the

Cranial nerves

Number	*Name*	*Type/activity*
1st	Olfactory	Sensory (smell)
2nd	Optic	Sensory (vision)
3rd	Oculomotor	Mixed. Motor (movement of eyeball, eyelid and pupil). Sensory (muscle sense)
4th	Trochlear	Mixed. Motor (eyeball movement). Sensory (muscle sense)
5th	Trigeminal	Mixed. Motor (chewing). Sensory (touch, temperature, pain)
6th	Abducent	Mixed. Motor (eyeball movement). Sensory (muscle sense)
7th	Facial	Mixed. Motor (facial expression, secretion of saliva and tears). Sensory (taste, muscle sense)
8th	Vestibulocochlear	Sensory (hearing, equilibrium)
9th	Glossopharyngeal	Mixed. Motor (swallowing, saliva production). Sensory (taste, blood pressure, muscle sense)
10th	Vagus	Mixed. Motor (swallowing, muscle movement). Sensory (from throat, lungs, heart, stomach, intestines)
11th	Accessory	Mixed. Motor (swallowing, head movement). Sensory (muscle sense)
12th	Hypoglossal	Mixed. Motor (swallowing, tongue). Sensory (muscle sense)

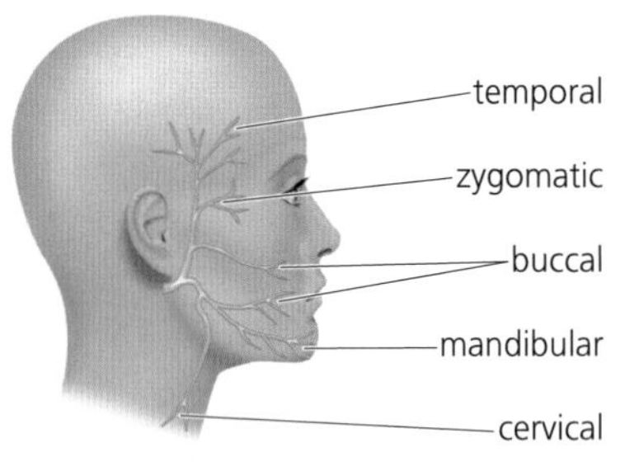

7th cranial nerve

ear muscle and muscles of facial expression, the tongue and the palate. This nerve has five branches:

1 temporal nerve – orbicularis oculi and frontalis muscles
2 zygomatic nerve – eye muscles
3 buccal nerve – upper lip and sides of nose
4 mandibular nerve – lower lip and mentalis muscle
5 cervical nerve – platysma muscle.

11th cranial nerve (accessory nerve) This nerve supplies the sternomastoid and trapezius muscles, and assists in moving the head and shoulders.

Spinal nerves

There are 31 pairs of spinal nerves. They are connected to the spinal cord and their names reflect the region from which they exit the spine:

- 8 pairs of cervical nerves
- 12 pairs of thoracic nerves
- 5 pairs of lumbar nerves
- 5 pairs of sacral nerves
- 1 pair of coccygeal nerves.

Each nerve divides and branches into smaller and smaller nerves to form a huge network that covers the entire body.

Neurones

All nerve tissue is composed of nerve cells or neurones. These cells connect parts of the body to the CNS and conduct impulses throughout these organs.

Sensory receptors

Found in many areas, including the dermis of the skin, muscles, tendons, joints, nose, mouth, eye, ear. When stimulated, impulses pass from the receptor along the fibres of a **sensory (receptor) neurone** – to the CNS. This gives the sensations such as smell, taste, touch and hearing. This information allows the body to make informed choices about which response is appropriate.

Motor (effector) neurones

These conduct impulses from the CNS to the muscles or glands. If the motor neurone initiates voluntary muscle contractions, it will form motor end plates on the muscle fibres. Each neurone can stimulate between 10 and 2000 muscle fibres, depending on whether the muscle action is very precise or more general.

Nerves

A nerve is a collection of single neurones covered in a protective sheath. There are two kinds of nerve:

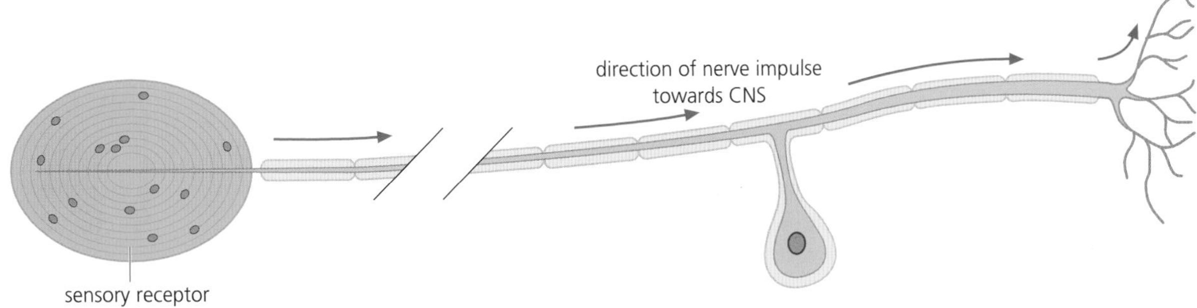

A sensory nerve

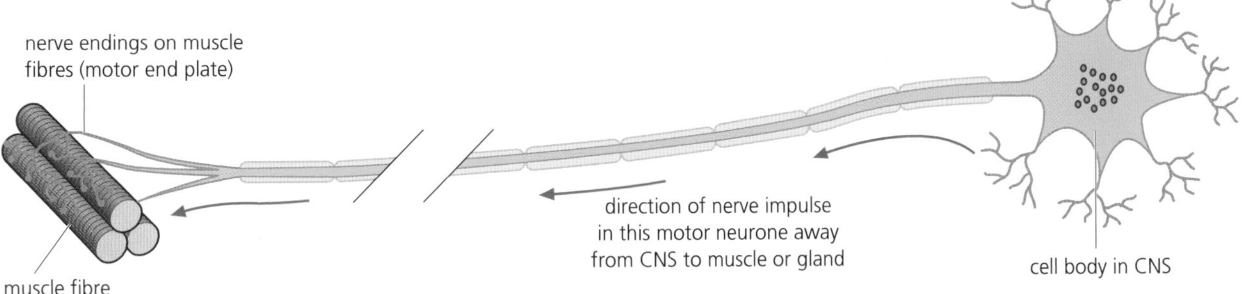

A motor neurone with detail of a motor end plate

1 Sensory nerve – these contain only sensory neurones. They receive information and pass it to the brain. Usually they are found near the surface of the skin, and respond to pressure, touch, temperature and pain.
2 Motor nerve – these usually are situated in muscle tissue, they act upon information received from the brain, causing a specific response, usually movement of the muscle.

Certain nerves are 'mixed' nerves, in that they contain both sensory and motor neurones.

Transmission of nerve impulses

Messages travel along nerve fibres as electrical impulses. The electrical impulses are a direct result of changes to the polarity of the membrane of the nerve fibre. A resting nerve fibre becomes polarized when there are more +ve ions present on the outer surface and more −ve ions present inside. When the neurone is stimulated, a wave of depolarization travels among the fibre as the charges become temporarily reversed.

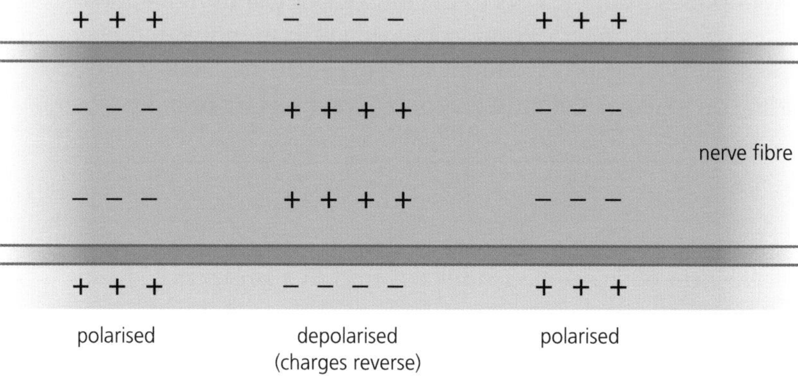

Conduction of nerve impulses

Passage of impulses between neurones

Information is passed from one neurone to another, even though they never touch. When an impulse comes to the end of a nerve fibre a chemical is released, called a **neurotransmitter substance**, e.g. acetylcholine. This

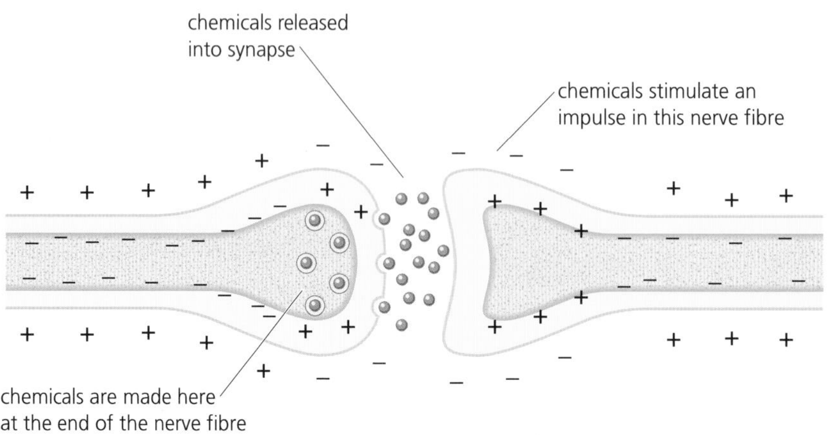

The passage of an impulse across a synapse

chemical passes across a tiny gap (synapse) and is taken up by the next neurone, generating an electrical impulse in that neurone.

Passage from a neurone to a muscle fibre

This is similar to the passage across the synapse between two neurones, and makes use of chemical transmitter substances. These chemicals are released at the end of a motor neurone into the muscle, so that all muscle fibres stimulated by that neurone will contract.

A muscle will only contract if it is stimulated by a motor nerve. The place at which a motor nerve enters a muscle is called a **motor point**. One neurone and the muscle fibres it stimulates is called a **motor unit**. The point of contact between the neurone and the muscle fibre is called the **motor end plate** or **neuromuscular junction**.

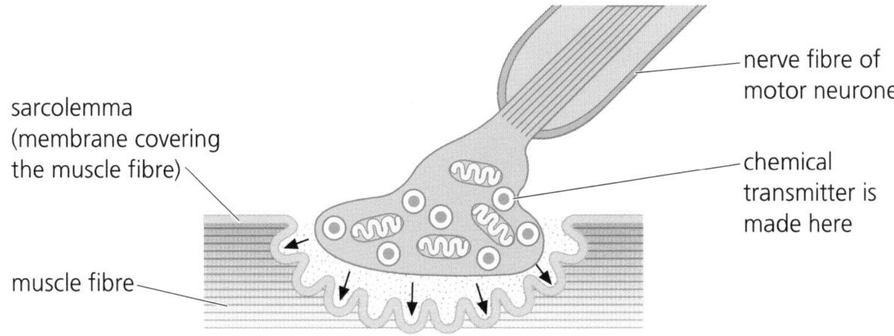
sarcolemma (membrane covering the muscle fibre)
muscle fibre
nerve fibre of motor neurone
chemical transmitter is made here

The synapse and neuromuscular junction (motor end plate)

Voluntary and reflex actions

Voluntary actions can be controlled, and are initiated by the brain, e.g. walking and throwing. A reflex action is a fast involuntary response to a stimulus, e.g. dropping a hot pan. This response happens because pain receptors in the hand are stimulated. Impulses are carried by sensory nerves to the spinal cord and are transmitted by relay neurones to motor neurones. Immediately, impulses pass to the arm muscles which are stimulated and contract and the pan is dropped. A reflex involving the spinal cord is called a **spinal reflex**. Impulses will also pass up the spinal cord to the brain, and

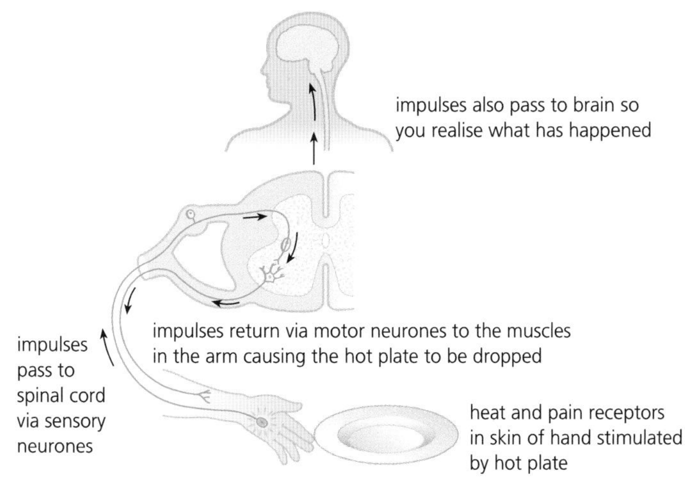
impulses also pass to brain so you realise what has happened
impulses return via motor neurones to the muscles in the arm causing the hot plate to be dropped
impulses pass to spinal cord via sensory neurones
heat and pain receptors in skin of hand stimulated by hot plate

A simple reflex arc

you become aware of what has happened. A secondary response could be to scream in shock at the hot pan. Other reflex actions involve the cranial nerves, such as swallowing, blinking, sneezing.

The autonomic nervous system

This system controls involuntary actions of smooth muscle, cardiac muscle and glands. It can regulate:

- pupil size
- vasodilation/vasoconstriction
- heart rate
- gut movements
- gland secretions.

The two divisions of the autonomic nervous system are listed in the table below:

Sympathetic division	*Parasympathetic division*
● Times of stress	● Times of peace/relaxation
● Stimulation	● Inhibition
● In periods of stress or danger it prepares the body for physical activity in case escape or fighting is necessary	● Stimulated in times of relaxation
● Increases rate/force of heartbeat	● Digestion stimulated and food absorbed better
● Dilates bronchioles of lungs	● Slows down body activity
● Dilates pupils of eyes	● After times of stress it will help the function of the organs to return to normal
● Increases sweating	
● Increases blood supply to muscles	
● Blood sugar levels rise	
● Non-essential activities are inhibited such as digestion/gut movement and urine production	

FACT

The urinary system is composed of:

- 2 kidneys
- 2 ureters
- the bladder
- the urethra.

THE URINARY SYSTEM

The function of the urinary system is to filter waste products, thereby regulating the composition, volume and health of blood.

- Waste is filtered from the blood, then excreted as a waste liquid – urine. The body has various ways of excreting waste products. **Excretion** is the term used to describe how the body eliminates waste.
- It regulates blood pressure and helps to control the pH of the blood.

The urinary system

Structure	*Description*
Kidneys	Bean-shaped organs located just above the waist at the back of the abdomen. They are responsible for filtering nitrogen-containing waste, such as urea, from the bloodstream. To ensure the body maintains the correct salt level, the kidneys regulate how much water is passed out of the body
Ureters	These are tubes leading from each kidney to the bladder. Waste is carried down the tubes to the bladder where it is stored as urine. The ureters have valves to prevent any backflow when the bladder is full
Bladder	Located in the lower part of the pelvic region. It is a reservoir for urine, which is capable of contracting and expanding depending on the amount of urine it contains
Urethra	The lowest part of the bladder, urine leaves the body via the urethra. A sphincter (circular muscle) keeps the urine within the bladder. When the bladder is full, the sphincter relaxes at the same time as the bladder wall contracts and the urine is expelled – urination

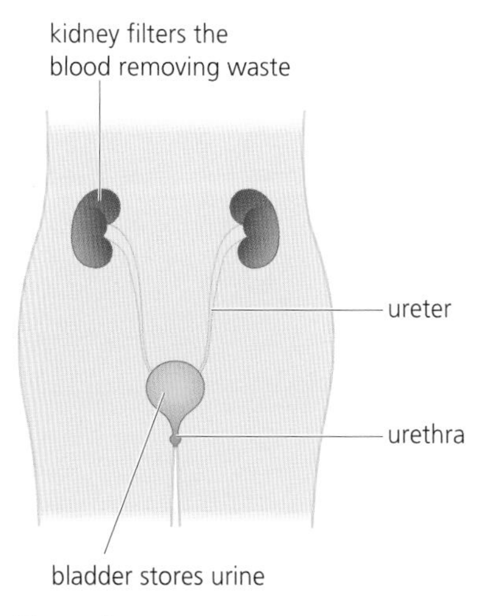

The urinary system

THE ENDOCRINE SYSTEM

The endocrine system is a very important body system and controls many of the body's functions and emotions. The endocrine system works very closely with the nervous system, and consists of endocrine (ductless) glands. These glands secrete chemicals called **hormones** directly into the bloodstream, they circulate around the body and affect specific organs. The organ that is affected by a particular hormone is referred to as a **target organ**. Whereas nerve stimulation tends to give a quick response, hormones are usually associated with more long-term processes such as metabolism, growth and development.

> **FACT**
>
> The **pituitary gland** is the master gland of the endocrine system. It is sometimes referred to as the 'gland of destiny' because of its importance in the body's overall development, and that it exercises control over most hormone systems.

Functions of the endocrine glands

Gland	*Hormones secreted*	*Function*
Thyroid gland	Thyroxine	Controls the rate of metabolism
Parathyroid gland	Parathormone	Controls blood calcium levels
Pituitary gland	Trophic hormones: – FSH (follicle stimulating hormone – LH (luteinizing hormone – ADH (anti-diuretic hormone)	Act on other endocrine glands – Controls reproduction – Controls reproduction – Affects water balance
Thymus gland (endocrine and a lymphatic gland)	Various hormones	Stimulates lymphoid cells responsible for antibody production against disease

continued

Pancreas (islets of Langerhans)	Insulin	Controls blood sugar levels
Adrenal (medulla)	Adrenalin Noradrenaline	Prepares the body for sudden stressful events ('fight or flight' hormones)
Adrenal (cortex)	Glucocorticoids (cortisol)	Reduce stress responses such as inflammation
	Mineralocorticoids (aldosterone)	Controls level of sodium and potassium in the blood
	Oestrogens and androgens	As other sex hormones
Ovary	Oestrogens and progesterones	Control female reproduction events including puberty, menstruation, pregnancy and the menopause
Testes	Testosterone (an androgen)	Controls male fertility

Effects of hormones on body shape, skin and hair

Gland	*Hormone*	*Effect*
Thyroid	Thyroxine	Excess causes warmth, moist skin with thin hair and loss of body weight A lack of thyroxine causes swelling and puffiness of the face, weight gain and muscular weakness
Parathyroid	Parathormone	Lack of hormone not only affects the bones, but also causes abnormal production of keratin, affecting hair, skin and nails
Pituitary	Growth hormone (GH)	Excess hormone in adults causes coarsening of skin, increased hair growth and more muscular appearance
Adrenal	Glucocorticoids	Excess causes Cushing's syndrome characterized by a redistribution of fat producing a 'moon face', 'bull back', large abdomen and thin limbs. Purple stretch marks and bruises may appear on the skin Deficiency causes Addison's disease with weight loss and darkening of the skin
	Aldosterone	Excess can cause oedema
	Corticosteroids (sex hormones)	Excess of androgens causes virilism in women (deepening of the voice, growth of facial and body hair, muscle development and sometimes male pattern baldness) Excess of oestrogens causes feminization in men – breasts will enlarge
Ovary	Oestrogen and progesterone	Influences the typical 'female' shape, encourages fat to be laid down around hips, thighs and breasts. Keeps skin and hair in good condition. Distribution of body hair at puberty
Testes	Testosterone	Causes muscular development influencing 'male' body shape. Encourages fat to be laid down around the waist and abdomen. Causes growth of facial and body hair at puberty

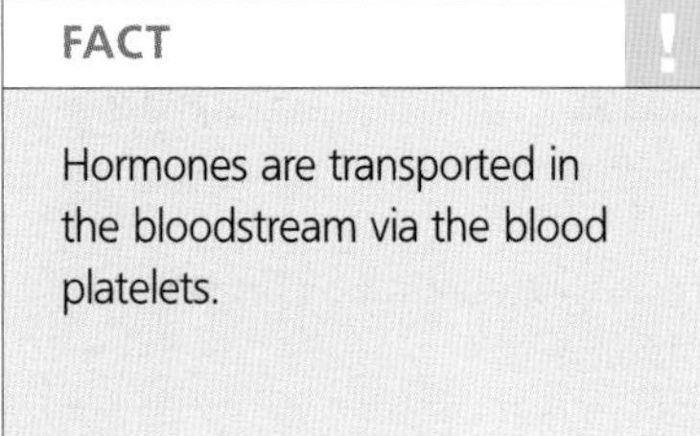

FACT

Hormones are transported in the bloodstream via the blood platelets.

FACT

Although it appears that the **endocrine glands** are independent of each other, they do work together very closely. Hormones from one gland often influence the output from another gland. Alongside the other components of blood, the secretions of these ductless glands provide a supportive medium for millions of body cells.

THE REPRODUCTIVE SYSTEM

Male reproductive system

Organs/structures	*Function*
Testes (male gonads)	A pair of oval glands, supported by the scrotum. They continually produce spermatazoa (sperm) from the age of puberty onwards. The male hormone testosterone is also produced
Ducts/glands ● vas efferentia ● vas deferens	These ducts store and transport sperm
Accessory glands seminal vesicles, prostrate gland, Cowper's gland	These all secrete fluids into the urethra, helping to make semen
Penis	Erectile tissue that dilates with blood when sexually stimulated. At ejaculation, during sexual intercourse, the sperm travel along the sperm duct, mix with secretions from the glands, and are deposited in the vagina of the female

Female reproductive system

Organs/structures	*Function*
Ovaries (female gonads)	Two walnut-sized structures, located on either side of the uterus in the pelvic cavity. Every 28 days they produce an ovum (egg), and also produce and secrete the female sex hormones progesterone and oestrogen that are essential to fertilization. The ovum travels down the oviduct, this is where it may be fertilized if sexual intercourse has taken place and sperm are present
Fallopian tubes	The ova enters the Fallopian tube, and passes down into the uterus
Uterus or womb	A fertilized ovum will embed in the wall of the uterus, where it will develop into an embryo. Birth is approximately 40 weeks later. An unfertilized ovum will travel through the uterus and be shed with the next menstrual flow
Vagina	A muscular tube which connects the internal and external sexual organs. The penis inserts into this tube during sexual intercourse, the menstrual flow passes down it and a baby is delivered through the vagina.
Mammary glands (breasts)	These are accessory glands. They start to develop at puberty and their main function is the secretion and ejection of milk

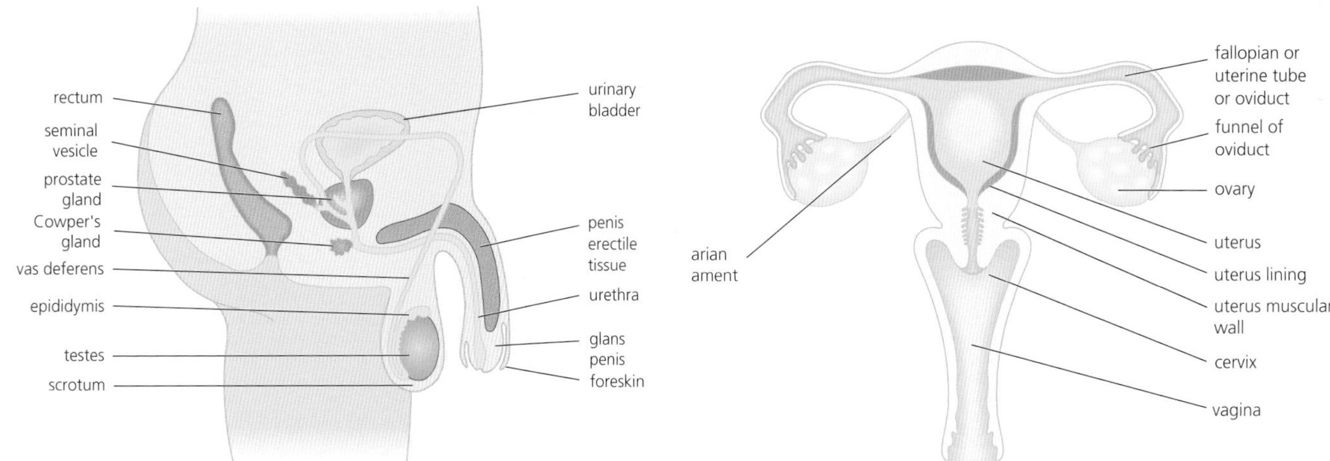

Male reproductive organs

Female reproductive organs

Reproduction

Reproduction refers to the process of producing life. Fertilization occurs when a single sperm penetrates the outer layer of an ovum and fusion takes place. A single nucleus is produced, which then starts to continually divide. Within 3 days the ovum will travel to the uterus and embed into the lining. The egg is nourished and a placenta forms. By week 12 the placenta is an independent organ allowing substances to pass between the mother and foetus. The umbilical cord attaches the foetus to the placenta. This cord is a route for nourishment and oxygen to feed the growing baby, as well as allowing waste products to be transported back to the mother. Pregnancy lasts for approximately 40 weeks, by which time the foetus is fully developed and ready to be born.

Menstruation

This cycle occurs from puberty until the menopause, approximately 35 years. The menstrual cycle lasts for an average of 28 days, and is a sequence of changes in a non-pregnant female to the endometrium (mucous membrane limning of the uterus).

The ovum is released by the ovary, and travels down the Fallopian tube to the uterus. If it becomes fertilized, it will embed into the wall of the uterus and receive nourishment and develop into an embryo. If it is not fertilized, the lining of the uterus falls away and is shed as the menstrual flow. The lining of the uterus is then replenished in time for the next ovum that is released.

Menopause

At the menopause, the menstrual cycle ceases, and the following changes can occur:

- The ovaries become inactive and atrophy.
- Ovarian production of the hormones oestrogen and progesterone stops.

Female reproductive disorders

Dysmenorrhoea	Painful menstruation. May be due to reproductive disorders, or hormone changes in young females
Amenorrhoea	Absence of menstruation. Extreme weight changes or excessive exercise can cause this
Ovarian cysts	Fluid-filled swelling on the ovary. Can be symptom-free, or cause problems and pain and need surgery
Pre-menstrual tension (PMT)	Symptoms that occur a few days before menstruation, including headaches, irritability and fluid retention

- Other reproductive organs begin to atrophy – uterus, vagina, oviducts, breasts.
- Bones become more brittle.
- Blood cholesterol levels increase.
- Risk of suffering a heart attack increases.

Hormone replacement therapy (HRT) can delay certain changes.

Breasts

The breasts or mammary glands are accessory glands of the female reproductive system. Their main function is to produce milk for the offspring. The secretion and ejection of milk is called lactation.

It is vital that all females are aware of any developments or changes to their breasts. As a spa therapist you should reinforce medical advice for individuals to be vigilant and able to self-examine. Breast tumours can be felt as lumps in the breast tissue. Benign tumours are common and often

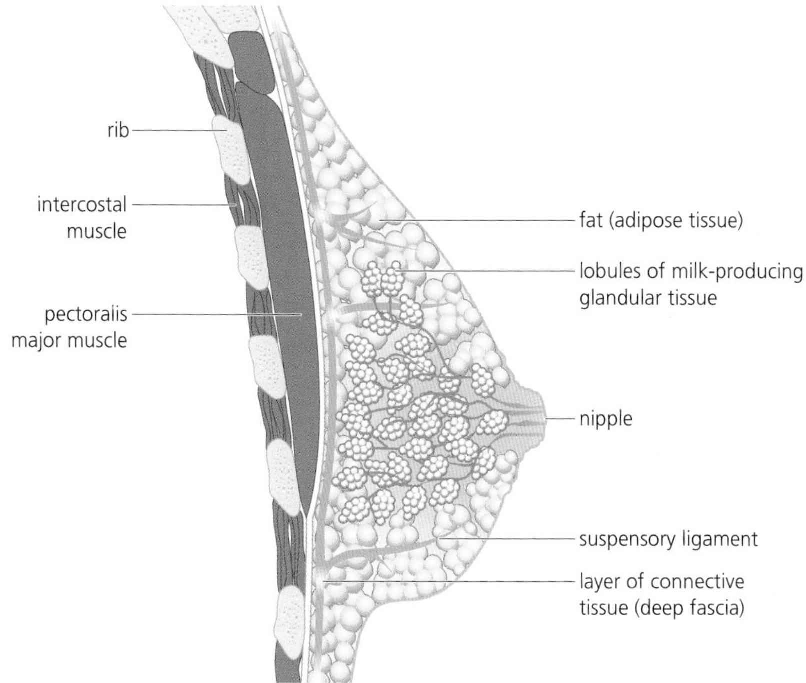

Vertical section showing breast tissues

The breast

Organ/structure	*Function*
Lobes/lobules	Each breast consists of 15–20 lobes. Each lobe is further divided into separate lobules, separated by adipose tissue. The amount of adipose tissue will determine the size of the breast. These lobules contain milk secreting cells called alveoli
Alveoli	These carry milk into a series of secondary tubules, which then pass into the mammary ducts
Mammary ducts	These are located close to the nipple. They form ampullae where milk is stored, then become lactiferous ducts which end at the nipple. Milk is produced under the influence of the hormone prolactin; it passes through the ducts to the nipple. During breastfeeding the milk is ejected in response to the hormone oxytocin, which is produced as the baby starts to suckle. Oxytocin is also responsible for contractions of the uterus, therefore breastfeeding helps the uterus return to its original size more quickly
Suspensory ligaments	The breast lies over the chest muscles (pectoral and serratus anterior) and is attached to them by a layer of connective tissue. The breast is anchored to the connective tissue by strands of tissue called the suspensory ligaments. These are not strong or robust ligaments, and the breast needs to be treated as fragile, and supported wherever possible

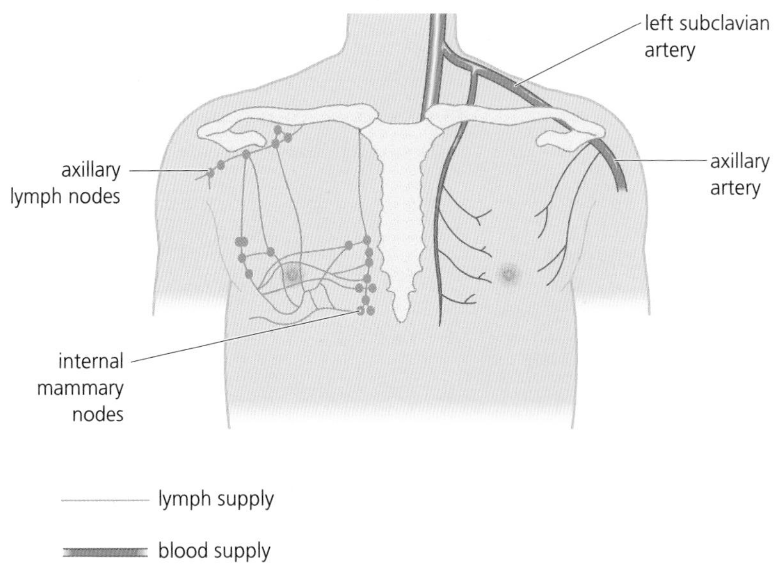

Lymph and blood supply to the breast area

self-contained and can be removed by minor surgery. Cysts are a hollow type of tumour, containing fluid. Fibroadenomas can feel firm and rubbery.

A malignant tumour can spread quickly to other tissues and areas of the body, often via the lymphatic system. Early detection and treatment is vital. The individual will probably not experience any pain or discomfort, so it is absolutely essential that they visit their doctor if they notice any changes such as: thickening, swelling, lumps, dimpling, puckering, scaliness, irritation, nipple change or discharge.

CELLS AND TISSUES

Cells

A cell is the basic unit of a living organism. There are hundreds of millions of cells in the body. Each cell has common features:

- Cell membrane – this surrounds the cell, forming a boundary between the cell and the environment. The membrane has a porous surface so soluble substances can pass through; for example, food enters and waste products leave the cell.
- Protoplasm – a colourless jelly within the cell membrane.
- Nucleus – a dense mass of protoplasm, containing chromosomes and genes vital for cell reproduction and cell functioning.
- Cytoplasm – the liquid within the cell membrane, surrounding the nucleus, contains the nutrients essential for growth and repair.
- Mitochondria – provide the energy for the cell to be able to perform its activities.

FACT

The process of cell division is called **mitosis**. The cell reproduces and two new identical cells are created.

TERMINOLOGY

Cells specialize in carrying out particular functions.

Tissues groups of cells that share the same purpose, function, shape, size or structure.

Organs tissues that group together to form a larger functional and structural unit.

Types of tissues

Tissue	*Function*	*Example*
Epithelial tissue	Protective covering for surfaces and linings. Can be: – simple – compound	● Skin epidermis ● Lining of heart, blood, lymph vessels ● Digestive/respiratory organs
Connective tissue	A structural tissue that provides support and protection, and 'connects' (binds) body tissues. Cells include: – plasma – macrophages – fibroblasts – melanocytes – adipose cells	● Bone ● Cartilage ● Mucous membranes ● Adipose tissue ● Collagen
Muscular tissue	Capable of contracting and providing the body with movement	● Cardiac (involuntary) ● Visceral (involuntary) ● Skeletal (voluntary)
Nerve tissue	Responds to stimulus, and communicates between the brain and other areas of the body	● Neurones
Blood tissue	A type of liquid 'connective tissue' which carries nutrients and waste products around the body	● Blood

THE SKIN

The skin is a very large organ, covering the entire body. It provides protection, and varies in thickness, texture, colour and sensitivity.

The skin has many functions:

1 Protection
  - the skin acts as a barrier and 'cushions' the underlying structures from physical injury
  - **sebum**, the skin's natural oil, provides a waterproof coating to the skin. This prevents the skin from losing vital moisture, and therefore prevents the skin from dehydrating
  - the outer surface of the skin is bactericidal, this helps to stop harmful micro-organisms from multiplying. The stratum corneum layer (outer layer) of the skin acts as a barrier and prevents many substances from being absorbed
  - the skin produces **melanin**, a pigment that absorbs harmful rays of ultraviolet light.

2 Excretion
   Perspiration is the term used to describe how the sweat glands excrete a range of waste products (water, salt, etc.).

3 Heat regulation
   The skin helps the body to control its temperature. If the body is too hot, capillaries in the skin are dilated to allow heat loss to the environment, plus sweating cools the body. If the temperature is too cool, the capillaries constrict to prevent heat loss, plus the hairs stand on end on the skin ('goosebumps') and trap air to act as an insulator.

4 Sensation
   The skin contains many sensory nerve endings, such as touch, pressure, heat, cold and pain. The nerves inform the brain of the sensations, which then sends impulses to the motor nerves and a reaction will take place. The skin is also sensitive to certain external and internal stimuli, and will become red, hot and irritated, this gives a 'warning' that something is wrong.

5 Vitamin production
   Ultraviolet rays act on a substance found in sebum and convert it into vitamin D. This vitamin is essential for the body to absorb calcium and phosphorous.

6 Moisture control/absorption
   The skin controls moisture from within the deeper layers of the skin. Because the skin has a waterproof barrier, absorption is very difficult. However, the outer layers of the skin absorb small amounts of creams and oils, used for very dry skin. A very limited amount of absorption can take place via the hair follicle.

Structure of the skin

The skin is divided into three main layers:

1 epidermis – the outer layer
2 dermis – the inner, main part of the skin
3 subcutaneous layer – consists of adipose tissue, muscles and veins.

The epidermis and dermis are bonded together by a special layer called the **basement membrane**. Should the two layers separate, fluid fills the space and a blister is created.

epidermis
basement membrane
dermis
subcutaneous layer

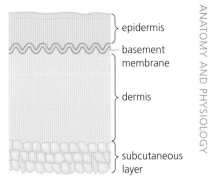

Layers of the skin

Epidermis

This is the outer layer of the skin, directly above the dermis. Its main function is to protect the deeper tissues and structures from harm.

The epidermis has five distinct layers, each one very recognizable because of the shape and function of its cells. The main type of cell is the keratinocyte. These produce a protein called **keratin** which is responsible for the toughness of skin, ensuring that substances cannot pass through the epidermis.

It takes approximately 4 weeks for a cell to travel from the bottom layer of the epidermis to the outer surface. The cell is formed in the bottom layer, and then moves through the different layers, changing its shape and structure. In the final stages it becomes an empty shell which is eventually shed from the skin's surface.

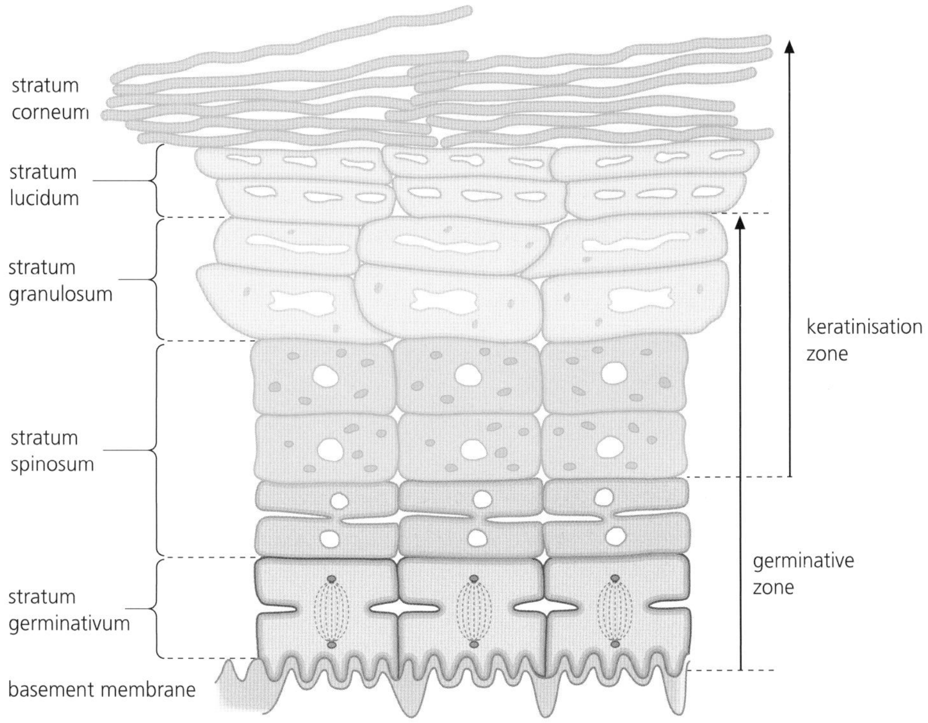

Layers of the epidermis

The epidermis

Layer of the epidermis	*Activity*
The germinative zone In this zone the cells of the epidermis are living cells	
Stratum germinativum (basal layer)	● The lowest level of the epidermis ● Formed from a single layer of column-shaped cells joined to the basement membrane ● Cells divide continuously and produce new epidermal cells (keratinocytes). Cell division is called mitosis
Stratum spinosum (prickle-cell layer)	● Formed from 2–6 rows of elongated cells ● The cells have spiky spines on their surface, which connect to surrounding cells ● Each cell has a nucleus and is filled with fluid
Stratum granulosum (granular layer)	● Composed of 1, 2 or 3 layers of cells which have become flatter ● The nucleus of each cell begins to break up, creating granules within the cell cytoplasm ● The granules are known as keratohyaline granules, which later become keratin
The keratinization zone This zone is where the cells begin to die and finally are shed from the skin. Cells become progressively flatter, and the cell cytoplasm is replaced with the protein keratin	
Stratum lucidum (lucid layer)	● Only seen in non-hairy areas of the skin, e.g. palms of hands and soles of feet ● Cells have a nucleus and are filled with a clear substance called eledin
Stratum corneum (cornified layer)	● Formed from several layers of flattened, scale-like overlapping cells, composed mainly of keratin ● The cells help to reflect ultraviolet light from the skin's surface ● It takes 3 weeks for a cell to reach this layer, after being formed in the stratum germinativum ● Cells are shed from the surface of the skin in a process known as desquamation

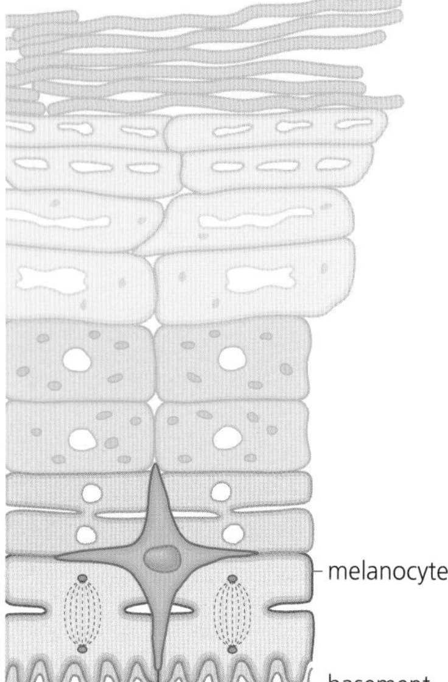

A melanocyte

Langerhan cells These cells are found in the germinative zone. They absorb and remove foreign bodies that enter the skin. Then they travel into the dermis, and finally enter the lymph system.

Melanocyte cells Melanocytes produce the skin pigment melanin. Approximately 10 per cent of the germinative cells are melanocytes. Ultraviolet rays stimulate the melanocyte to produce melanin. Their function is the protect the other epidermal cells from the harmful effects of ultraviolet radiation.

Dermis

The dermis supports the epidermis, is composed of dense connective tissue and is responsible for the elasticity of the skin. The dermis contains many appendages:

- nerve endings
- blood and lymph vessels
- hair follicles
- sweat and sebaceous glands.

The tissue of the dermis is composed of:

- collagen – for support
- elastin – for elasticity
- fibroblast cells – manufacture collagen and elastin.

The dermis provides the epidermis with nourishment; it has two main layers:

Papillary layer This is the upper part of the dermis, and is a very important layer. It is irregular in shape, with protrusions called papillae into the epidermis. A network of fine capillaries provide oxygen and nourishment to the skin and take away waste products. A variety of nerve endings are situated in this layer; touch, cold, heat and pain.

Reticular layer This is the lower part of the dermis, below the papillary layer. Collagen and elastin fibres interweave to form a resilient network. Yellow elastin fibres give the skin its elasticity, and white collagen fibres give it strength. Both fibres are produced by cells called fibroblasts, and are supported in a gel called **ground substance**. In young skin the network of fibres is strong, and the skin appears youthful, toned and firm. With age, the fibres harden and fragment, and the network begins to break down and loses its elasticity and suppleness. The skin will then visibly show signs of age.

Also in this layer are the sweat and sebaceous glands, and the erector muscles – pili. Arterioles and venules are present in the area, and they link up with fine capillaries.

Subcutaneous layer

This layer is situated below the dermis, and can be referred to as the **hypodermis**. The fat layer within this area consists of cells called adipose cells. The thickness of the fat layer varies in different areas of the body, e.g. around the eyes it is very thin.

The fatty layer acts as:

- protection, giving rounded contours to the body
- an insulator to conserve body heat
- a cushion to prevent bone and muscle injury
- an energy store, as the fat can be used when needed.

Skin appendages

Sweat glands

These glands are called **sudoriferous glands** and are found all over the body, with most concentrated on the palms of the hands and soles of the feet. The main function is to regulate body temperature through the evaporation of sweat from the skin's surface. Their structure is a coiled base in the dermis,

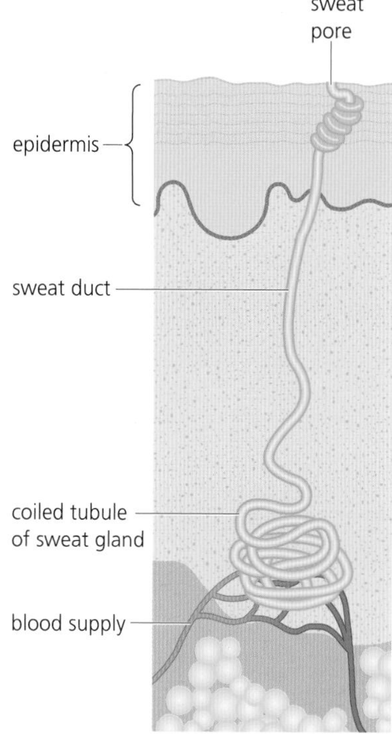

Eccrine sweat gland

which leads to a tube that leads to the epidermis and ends with a sweat pore on the surface of the skin. There are two kinds of sweat gland:

Eccrine glands Found all over the body and respond to heat to maintain the body temperature. They continuously secrete small amounts of sweat, even when it is not noticeable.

Apocrine Found in the armpit, groin and nipple areas of the body, usually attached to a hair follicle, and are larger than the eccrine glands. They are regulated by hormones, are activated at puberty and can react to situations such as stress, anxiety and excitement. They secrete a thicker fluid than the eccrine glands, which contains substances such as fats, sugars and proteins. They are associated with sexual attraction because there are slight amounts of aromatic molecules called **pheromones** in the sweat.

Hair

Hair is a long thin filament-type structure that grows from a follicle in the skin. Hair covers most of the body, except the palms of the hands, soles of the feet and lips.

The hair is made up of epithelial cells, in three distinct layers:

1 Medulla
The central part or core of the hair. The cells contain soft keratin, and often granules of pigment. Very thin hair may not have a medulla.

2 Cortex
This is the largest part of the hair and consists of layers of tightly packed elongated cells. These contain hard keratin and granules of pigment. It is the pigment that gives the hair its colour. When the production of pigment stops, the hair turns white. Collectively on the head, hair may appear grey, but in fact hair is either coloured or white.

Hair

Type	*Function*
Body hair	Provides insulation, has a sensory function and assists with the flow of sebum onto the skin's surface
Scalp hair	Protects the head against injury and sun-burn, and insulates against cold temperatures
Eyelashes	Prevents foreign particles, such as dust entering the eye
Eyebrows	Protects the browbone form injury, and prevents sweat running into the eyes
Ear hair	Protects the ear canal, preventing foreign particles from entering
Nostril hair	Prevents inhalation of foreign particles, such as dust

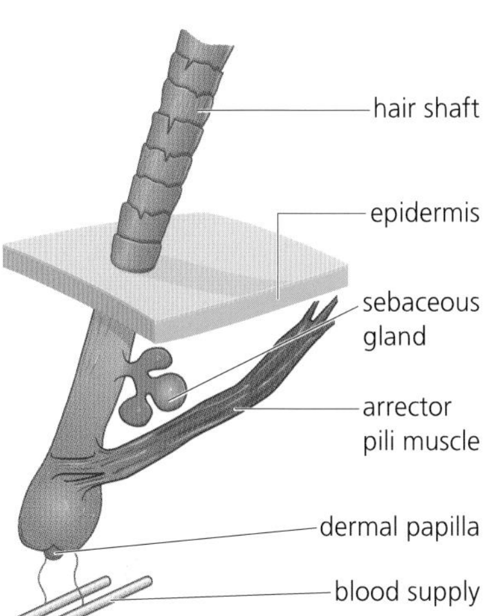

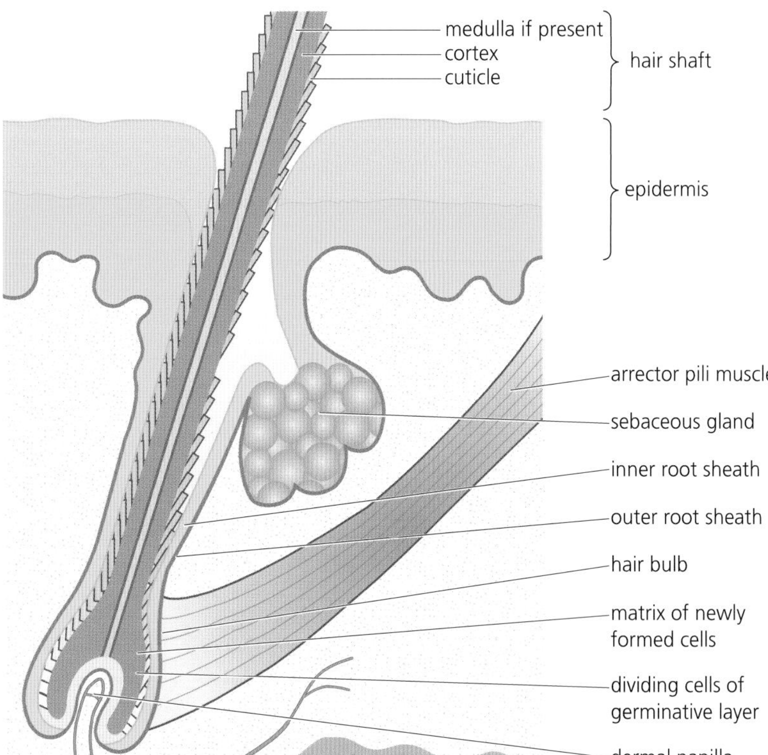

Cross-section of the hair follicle and hair

3 Cuticle
The outer layer of the hair and provides protection. The cells are thin, flat and unpigmented. They overlap with each other to form a protective layer.

Hair is structured in three distinct parts:

1 root – the part that is in the follicle
2 bulb – the rounded part at the bottom of the root
3 shaft – the part of the hair extending above the surface of the skin.

Skin appendages and hair follicle

Structure	*Description*
Hair follicle	Tube shaped indentation in the epidermis
Arrector pili muscle	A muscle that is attached to the base of the hair follicle. It is stimulated by cold, fright or aggression, and pulls the hair into an upright position, which then traps air, causing 'goosebumps'
Sebaceous gland	Attached to the upper part of the hair follicle. The gland produces sebum and via a duct this is secreted directly onto the hair follicle. Sebum is an oily substance, which softens and lubricates the skin and hair. It 'waterproofs' the skin and protects it against fungal and bacterial infections
Sudoriferous (sweat) glands	There are two types: 1 eccrine – sweat glands found all over the body, respond to heat 2 apocrine – larger, attached to a hair and found in areas such as the armpit and groin

continued

Dermal papilla	A small organ, made up of a sheath of connective tissue, which is surrounded by the hair bulb. It has a strong blood supply which is vital to feed the hair and promote growth
Bulb	At the bottom of the hair root, the rounded part. Within the hair root is a cavity in which the dermal papilla is located. The lower area of the bulb contains cells that are constantly dividing and creating the hair (matrix). The hair constantly develops on its upward journey to the surface of the skin
Matrix	Lower part of the bulb, where cells constantly divide to create the hair
Hair follicle	Made up of three sheaths: 1 inner epithelial root sheath 2 outer epithelial root sheath 3 connective tissue sheath
Nerve supply	Type and number of nerves vary depending on the type of hair

Three types of hair

Terminal	Long, coarse and pigmented. Vary in shape, length, colour and texture. Their follicles are deep with well-defined bulbs
Vellus	Soft, fine and downy hair located on the face and body. Usually short, unpigmented and without a medulla. Their follicles are shallow, with a poorly defined bulb
Lanugo	Fine, soft, unpigmented and found on foetuses. They develop at month 3–5 of the pregnancy, and are replaced by vellus hairs in the final stages of pregnancy. Lanugo hairs on the scalp and eyebrows/eyelashes develop into terminal hairs

FACT

The shape of the hair follicle affects the type of hair. Angled and bent follicles produce curly hair.

TERMINOLOGY

Acid mantle because of sweat and sebum, the skin is slightly acidic (pH 5.5–5.6). This is called the 'acid mantle' and it discourages bacteria or fungal infections.

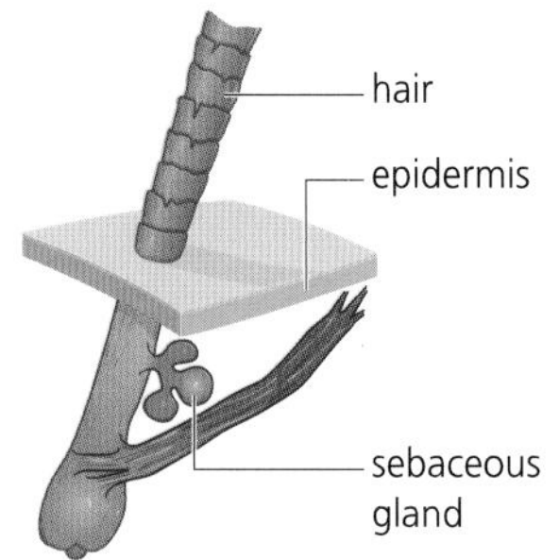

A sebaceous gland

Hair growth

Hair grows in a cycle, in three stages:

Anagen	Actively growing stage: – follicle forms, hair bulb develops, nourished from the dermal papilla – new hair grows from the matrix in the bulb
Catagen	Changing stage: – hair separates form the papilla – continues to move up the follicle – can rest around the base of the sebaceous gland until it becomes loose or is pushed out by a new hair
Telogen	Resting stage: – some follicles do not go through this stage – hair may stay loosely connected in the follicle

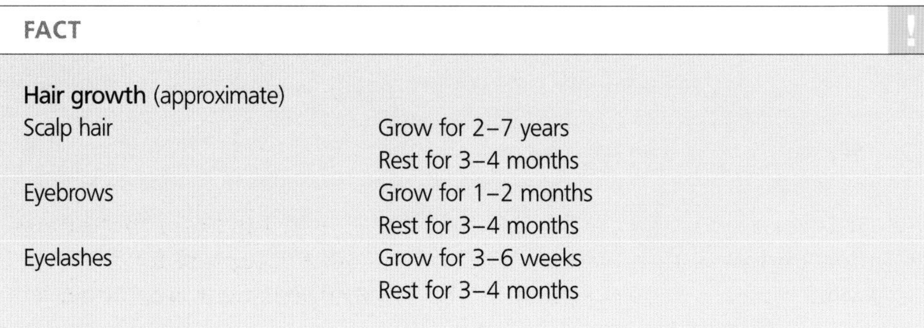

FACT

Hair growth (approximate)

Scalp hair	Grow for 2–7 years Rest for 3–4 months
Eyebrows	Grow for 1–2 months Rest for 3–4 months
Eyelashes	Grow for 3–6 weeks Rest for 3–4 months

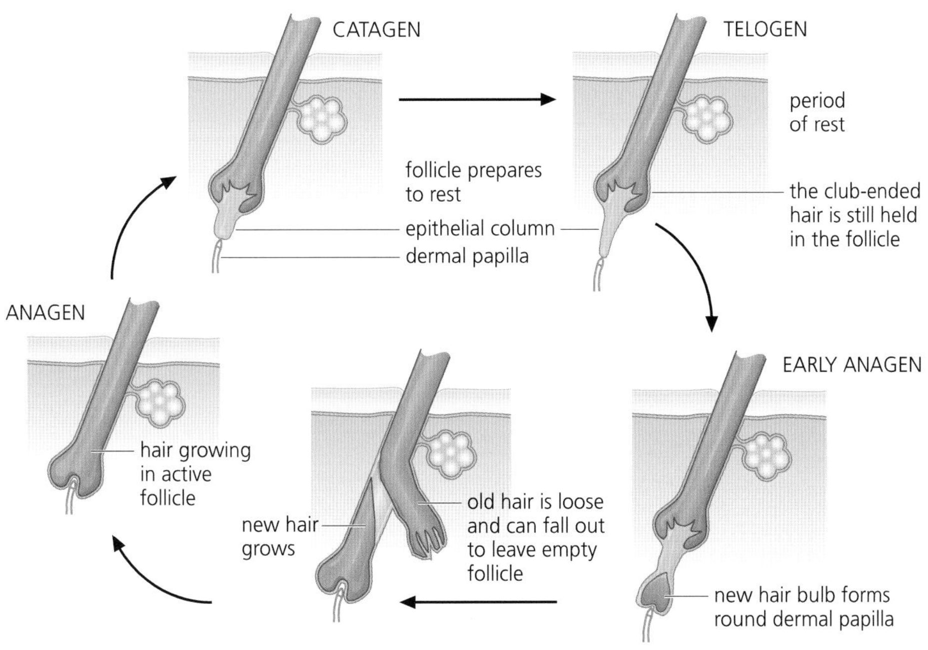

The hair growth cycle

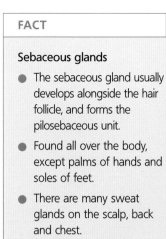

> **FACT**
>
> **Sebaceous glands**
>
> - The sebaceous gland usually develops alongside the hair follicle, and forms the pilosebaceous unit.
> - Found all over the body, except palms of hands and soles of feet.
> - There are many sweat glands on the scalp, back and chest.
> - At puberty the male hormone (androgen) stimulates the glands into action, with men secreting slightly more. The activity of the glands usually slows down in adulthood.
> - Sebum keeps the skin soft and supple and prevents moisture loss and dehydration.
> - Sebum is made of waxes and fatty acids. It has bactericidal and fungicidal effects.

THE FIVE SENSES

Sight

Sight is one of the body's main methods of interpreting the world. The organs of sight are the eyes, located in the orbital cavity and supplied by the optic nerve. The eye area has various parts that are for protection. The eyelids are fringed with eyelashes to help collect dust. The eyebrows help prevent sweat from running into the eyes. The conjunctiva is a membrane that covers the front of the eye, this protects the eye, but also prevents friction and allows the lids to open and close easily. The tear producing glands also perform a protective function, as tears wash away foreign particles and kill bacteria.

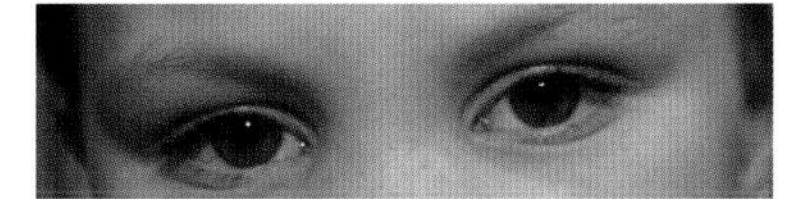

The cornea is the outer coating of the eye, and is very important for giving a focussed image. The pupil is a circular opening in the iris, which controls the entry of light as it can change diameter. Light then penetrates the lens and passes through the clear jelly (vitreous humour) that fills the eyeball, and then falls on the retina. The retina contains photo-receptor cells, the rods and cones. As a result, nerve impulses are generated which pass to the brain for interpretation as vision.

Sound

The ear is the organ responsible for hearing. It is divided into three parts: the outer, middle and inner ears. The ear contains receptors for balance and sound waves, and is supplied by the vestibulocochlear cranial nerve.

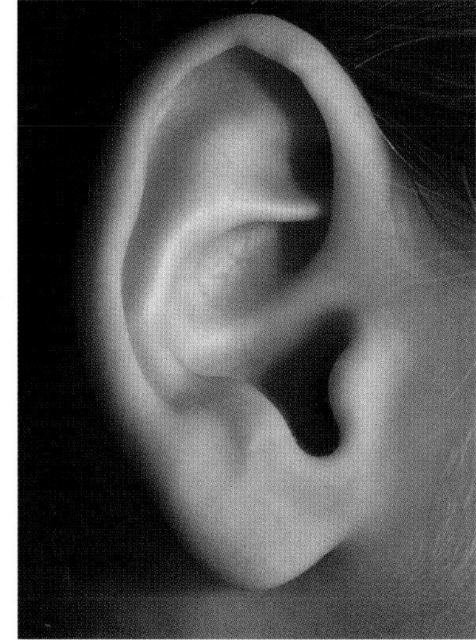

The ear

Part of ear	*Function/activity*
Outer ear	Collects the sound waves, they are then directed inwards to the eardrum in the middle ear. There is an auditory canal in the external ear that equalizes air pressure
Middle ear	At the end of the auditory canal lies the eardrum or tympanic membrane. On the other side is the cavity of the middle ear, which communicates with the back of the throat through a canal known as the Eustachian tube. This opens into the nose and throat and provides a complementary flow of air from the inside to match the pressure of air on the outside of the eardrum. Across the cavity of the middle ear, linking the eardrum with the inner ear, there are small bones; the hammer, the anvil and the stirrup. These are the smallest bones in the body, and they transmit the vibrations of the eardrum to a membrane
Inner ear	Contains the organs of balance and hearing. There is a fluid-filled coiled tube, resembling a snail's shell, called the cochlea. Here the vibrations are converted to nerve impulses that the brain perceives as sound

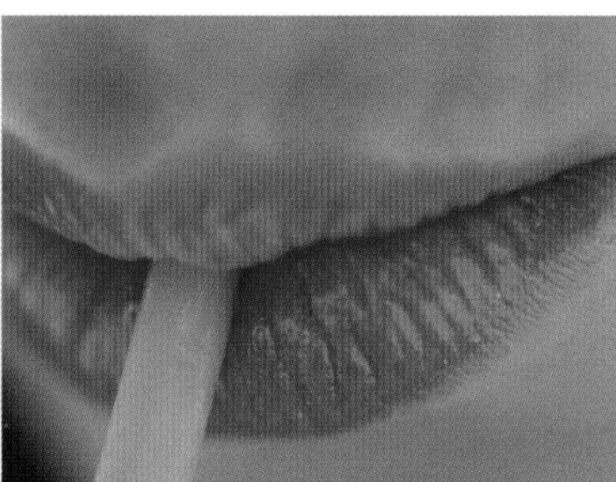

Taste

Taste is closely linked with smell, both senses sample experiences and report back to the brain. They are both chemical senses and taste is the weaker, often depending on the sense of smell to enhance it.

The sense of taste allows the body to appreciate food and drink, and also warn if food has gone stale or bad. The main organs of taste are microscopic nerve endings called 'taste buds'. These are located on the tongue, and to a smaller extent on the other surfaces of the mouth.

Taste buds register only four basic sensations: sweet, salt, sour and bitter. Most tastes are combinations of these four basic sensations. Different parts of the tongue are sensitive to different tastes, with the centre having no sense at all and most of the taste buds being concentrated towards the back. Taste buds cannot detect dry or solid tastes, so the saliva is very important, as it dissolves the chemicals and washes them over the taste buds. The receptor cells are stimulated and they send signals to the taste centres in the brain.

Smell

Smell is closely linked with taste. A foul smell can often leave a nasty taste in the mouth, and if you have a 'stuffed nose' you often cannot taste your food. Enjoyment of food is a combined sensation from the tongue, palate and nose. The nose is the main organ of smell, it has two functions: respiration and sense of smell.

Smell is not as sensitive in humans as in animals; evolution has decreased the importance of smell, as man has come to rely more on sight and

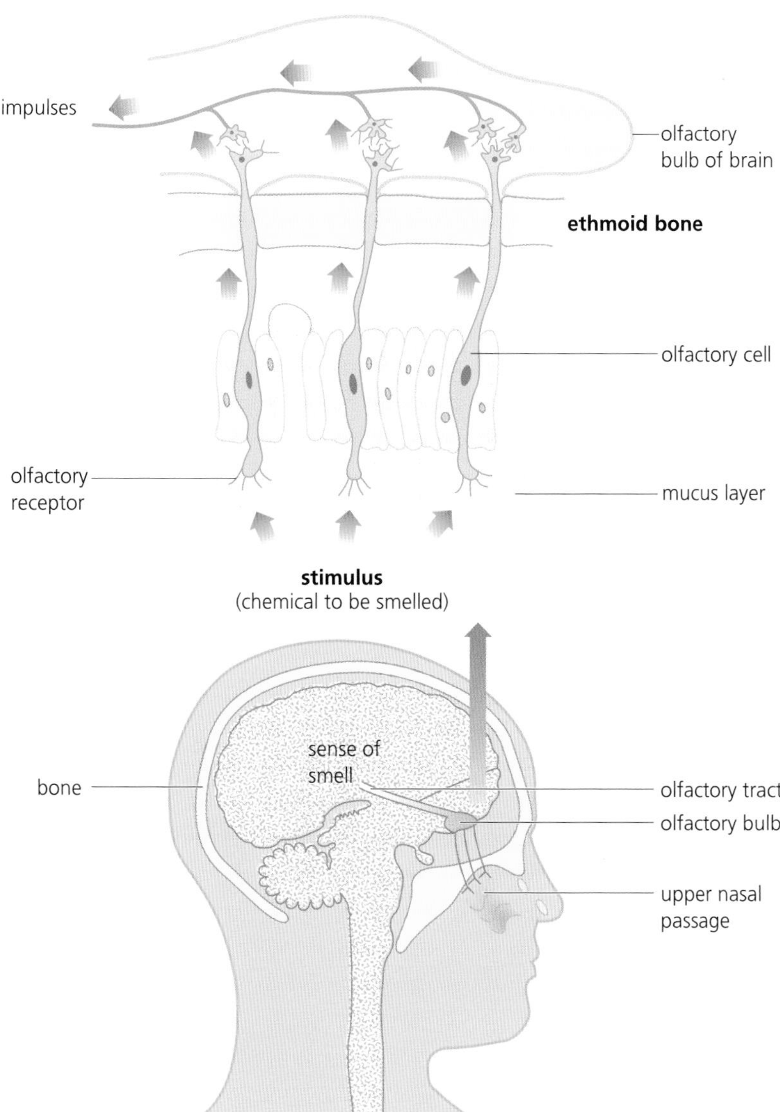

The position of the olfactory centre, and olfactory nerve and receptors

> **FACT**
>
> The **limbic system** is an area of the brain that deals with memory, moods, emotions, motivation and creativity. This area of the brain is very closely associated with the area that receives messages from the olfactory cells in the nose. This connection explains why smell is so evocative, and can instantly bring back very vivid memories. Within the spa sector, a client may use a retail product at home, and the smell can instantly take them back to the treatment they enjoyed on their last visit to the spa. The smell can ease stress and increase relaxation as it is so clearly associated in the client's mind with the spa treatment and the entire spa environment. This is very powerful, and an invaluable benefit for your retail recommendations.

hearing. The first cranial nerve is called the olfactory nerve because it is the sensory nerve responsible for the sense of smell. In the upper nasal passages, olfactory receptors are present, covered in a thin mucous. Certain chemicals dissolve in the mucous and stimulate the receptors of the sensory cells. Nerve fibres from the receptors group together to form the olfactory nerves, which then pass through the ethmoid bone into the olfactory bulbs. These bulbs are located below the frontal lobes of the cerebrum.

Touch

The brain is constantly fed a stream of information about the sensations of touch, pressure and temperature. These stimuli originate in the skin, which is the body's main contact with the external environment. The skin has very sensitive sensory equipment, so that all physical sensations can be detected.

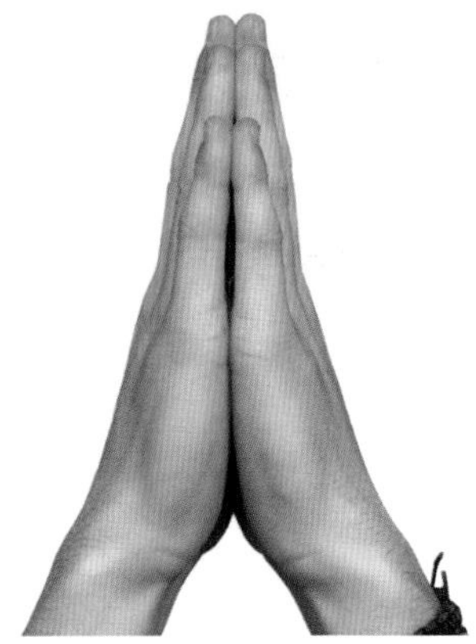

Sensitivity to a stimulus is not uniform all over the body. Sometimes receptive fields overlap and boost the level of sensation. For example, there are more touch receptors on the tongue and fingertips than on the back. Many receptors adapt to unimportant stimuli; for example, we do not continuously feel the shoes on our feet.

The various stimuli are converted to nerve impulses and travel via the spinal cord to an area in the brain known as the thalmus. It groups together impulses of the same nature and transmits this to the sensory cortex, which analyses the sensations.

Touch

Sensation	*Description*
Pressure/touch	Pressure receptors are known as Pancian corpuscles. They are mainly found in the dermis of the skin, and also respond to stretch and vibration. They are distributed over the body, and are abundant in hairless areas, such as the palms and soles
Heat/cold	Two kinds of skin receptors specialize in thermal changes. The Kraus end bulbs respond to cold, and Ruffini corpuscles react to heat
Pain	Pain can be both physical and psychological. Physiologically it originates from sensory receptors all over the body. However, psychological and cultural attitudes can override the most powerful pain stimuli
Itch	Mild stimulation of the pain receptor
Tickle	Light agitation of touch receptors
Vibration	Felt via pressure receptors

Assessment of knowledge and understanding

When you have some free time, test your understanding and knowledge by answering the following questions. Do this at regular intervals and it will reinforce your learning and help you retain the knowledge, so you are able to perform better in your assessments.

Bones and joints

1 What does lateral mean?
2 What is the axial skeleton made up of?
3 How many lumbar vertebrae are there?

Muscular system

1 Describe muscular fatigue?
2 What is the action of the occipito-frontalis muscle?
3 What is the name of the muscle on the posterior aspect of the upper arm?

Cardiovascular system

1 List the four main functions of blood.
2 Describe three difference between a vein and an artery.
3 Which artery supplies the muscles and tissues of the face?

Lymphatic system

1 List three functions of the lymphatic system.
2 Name the lymph nodes in the armpit?
3 Name three lymph organs.

Digestive system

1 List the four stages of digestion.
2 What is peristalsis?
3 Name the finger-like projections that are found on the lining of the small intestine.

Respiratory system

1 Describe three functions of the respiratory system.
2 What is a bronchiole?
3 What is the name of the muscles that lie between the ribs?

Nervous system

1 What does the central nervous system consist of?
2 What is the name of the 7th cranial nerve?
3 List three things that the autonomic nervous system regulates?

Urinary system

1 List three functions of the urinary system.
2 List the four parts of the urinary system
3 What is the function of the kidneys?

Endocrine system

1 List three functions of the endocrine system.
2 What hormone does the thyroid gland secrete?
3 List the two hormones produced by the ovaries.

Reproductive system

1 What is the function of the testes?
2 What is the function of the ovaries?
3 What is amenorrhoea?

Cells and tissues

1 What is the function of connective tissue, and give an example.
2 What characteristics does muscular tissue have? Give three examples.
3 What is mitosis?

Skin

1 List four functions of skin.
2 List the five layers of the epidermis.
3 Describe the two types of sweat glands

The five senses

1 What is the function of the conjunctiva of the eye?
2 List the three parts of the ear.
3 List the four basic sensations that your taste buds can detect
4 Which sensory nerve is responsible of the sense of smell?

SPA PROFILE

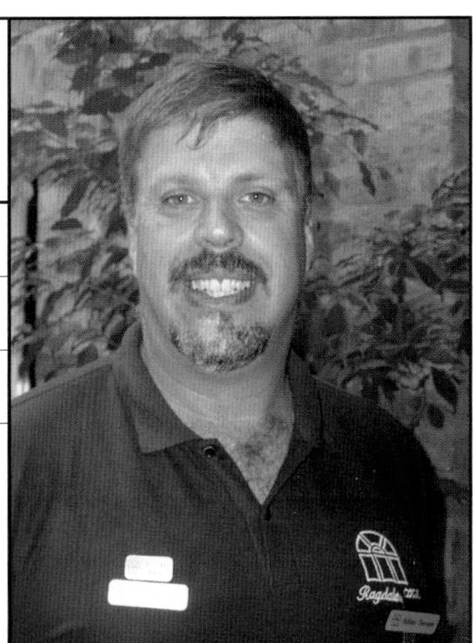

Name: David Pike

Position: Senior Holistic Therapist

Establishment: Ragdale Hall Health Hydro, Leicestershire

Training/experience: Completed 2 years at Midlands School of Massage and then went on to do an Osteopathy Degree at Oxford Brooks University. Worked for himself doing remedial massage and for an Osteopath for 2 years. Has now worked at Ragdale for 5 years in which time he has been trained to carry out La Stone Therapy and has helped to develop Wave Translator treatments, Chirotherapy and Reiki further. David started off at Ragdale as a massage therapist and has worked his way up to Senior Holistic Therapist.

Treatments carried out: La Stone Therapy, Reiki, Chirotherapy, Chakra Journey on Wave Translator (Sound Massage Bed)

Main responsibilities: To treat guests, work as a team member, guide junior therapists and provide motivation and encouragement (he calls it bear hugs!).

Best parts of the job: 'Working with the guests and helping them to relax. Making a difference to people's lives. Supporting other therapists in the salon.'

Secrets of a successful Spa Therapist: 'To know what your customer wants/needs and act on that. Being in tune with people and bringing the best out of people. Experience of life. Being empathetic towards clients. Going that extra mile.'

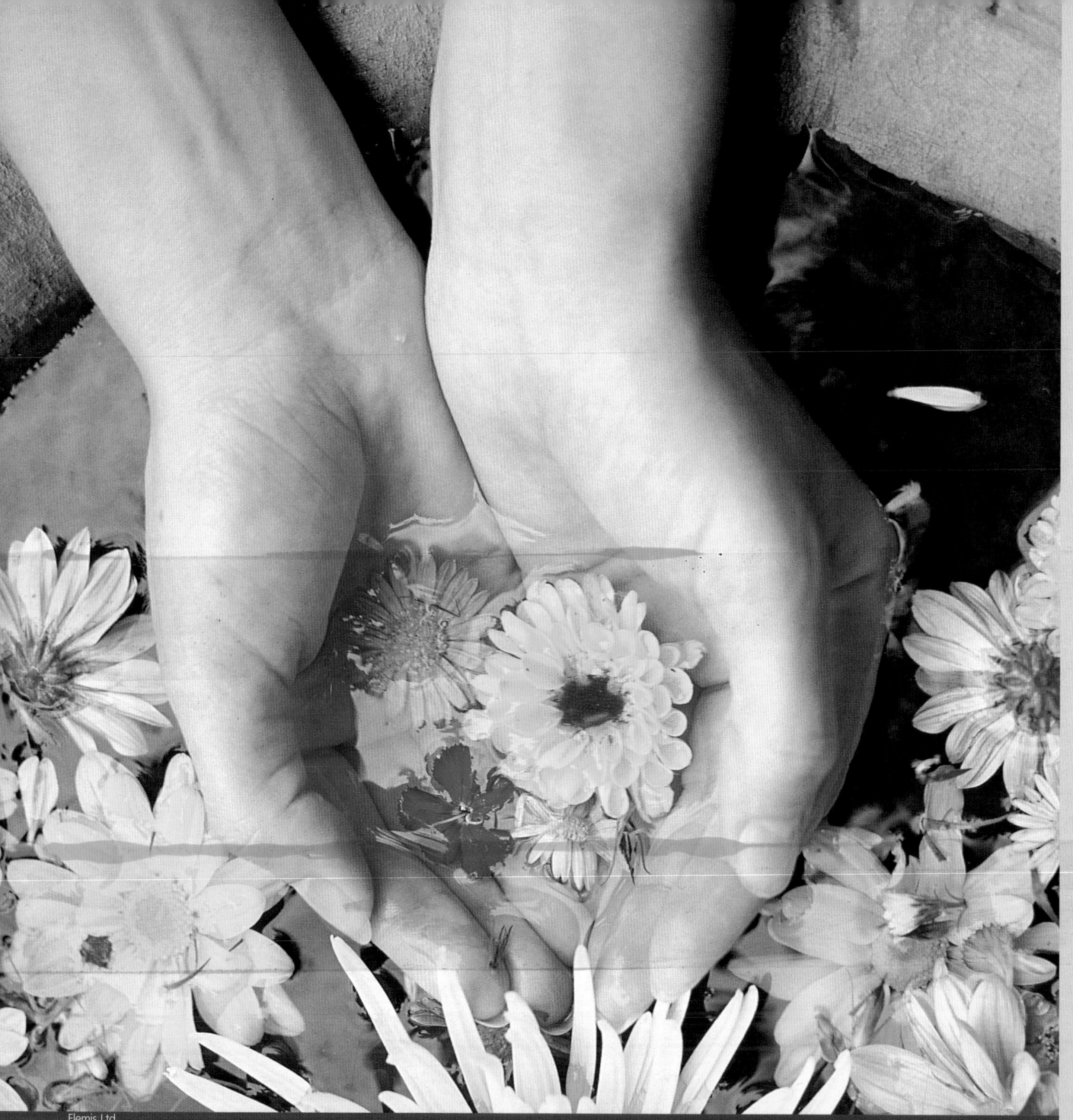

Elemis Ltd

The spa industry now greets a ***much wider audience****. It embraces a variety of cultural therapies, demanding that we meet the client's* ***expectation of quality****, taking them* ***on a journey*** *of touch, experience, knowledge and great results, all delivered in a* ***beautiful, luxurious****, almost like 'coming home',* ***non-intimidating*** *and* ***unisex*** *environment. What more does any therapist want as the spa industry presents them with the* ***perfect playground*** *to learn, to create, to be innovative and to use their education to its highest level.*

NOELLA GABRIEL, DIRECTOR OF TREATMENT AND PRODUCT DEVELOPMENT, ELEMIS

4 SENSATION

Whatever the treatment, whatever the product, the unique culture of spa and wellbeing is helping the populace to take time out, count the daisies and rejuvenate. Spas are where 'magic' happens; this is where time has no place, this is where one's mind, body and soul receives nurturing, solace and tranquillity; this is where one can experience the wonder of one's own moment in time.

CAROL FLEMING – EXCLUSIVE SPAS AUSTRALIA, OWNER/OPERATOR OF THE SEBEL REEF HOUSE SPA, PALM COVE, QUEENSLAND, AUSTRALIA

The spa industry is a young and fast growing industry with lots of new ideas, changes and development – this brings a lot of variety to the role. I enjoy cooperating with people: to have personal contact with our guests, and leading my spa team gives me a good feeling every day. We are doing something positive: the guests are leaving us in a better shape, better mood and better spirit than they arrived. What could you imagine to do more satisfying?

JUERG SCHUEPBACH, SPA DIRECTOR, VICTORIA-JUNGFRAU GRAND HOTEL & SPA, SWITZERLAND

chapter 7

Heat treatments

BT29

Provide specialist spa treatments

BT15

Assist with spa treatments

Learning objectives

This unit covers the skills a spa therapist needs to provide heat treatments.

It describes the skills and knowledge necessary to enable you to:

- **prepare, clean and maintain the spa environment**
- **consult with and prepare the client for treatment**
- **monitor the heat treatments**
- **provide aftercare advice**

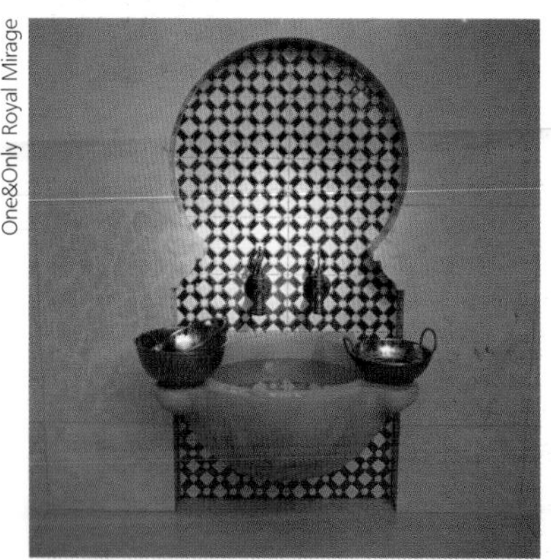

One&Only Royal Mirage

Basin in a hammam

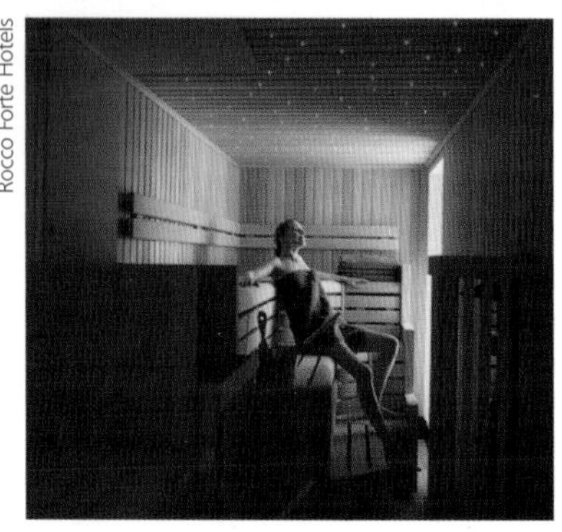

Rocco Forte Hotels

Heat treatment

When providing heat treatments it is important to use the skills you have learnt in the following core units:

G1 Ensure your own actions reduce risks to health and safety

G6 Promote additional products or services to clients

G11 Contribute to the financial effectiveness of the business

INTRODUCTION

There are many different types of heat treatments on offer in spas. They may be used as a stand-alone treatment, or often to enhance the benefits of other treatments, such as massage. The larger spas may offer the full range of heat treatments, whilst a smaller day spa with restricted space could decide to just concentrate on an individual steam bath.

The more popular heat treatments include:

- sauna baths
- steam baths
- infra-red
- spa baths/whirlpool baths
- foam/aerated baths.

This chapter focuses on the main heat treatments. Water-based treatments, such as the whirlpool baths, are covered in detail in chapter 9.

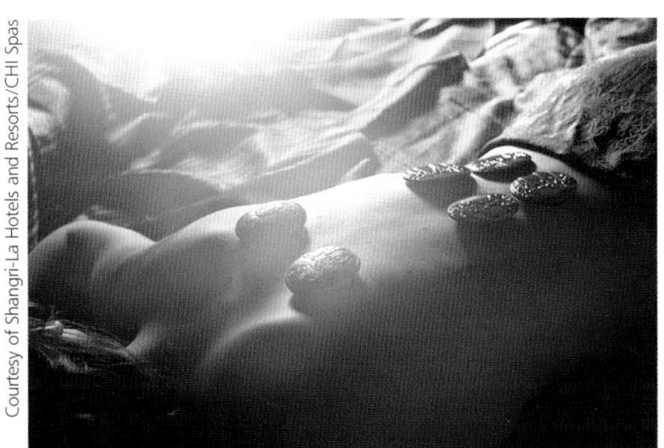
Courtesy of Shangri-La Hotels and Resorts/CHI Spas

Heat can relax tense, tight muscles

SPA TIP 

When purchasing heat equipment, consider the space you have available, the treatments you want to offer, your clientele and whether you have shower facilities. A **sauna** is a large investment, and needs quite a lot of space, so do your research first and then you will not make any costly mistakes.

FACT

During a heat treatment the body temperature can rise by 1–2 °C.

GENERAL EFFECTS OF HEAT ON THE BODY

Heat treatments raise the body temperature and have a wide range of effects:

- Blood circulation is increased, the temperature of the body is raised.
- Superficial capillaries dilate in an attempt to cool the body. This vasodilation means an increase in the blood flow to the area, nourishing every cell.
- Hyperaemia is produced, the skin reddens and warms. The overall skin colour can be improved.
- Blood pressure is lowered as a result of the vasodilation.
- The increased body temperature causes an increase in the heart rate and the pulse rate quickens.
- Lymphatic circulation increases, speeding up the removal of waste products and toxins.
- Sensory nerve endings are soothed, and the client feels relaxed.
- Tense, tight muscles relax. After exercise, heat treatments can prevent a build-up of the lactic acid which causes stiffness.
- Sudoriferous glands are stimulated, and produce more sweat as a means of cooling the body. Waste products are removed, which has a skin cleansing action.
- Sebaceous glands are stimulated and produce more sebum, which helps to keep the skin soft and supple.
- Metabolism increases slightly, and a feeling of wellbeing is produced. Clients often feel glowing, clean and invigorated after treatments such as saunas and steam baths.

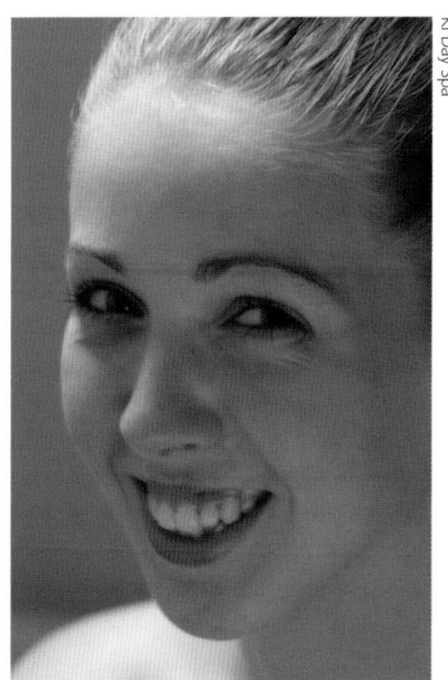
Ki Day Spa

Clients feel glowing, clean and invigorated after a heat treatment

USES OF HEAT TREATMENTS

Heat can be used in a variety of ways and for many reasons:

- To relax a stressed, anxious client.
- To relax tense, tight muscles before a body massage. The heat will start the relaxation process, and the massage is then more effective.

SPA TIP 

If you do not have access to a heat treatment in the spa, advise the client to take a warm shower as this will be very relaxing and help enhance the treatments that follow.

FACT

Lactic acid is a by-product of metabolism. This can cause stiffness in muscles after exercise. Heat treatment and massage can help relieve stiffness and relax tense and tight muscles.

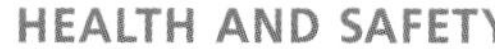

HEALTH AND SAFETY

Blood shunting is where the body directs blood to the area it is most needed; e.g. after a meal, blood is 'shunted' towards the organs of digestion. Care should be taken when giving heat treatments, as the blood is 'shunted' away from other organs and is directed to the skin to regulate body temperature. This could lead to problems with digestion if a client has a heat treatment immediately after eating.

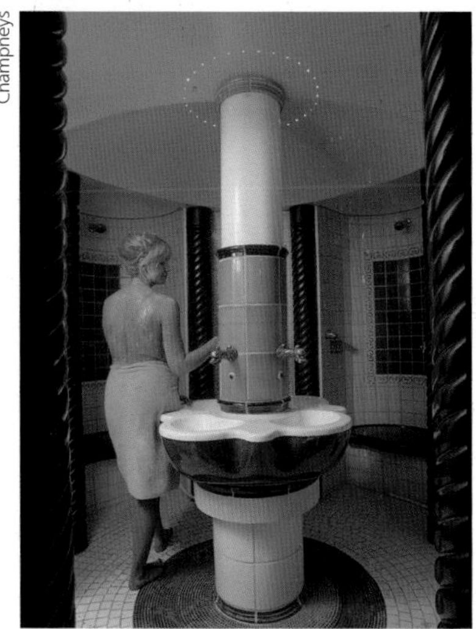

Champneys

Heat treatments can be deep cleansing and detoxifying, clients feel the body has been purified and cleansed of impurities

- To soften the tissues so they are more receptive to other treatments, such as G5 or body massage.
- After exercise to help prevent the build-up of lactic acid in muscles.
- Can be part of a 'client package/journey' to give a general sense of wellbeing.
- Deep cleansing and de-toxifying, clients feel the body has been purified and cleansed of impurities.

CONSULTATION

As outlined in chapter 15, a full consultation should be carried out to make sure the treatment is safe and effective and every stage of the consultation checklist should be checked prior to treatment.

RECEPTION

Heat treatments are usually combined with at least one other treatment and the receptionist should be aware of bookings so that the facility is not overbooked and clients are not left disappointed. The length of a heat treatment will depend on your consultation with the client and their individual needs. The first treatment is always short, maybe only 5 minutes, so that the client can get used to it gradually and any adverse reactions can be monitored.

CONSULTATION CHECKLIST

Heat treatments

- Quiet private area
- Client privacy
- Plenty of time
- Client comfortable and at ease
- Aims of treatment/outcome
- Treatment plan
- Postural check
- Fill in record card
- Client signed record card
- Check contra-indications
- Skin/sensitivity tests
- Explain contra-actions
- Client questions

TERMINOLOGY

Humidity refers to the amount of moisture in the air.

Relative humidity is the measurement of moisture content as a percentage of the maximum it can hold at that temperature. The maximum capacity of moisture in the air is 100%. Dry heat treatments such as saunas have a low humidity, often as low as 10%. Whereas wet heat treatments like steam baths have high humidity, often as high as 90%. Humidity is measured by a hygrometer.

Treatment	*Average treatment length*	*Frequency*
Sauna	15–20 mins	2–3 times per week
Steam bath	10–15 mins	2–3 times per week

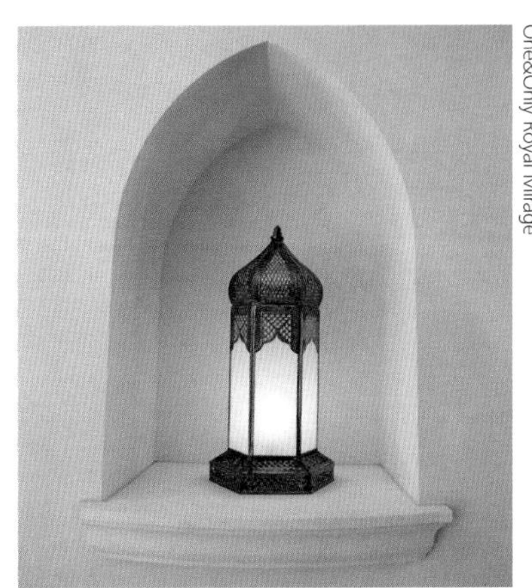
One&Only Royal Mirage

Comparison of temperatures and humidity levels

Heat treatment	*Approximate temperature °C*	*Approximate humidity (%)*
Dry heat		
Finnish sauna	70–100	10
Aromatic herb bath	60	15
Laconium sauna	45–60	15–20
Moist heat		
Steam bath	55	90
Caldarium	40–45	Variable
Turkish hammam	60–80	Variable
Rasul	42	Variable
Serail mud chamber	35–45	Variable
Japanese salt room	45–48	variable

CONTRA-INDICATIONS

The therapist must be aware of all the contra-indications to heat treatment, so that the treatment is carried out with full regard for the client's safety and wellbeing. The following conditions prevent the client from having a heat treatment:

- pregnancy
- recent scar tissue
- under the influence of alcohol or drugs
- first 2 days of menstruation
- after a heavy meal
- severe exhaustion
- severe bruising
- hepatitis
- migraine.

The following conditions are also contra-indicated, but the client can seek medical advice so their doctor can give permission for treatment to go ahead:

- high or low blood pressure
- cardiovascular conditions
- respiratory conditions

TERMINOLOGY

Contra-indication is a condition of the body that prevents a treatment from being carried out.

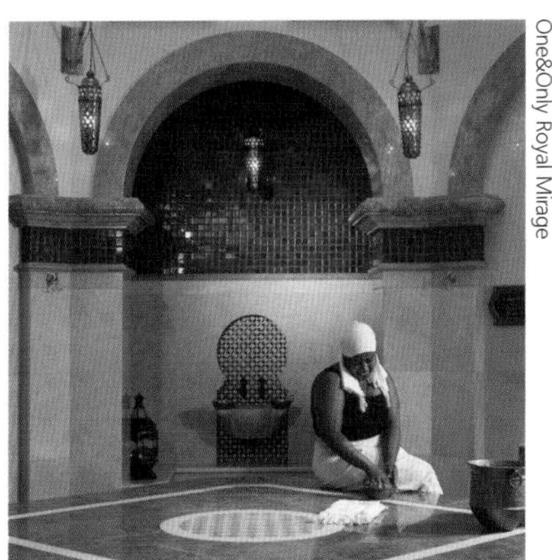
One&Only Royal Mirage

Ensure you check all contra-indications so that it is safe for the client to have the heat treatment

- diabetes
- liver/kidney/pancreatic disorders
- psoriosis
- viral conditions, e.g. verruca
- bacterial conditions, e.g. impetigo
- fungal conditions, e.g. tinea
- contagious diseases.

SIGNATURE TREATMENT S

Champneys Health Resorts

'Wax Bath: Give yourself a treat and experience a Champneys Henlow Wax Bath. Warm paraffin wax is whisked and applied all over the body, blankets are wrapped around you to retain temperature and body heat. As you relax, the wax will soften dead skin cells and help draw out excess fluid, the result is softer, smoother and conditioned skin.'

SAUNA

The sauna is a dry heat treatment and the main types include:

- traditional Finnish or Tyrolean sauna
- laconium sauna

Effects of sauna

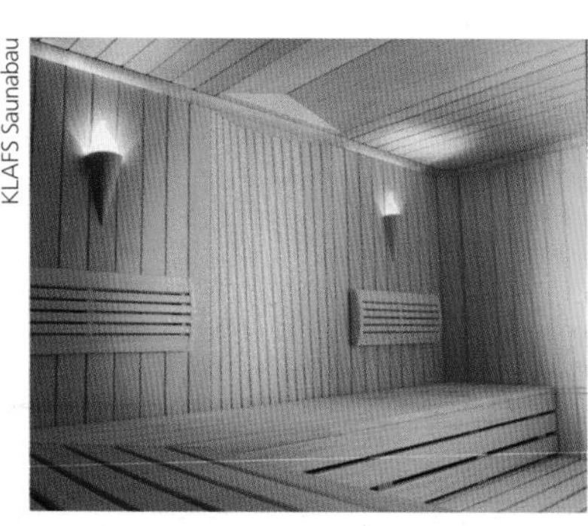

KLAFS Saunabau

Saunas need careful preparation

- Temperature of the body rises.
- The metabolic rate is slightly increased.
- Blood pressure drops slightly (by 10–15 per cent), the pulse rate quickens to compensate.
- Increased blood and lymphatic circulation. A hyperaemia (reddening) is produced, leading to increased nourishment and a healthy pink glow.
- Sudoriferous (sweat) glands are stimulated. Pores are opened and sweating occurs, removing waste products and generally cleansing the body.
- Slight increase in the activity of the sebaceous glands.
- Mental and physical relaxation. Very soothing effect of heat on the nerve endings. The muscles are warmed and relaxed.
- A feeling of invigoration and refreshment – 'wellbeing'.

EQUIPMENT LIST

- sauna bath
- ventilation
- shower
- shower products
- water in wooden bucket, with wooden ladle
- record cards
- towels
- bath robes
- disposable footwear/flip flops

Preparation of the sauna and treatment area

- Switch the sauna on, select the temperature (70–100 °C for a Finnish sauna, 55 °C for a laconium sauna) and allow to heat up for at least 45 minutes.
- Fill a wooden bucket with water.
- Place clean towels on the wooden benches and on the wooden duckboards in the sauna and leading to the shower.
- The shower should be checked to ensure it is disinfected, has shower products (no soap on the floor!) and the temperature is easy to control.
- Make sure air vents are open.
- Provide plenty of clean towels and an empty laundry/linen basket.

Preparation of the client

During the consultation, the spa therapist must follow all of the general steps described in chapter 15 and, in particular for a heat treatment, be sure to:

- Fill in the record card and check for contra-indications.
- Explain the treatment, effects and sensations. Encourage the client to ask questions so they are fully briefed and are not nervous.
- Carry out the thermal skin sensation test to check that the client is sensitive to heat, otherwise they could burn and would not be aware.
- The client removes all clothing. A dressing gown, disposable slippers and paper briefs can be provided.
- The client must remove jewellery, contact lenses and spectacles. A locker should be provided for personal possessions.
- The client showers prior to heat treatment to make sure products such as deodorant and perfumed body lotion are removed. Prepare the shower so that it is at the correct temperature before the client enters.

HEALTH AND SAFETY !

Thermal sensitivity test Two test tubes are used, one filled with hot water and one with cold water. The client closes their eyes, and, at random, the therapist places the test tubes on the skin. The client has to distinguish which is hot and which cold. If the client cannot tell the difference, the treatment is contra-indicated.

Treatment procedure

- Check the temperature (thermometer) and humidity (hygrometer) of the sauna.
- Client enters sauna, and is advised that it is wise to start by using the cooler lower benches.
- Constantly monitor the client's progress, stay within the area and make regular checks through the glass in the sauna door.
- After 10 minutes, escort the client to the shower. The shower will cool the body and remove perspiration.
- If it is not the client's first treatment, they return to the sauna for a further 10 minutes and then shower again. This can be repeated at intervals, with a normal treatment time lasting approximately 20 minutes.
- The client finishes the treatment with a final shower.
- To ensure the body cools and returns to normal, the client must rest for at least 15–20 minutes and have a drink of water. It may be that they are having a **linked treatment**, such as a massage, and this encompasses the rest period.

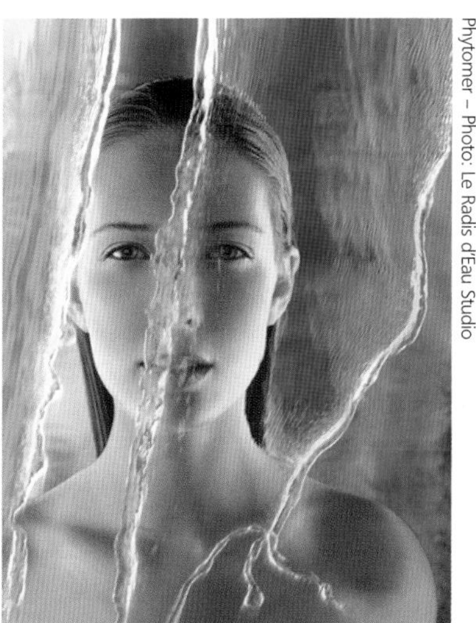

Phytomer – Photo: Le Radis d'Eau Studio

The sauna treatment finishes with a shower

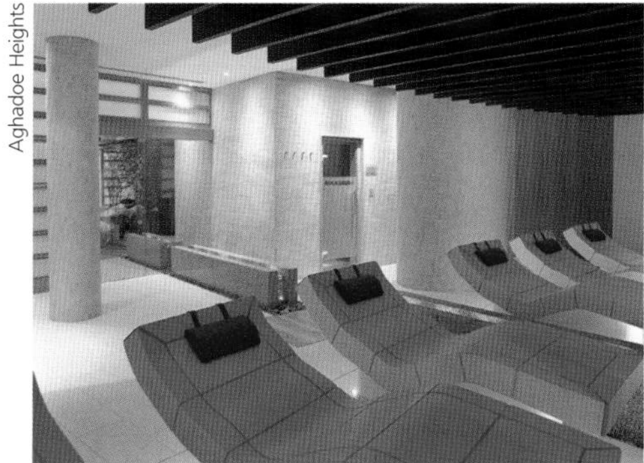

Aghadoe Heights

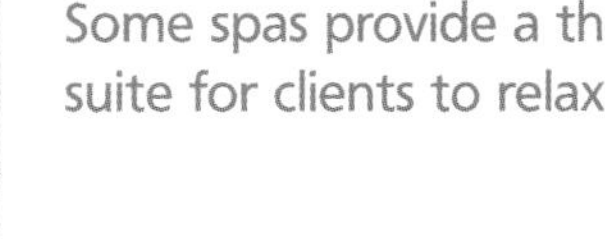

Some spas provide a thermal suite for clients to relax in

HEALTH AND SAFETY

The client's pulse can be taken before and after the sauna treatment, to ensure it is initially normal and returns to normal afterwards.

ACTIVITY

Make a list of all the precautions for a sauna bath treatment, and alongside each precaution list the danger and the reason why it is necessary.

HEALTH AND SAFETY

Always explain to the client that if at any time in the sauna they feel faint they must inform the therapist. For this reason they must never be left unattended.

FACT

Traditionally in Scandinavian countries, sauna users would tap their skin with supple and flexible birchwood twigs to increase the blood circulation.

FACT

Pine wood is ideal for the construction of saunas as it can breathe (exchange of oxygen through the wood) and is a 'low sap' variety that does not warp when heated. The wood needs to be capable of removing all the moisture from within the bath so the air does not become stale or unhygienic, with an unpleasant smell. The natural essence of pine also adds an authentic aroma to the treatment.

ACTIVITY

Make a list of all the differences between a sauna bath and a steam bath treatment.

- Fill in the record card with details of the treatment (time, temperature, etc.).
- Provide aftercare advice.

General precautions

- Fully explain the 'sauna routine', including how to put water on the coals at arms length to avoid scalds.
- Explain to the client that the lower benches are cooler, and it is recommended that they start the treatment on these.
- To avoid slipping, wooden duckboards can be placed on the floor of the sauna and en route to the shower.
- Make sure the air vents are open to ensure good ventilation.
- To ensure the treatment is hygienic, regularly scrub and disinfect using products recommended by the manufacturer.
- The client should wear disposable footwear to prevent the spread of contagious conditions, e.g. verrucas. A footbath can also be provided to avoid cross-infection.
- Leave the door open at the end of the working day, so fresh air can circulate and stale odours are avoided.

Traditional Finnish or Tyrolean sauna

A sauna bath has been established in Finland for over 1000 years. The sauna may be in a separate building, or installed within a room. Traditionally in Scandinavian countries, a pine log sauna is located near a lake. This makes it easy to take a plunge in the icy-cold lake at frequent intervals during the sauna. Today's sauna baths are based on the Finnish model of log cabins heated by stoves to produce dry heat effects.

The sauna is made from solid wood (usually pine wood) or panels of wood packed with insulated material to contain more of the heat within the bath.

Sâmas

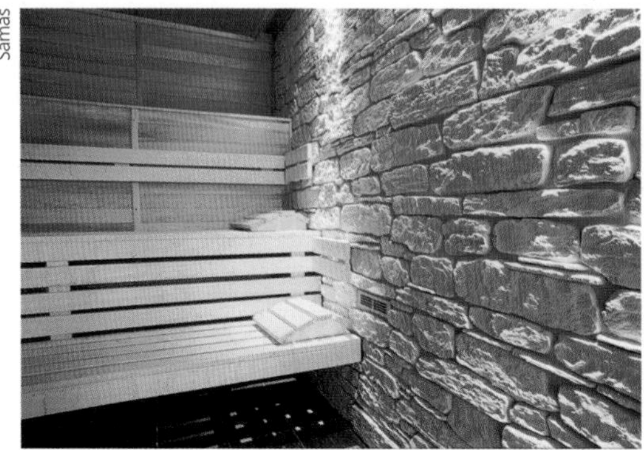

A sauna

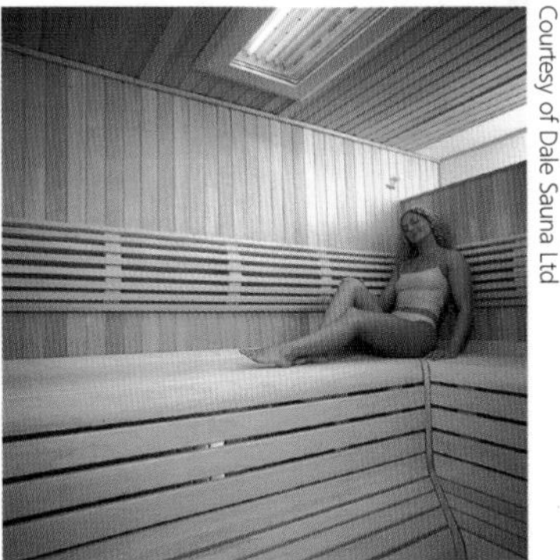

Courtesy of Dale Sauna Ltd

A traditional pine sauna

In a sauna there are flat wooden benches at different levels on which the client relaxes. Clients often start on the cooler lower benches and gradually move to the higher ones as they get used to the heat. An electric stove heats coals or rocks to give off heat, and water can be poured on to the rocks to increase the humidity level. The temperature ranges between 70 and 100 °C, depending on the client's preference.

The humidity level is low, sometimes as low as 10 per cent. The client can tolerate higher temperatures with 'dry' heat because the sweat can evaporate, therefore cooling the body down.

HEALTH AND SAFETY !

Saunas usually take at least 30 minutes to heat up. When at the correct temperature, it turns itself off (thermostatically controlled) but the heat increases as the temperature of the wood continues to increase and radiate back into the cabin, giving a build-up effect. For this reason, do not set the initial temperature too high.

Laconium sauna

This is a much cooler, gentler type of sauna, with the heat evenly distributed. Many clients will prefer this type as opposed to the often extreme heat in the traditional Finnish sauna. The relaxing atmosphere is further enhanced by aromatic essence to create a 'Roman sauna' atmosphere, as opposed to the Finnish pine wood environment. The average temperature is 55 °C, as opposed to a traditional sauna which is 70–100 °C. The laconium is heated usually by underfloor heating, and not by a stove. The cleansing effects are the same, but milder. Clients who cannot tolerate extreme heat or who have sensitive skin find the laconium sauna suits their needs.

HEALTH AND SAFETY !

Ensure there is sufficient space around a sauna for air to circulate. Usually, there are air vents (inlet) at floor and ceiling. There should be a constant air exchange in the sauna, at least 7–8 times each hour.

Aromatic herb bath

An 'aromatic herb bath' is a very mild sauna with low humidity, but with the addition of aromatic herbal steam. Periodically, water is released on to a tray of warm herbs (e.g. lavender, chamomile, rosemary). This produces a pleasant, fresh, alpine aroma that helps clients relax. This treatment can be used at the beginning or end of the spa experience, and a Kneipp hose can be provided to cool the client when necessary.

HEALTH AND SAFETY !

A **laconium sauna** can have a water fountain to make the atmosphere more pleasant and to prevent static air build up. Also, a Kneipp hose can be provided to cool the body down and refresh the client so they can stay in the laconium longer.

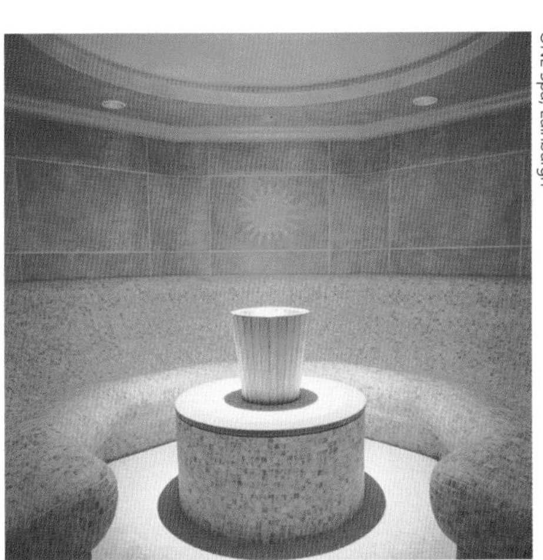

ONE Spa, Edinburgh

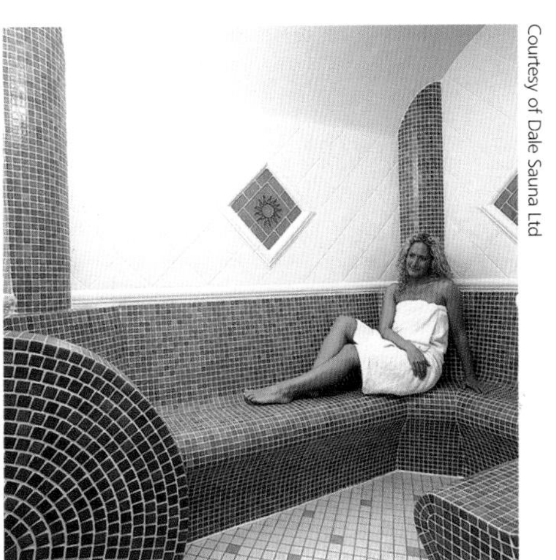

Courtesy of Dale Sauna Ltd

Laconium saunas

Courtesy of the Detox Box

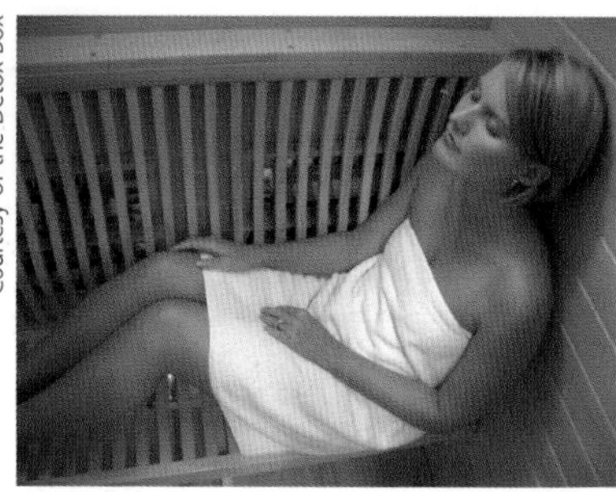

An infra-red sauna

Infra-red sauna

This type of sauna uses infra-red heat, and is less oppressive than a traditional sauna. The rays penetrate the body to a depth of 45 mm and stimulate deep tissues and organs. In addition, the heat can relax muscles, relieve pain and increase the metabolic rate, and the sweating cleanses the body and removes toxins. Colour therapy is used to enhance the treatment. The whole spectrum of light can be used with attendant benefits, e.g. red light increases energy and vitality, and blue/violet light reduces anxiety and stress.

SIGNATURE TREATMENT S

Aghadoe Heights, Ireland

'Up To Par Golfers: Begin your relaxation in the Thermal Suite where you have the opportunity to use our dry heat and wet cabins (rock sauna, laconium, hammam, serial, Irish mist and tropical rain showers, delunge shower, and heated loungers). Followed by a deep tissue massage targeting specific muscle groups. It warms and treats the muscles to give intense relaxation and relief of aches and pains associated with over strain tiredness. 2 hrs'

Vibratory sauna

A 'vibratory sauna' combines heat with vibration to enhance relaxation and is ideal for those who do not like heat on their faces (sensitive skin) or find it uncomfortable breathing in hot air. The client lies down in a long cabinet on a vibrating couch while the therapist controls the temperature, time and strength of vibration (the client themselves can also alter the temperature from inside). The personalized temperature makes this a very private treatment and is very effective at treating muscular aches and pains.

STEAM BATH

The steam bath originates from ancient Turkish baths or steam rooms and is one of the most popular forms of pre-heating the body in the spa.

The steam bath is usually constructed of fibre-glass or metal. The cabinet permits one person to sit comfortably with their head placed through the opening in the top. The height of the seat can be varied to suit the client. Metal baths are durable, but they get very hot and need a lot of towels to protect the client. Fibre-glass models are more attractive, are easier to clean and, as they do not get very hot, require fewer towels to protect the client.

Courtesy of Dale Sauna Ltd

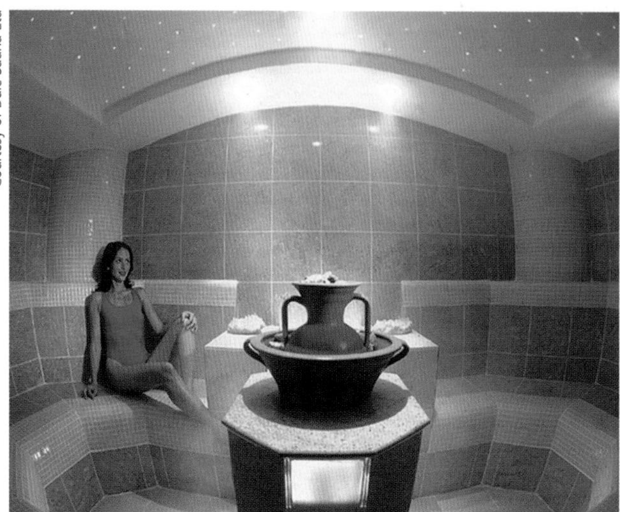

A steam room

The temperature in a steam bath ranges between 50 and 55 °C, depending on the client's preference. Steam is produced by an electrical element that heats water in a bath under the seat. This is controlled by a thermostat. The water tank should be rust-free, and the design of the bath usually includes protection for the legs. The steam should be able to circulate freely and not accumulate as this may scald the skin.

Effects of steam baths

- Temperature of the body rises.
- Slight increase in metabolic rate.
- Blood pressure drops slightly (10–15 per cent) and pulse rate quickens to compensate.
- Increase in lymphatic circulation, helps remove waste products and toxins.
- Increased blood and lymphatic circulation. A hyperaemia (reddening) is produced, leading to increased nourishment and a healthy pink glow.
- Increased activity of the sudoriferous (sweat) glands.
- Steam settles on the outer layer of the skin, softens the horny layer, dead skin is released. The skin is more easily desquamated.
- Mental and physical relaxation. Very soothing effect of heat on the nerve endings. Plus, the muscles are warmed and relaxed.
- A feeling of invigoration and refreshment – 'wellbeing'.

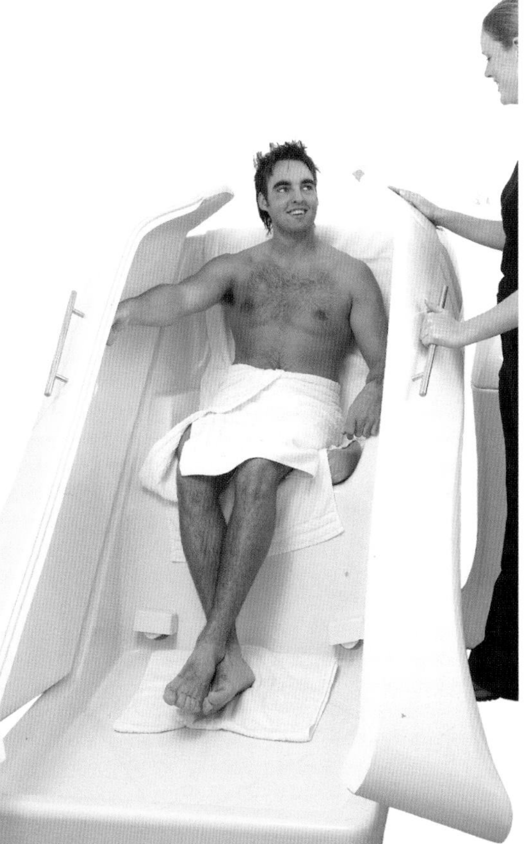

Courtesy of OxygenPowerProducts

Equipment is available that uses an automated system to enrich the steam with oxygen. 'Activated' oxygen is used, leaving the body clean, refreshed and with increased energy levels

SPA TIP 

When purchasing a steam bath, consider the size of the water bath as this depends on how frequently the bath will be used. A large water bath has capacity for 6–10 baths without needing to be refilled; this will save time.

SPA TIP 

Because the head is free from the heating effect, a steam bath is much better for clients with dry, sensitive skin on their faces as it is less likely than a sauna to cause dilated capillaries.

EQUIPMENT LIST

- steam bath or room
- ventilation
- distilled water
- shower
- shower products
- record cards
- towels
- bath robe
- disposable footwear/flip-flops

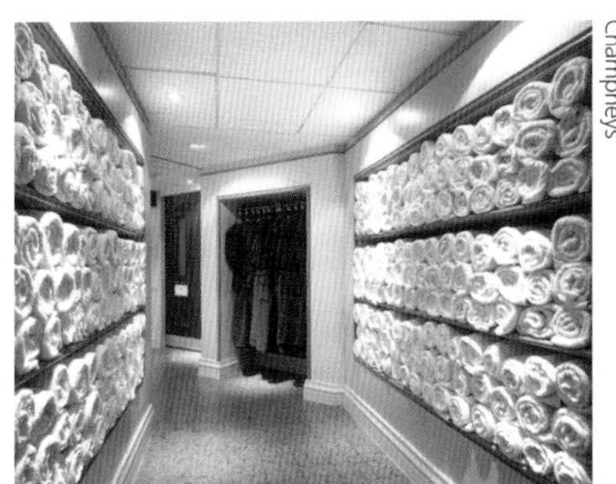

Champneys

A huge amount of robes and towels are needed when offering spa treatments

ACTIVITY

Make a list of everything you could do to make sure the steam bath is a truly relaxing, luxurious treatment.

ACTIVITY 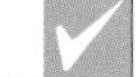

Some clients may be apprehensive before their first steam bath treatment. Make a list of the factors that will inspire confidence, e.g. a full explanation of the treatment.

HEALTH AND SAFETY 

If it is the client's first steam treatment, limit the treatment to 10 minutes. An average treatment is approx 15–20 minutes, with a maximum length of 30 minutes.

HEALTH AND SAFETY 

After the steam treatment the client's skin is sensitized and therefore they cannot have treatments such as infra-red, ultraviolet/tanning, waxing, etc.

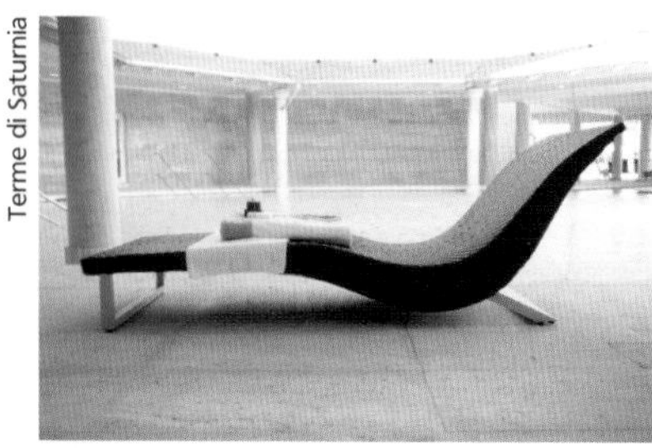

Terme di Saturnia

Provide an area for the client to relax after the steam treatment

Preparation of the steam bath and treatment area

- Disinfect the steam bath.
- Fill the water tank ⅔rds full of water. Hot water can be used to speed the heating process up.
- Place clean towels over the seat and floor.
- Place a towel over the opening of the steam bath to allow heat to build up inside.
- Plug the steam bath into the electricity mains socket and set the timer and temperature control.

Preparation of the client

See preparation for sauna bath.

Treatment procedure

- Check the temperature of the steam bath, and that it is thermostatically controlled.
- Client enters the steam bath. They can discreetly remove their towel or gown and pass it to the therapist. Tuck a towel around their neck to prevent steam escaping. Their shoulders can be protected with a towel, and ensure their hair is covered with a towel or cap.
- Stay with the client constantly in order to monitor their progress. Do not leave the client unattended, as they may panic thinking they cannot get out of the bath and become distressed.
- After 10 minutes, escort the client to the shower. The shower will cool the body and remove perspiration.
- If it is not the client's first treatment, they may return to the steam bath for a further 10 minutes and then shower again. This can be repeated at intervals, with a normal treatment time lasting approximately 15–20 minutes.
- The client finishes the treatment with a final shower.
- To ensure the body cools and returns to normal, the client must rest for at least 15–20 minutes and have a drink of water. It may be that

HEALTH AND SAFETY

Check that the steam bath is:

- maintained well and serviced regularly
- take all general electrical precautions
- follow the manufacturer's instructions
- clean and disinfect the steam bath before every client
- make sure the water bath is ⅔rd full, check during treatment that the water is not getting too low
- fresh, clean towels on the seat, floor
- check the thermostat is working, and the temperature is suitable for the client.

they are having a **linked treatment**, such as a massage, and this encompasses the rest period.

- Fill in the record card with details of the treatment (time, temperature, etc.)
- Provide aftercare advice.

General precautions

- Fully explain the 'steam bath routine'. Explain that they are not trapped inside the bath. To avoid feelings of claustrophobia, show the client how easily the door opens.
- To avoid slipping, wooden duckboards can be placed on the route from the steam bath to the shower.
- To ensure the treatment is hygienic, clean and disinfect before each client, using products recommended by the manufacturer.
- The client should wear disposable footwear to prevent the spread of contagious conditions, e.g. verrucas. A footbath can also be provided to avoid cross-infection.
- Leave the door of the steam bath open at the end of the working day, so fresh air can circulate and stale odours are avoided.

STEAM ROOM

Steam rooms originate from the Turkish baths of many thousands of years ago. Turkish baths usually consist of a series of rooms filled with steam, all at different temperatures. Rooms are entered from the coolest to the hottest, and then slowly back through to the coolest room again. Cold plunge pools can be situated at various stages.

In spas, rather than having small steam baths, it is more efficient and effective to provide one large steam room. A hidden boiler produces the steam which is then directed into the room by tubes or pipes. The water vapour (steam) circulates inside the steam room, and ventilation is important to ensure the environment is pleasant and not too hot and uncomfortable.

The main types of steam treatment include:

- steam bath/cabinet
- caldarium and tepidarium
- rasul

Caldarium

This is an 'aromatic' steam room. Herbal or aromatic essences are added to the steam for therapeutic benefits, e.g. rose, jasmine or lavender. In some caldariums, light and sound effects can be used to enhance the relaxing effect of the treatment. A Kneipp hose can be provided so the client can cool down throughout the treatment.

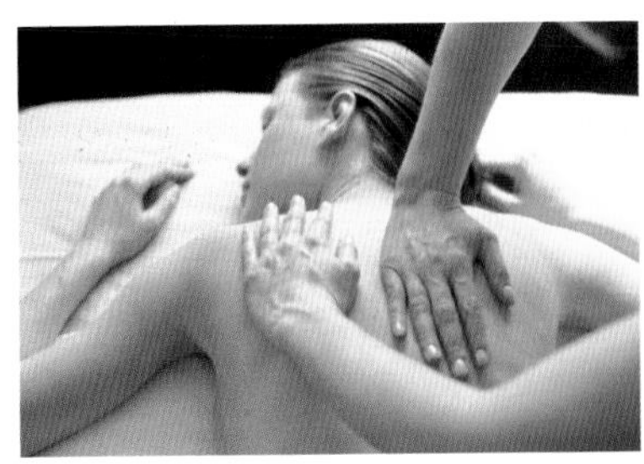

Terme di Saturnia

Massage is an ideal 'linked treatment following a steam bath'

ACTIVITY

Make a list of all the precautions for a steam bath treatment, and alongside each precaution list the danger and the reason why the precaution is necessary.

HEALTH AND SAFETY

Make sure the shower is safe and hygienic:

- check the temperature before the client enters
- non-slip base to the shower
- wooden duckboards en route to the shower
- soap in a holder or dish
- clean, disinfected shower
- can provide a footbath facility.

HEALTH AND SAFETY

Do not add any essential oils or products to the water bath as this may lead to problems, such as spitting, which could scald the client.

FACT

1200 AD Britons discover **Turkish baths** during the Crusades. This may have led to the development of **sweat houses** in London.

FACT

80 AD The Romans associated personal hygiene with health, and the bathing ritual became the focus for their social life. Advanced facilities were built including **caldariums** (hot/steam baths), **tepidariums** (warm bath) and **frigidariums** (cold plunge pools).

SPA TIP

Steam cabins/cubicles are adaptions of the steam bath, often with aromatic oils used for various effects. The client sits within the cabinet, head included. Music or motivational tapes can be played to suit the client's requirements.

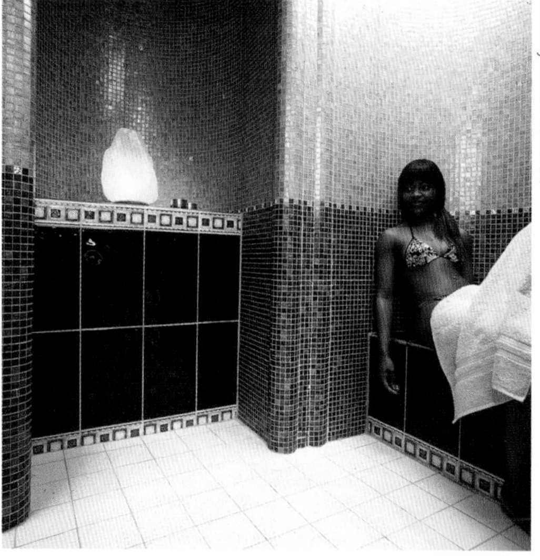
Courtesy of Dale Sauna Ltd

A caldarium

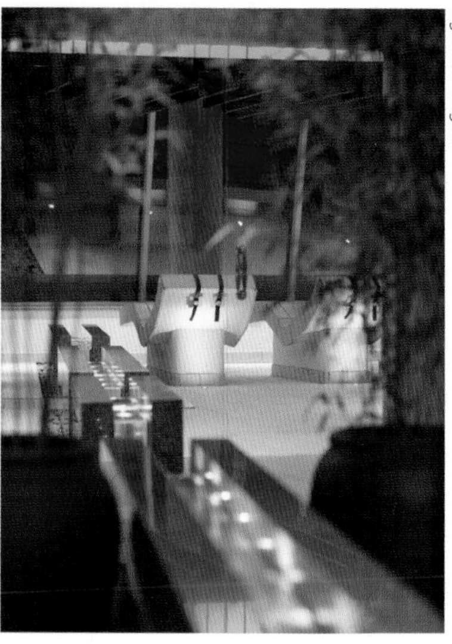
Aghadoe Heights

A thermal suite

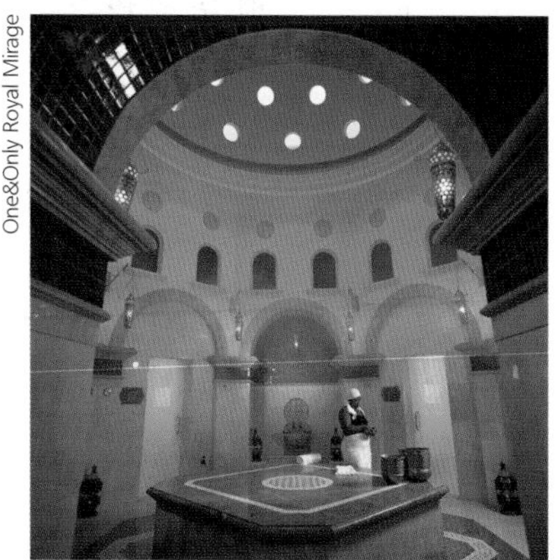
One&Only Royal Mirage

An oriental hammam

Tepidarium

A very mild steam room, that acts as a relaxation area. The body is kept warm to allow the client to relax after or between treatments. During this time, the body temperature, pulse and blood pressure slowly return to normal.

Hammam

Traditionally a 'bath house', often with a dome-shaped central chamber, with other rooms or chambers leading from it. It produces a hot, moist aromatic effect, with the hottest room having underfloor heating. In some hammams, light and sound effects are used to enhance the relaxing effect of the treatment. A Kneipp hose can be provided so the client can cool down throughout the treatment. The walls, floor and benches are usually tiled, often in a Roman or Turkish style.

Rasul

This is a treatment that combines herbal steam, mud and showers. The rasul is becoming increasingly popular. It is a treatment designed to:

- smooth the skin
- cleanse the respiratory system
- detoxify the body
- revitalize energy levels.

A tiled room, with heated walls and floor, is heated to approx 42 °C. Often the room has a planetarium ceiling, or night-time sky effect with stars. Herbs are used to produce a gentle aromatic steam effect. The client enters the rasul, and a dry heat is used to warm and relax the client. Next, the spa therapist will show the client how to apply the mud to their body. Chakra-balancing medicinal muds are applied to various parts of the body. The different coloured muds have healing properties and are unchanged since the days of the ancient Greeks. The mud manufacturer's instructions should be followed, but usually they are as follows:

- Bolus alpha – a creamy white medicinal mud for the face and sensitive areas of the body.
- Bolus beta – a yellow creamy medicinal mud with gentle peeling properties.
- Bolus delta – a blue medicinal mud that absorbs toxins and exfoliates.

Once the mud has been applied, the client relaxes in the dry heat. The mud starts to dry, and the client can massage the mud on their skin to help exfoliation and the detoxification effect of the mud. Then aromatic steam (lemon grass, lavender, etc.) is produced in the chamber, usually by controlled shots, and the temperature and humidity rise. The mud starts to liquify on the skin, which tingles as the mud begins to be absorbed. Finally, an automatic shower is activated, taking the form of a warm tropical rain shower. The client bathes in the shower, and washes away any excess mud; this helps exfoliation and stimulates the blood supply, leaving a glowing complexion.

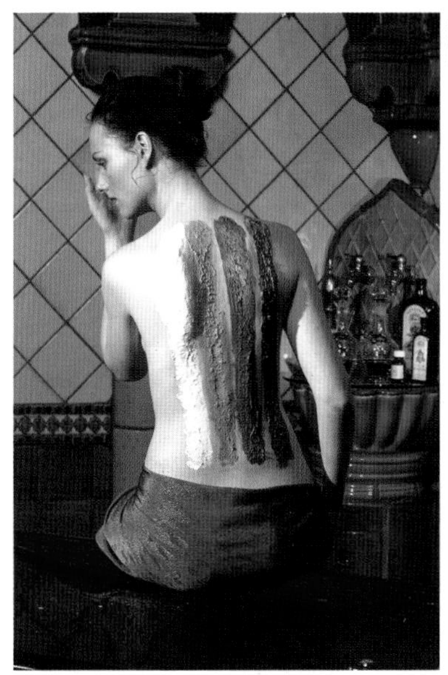
Kurland

The different types of rasul mud

Serail mud chamber

Similar to a rasul, the 'serail' is tiled with showers around the chamber, with seating and a central basin. The client enters the serail, and dry air warms the body. Therapeutic mud is applied to the body, and the client relaxes on the bench seats. After 15 minutes, herbal steam is released in the chamber, and the temperature reaches 45 °C. Once the mud has started to liquify, the client can massage the mud into the skin, helping to exfoliate and remove toxins. The body starts to perspire, and the client can either use a central basin or a Kneipp hose to refresh themselves. After 15 minutes, the herbal steam ceases, and the client can remove the mud using showers directed from above and then from the side. The client is advised to relax in the tepidarium/relaxation area after the treatment until the body has normalized.

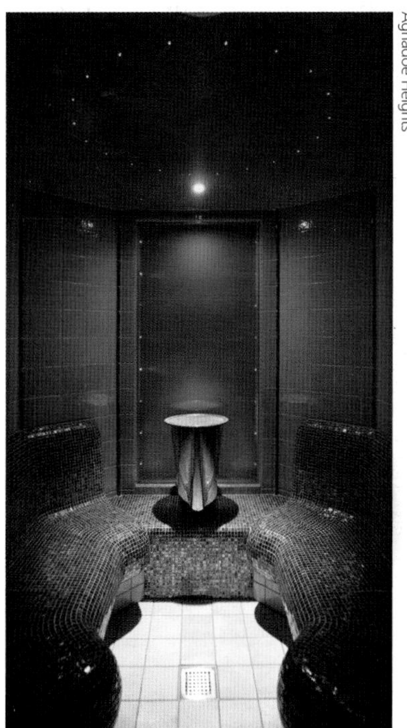
Aghadoe Heights

A serail mud chamber

Japanese salt room

A fully tiled chamber, with individual reclining seats/loungers with foot rests. Some salt rooms have a rose quartz crystal in the centre of the room. The temperature is approximately 45–48 °C and the treatment is recommend for 15–20 minutes. Steam, essential oils and salt combine to produce an atmosphere that resembles sea air. Essences, such as menthol, help sinus problems and improve breathing. The client must be advised to shower thoroughly after this treatment, so any remaining salt does not dry the skin or cause irritation.

Kraxenstove

Alpine farmers discovered that hay produces a spicy herbal aroma when placed in a farmhouse stove. The treatment is very relaxing, and can help dilate arteries

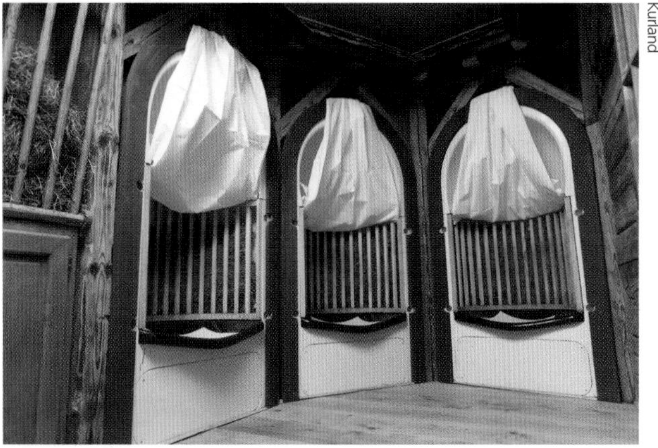
Kurland

Kraxenstove

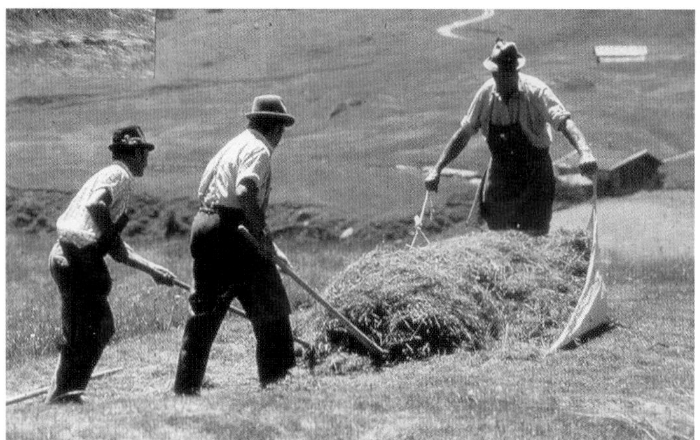
Kurland

Hay is used in a kraxenstove

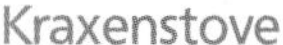

and lower blood pressure. With this heat room, the aroma is not produced by concentrated essences but by real alpine hay. The hay, containing alpine flowers, is built into the backrests of the seats in the heat room. Steam is passed through the hay at intervals, and warms and relaxes the back muscles.

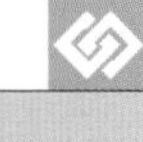

LINKED TREATMENTS

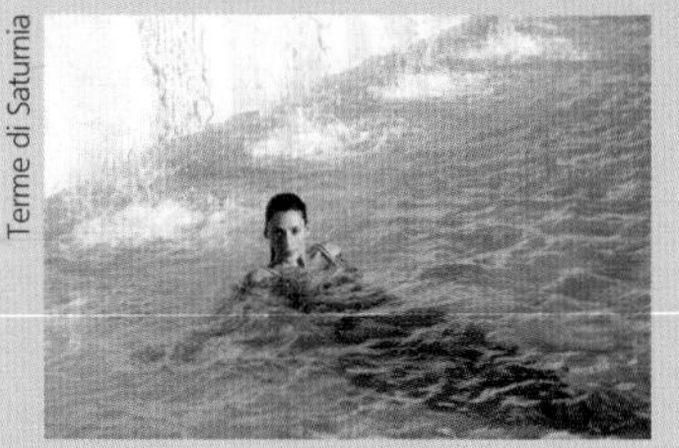
Terme di Saturnia

Water treatments link well with heat treatments

Heat treatments in a spa are one of the 'core' treatments, and can readily be combined with a huge range of other treatments, including:

- water treatments, e.g. spa pool, jet massage, flotation
- massage treatments, e.g. body massage, Indian head massage, massage with pre-blended oils, Thai massage, Balinese massage, remedial massage
- body envelopments, wraps, scrubs, exfoliation
- relaxation, e.g. sound therapy, tepidarium.

AFTERCARE AND TREATMENT ADVICE

At the end of the heat treatment, it is important that the client does not quickly get up and start getting dressed. Let the client relax, either in a relaxation room or on the treatment couch. Ensure it is not too cool.

Explain that they need to rest for at least 20–30 minutes, to allow the body temperature and blood pressure to return to normal. If they are too quick and rush, they may feel faint and dizzy, as the blood rushes from their head. After lying down and having a heat treatment, the body needs slowly to get used to being cool and upright again.

Whilst the client is resting, you have the opportunity to go through the aftercare and treatment advice. Offer the client a glass of water or fruit juice,

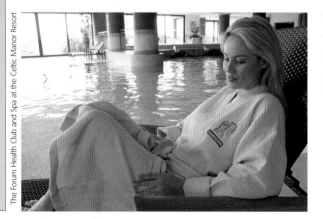
The Forum Health Club and Spa at the Celtic Manor Resort

The client needs to avoid further heat treatments, and must take it easy for a few hours after treatment

and advise them to drink plenty of water during the next few hours. The client must avoid further heat treatments, especially infra-red or ultraviolet, as the skin is sensitized.

Furthermore, to ensure they maximize the effectiveness of the treatment, advise the client to take it easy for a few hours after treatment, and avoid eating a heavy meal or drinking alcohol.

AFTERCARE AND TREATMENT ADVICE

After-treatment advice	✔ Shower ✔ Rest period 20–30 minutes ✔ Monitor reactions ✔ Drink water/fruit juice ✔ Avoid stimulants ✔ Avoid further radiation treatments, e.g. infra-red and ultraviolet/tanning
Products used during the treatment	✔ Explain details of products ✔ Homecare recommendation ✔ How to use the products ✔ Written prescription ✔ Additions – candles, body brush, eye mask, etc.
Contra-actions	✔ Explain possible reactions to heat ✔ Advise on recommended action
Posture	✔ Posture awareness ✔ Postural advice
Lifestyle pattern	✔ Dietary and fluid intake ✔ Exercise habits ✔ Smoking habits ✔ Sleep patterns ✔ Hobbies/interests ✔ Means of relaxation
Further heat treatment	✔ Benefits of continuing treatments ✔ Courses/financial incentives
Linked treatments	✔ Benefits of combining with other treatments, e.g. massage, water treatments, wraps
Frequency of treatments	✔ Recommended frequency and time intervals

LINKED PRODUCTS

Below is a list of products, linked to **heat**, that should be available for the client to purchase in the spa:

- body wash/foam
- body scrub
- body brush
- loofah mitt
- body oil/cream
- available from reception: bath robes, slippers towels, eye masks, toilet bags, oil burners, candles, vitamins, etc.

CONTRA-ACTIONS

Feeling faint, nauseous

Low blood pressure and loss of water from the body can lead to dehydration. This may cause the client to feel faint or nauseous or get a headache. If the humidity is too low and the air is very dry, the client may find it difficult to breathe.

Action

- A drink of water should be given to rehydrate the body.
- The client should lie down and rest.
- A cool compress can be placed over the forehead.

Skin irritation

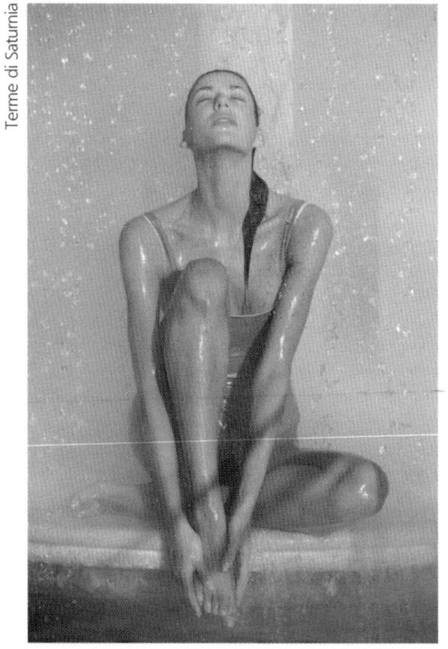

Terme di Saturnia

A shower can help skin irritation

High temperatures can cause some sensitive skins to be irritated and react adversely, especially in the dry heat of a sauna.

Action

- The client needs to lower their body and skin temperatures by taking a cool shower.
- A soothing cream can be applied to reduce any reaction or irritation.
- If the irritation continues, the client must seek medical advice.

Heat exhaustion

This is caused by the loss of body fluids and salt – the client has perspired too much! The loss of body fluid leads to headaches, nausea, dizziness, sickness and fainting.

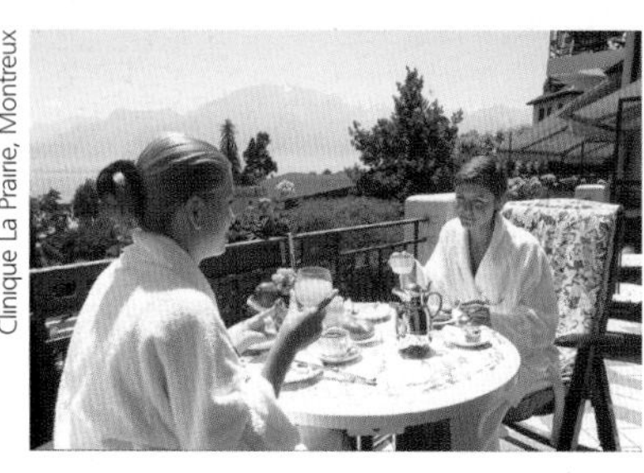

Clinique La Prairie, Montreux

If suffering from heat exhaustion, the client needs to drink fruit juice to rehydrate the body

Action

- The client should drink fruit juice or a specialist drink for rehydration.
- The client should rest lying down; legs may be raised to prevent fainting.
- A cool compress may be applied to the forehead.
- If the symptoms continue, the client must seek medical advice.

Muscle cramp

This is usually caused by excessive sweating.

Action

- The client must drink water to rehydrate the body. A little salt may be added to help replace salts lost in perspiration.
- The muscle can be gently stretched and massaged to help ease the cramp.

Burn/scald

A scald may be caused by the client pouring water on the coals in the sauna and not using an outstretched arm. The steam from the coals will rise quickly and scald the skin. Also, a shower that is too hot may scald the client. A burn may occur if the client leaves jewellery on, or touches any metal exposed in the sauna.

Action

- Run cold water over the area immediately.
- Apply a sterile dressing that will not adhere to the skin and cause further damage. This will prevent any infection from entering the skin.
- If the burn is severe, or does not heal, the client must seek medical advice.

Nose bleed

In some clients, the high temperature may irritate the mucous membrane in the nose and can lead to a nose bleed.

Action

- The base of the nose can be pinched for 10–15 minutes.
- The client will need to breathe through their mouth during this time.
- If the nose bleed does not stop after 30 minutes, the client must seek medical advice.

HEALTH AND SAFETY !

Always prepare the shower for the client, if you can.

FACT !

A **scald** is always from wet heat, a **burn** from dry heat

SIGNATURE TREATMENT S

Champneys Henlow

'Wax Bath treatment: Warm paraffin wax is whisked and applied all over the body, blankets are wrapped around you to retain temperature and body heat. As you relax, the wax will soften dead cells and help draw out excess fluid. The result is softer, smoother and conditioned skin. 45 minutes (For the Complete Wax Experience, enjoy a full body scrub with the "Citrus Glow Body Scrub" followed by the wax bath as described above).'

SPA PROFILE

Name: Sobat Ali Din

Position: Senior Therapist

Establishment: Sequoia at The Grove

Products used: ESPA, OPI.

Number of staff/roles: 60+ staff in total, including 20–25 therapists.

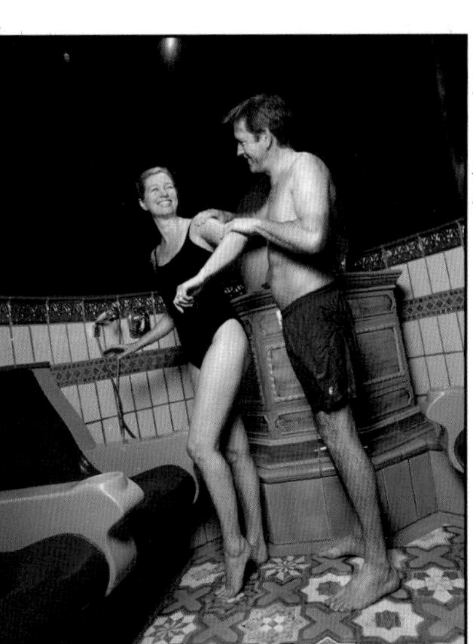

Courtesy of Champneys

Courtesy of Sequoia at the Grove, Herts

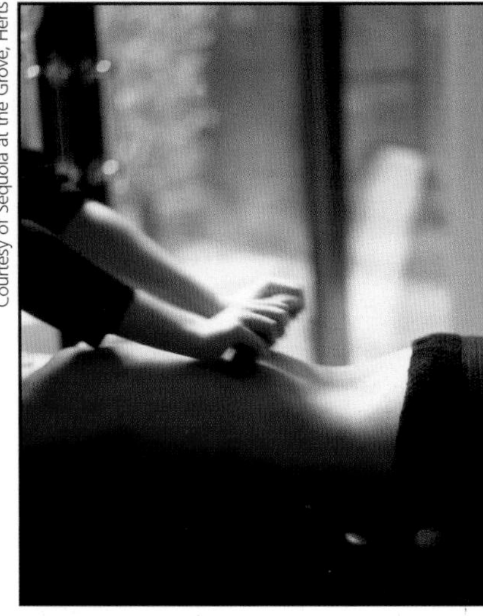

Training/experience: Trained at the British School of Complementary Therapies in massage. Trained at the College of Psychic Studies for five years. Trained at Barnfield College Luton in sports massage and remedial sports massage.

Main responsibilities: Checking room standards of all treatment rooms. Training of the spa attendants.

Best parts of the job: Looking at the reaction on people's faces after a treatment. Giving your time and energy to people who really need a treatment. Having that coffee before the shift starts in the morning.

Secrets of a successful spa therapist: Grounded; organized; flexible/versatile; sense of humour; maturity; be aware of the client's needs, i.e. be in tune with their 'energy'.

SPA PROFILE

Name: Michelle Young

Position: Spa Director, The Fairmont Empress, Victoria, BC

Establishment: Willow Stream Spa at the Fairmont Chateau, Victoria, Canada

Products used: Willow Stream Spa range created for the spa by Warren Botanicals, Kerstin Florian International Products and Aromatherapy Associates.

Number of staff/roles: 43 in total including Spa Manager, body therapists, aestheticians, receptionists.

Training/experience: Aveda Institute in Victoria, Canada; Esthetician Diploma BC.

Main responsibilities: 'Recruitment and developing the team. Meeting with the media to help market the spa, such as corporate packages, spa sampler evenings. Financial management of the spa, making sure that staff meet targets that are set. Arranging team and management meetings within the spa. Regular meetings held with the hotel to ensure the spa is following their corporate direction.'

Best parts of the job: 'Putting together the team has been one of the most important things I have achieved since becoming Spa Director, making sure that their professional philosophies reflect their personal philosophies. I enjoy sharing ideas with staff and working with the Willow Stream high standards of spa service and their values – "food, water and rest" is important for the clients and the staff.'

Secrets of a successful spa therapist: 'Do their personal philosophies fit into the spa's concept, and I always question what do they want to do or where do they want to be? They must have a passion for the job and for what the spa is about. When interviewing a new member of staff I always think of what personality is missing in the team, how will this person fit into the team and what knowledge and skills can they bring with them that we may be missing.'

Assessment of knowledge and understanding

When you have some free time, test your understanding and knowledge by answering the following questions. Do this at regular intervals and it will reinforce your learning and help you retain the knowledge, so you are able to perform better in your assessments.

Organizational and legal requirements

1 Why is it important to maintain high standards of hygiene? List the hygiene precautions that must be taken when the client is having a sauna treatment.

2 Why is it recommended that written instructions for equipment should be clearly displayed?

3 What would you do to ensure the 'ambience' of the spa environment is ideal for heat treatments.

Client contact and consultation

1 Why would you encourage and allow time for questions during the initial consultation?

2 Why must you never leave a client unattended during a steam bath treatment?

3 Why is it important to protect a client's modesty and privacy during a heat treatment?

4 List five contra-indications that would prevent a client from having a heat treatment.

Equipment and materials

1 Give three reasons why pine wood is often used to make saunas.

2 How would you prepare a steam bath for treatment?

3 What is the normal temperature range for a traditional sauna bath?

4 What is a laconium sauna, and what is the approximate humidity level during this treatment?

5 Describe the thermal sensitivty test; why must this be carried out prior to a heat treatment?

6 What is the approximate temperature for a steam bath treatment?

7 What is an infra-red sauna? And what effect does it have on the body?

8 What is the approximate humidity level in a sauna?

9 Describe a caldarium.

10 Describe a rasul treatment.

Heat treatments

1 What is the average treatment time for a sauna treatment and a hammam treatment?

2 List five effects of a sauna bath on the body.

3 Describe three possible contra-actions of a heat treatment, and what action should be taken.

4 Why is it important to shower, rest and drink water after a heat treatment?

Aftercare advice

1 What treatments must you advise the client to avoid after a heat treatment?

2 List four other treatments you could promote and 'link' with a heat treatment.

3 List five products you could suggest for use at home that would benefit the client having a heat treatment.

chapter 8

Chill treatments

BT29

Provide specialist spa treatments

Learning objectives

This chapter covers the skills a spa therapist needs to provide chill or cold spa treatments. It describes the skills and knowledge necessary to enable you to:

- **prepare, clean and maintain the spa environment**
- **consult with and prepare the client for treatment**
- **monitor the chill treatments**
- **provide aftercare advice**

When providing chill treatments it is important to use the skills you have learnt in the following core units:

G1 Ensure your own actions reduce risks to health and safety

G6 Promote additional products or services to clients

G11 Contribute to the financial effectiveness of the business

INTRODUCTION

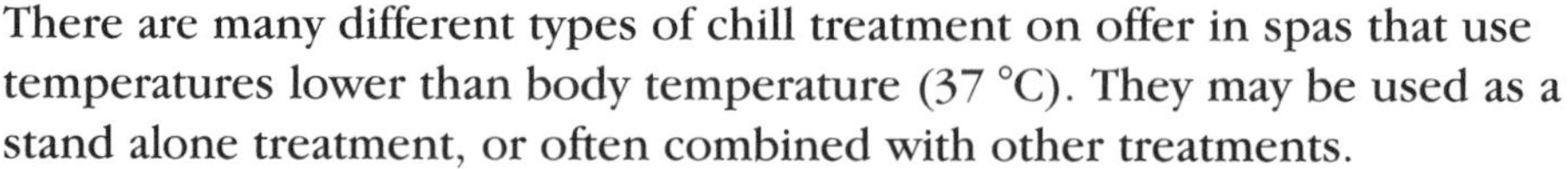

There are many different types of chill treatment on offer in spas that use temperatures lower than body temperature (37 °C). They may be used as a stand alone treatment, or often combined with other treatments.

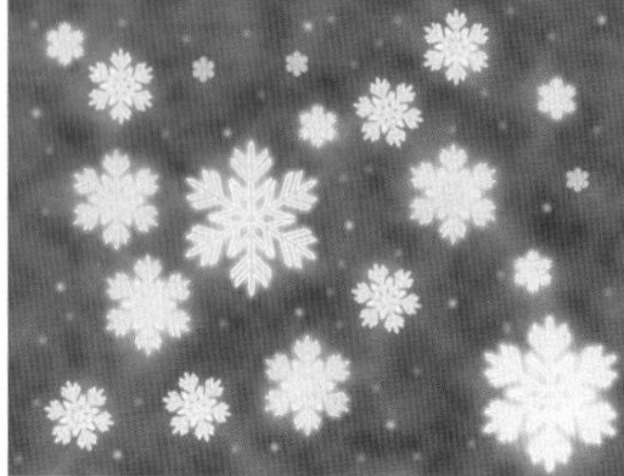

FACT

Babylonians discovered the benefits of cold compresses in 1800 BC.

There are a variety of chill treatments, such as:

- ice room (frigidarium)
- ice fountain
- cold bath
- cold affusions
- cold plunge pool
- cold footbath
- cold shower (and alternating showers)
- Vichy shower (see chapter 9)
- cool moist blanket body wrap
- cold compress

- snow walking
- snow cabin/snow paradise
- ice cave/ice igloo.

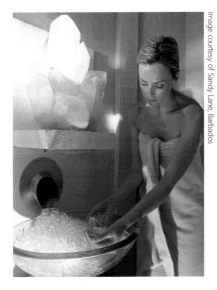

TERMINOLOGY

Chill treatments are also sometimes referred to as 'cold' treatments.

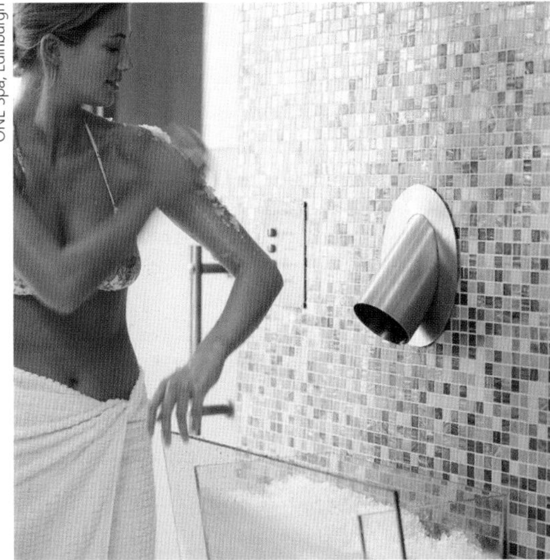
ONE Spa, Edinburgh

An ice shower

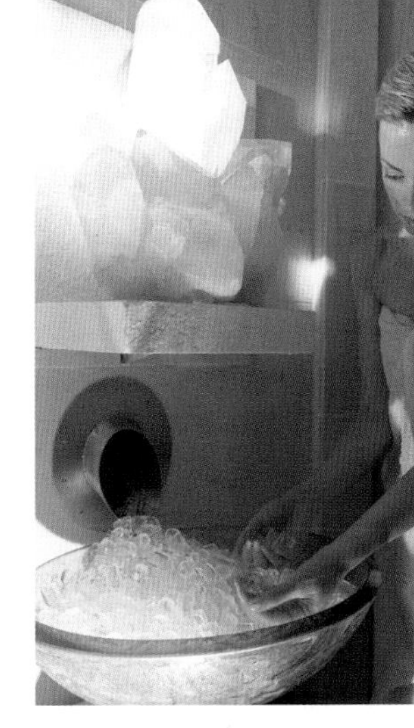
Image courtesy of Sandy Lane, Barbados

An ice room

FACT

In ancient Greece (600 BC) Spartan warriors kept fit by bathing each day in cold water. This also helped reduce inflammation and heal injuries sustained in battle.

EFFECTS OF COLD ON THE BODY

Chill treatments lower the body temperature and have the following effects on the body:

- Blood circulation is decreased, the temperature of the body lowered.
- Superficial capillaries constrict in an attempt to conserve body heat – **vasoconstriction**. Blood circulation is decreased to the area.
- The skin goes pale, as the capillaries constrict.
- Analgesic effect on superficial nerve endings – blocks out pain impulses, numbs the area.
- Tightening effect on the skin, helps prevent stretch marks and can help skin tone when loosing a large amount of weight.

HEALTH AND SAFETY

Be careful about checking contra-indications thoroughly, as chill treatments can be a shock to the system. Clients with a history of coronary disease or strokes should not use the chill facilities or equipment.

FACT

In 200 AD a famous doctor called **Galen** recommended that his patients bathe in baths of differing temperatures, especially alternating hot and cold baths to stimulate blood circulation.

FACT

Hippocrates recommended cold baths, but only for those used to them. He found that cold water poured over the head could induce sleep and helped reduce pain in the ears and eyes.

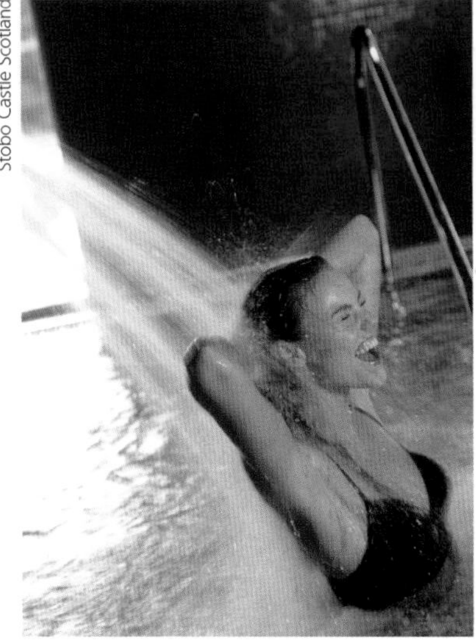

Cold water gives a general feeling of invigoration and energy – it's good for lethargic and tired clients

- Metabolism can be increased if the client is cold for a period of time, as shivering occurs to try and increase the body temperature. The arrector pili muscles attached to body hairs bring about 'goosebumps' in an attempt to trap air and warm the body.
- General feeling of invigoration and energy, good for lethargic, tired clients.

USES OF CHILL TREATMENTS

- To cool the body during heat treatments; e.g. during a sauna, the client can intermittently use a chilled plunge pool.
- To cool and reduce heat in hot, inflammed joints.
- To reduce the inflammation in an area, e.g. immediately after a sprain or strain to muscle tissue.
- To relieve pain, due to the analgesic effect on superficial nerve endings.

FACT

Cryotherapy does not mean 'cold' therapy or chill treatments. It is a term used to describe a procedure carried out by a doctor where liquid nitrogen freezes and removes body tissue, e.g. warts, skin growths or skin lesions.

CONTRA-INDICATIONS

As a therapist you must be aware of all the contra-indications to chill treatments, so that treatments are carried out with full regard for the clients' safety and wellbeing. Contra-indications to chill treatments include:

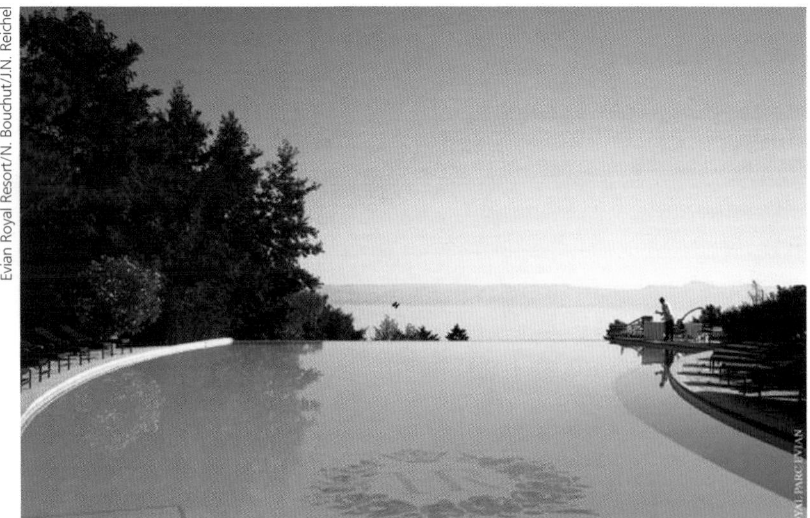

Swimming in cold water can have a tightening effect, helping to improve the condition and tone of the skin

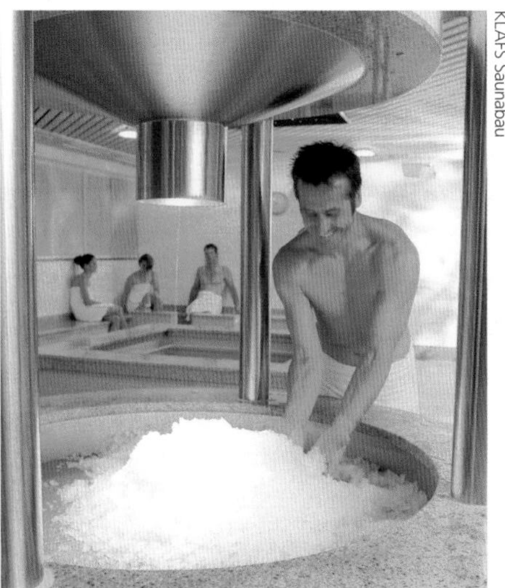

Chill treatments are invigorating and stimulating. Ensure you check the client for contra-indications on every visit to the spa, in case their health or circumstances have changed

- high or low blood pressure
- heart disorders/disease
- circulatory problems
- strokes
- respiratory problems, e.g. asthma
- fever
- pregnancy
- epilepsy
- open wounds
- infectious conditions.

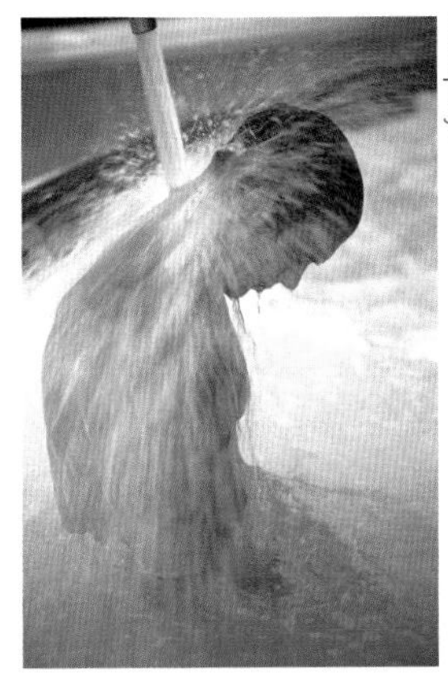
Champneys

A cold shower is very invigorating

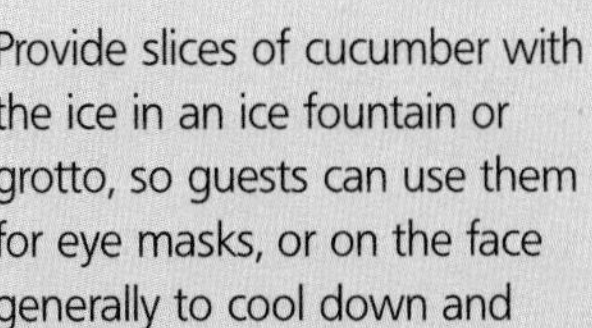

SPA TIP

Provide slices of cucumber with the ice in an ice fountain or grotto, so guests can use them for eye masks, or on the face generally to cool down and soothe the skin.

FACT

In the Roman ruins at Bath, a half-circle bath can still be seen. This type of bath dates back to the time of Celsus (30 AD) when he immersed his patients up to the neck in cold water to cure swelling of the body and legs.

CONSULTATION

As outlined in chapter 15, a full consultation should be carried out to make sure the treatment is safe and effective and every stage of the consultation checklist should be cleared prior to treatment.

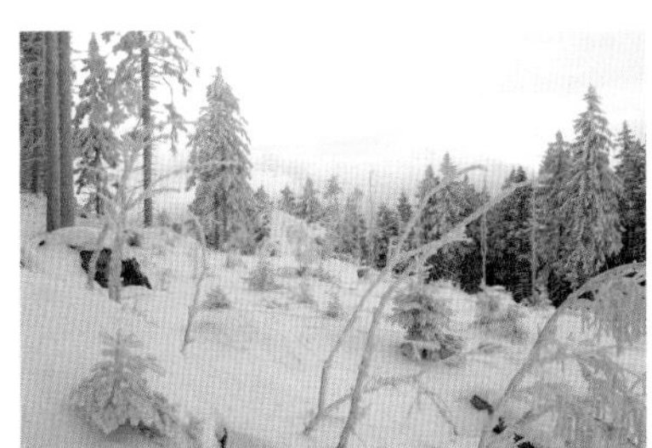

TYPES OF CHILL TREATMENTS

Ice room (frigidarium)

An ice grotto or ice room usually operates at 15 °C or less. The room is usually fully tiled and air-conditioned. Clients can use the ice room to stimulate the blood and lymph circulation, especially when alternated with a sauna or other heat treatment.

The client rubs the crushed ice all over their body, cooling it down and leaving them feeling invigorated and alive. They can then choose to rest in the relaxation area for 20 minutes, before continuing to another spa treatment. If it is the final treatment, the client should rest for 20 minutes, preferably wearing a warm gown, and drink plenty of water to re-balance the body.

The ice room must be looked after carefully to ensure it is well maintained and operates efficiently. Always:

- Follow the manufacturer's instructions.
- Disinfect regularly all surfaces of the ice room to ensure a hygienic environment and prevent possible spread of infection.
- Make sure the floor is clean and dry – if there is water on the floor the client may slip.
- Provide clean towels on any seating areas.
- Ventilate in the ice room by leaving the door open at the end of the working day.

CONSULTATION CHECKLIST

CHILL TREATMENTS

- Quiet private area
- Client privacy
- Plenty of time
- Client comfortable and at ease
- Aims of treatment/outcome
- Treatment plan
- Postural check
- Fill in record card
- Client signed record card
- Check contra-indications
- Skin/sensitivity tests
- Explain contra-actions
- Client questions

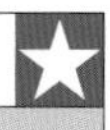

SPA TIP

To get an invigorating and fresh sensation, encourage guests to rub ice all over their bodies to cool down.

FACT

Cooling down after using a heat experience such as a sauna is vital to decrease the body temperature, clean the skin of sweat and encourage feelings of wellbeing. Spas have used showers for this purpose for many years, but manufacturers have now developed new and exciting ways to cool down, such as 'ice caves' and 'snow paradise'.

FACT

One of the most famous cold water cures happened in 23 AD when Antonius Musa cured the 'diseased liver' of Emperor Augustus simply by repeated cold baths.

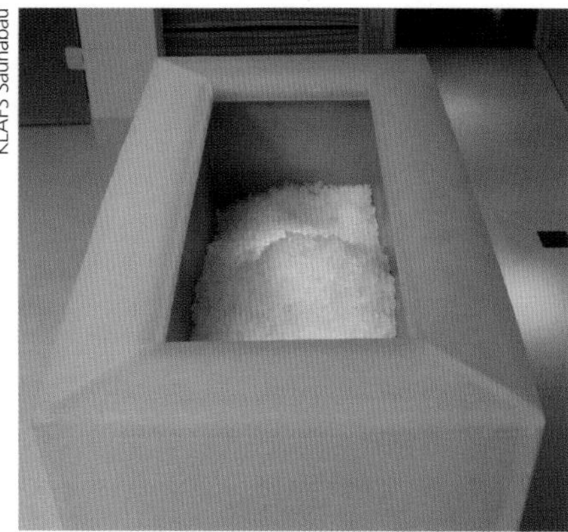

KLAFS Saunabau

An ice fountain in an ice room, KLAFS

Ice fountain

An ice fountain has similar benefits to an 'ice room' but it is usually a free standing piece of equipment that dispenses crushed ice automatically. The ice fountain is usually positioned close to a plunge pool, sauna or steam room. The client can either add ice to the plunge pool, or rub the crushed ice all over the body. The effects are identical to those of the ice room.

Cold bath

The cold bath is very stimulating and is offered in some traditional spas to help circulation, fever and to cool the body after a strong heat treatment. The temperature is approximately 75 °F/24 °C. The client should be very healthy, with no contra-indications. Usually the spa therapist assists the client into the bath, and they then only stay in the bath for a very short time. Whilst in the bath an exfoliating glove can be used.

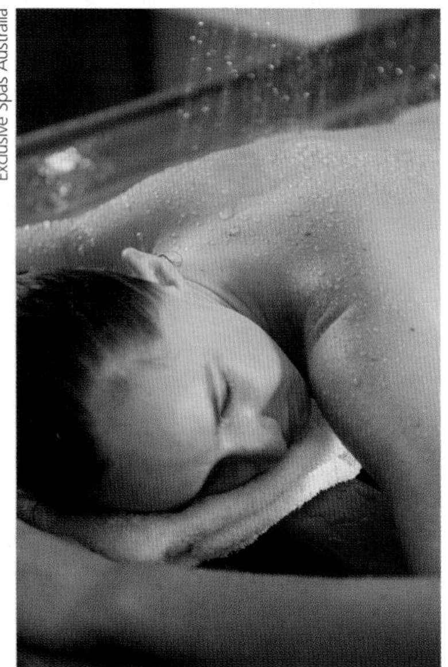

Exclusive Spas Australia

A cold affusion shower is very refreshing and can help tiredness and fatigue

Cold affusions

A cold affusion shower is very refreshing and increases blood circulation and metabolism. Overall, it can help tiredness and fatigue and those clients with a weak immune system. The treatment can be given to the whole of the body, or to specific body parts such as the chest. A shower hose is used, and the body is treated using a specific sequence, moving from one area to another systematically. After the treatment the client can rest for up to an hour.

Cold plunge pool

This is usually quite a small deep pool situated close to the sauna and steam rooms. Clients can plunge or jump into the pool intermittently during a heat treatment. This is usually quite a shocking experience, and many clients choose to enter slowly. The cold temperature in the pool quickly cools the body, and stimulates the blood circulation. The 'contrast' in temperature between the hot and cold can be beneficial to the body, as the circulation is increased. Often, there is an ice-machine next to the plunge pool, with ice added to ensure the water remains refreshingly 'chilled'.

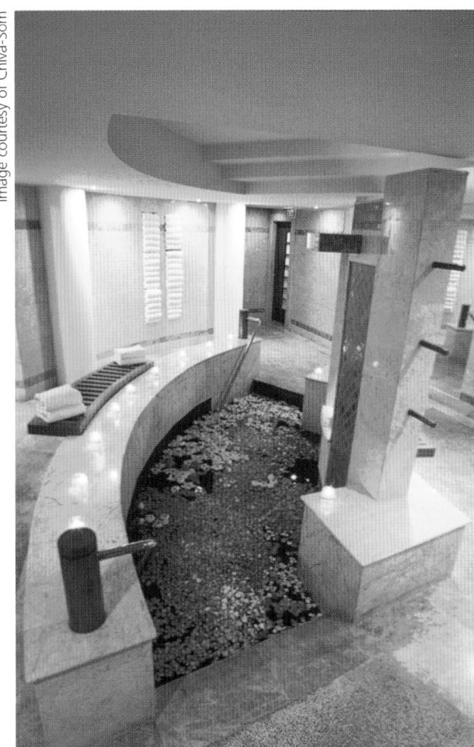

Image courtesy of Chiva-Som

A cold plunge pool, ice can be added periodically to keep it chilled, Chiva-Som

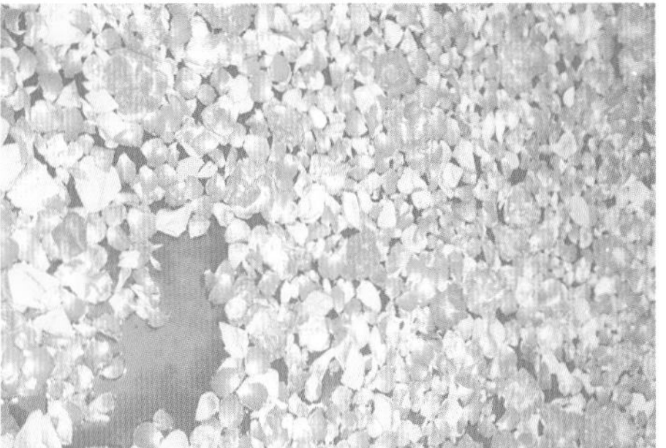

Cold footbath

A cold footbath can be used to help circulatory disorders and tired feet. The blood circulation is increased, metabolism is stimulated and it can help insomnia. The temperature of the footbath is approximately 54 °F/12 °C. The client can soak the feet in the bath for up to a minute.

Alternating warm and cold footbaths can be very stimulating. Blood circulation is increased, and the body's heat regulatory system is improved. The warm footbath is approximately 100 °F/37 °C, and the cold approximately 54 °F/12 °C. The client alternates between the two baths, spending 5 minutes with both feet in the warm bath, then 15 seconds in the cold bath – this can be repeated 2 or 3 times.

Cold shower (and alternating showers)

A cold shower can be used to reduce body temperature after a heat treatment, to overcome tiredness and fatigue, and generally to provide a tonic effect on the entire body. The client showers in as cold a temperature as they can tolerate, and for as long as possible. The tolerance to the cold quickly increases, and the client finds they get used to it and over a period of time can spend longer in the shower.

With 'alternating' showers, the client should start with a warm shower, then slowly decrease the temperature to cold. This can be repeated 2–3 times, depending on the client's tolerance. This treatment hardens the body, and has a toning effect on the skin.

FACT

In the 1680s Sir John Floyer found that bathing in cold water stimulated the circulation and induced sleep. He was also the first person to recommend 'plunging the part into cold water' for burns and scalds.

TERMINOLOGY

A **sitz bath** is a chair-like bath, with the hips immersed in hot water, and the feet immersed in alternate hot and cold water. This is very stimulating, and can help the immune system.

FACT

Around 1680 Dr Joseph Browne believed that cold water bathing cured tuberculosis, dropsy, tinnitus, gut problems and 'strange imaginings'. He also felt that the 'muscles of the heart become stronger by cold bathing'.

TERMINOLOGY

A **Scottish douche** is where the client stands and the spa therapist directs a high pressure hose of alternating warm and cold water. **Very bracing.**

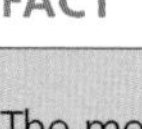

TERMINOLOGY

Tonicite a very 'bracing and toning' effect.

FACT

The methodist clergyman John Wesley (1703–91) believed that cold bathing prevented many diseases, and furthermore that it helped prevent people from catching cold. He strongly felt that it helped many conditions, such as asthma and tetanus.

Cool moist blanket body wrap

This is a treatment that is very effective in helping to detoxify the body, treat fevers, cool the body and improve chronic diseases. It should be carried out under medical supervision. The client has a hot bath, in which there may be mineral salts or aromatherapy oils for detoxification. The client then lies on the bed and is wrapped in a sheet that has been soaked in cold water and wrung out. Once wrapped in the cold sheet, warm blankets cover the client. At the end of the treatment, the different parts of the body can be washed with diluted vinegar (ablution). The skin is dried, and the client can then rest and rehydrate with refreshing drinks.

Cold compress

This would usually be performed in a spa with medical supervision. The cold compress reduces inflammation and can promote digestion. Often a linen sheet is immersed in cold water, wrung out and applied to the abdomen. The client is then wrapped in a warm blanket, and rests.

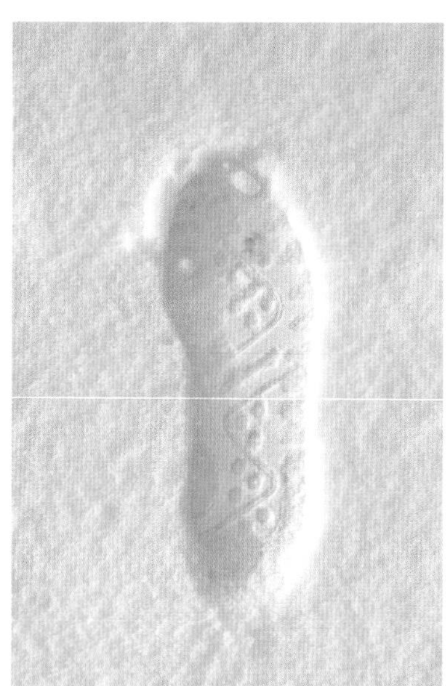

Snow walking

This unique treatment stimulates circulation and refreshes the body. Some spas, under medical supervision, may use this activity to treat tiredness and fatigue, chronic headaches and clients prone to infection. The client must be checked for contra-indications, and, if given the go-ahead, initially walks in the snow for only a few seconds, but slowly builds up to 3 minutes. Immediately after the snow walk, the feet need to be warmed up by brisk walking, massaging/rubbing and wearing warm socks/bootees.

Snow cabin/snow paradise

The ultimate way to cool down. The cabin temperature is maintained at approximately −15 °C and filled with real snow. The interior surface is designed to create a rock face which allows the snow to settle around the cabin. The guest would normally only be in the cabin for a few minutes and could place the snow on the body to speed the cooling process.

ACTIVITY

Write down a list of 3 features and 3 benefits of 'chill' treatments. If needs be, word-process and laminate. Keep this card close at hand, and learn off by heart, so that should a client ask you about chill treatments, you are prepared and can give excellent advice.

FACT

Vincenz Priessnitz (1799–1851) was badly injured, but cured himself by repeated applications of cold wraps and blankets. He developed the regime by combining cold baths, wraps, fresh air, exercise and diet, and it became widely known as the 'Priessnitz cure'.

HEALTH AND SAFETY

Certain companies produce cold packs that can reach −20 °C. Follow the manufacturer's instructions carefully, limit the time and use a protective sheet between the pack and the skin to avoid burning and frostbite.

A snow cabin treatment, KLAFS

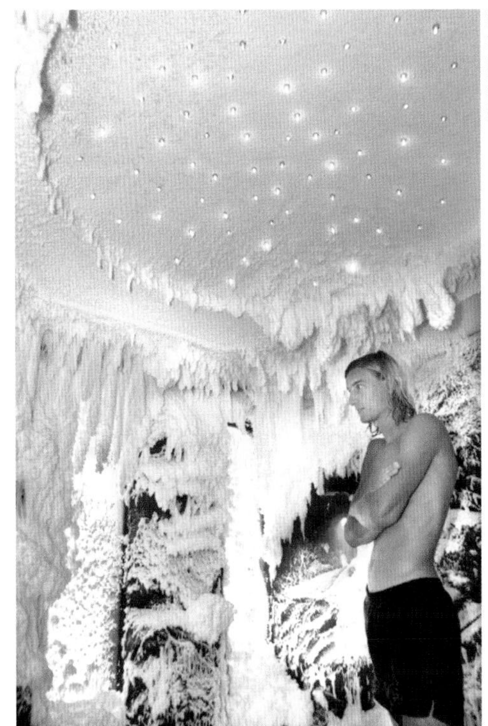

KLAFS Saunabau

Ice cave/ice igloo

The cabin is cooled to 5 °C to allow the guest to cool down relatively gently. There is normally an ice fountain within the cabin which provides the guest with crushed ice to place on the body to enhance the cooling process. The interior design of these cabins can be a craggy rock face or be tiled with a domed roof similar to an Eskimo igloo.

AFTERCARE AND TREATMENT ADVICE

At the end of the chill treatment, it is important that the client does not quickly get up and start getting dressed. Let the client relax either in a relaxation room or on the treatment couch. Ensure it is not too cool. Explain that they need to rest for at least 20–30 minutes to allow the body temperature and blood pressure to return to normal. If they are too quick and rush things, they may feel faint and dizzy, as the blood rushes from their head. After having a cold/chill treatment, the body needs slowly to get used to being warm again.

Whilst the client is resting, it gives you an opportunity to go through the aftercare and treatment advice. Offer the client a glass of water or fruit juice, and advise them to drink plenty of water during the next few hours.

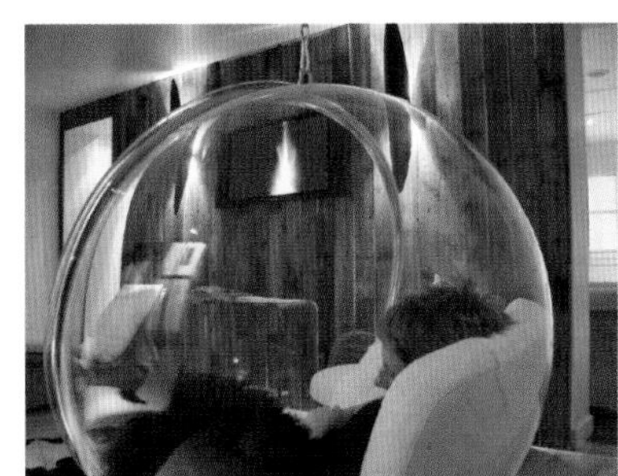

Cowshed Spa. Photographs provided for use, by kind permission of the Scotsman Hotel, Edinburgh

After the cold/chill treatment it is important that the client relaxes for 20–30 minutes, to allow the body temperature and blood pressure to return to normal

SIGNATURE TREATMENT S

Mandara Spa

'Mandara Massage: Mandara Spa Signature, performed by two therapists working together in rhythmic harmony. This massage combines 5 different massage styles, Japanese Shiatsu, Thai massage, Lomi Lomi, Swedish and Balinese which promote pure pleasure in mind. Shower, Floral Foot Bath, Mandara Massage, Refreshment. 60 minutes'

LINKED TREATMENTS

Cold/chill treatments in a spa are usually combined with a huge range of other treatments. The following treatments can 'link' with chill experiences:

- heat treatments, e.g. sauna, steam, hammam, rasul, etc.
- water treatments, e.g. spa pool, jet massage, flotation
- massage treatments, e.g. body massage, Indian head massage, pre-blended oils massage, Thai massage, Balinese massage, remedial massage, leg massage
- body envelopments, wraps, scrubs, exfoliation
- relaxation, e.g. sound therapy, tepidarium.

Seaham Hall

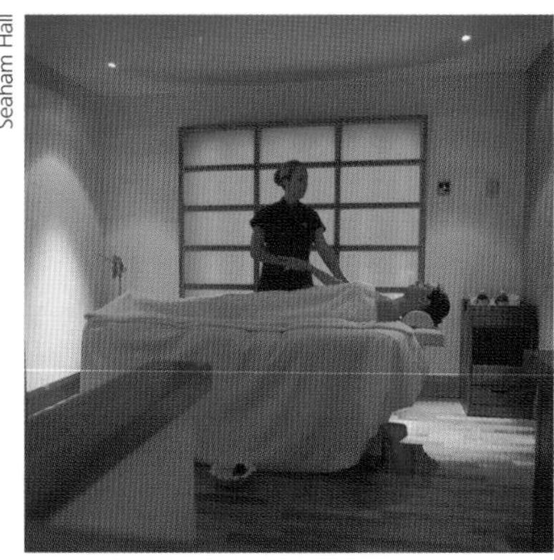

Massage 'links' well with cold/chill treatments

AFTERCARE AND TREATMENT ADVICE

After-treatment advice	✔ Shower ✔ Rest period 20–30 minutes ✔ Monitor reactions ✔ Drink water/fruit juice ✔ Avoid stimulants
Products used during the treatment	✔ Explain details of products ✔ Homecare recommendation ✔ How to use the products ✔ Written prescription ✔ Additions – candles, body brush, eye mask, etc.
Contra-actions	✔ Explain possible reactions to cold/chill ✔ Advise on recommended action
Posture	✔ Posture awareness ✔ Postural advice
Lifestyle pattern	✔ Dietary and fluid intake ✔ Exercise habits ✔ Smoking habits ✔ Sleep patterns ✔ Hobbies/interests ✔ Means of relaxation
Further cold/chill treatment	✔ Benefits of continuing treatments
Linked treatments	✔ Benefits of combining with other treatments, e.g. heat, massage, water treatments, wraps
Frequency of treatments	✔ Recommended frequency and time intervals

SPA PACKAGE

- experience shower
- Turkish hammam
- ice room
- massage with pre-blended oils
- Zen garden
- relaxation.

LINKED TREATMENTS

See chapter 11 for full details of 'linking' products with treatments. A client will usually combine a chill treatment with other spa routines and experiences such as heat. Please refer to chapter 7 for descriptions of products that can be linked to heat treatments as they would equally well suit the client who has combined heat with chill experiences.

SPA PROFILE

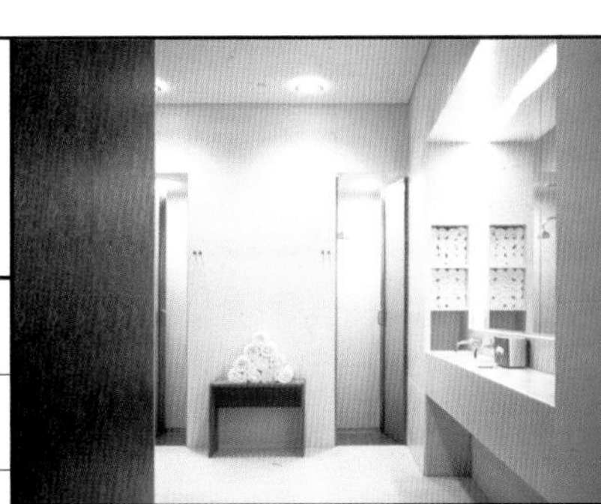
Courtesy of Bliss Spa

Name: Kate Hudspith

Position: Bliss Spa Technician

Establishment: Bliss, London

Products used: Bliss, Laboratoire Remede, Poetic and Diamancel bath, body, skincare + grooming.

Number of staff/roles: There are between 60 and 70 staff in the United Kingdom covering all areas of Bliss.

Training/experience: I spent 3 years training at the London College of Fashion, completed an NVQ level 2 and a BTEC National Diploma in Beauty Therapy and then studied holistic training for a year – covering reflexology, aromatherapy and Indian head massage. Whilst at college, and for about a year after, I worked in a small salon. Before starting at Bliss I worked on cruise ships, in a spa in the USA and at Selfridges in London.

Main responsibilities: Performing spa treatments (such as facials and waxing). I also train new staff members.

Best parts of the job: I love learning, I love making our guests feel good, and I love to motivate people and make their experience one they'll remember.

Secrets of a successful spa therapist: Bliss is successful, I think, because we really have our own personality. Not only are Bliss treatments of incredible quality, our facilities are always supremely clean, our technology is cutting edge, our service menu is fun to read, and our staff members are fun and FRIENDLY. We welcome everyone (not only the fancy and the famous), love our jobs, use great products, and constantly look for new ways that we can make our offerings more interesting for our clientele. We also make sure to interject all of our communication pieces with a hint of humour (without being cheesy, of course). It's a special Bliss branding – being funny, to make you laugh a little, which is really the best way to relax.

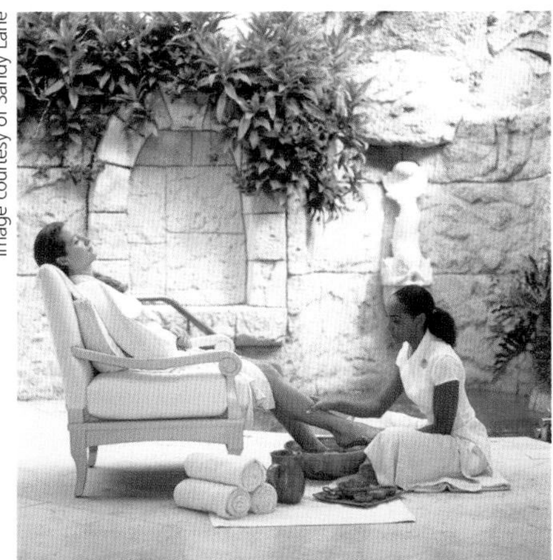
Image courtesy of Sandy Lane

After a cold/chill treatment the legs will be refreshed and stimulated. A leg and foot massage can follow to relax muscles and nourish the skin

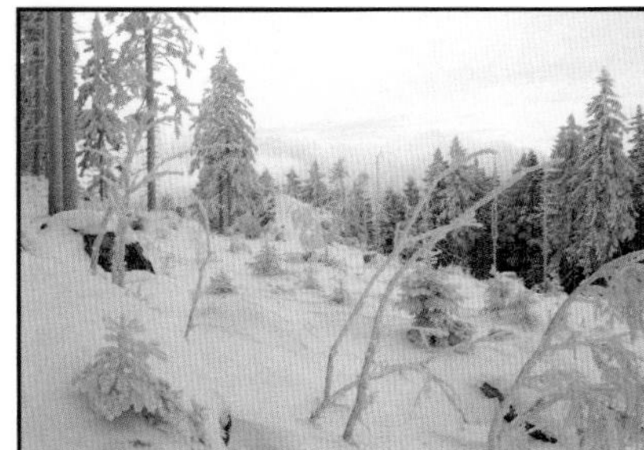

SPA PROFILE

Name: Fiona Caldwell

Position: Aesthetician

Establishment: Vida Wellness Spa, Fairmont Chateau, Whistler, Canada

Products used: Dermalogica, Vida Ayurvedic Treatment products.

Number of staff/roles: 70 in total including Spa Director, Spa Manager, supervisors, dispensary assistants, aestheticians, massage therapists

Training/experience: Abraham Moss College, Manchester, UK; BTEC National Diploma in Beauty Therapy; Diploma in Aromatherapy, Reflexology, Massage Therapies (studied in New Zealand).

Main responsibilities: 'As a therapist I do Dermalogica facials, manicures/pedicures, waxing and self-tanning treatments. It is my job to make sure that the client receives the best treatment they have had with a high standard of customer care that reflects Vida's philosophies.'

Best parts of the job: 'Vida is about educating the guest as well as having treatments, to enhance their lifestyle, diet, skin, posture/exercise. The client is given information sheets to take home about lifestyle and homecare, which follow the Ayurvedic principles of the spa. I also enjoy working with therapists who have backgrounds in holistic treatments and share the same beliefs about therapies that I have.'

Secrets of a successful spa therapist: 'It is important that they have the subject knowledge and a skill to connect with each guest on an individual level.'

Assessment of knowledge and understanding

When you have some free time, test your understanding and knowledge by answering the following questions. Do this at regular intervals and it will reinforce your learning and help you retain the knowledge, so you are able to perform better in your assessments.

Organizational and legal requirements

1. Why is it important to maintain high standards of hygiene when the client is undertaking chill/cold treatments?

Client contact and consultation

1. Why would you encourage and allow time for questions during the initial consultation?
2. Why is it important to protect a client's modesty and privacy during a cold/chill treatment?
3. List five contra-indications that would prevent a client from having a cold/chill treatment.

Equipment and materials

1. How would you recommend an 'ice room' is maintained?
2. What is the normal temperature range for an 'ice room'?
3. What is the approximate temperature for a 'cold bath'?
4. What is a cold affusion? And what effect does it have on the body?
5. What is the approximate temperature of a cold footbath? And what is the effect on the body?
6. Describe an 'alternating footbath'?
7. What effect does a cold shower have on the body?
8. Describe an ice igloo. What effect does it have on the body?
9. Describe a snow cabin. What effect does it have on the body?

Cold/chill treatments

1. List five effects of a cold/chill treatment on the body.
2. Describe three uses of a cold/chill treatment.
3. Why is it important to shower, rest and drink water after a cold/chill treatment?

Aftercare advice

1. List four other treatments you could promote and 'link' with a cold/chill treatment.
2. List five products you could suggest for use at home that would benefit the client having a cold/chill treatment.

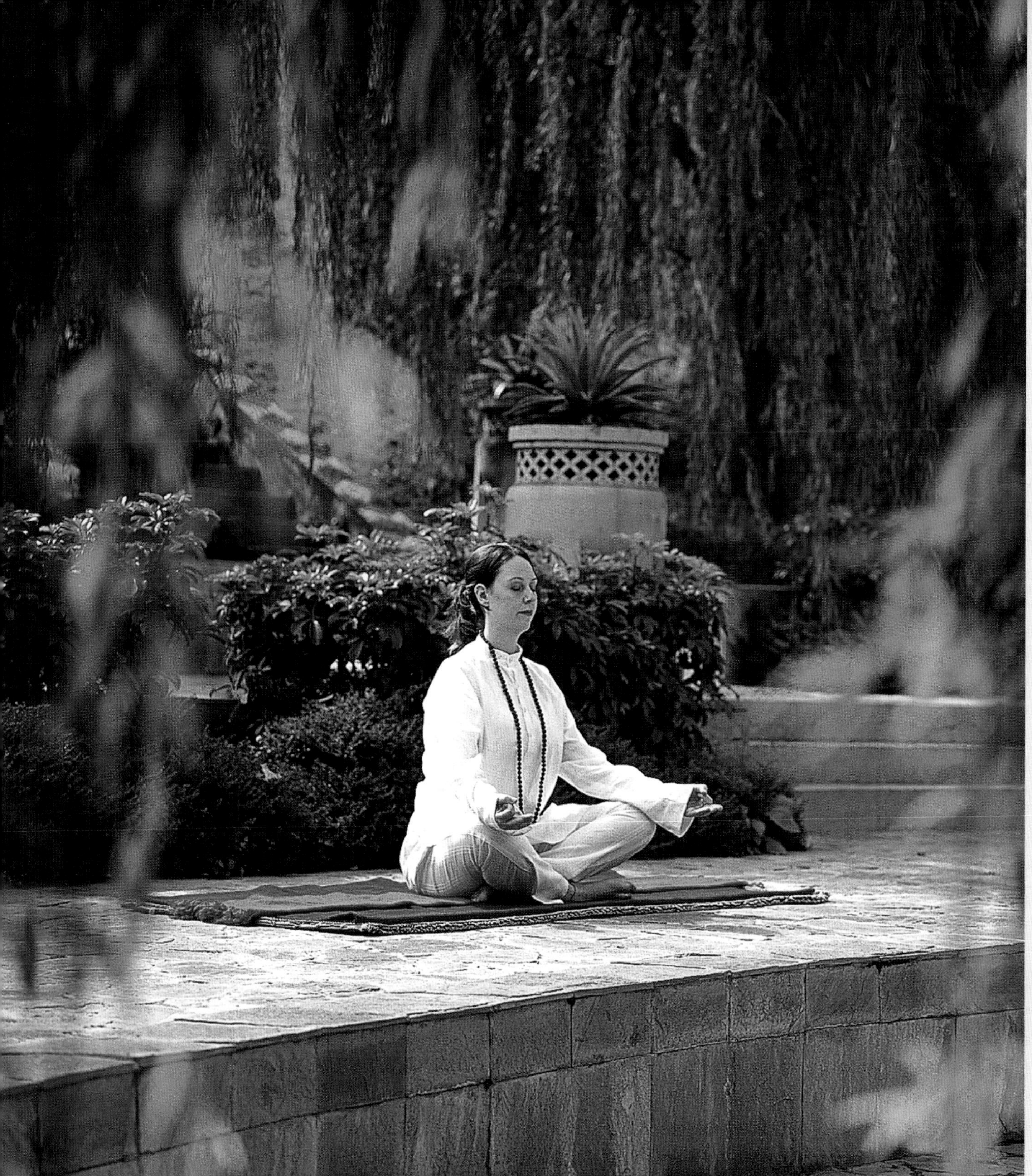
Ananda – In The Himalayas

*Spas are **hot**; the industry is **thriving**! If we unite to deliver **quality** to the consumer the spa industry will continue to **grow**, providing decades of secure rewarding employment for **millions** across the globe. Join us, there is no business like the spa business!*

COLIN GARY HALL, SPA DIRECTOR, ANANDA – IN THE HIMALAYAS, INDIA

5 SPLASH

The potential for a career in the spa industry is only just being realized: with a combination of increased awareness within societies for total wellbeing, a product that is only at the beginnings of its lifecycle with regards to growth, the variety of career paths that can be taken, and the global opportunities for employment that are available – I cannot think of another industry that offers such vibrant prospects.

EMLYN BROWN, SPA DIRECTOR, ASSAWAN SPA, BURJ-AL-ARAB, DUBAI, UAE

A few years ago, many people equated 'spa' with only running sulfur waters and sheep cell injections. Now, 'spa-ing' is no longer considered to be uncommon – there are more spas popping up every day, in many different types of neighbourhoods. Spas are no longer only for the 'elite', they're for everybody.

MARCIA KILGORE, FOUNDER OF BLISS

chapter 9

Water treatments

BT15

Assist with spa treatments

BT29

Provide specialist spa treatments

Learning objectives

This chapter covers the skills a spa therapist needs to provide water treatments.

It describes the skills and knowledge necessary to enable you to:

- **consult with and prepare the client for treatment**
- **provide flotation treatments**
- **provide hydrotherapy treatments**
- **monitor water, temperature and spa treatments and environment**
- **provide aftercare advice**

When providing water treatments it is important to use the skills you have learnt in the following core units:

G1 Ensure your own actions reduce risks to health and safety

G6 Promote additional products or services to your clients

G11 Contribute to the financial effectiveness of the business

INTRODUCTION

The use of water in a spa was the original base for natural treatments thousands of years ago. In today's spa it has a vital role to play in the treatments offered – spa baths, showers, pools – and the water used, whether mineral-enriched or ordinary, can be used for therapeutic benefits and to the relax the mind and body.

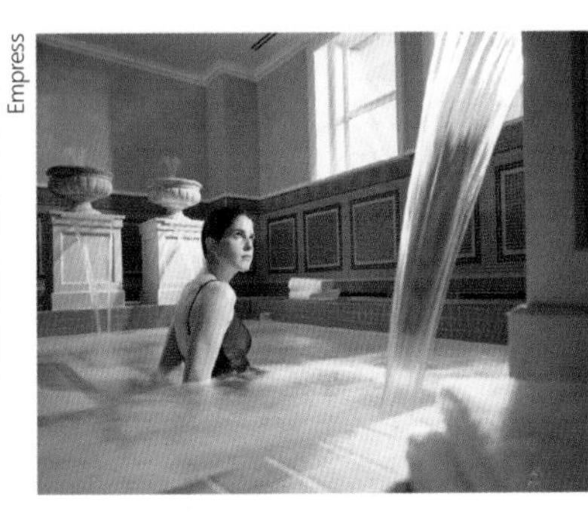

Willow Stream Spa at The Fairmont Empress

Hungarian Mineral Pool, Willow Stream Spa at The Fairmont Empress

The use of water-based therapies in spas set them apart from traditional beauty salons and leisure clubs and natural sources of water were the reasons for the original spas centuries ago.

Historical records depict the use of water for its healing properties from the time of the Egyptians, Romans, Greeks and Turks, but it was the Romans who are credited with introducing spa baths into Europe. Towns developed around these spa baths, which for hundreds of years became retreats and holiday destinations for people to bathe, sample the healing properties of the water and to convalesce after illness. These spa towns are still popular tourist centres today – Cheltenham, Bath, Buxton, Harrogate in the United Kingdom, Baden-Baden in Germany – with Bath and Baden-Baden re-developing their spa facilities to accommodate a new spa clientele.

In European spas the use of water is seen as the main part of the spa experience and is used for a variety of medical conditions. France, for example, is renowned for its thalassotherapy centres using seawater and seaweed products to mineralize and detoxify the body. Water treatments are also rapidly growing in popularity in Asia and the United States where they are used alongside more traditional pampering treatments.

USES OF WATER TREATMENTS

As mentioned previously, water has been used for its therapeutic qualities for centuries. It is still used today in spas for this purpose, but many clients also use hydrotherapy to help relax, for stress relief, to improve skin conditions and to relieve muscular aches and pains. The use of hot and cold water in a treatment is also extremely beneficial in stimulating the circulation and leaving the client feeling invigorated.

Water treatments have many physical and psychological benefits and these are tabulated below.

Physical	*Psychological*
Induces relaxation – by soothing sensory nerve endings, increasing blood to the muscles and warming the body (heat treatments)	Relaxes the mind – as the body relaxes and nerves endings are soothed
Stimulates the immune system – by removing local toxins and waste products	Improves sleep patterns as the body is relaxed
Improving muscle condition – by relaxing the muscles (heat), stimulating muscle tone (hot and cold) and removing lactic acid from the muscles, particularly after muscular activity	Stimulates energy levels – as toxins are removed from the body
Metabolism may be increased, particularly if using seaweed in the treatments or using stimulating treatments	Uplifting and a feeling of wellbeing – nerve endings can be stimulated as well as soothed
Lymphatic circulation is increased – beneficial for areas of oedema or fluid retention	
Increases the flexibility in joints by removing excess toxins, reducing swelling	
Skin is nourished and its condition is improved due to the mineral-rich properties in the water	

TERMINOLOGY

Hydrotherapy the therapeutic use of water in treatments, which includes underwater massage, jet blitzes, baths, steam baths, showers.

Thalassotherapy from the Greek 'thalassa' for sea and 'therapia' for treatment. All the treatments use seawater, seaweed and algae and exploit the sea's mineral properties for curative and preventative purposes.

Balneotherapy employs hot water springs, mineral water or seawater to bathe in, or incorporates underwater massage using localized jets to stimulate aching muscles.

HEALTH AND SAFETY

If bathing in seawater with high concentrations of salt, such as the Dead Sea, you need to cover up any cuts or rashes as they will sting terribly on contact (even though they will heal quickly as a result), and avoid getting any of the water in your eyes.

FACT

The **Dead Sea** is a popular destination for those seeking the mineral rich qualities of the salt water, which have proven beneficial for treating skin conditions such as eczema and psoriasis and aliments such as arthritis and rheumatic conditions.

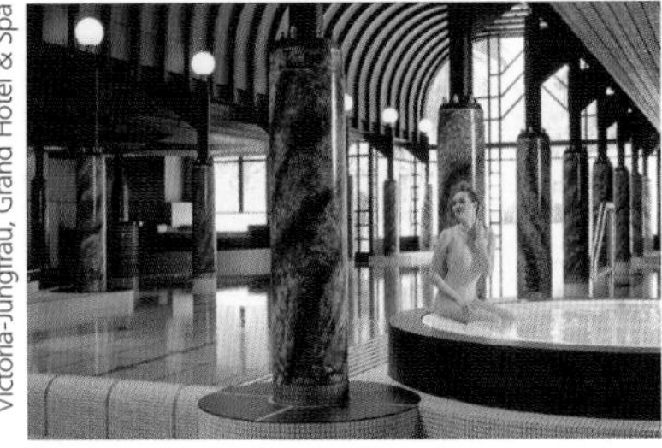

Spa pool, Victoria-Jungfrau, Switzerland

Conditions/clients that benefit from the use of water treatments are:

- stress
- arthritis/rheumatism
- rehabilitation from illness
- sports injuries
- fluid retention
- skin problems – eczema, psoriasis
- clients de-toxing/dieting
- elderly clients – water acts as a buoyancy.

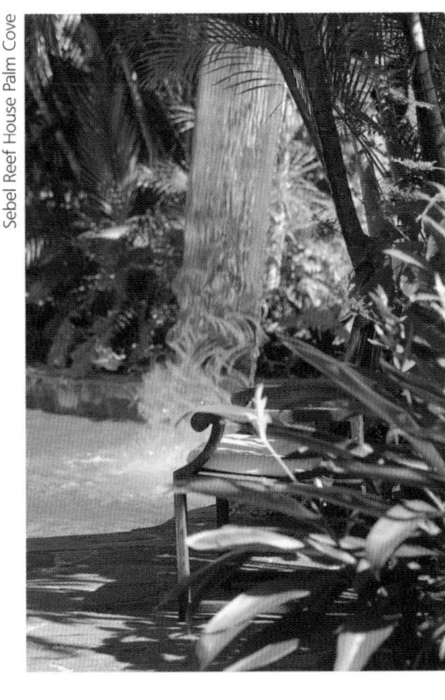

WATER TREATMENT TYPES

There are many water therapies available in today's spas, some of them are signature treatments to the particular spa. In this chapter we are concentrating on six of the most widely available water treatments offered in spas:

1 spa pool
2 hydrotherapy bath
3 flotation
4 Blitz/Scotch shower
5 Swiss/Vichy shower
6 Kneipp therapy

as well as swimming pools and watsu.

In chapters 7 and 8 there are features on other spa treatments that use water, including sauna, steam and frigidarium. There are a number of contra-indications and restrictions to water therapy treatments.

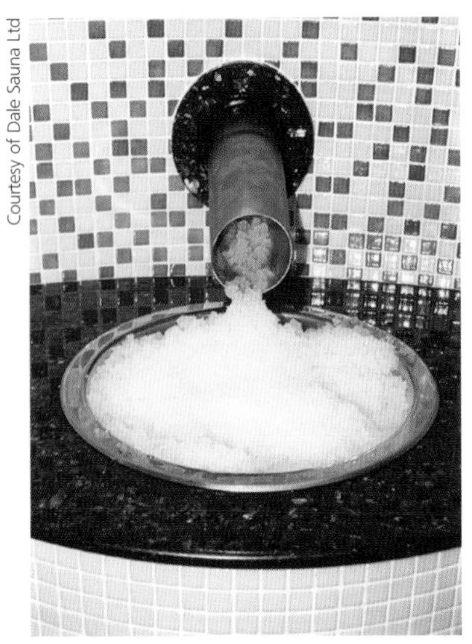

Ice room

CONTRA-ACTIONS FROM WATER THERAPY

Due to the temperatures used in water-based treatments and the stimulation of circulation there are a few adverse reactions the client may experience afterwards:

- Client may feel faint – this could be caused by dehydration and by treatment duration being too long. Make sure they rest and drink plenty of water.
- Nausea – this may again be caused by dehydration and also the water motion in the spa/hydrotherapy pool. Clients must rest and drink plenty of water.

- Headaches – dehydration or heat exhaustion. Drink plenty of water and use a cool cloth on the forehead.
- Skin irritation – due to chemicals in the spa pools or products used in the treatment. Get the client to shower immediately to remove the products and a soothing cream may be used.

Total contra-indications	*Contra-indications that may restrict treatment*
High temperature	Varicose veins – jet massage
Contagious or infectious diseases	Severe bruising
Under the influence of drugs or alcohol	Sunburn
Recent operations or radiotherapy/ chemotherapy treatment	Recent waxing, epilation, skin peels – avoid for 24 hours
Any severe kidney disorders	Cuts and abrasions – area must be protected
Severe urinary infections	Perforated eardrums – must use ear plugs
Pregnancy – seek doctor's approval	Immediately after a heavy meal
Medical oedema – seek doctor's approval	
Epilepsy – seek doctor's approval	
Sensitivity to pool chemicals	
Claustrophobia – flotation treatment	
Circulatory disorders – seek doctor's approval	
Osteoporosis – seek doctor's approval	
Patients who are incontinent – in pool treatment	
Asthma – seek doctor's approval	

SPA HYGIENE 

- All towels and bed linen should be washed in very hot, soapy water in order to remove any oil.
- All work surfaces should be cleaned daily with a disinfectant spray.
- All floors should be cleaned daily and in between treatments if there is a lot of water on them.
- Use fresh towels/gowns for each client.
- All hydrotherapy equipment should be cleaned according to manufacturers' instructions.

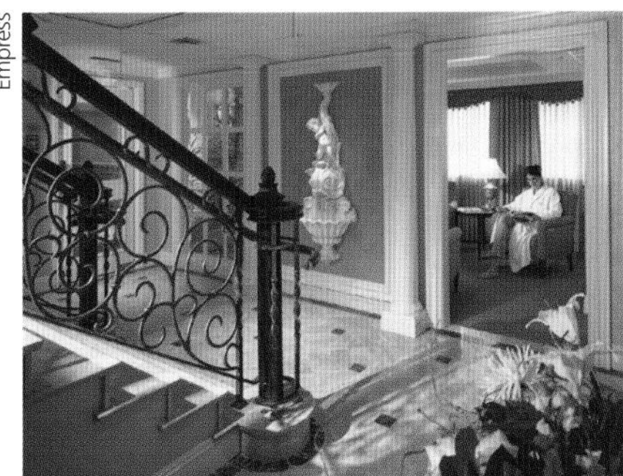

Willow Stream Spa at The Fairmont Empress

Lounge, Willow Stream Spa at The Fairmont Empress

HEALTH AND SAFETY

If a client has a suspected allergy to a product used in a water treatment then a patch test must be carried out first. Apply the product behind the ear or in the crease of the elbow and leave for 24 hours. If the client has an allergy, then they may have itching, redness, swelling in the area. Avoid the treatment and record any reaction on the client's record card.

PREPARE FOR TREATMENT CHECKLIST Water treatments

✔ Correct environment	✔ Bathrobe
✔ Be safe . . .	✔ Help client onto/into equipment
✔ Hygiene	✔ Correct client positioning
✔ Professional appearance	✔ Client warm, relaxed and comfortable
✔ Equipment/products/consumables	✔ Wash hands
✔ Record card	✔ Cleanse skin, if appropriate
✔ Private changing facilities	✔ Select treatment products, if being used

FACT

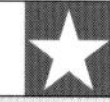

In Japanese hot pools, a wet towel placed over the client's head, which is believed to prevent them from passing out.

SPA TIP

Next to hydrotherapy pools place a bucket of iced water containing face cloths with slices of cucumber on top to refresh/cool the client.

SPA POOL

Also known as jacuzzi or whirlpool, the client sits or lies in a bath or tub of hot water which has high-pressure jets on the sides and bottom that circulate the water around the body. Warm air is injected into the water by propellers, which pass air through small nozzles/jets creating bubbles. The baths can be made out of shaped, durable acrylic, but they are not as strong as the hydro baths, which provide direct underwater massage.

Products used

Essential oils, mineral salt products and milk whey powder/bath cream can be used in the pool to aid relaxation, de-stressing and for alleviating

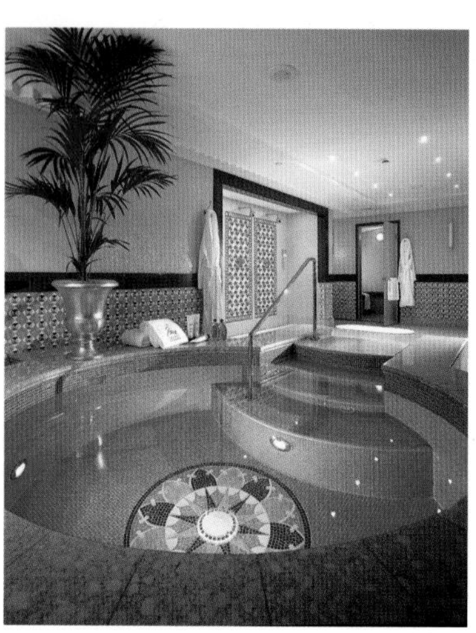

Jacuzzi, Burj-Al-Arab, Dubai

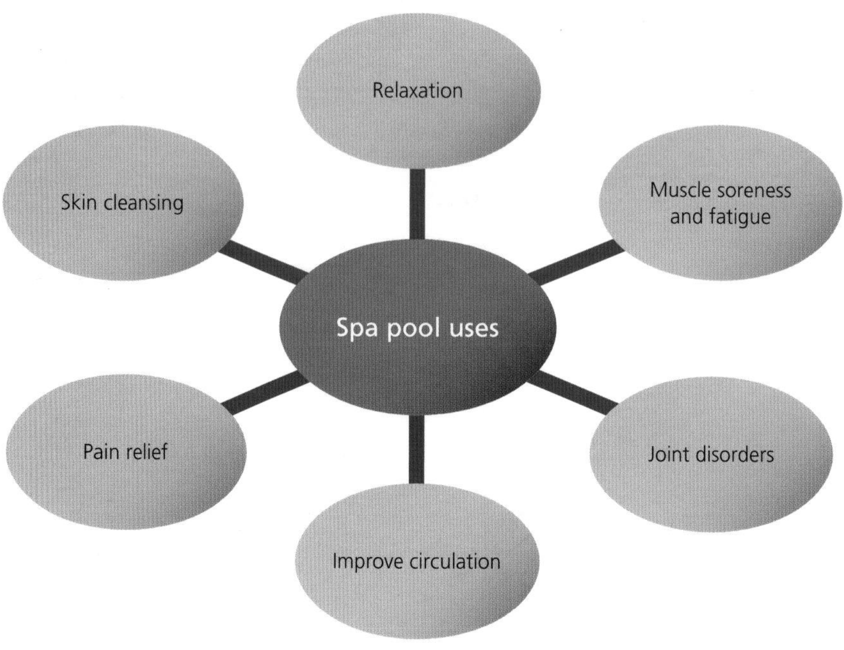

SIGNATURE TREATMENT

Sheraton Grand Hotel & Spa, Edinburgh, Scotland:

'**Escape at One**: This involves a series of "hands-off" treatments, designed to relax the mind and rejuvenate the body.

- **The Thermal Suite** has a range of heat and cooling experiences which cleanse the body and soothe aching muscles
- **The Rooftop Hydropool,** which has both indoor and outdoor areas, incorporates a variety of body jets providing mineral rich waters at the optimal temperature for the body to rebalance

Escape at One also incorporates the 19 m Swimming Pool, Cleopatra Baths and Gym'

HEALTH AND SAFETY

The water temperature in the spa pool should ideally be between 34 and 38 °C.

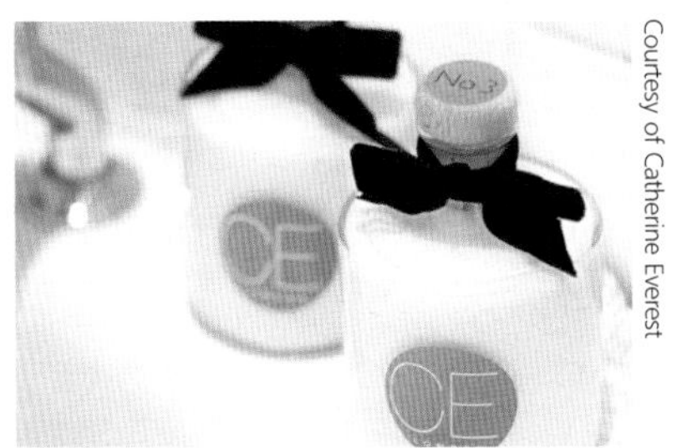
Courtesy of Catherine Everest

Bath milk

muscular aches and pains. Depending on the spa products used within the spa this may differ, and each spa will have certain rituals created into their treatment menu to incorporate this.

Consultation

Follow the general consultation steps outlined in chapter 15, concentrating on those contra-indications which are specific to water-based treatments. Spa pool treatments are often used with other body treatments to increase their therapeutic effects. If the client is using a jacuzzi or whirlpool, recommend that the client brings a swimming costume to maintain their modesty as there may be other people in the pool. Treatment should last approximately 15–20 minutes and may be given daily, depending on the other treatments the client is receiving.

FACT

In Japan they take seasonal baths using mandarin orange peel baths in the autumn and warming ginger baths in the winter.

Preparing the treatment room or spa pool area

If the spa pool is individual for the client in a treatment room, then the ambience should be the same as for all spa treatments and be set to the standard required by the spa. If it is a communal pool then ambience is harder to create, but there are still standard procedures to be followed:

- Turn on the spa pool according to manufacturer's instructions.
- Fill the pool/bath with water and check the temperature.
- Test the water regularly to make sure that it has a balanced pH of 7.2–7.8.
- Add any appropriate products to the water as the pool is filling up.
- Make sure the area around the pool is clean.

HEALTH AND SAFETY

A communal spa pool will not be drained after each client, so it is important that the water is continually filtered and treated. All spa pools should be cleaned thoroughly at the end of each working day to remove any residue or product left in the bath that would make the water look unclean. See chapter 10 on testing and monitoring spa water.

EQUIPMENT LIST

- spa pool
- water testing equipment
- clean towels – small hand and large bath sheets
- shower
- skin cleansing products
- treatment products for the bath
- aromatherapy burner – if in a small room, can create a nice aroma
- candles – can be used in the room for subtle lighting, if appropriate
- water and glass tumblers – for the client

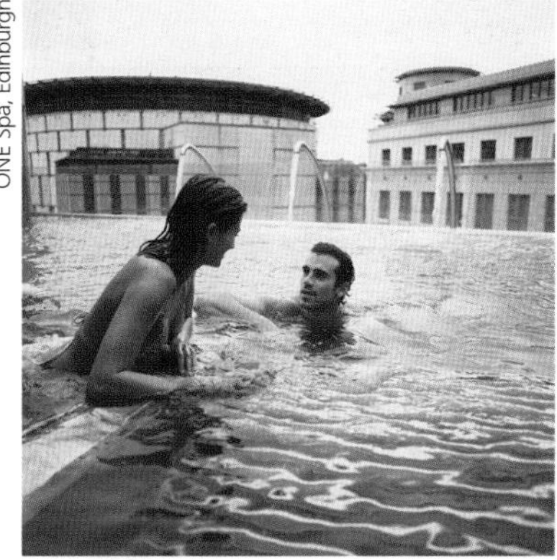
ONE Spa, Edinburgh

Hydropool

SIGNATURE TREATMENT S

La Costa Spa and Resort, Carlsbad California

'AGUA de la VIDA: With soothing whirlpools, thundering Roman Waterfalls, a purifying steam room and more. AGUA de la VIDA "the water of life", is an experience unique to La Costa. A series of water elements combined with a professional exfoliating scrub. It is the perfect prelude to a spa treatment, or an exhilarating journey all on its own.'

Preparation of the client

- The client should remove all clothing, jewellery, contact lenses and spectacles and wear a swimming costume or bikini when using a communal pool.
- Remove any make-up the client may be wearing using appropriate cleansing products.
- It is advisable that the client has a shower before a treatment to warm the muscle tissues and cleanse the body.
- Disposable slippers may be given to the client to wear when walking from the shower to the pool.

Treatment application

1. Assist the client into the pool, making sure that they are comfortable with the temperature.
2. Start the pool and allow the client to relax.
3. Keep checking with the client throughout to make sure they feel ok.
4. Leave the client for a maximum of 20 minutes.
5. Assist the client out of the pool and wrap them in either warm towels or a warm robe.
6. Encourage the client to take a shower, unless their treatment has included specific treatment products.
7. Allow the client to relax for 10–15 minutes with a glass of water.
8. Provide aftercare advice to the client, including further treatments and product use.
9. Record any comments or reactions on the record card.

HYDROTHERAPY BATH

This is similar to the spa pool but with the added benefits of various high-pressure jets, which can be directed at specific areas of the body, and a hand manipulated hose incorporated into the bath can also be used to direct water onto target areas of the body. Water used in the bath is commonly heated to temperatures of 34–38 °C. Seawater may be used, or the water may be infused with essential oils or mineral salts.

Hydrotherapy baths are a popular enhancement to treatments offered in a spa. As the baths fit the shape of the body, specific areas of the body can be massaged with these high-pressure jets and lymphatic drainage can be given through the therapist using the hose to target specific areas on the client.

As the bath is computer controlled it allows for preset massage programmes and sequences and maintenance of a constant temperature, and each of the jets can be automatically re-directed so as to create the benefits of a traditional massage.

FACT !

One of the signature treatments of a spa in France that specializes in water therapies involves lying in a warm bath in which 180 water jets are let loose on every part of the body, from the soles of the feet to the nape of the neck, leaving the client feeling energized but relaxed.

Anassa

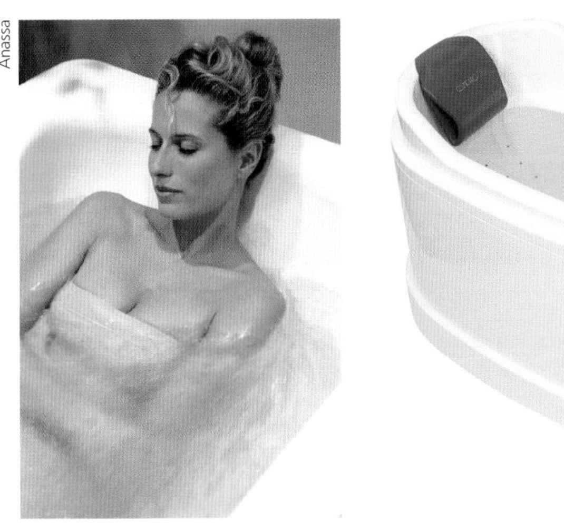

Hydrotherapy bath

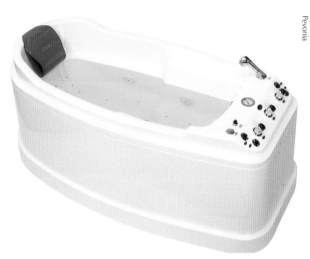

Pevonia

Hydrotherapy bath

SPA TIP

An example of how traditional massage movements can be replicated in the bath is simulating petrissage movements on the back by boosting the jets either side of the spine, starting from the lower back and moving upwards towards the shoulders.

HEALTH AND SAFETY

Baths should be cleaned thoroughly after each client and the jets cleaned through every morning to prevent them getting clogged with residue from products.

Products used

The same as in spa pools, but can be targeted more to the client's individual needs. If the spa specializes in thalassotherapy treatments then seawater may be used in the bath, but always check the manufacturer's guidelines first.

Consultation

Follow the general consultation steps outlined in chapter 15, concentrating on contra-indications specific to water-based treatments. Hydrotherapy

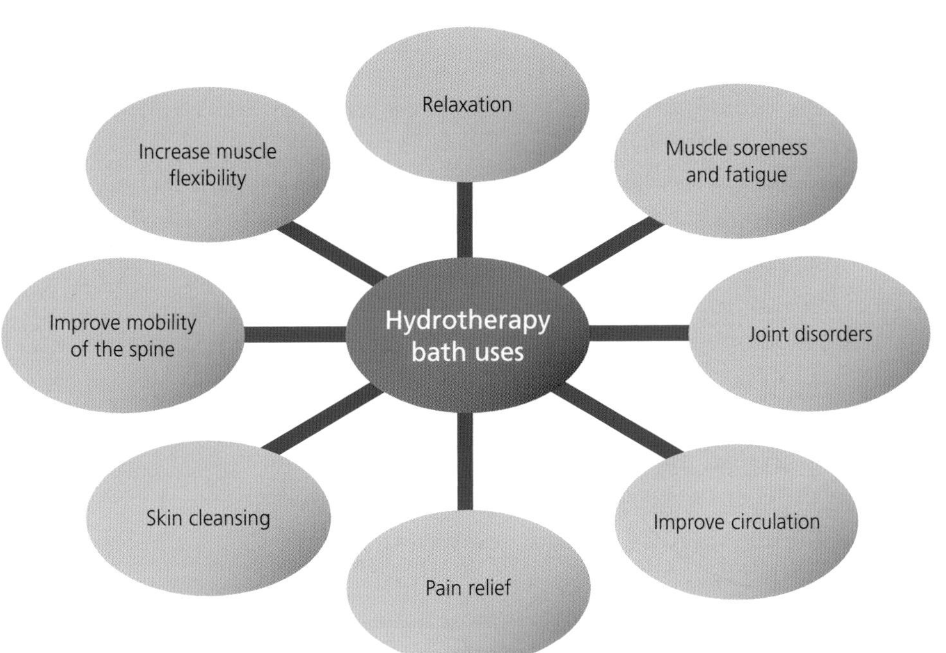

treatments are often used with other body treatments to increase their therapeutic effects. Treatment should last approximately 15–20 minutes and may be given 2–3 times per week, depending on the other treatments the client is receiving.

EQUIPMENT LIST

- hydrotherapy bath
- clean towels – small hand and large bath sheets
- shower
- skin cleansing products
- treatment products for the bath
- aromatherapy burner – can create a nice aroma
- candles – can be used in the room for subtle lighting, if appropriate
- subtle music – to assist clients relax
- water and glass tumblers – for the client after the treatment

Preparing the treatment room

The ambience should be the same as for all spa treatments and be set to the standard required by the spa. There are standard procedures to be followed for preparation of a hydrotherapy bath:

- Turn on the bath according to manufacturer's instructions.
- Fill the bath (no higher than the client's shoulders) with warm water and check the temperature.
- Turn on the jets to clear.
- Add any appropriate products to the water as the pool is filling.
- Check the programme for the jets is set to the client's needs.

Preparation of the client

- The client should remove all clothing and jewellery.
- Remove any make-up the client may be wearing using appropriate cleansing products.
- It is advisable that the client has a shower before a treatment to warm the muscle tissues and cleanse the body.
- Disposable slippers may be given to the client to wear when walking from the shower to the bath.

Treatment application

1 Assist the client into the bath, making sure that they are comfortable with the temperature.
2 Ensure that they are positioned correctly and aligned with the jets appropriate for that body area (spine, neck, feet).
3 Start the bath, set the appropriate programme and allow the client to relax.
4 If incorporating the manual hose, direct the water on the appropriate areas for deep tissue massage and lymphatic drainage.
5 Keep checking with the client throughout to make sure they feel ok.
6 Leave the client for a maximum of 20 minutes.
7 Assist the client out of the bath and wrap them in either warm towels or a warm robe.
8 Encourage the client to take a shower, unless their treatment has included specific treatment products.

HEALTH AND SAFETY !

If using the manual hose make sure it always remains under the water when massaging the client, otherwise water could end up all round the room!

HEALTH AND SAFETY !

If the client has severe varicose veins avoid using the manual hose on the affected area.

9 Allow the client to relax for 10–15 minutes with a glass of water.

10 Provide aftercare advice to the client, including further treatments and product use.

11 Record any comments or reactions on the record card.

FACT

Dr John Lilly designed the first isolation tank in 1954. The tank was an enclosed chamber filled with approximately 10 inches of warm saturated solution of Epsom salts, dense enough for a person to float. He found that whilst he was in the tank he could relax his mind without distraction or loosing consciousness.

FLOTATION

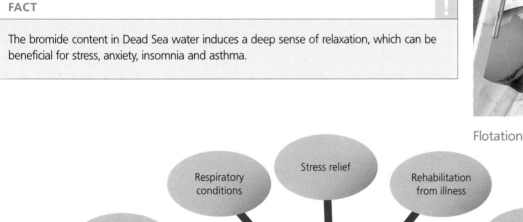

Flotation therapy is carried out in an enclosed tank or bath where the client floats in salt- and mineral-enriched warm water.

Today's flotation tanks are made from fibreglass, with the inside lined with plastic resin.

Flotation may be carried out in complete silence and in darkness or with lights and music, depending on the client's preference. Saturated mineral solutions are still used in flotation tanks, with companies like Finders using the added benefits of Dead Sea salts, which have beneficial effects on dry skin, eczema and psoriasis. Dry flotation is now commonly available in spas.

FACT

The bromide content in Dead Sea water induces a deep sense of relaxation, which can be beneficial for stress, anxiety, insomnia and asthma.

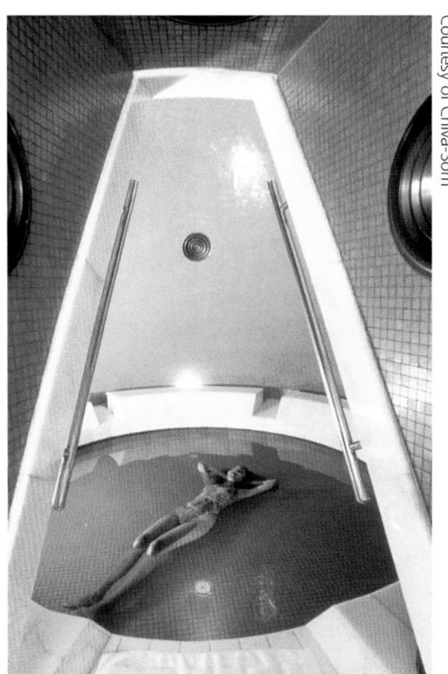

Courtesy of Chiva-Som

Flotation

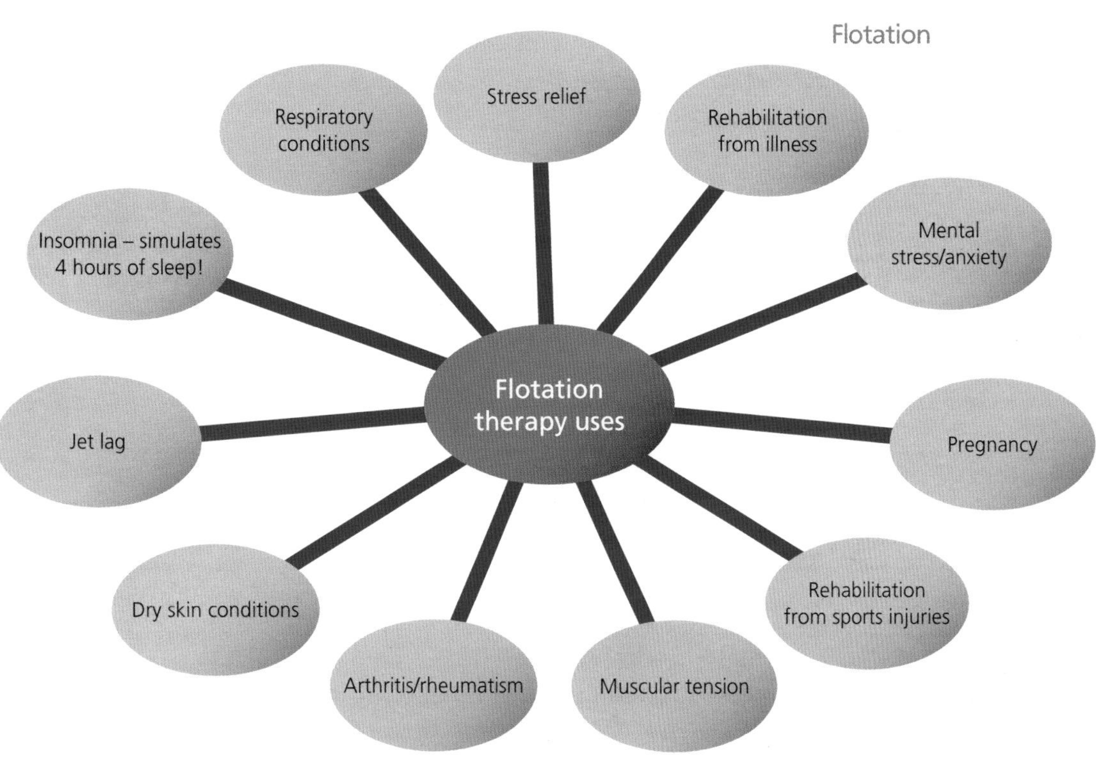

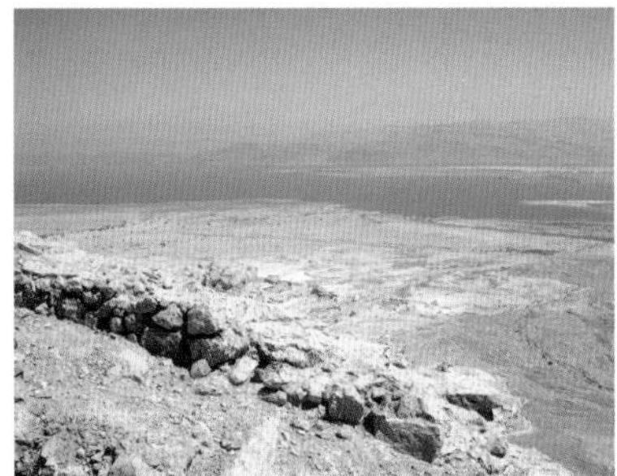

Dead Sea, Israel

HEALTH AND SAFETY

For clients who are claustrophobic the door can be kept open on an enclosed tank and a panic button is incorporated on the inside of the tank. New flotation pools are now becoming available in spas.

Products used

As mentioned earlier, the client lies in mineral-enriched water, which has numerous therapeutic qualities, so there is no need to add any additional products for the treatment, apart from the benefit of Dead Sea salts and similar products.

EQUIPMENT LIST

- flotation tank/bath
- epsom salts or mineral salt product
- chemicals to clean water
- clean towels – small hand and large bath sheets
- shower
- skin cleansing products
- petroleum jelly – to cover any cuts
- ear plugs – to prevent water in the ears
- aromatherapy burner – can create a nice aroma
- candles – can be used in the room for subtle lighting, if appropriate
- subtle music – to assist clients relax
- water and glass tumblers – for the client after the treatment

TERMINOLOGY

Buoyancy in water is when the body is balanced and held still in water through two opposing forces: buoyancy and gravity. Buoyancy in an upward direction and gravity in a downward direction.

Consultation

Follow the general consultation steps outlined in chapter 15, concentrating on those contra-indications specific to water-based treatments. Be particularly aware of clients who are claustrophobic or suffer from panic attacks, as the treatment will need to be adapted for them. A treatment usually lasts between 30 and 60 minutes and is given 2–3 times a week; some spas recommend a longer treatment to appreciate the full effects of a flotation treatment.

Preparing the treatment room

The ambience should be the same as for all spa treatments and be set to the standard required by the spa. Make sure the room is dimly lit and relaxing music is played. There are standard procedures to be followed for preparation of a flotation tank/bath:

- Fill the tank/bath to about 25 cm with warm water adding the Epsom salts or mineral salt products according to the manufacturer's instructions.
- Check the temperature is between 34 and 36 °C.
- Continually check the water between treatments to ensure it has a balanced pH of 7.2–7.4.
- The water should also be filtered between clients to remove any residue and be perfectly clear.

Preparation of the client

- The client should remove all clothing and jewellery.
- Remove any make-up the client may be wearing using appropriate cleansing products.
- It is advisable that the client has a shower before a treatment to warm the muscle tissues and cleanse the body.
- Disposable slippers may be given to the client to wear when walking from the shower to the tank/bath.
- Advise the client to use the toilet before flotation so they can fully relax.

Treatment application

1. Explain to the client how to operate the facilities in the flotation tank – lights, music, panic alarm, door (if there is one).
2. Assist the client into the tank, making sure that they are comfortable with the temperature.
3. Ensure that they are positioned correctly.
4. Ask the client to put in ear plugs, if required.
5. Keep checking with the client throughout to make sure they feel ok – particularly if they are nervous or it is their first treatment.
6. The treatment can last from 20 minutes to 1 hour.
7. Assist the client out of the tank and wrap them in either warm towels or a warm robe.
8. Encourage the client to take a shower to remove salts from the skin.
9. Allow the client to relax in a quiet area for 10–15 minutes with a glass of water.
10. Provide aftercare advice to the client, including further treatments and product use.
11. Record any comments or reactions on the record card.

HEALTH AND SAFETY !

Clients who are receiving flotation therapy for the first time must be given clear instructions before treatment begins, with a thorough explanation of the therapy. This is to alleviate any fears they may have, so that they enjoy their first experience of floating.

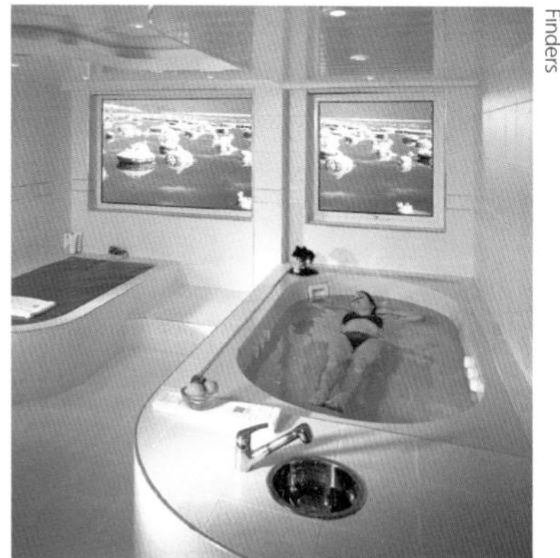
Finders

Hydrafloat flotation bath

BLITZ/SCOTCH SHOWER

This treatment involves a high-pressure shower jet directed at the body from various heights by a therapist who stands about 3 metres away from the client. The shower hose has a narrow jet nozzle, which forces the warm water out. The jet can be directed at different areas of the client's body to stimulate circulation and relieve tension in muscles, and different techniques can be performed to encourage lymphatic drainage. The temperature of the water can be changed from hot to cold should a more stimulating treatment be required.

Scotch shower uses:

- Muscle tension
- Stress
- Mild circulatory problems
- Cellulite
- Arthritis
- Overweight clients
- Clients on a detox programme

SPA TIP 

Blitz/Scotch shower treatment is now available in a stand-up shower, which can be used in the home or built into a treatment room. It has a digital control panel to programme the duration, temperature and variation of the sequence/ alternation of jets.

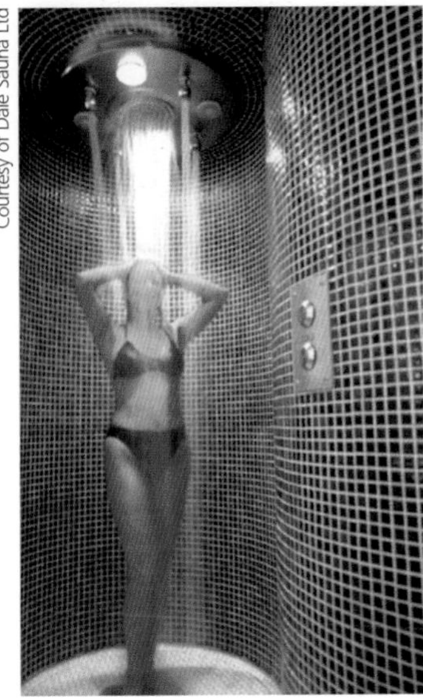
SPLASH Courtesy of Dale Sauna Ltd

Client showering

Products used

This treatment is usually used in a combination with other spa/hydrotherapy treatments, such as exfoliation, massage, steam and thalassotherapy. Seawater may be used in the jets, depending on the spa, instead of just hot and cold water.

Consultation

Follow the general spa consultation steps outlined in chapter 15, concentrating on contra-indications specific to water-based treatments. In particular, heart conditions, severe varicose veins and fragile bones must all be avoided with this shower. This treatment usually lasts between 15 and 20 minutes and can be given 2–3 times a week or, depending on the spa and treatment plan for the client, it may be given every day for 4–5 days.

Preparing the treatment room

The ambience should be the same as for all spa treatments and be set to the standard required by the spa. Ensure the shower is clean and that the floor is dry so that the client does not slip. Set the water to a warm temperature of approximately 34 °C.

Preparing the client

- The client should remove all clothing and jewellery – they may wear a bathing costume during the treatment.
- Remove any make-up the client may be wearing with appropriate cleansing products.
- Explain the procedure of the jet shower treatment to the client.
- Disposable slippers may be given to the client to wear when walking into the shower.
- Advise the client to use the toilet before the treatment as the shower jet may be uncomfortable if they have a full bladder.

EQUIPMENT LIST
blitz/Scotch shower hose
disposable foot wear – to prevent cross infection in the shower
warm towels – bath sheets
treatment gown
facial cleansing products – to remove any make-up
body treatment products – which may be applied after the treatment
jug of water and glass tumblers – for the client to rehydrate after the treatment

Treatment application

1. Ensure that the client is facing the back of the shower, with their back to the therapist.
2. They should be about 3 metres away from the therapist.
3. The jet must not be directed straight at the client to begin with.
4. Switch on the water and begin by breaking the spray by pressing the fingers into the jet at the nozzle.

5 Direct the spray at the client and after a few minutes apply the direct jet, starting at the ankles and working up the body, targeting specific areas if needed.
6 Ask the client to turn around, working on the sides of the body.
7 Then start on the front, directing the jet at the ankles and working up the body, finishing on the shoulder area – avoid the face.
8 For the last 2–3 minutes of the treatment conclude with a full body spray with warm water.

   Note: the temperature of the water from the jets can be alternated from hot to cold throughout the treatment if required.
9 Assist the client out of the shower and wrap them in warm towels or a gown.
10 Allow the client to relax in a quiet area for 10–15 minutes with a glass of water.
11 Products may be applied to the skin, such as body cream/oil.
12 Provide aftercare advice to the client, including further treatments and product use.
13 Record any comments or reactions on the record card.

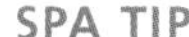

SPA TIP

At the Anassa Spa in Cyprus a blitz shower treatment is finished with an icy blast of marine water to invigorate and tone the muscles.

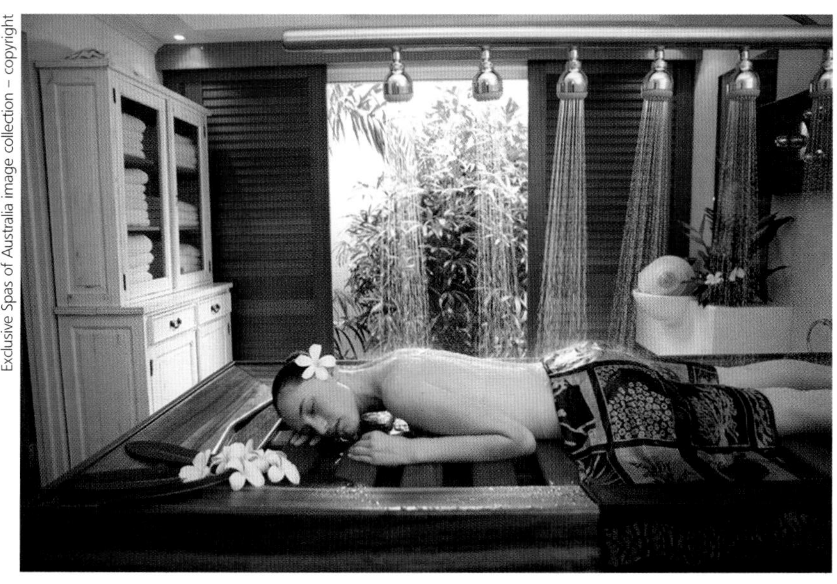

Exclusive Spas of Australia image collection – copyright

Swiss/Vichy shower

SWISS/VICHY SHOWER

Also known as the rain or affusion shower, this involves a cascading spray of water from five or more shower jets fixed to a horizontal shower bar. The client lies on a table below whilst the entire body is covered with a gentle shower of water. Massage and exfoliation treatments can be incorporated as the client lies on the bed and aromatic oils and other products can be introduced through the shower water. The water pressure and temperature can be adjusted to suit the client's needs,

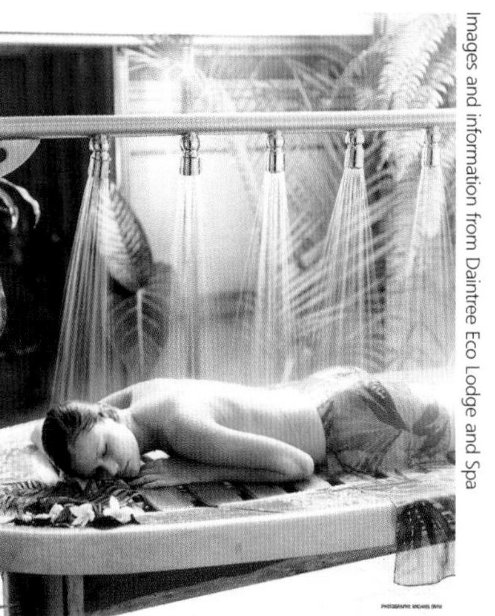

Images and information from Daintree Eco Lodge and Spa

Swiss shower table

SPA TIP

The **affusion shower** can use warm seawater and be combined with a deep tissue massage using essential oils as part of a treatment.

SIGNATURE TREATMENT

Danubius Health Spa

'Medicinal Water bathing: Rich in minerals and warmed by the heat of the earth's interior, thermal spring water is probably the most important natural remedy known to mankind. The spa water in Hungary is particularly effective in the treatment of rheumatism and disorders of the locomotor system and is effective in rehabilitation programs. Relaxing in thermal water is also a perfect way to release the stresses and strains of modern life. Visiting a Thermal Bath is part of everyday life for many Hungarians. Most guests will be advised to use the thermal waters as part of their program for a period of 20 minutes per day.'

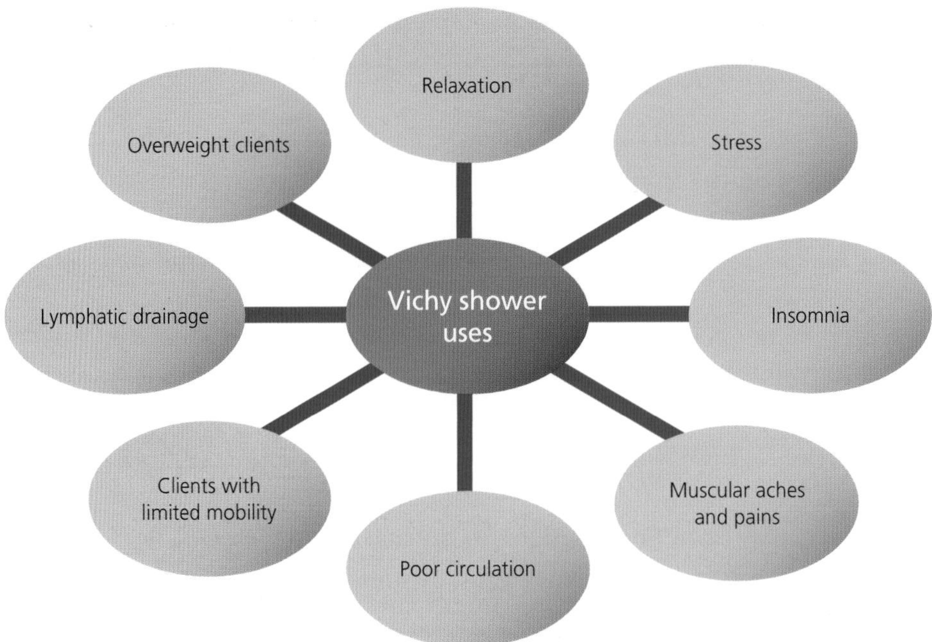
Vichy shower uses
Relaxation
Stress
Insomnia
Muscular aches and pains
Poor circulation
Clients with limited mobility
Lymphatic drainage
Overweight clients

though the general temperature of the water is usually about 38 °C. The anterior and posterior of the body are both treated in this form of hydro massage.

Products used

This treatment is usually used in a combination with other spa/hydrotherapy treatments such as exfoliation, massage and body wraps. Water-based aromatic products and oils can be introduced through the shower water to create a relaxing therapeutic treatment. Seawater may be used in the jets, depending on the spa, instead of just hot and cold water.

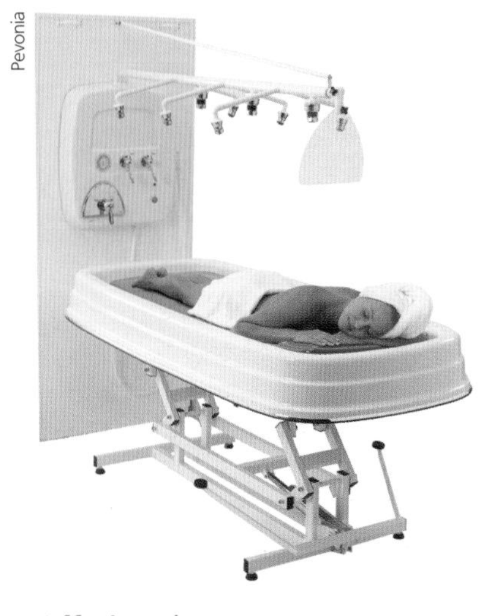
Pevonia

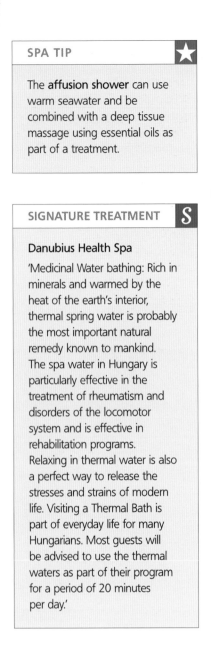

Affusion shower

Consultation

Follow the general consultation steps outlined in chapter 15, concentrating on contra-indications specific to water-based treatments. Consult on the treatment plan and how this form of shower can be incorporated with other spa treatments to increase the benefits. The treatment usually lasts about 20 minutes and can be given 2–3 times a week.

Preparing the treatment room

The ambience should be the same as for all spa treatments and be set to the standard required by the spa. Ensure the shower filters are clean and that the waterproof sheet on the table has been cleaned with appropriate products (the shower heads should be cleaned once a week).

Set the water to a warm temperature of approximately 38 °C and add any aromatic products to the diffuser in the shower system according to manufacturer's instructions.

Preparing the client

The client should be prepared the same as in the blitz/Scotch shower, making sure the client has received a full explanation of the treatment.

Treatment application

Assist the client to lie on the bed/table, face down to start the treatment.

1 Turn on the warm water with the spray facing away from the client and gradually move it across onto the client's body.
2 Leave the client to relax under the shower for 10 minutes before turning them over onto their back for a further 10 minutes.
3 If the treatment is being incorporated with a massage leave the client under the shower for 5 minutes to relax before starting the massage movements, and complete the massage with the client having a further 5 minute treatment under the shower.
4 Turn off the shower, moving the jets away from the client and helping them off the bed. Wrap in warm towels or a gown.

   Note: the temperature of the water from the jets can be alternated from hot to cold throughout the treatment if required.
5 Allow the client to relax after treatment in a quiet area for 10–15 minutes with a glass of water.
6 Provide aftercare advice to the client, including further treatments and product use.
7 Record any comments or reactions on the record card.

EQUIPMENT LIST

- Swiss/Vichy shower – combined with bed/table
- aromatic products for use with the shower
- warm towels – bath sheets
- treatment gown
- facial cleansing products – to remove any make-up
- body treatment products – which may be applied after the treatment
- jug of water and glasses – for the client to rehydrate after the treatment

KNEIPP THERAPY

This therapy uses hot and cold hydrotherapy treatments, along with herbs and minerals to help increase circulation. Popular in European spas, Kneipp therapy is most widely used in the form of treatment baths and showers using water of varied temperatures and incorporating the use of plant herbs.

FACT

A Bavarian priest, Sebastian Kneipp, pioneered Kneipp therapy at his treatment centre in 1889. In his cold baths the body could be immersed for between 30 seconds and 3 minutes to stimulate the nervous and circulatory systems. He also recommended walking barefoot in wet grass or snow for up to half an hour a day.

SPA TIP

At Chiva-Som Spa in Thailand, Kneipp therapy is incorporated into a footbath where the client walks calf-deep through a corridor of cold water with a bed of stones. Once the client is out of the water they are encouraged to have a hot steam bath.

Kneipp therapy uses:

- Muscle tension
- Stress
- Mild circulatory problems
- Cellulite
- Arthritis
- Lymph oedema
- Clients on a detox programme
- High blood pressure
- Headaches
- Fatigue

SPA TIP 

At the Capri Palace Hotel in Italy they have developed a 'seven day leg school programme' where, as part of the daily routine, clients can wade through hot and cold lanes of water in its 'Kneipp Vascular Pathway'.

Products used

Kneipp baths may use traditional herbs, such as chamomile, lavender, pine needle, rosemary and balm mint. Some spas may use herbs and spices that are native to their locality or products that have been pre-blended by a beauty/spa company and are individual to the type of spa and the treatments that are on offer. Kneipp therapy can be used alongside other spa treatments, such as massage, sauna, steam, thalassotherapy, exfoliation and body wraps.

Consultation

Follow the general spa consultation steps outlined in chapter 15, concentrating on contra-indications specific to water-based treatments. As the treatment sometimes involves extremes of temperature then particular attention must be paid if the client has any heart condition or history of blood clots, and it must not be given to pregnant clients.

SIGNATURE TREATMENT S

Danubius Health Spa

'Kneippness: Our treatments integrate the traditional Kneipp methods with the fundamentals of wellness, that is why they are called KNEIPPNESS. Kneipp treatments are applied onto the skin, or largest organ. They stimulate the nervous system which controls our inner organs. Treatments include pouring cold and warm water and jets of water on the various body parts, as well as packing, washing down, wrapping in herb infusions and aroma baths. In order to reach the correct balance between our body and soul, traditional Chinese and Indian therapies are applied (t'ai chi, yoga, etc.) along with walking or jogging bare foot in dewy grass or snow. This is supplemented by lifestyle and medical advice. Meals are composed mainly of vegetables, herbs and fresh bakery products. A medical examination is needed beforehand to determine the quantity and type of the treatments. The optimal duration of a cure is 2–3 weeks.'

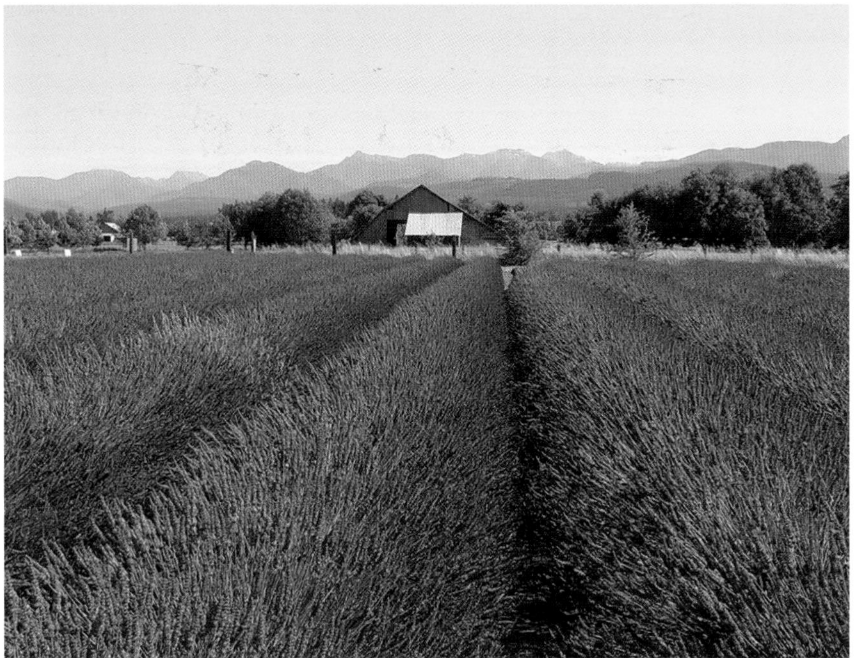

Lavender farm

HEALTH AND SAFETY

If the client is frail or elderly they may feel dizzy if the water is too hot and must be watched throughout the treatment.

SPA TIP

At the Willow Stream Spa in Banff, Canada, they incorporate the use of pine from the local pine forests into their signature pine herbal bath. They also use Hungarian minerals to aid detoxification and wildflower oils for aching muscles.

Treatment application

There are various ways in which treatments can be given, some forms employ powerful jets, such as the Blitz shower, where powerful jets of water massage the body using alternate hot and cold water to stimulate or, following the same procedure as in the Swiss shower, alternating the temperature of the water to invigorate the body. Using a bath is popular as this makes it easier to incorporate natural herbs:

- Arm/foot bath – can use both hot and cold water. If using cold water immerse the limbs for no more than 1 minute – depending on the client's tolerance of the temperature. If using warm water, 15–20 minutes.
- Hip bath (sitz) – again treatment can be with both hot and cold water using the same time guides as above for the different temperatures.
- Full bath – cold water: use only when clients are in good health for a maximum of 10 seconds. A warm/hot bath can be given for between 10–20 minutes.

During these treatments the client must be monitored at all times. Stop the treatment if the client feels either dizzy, faint or nauseous.

After the treatment the client should be wrapped in warm towels or a warm robe and allowed to relax for 15–20 minutes.

Encourage the client to drink plenty of water to re-hydrate.

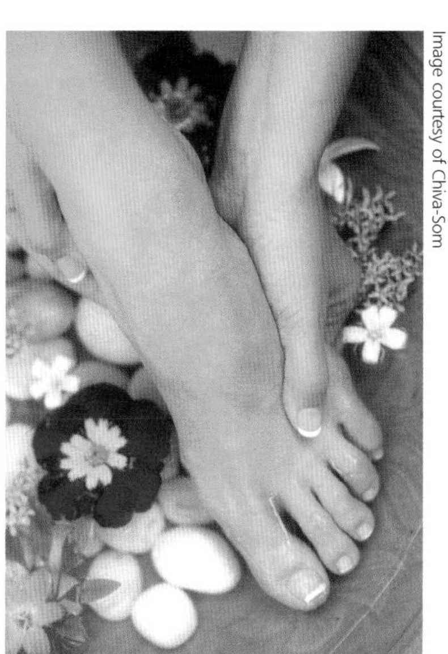

Image courtesy of Chiva-Som

Foot treatment, Chiva-Som

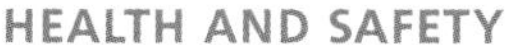

HEALTH AND SAFETY

If you are increasing the temperature from warm to hot then this must be done very gradually, otherwise the client may feel faint/dizzy.

HEALTH AND SAFETY

If the client is having a cold bath, splash cold water onto their forehead and check first to adjust the body to the temperature.

FACT

Where natural springs bubble up through the ground, the water can be diverted and used in thermal pools, which are beneficial for sufferers of arthritis, rheumatism and chronic joint and muscle disorders. Some spas in Germany and Hungary are used solely as thermal pools without any of the ultra-modern treatments available at other spas.

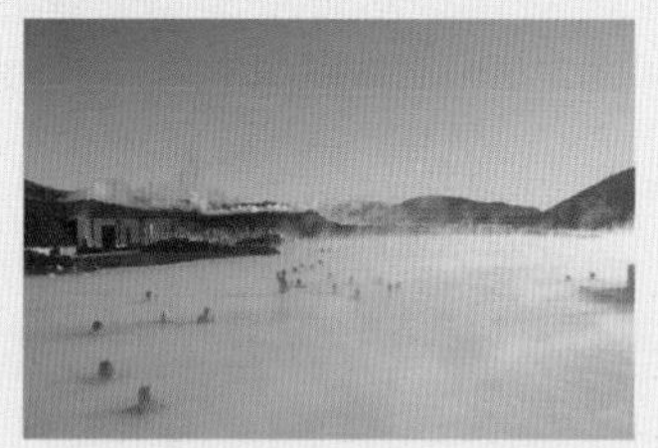

SPA HYGEINE

At the end of a treatment it is important that the spa area is cleaned in accordance with hygiene regulations and that equipment is closed down according to manufacturers' guidelines at the end of the working day. For more information on regulations, hygiene, monitoring spa water treatments and turning off spa equipment refer to chapter 10.

FACT

Water shiatsu was developed in the early 1980s by Harold Dull at Harbin Hot Springs, California.

SWIMMING POOLS

These are sometimes the focal point of a spa and are carefully incorporated into the whole design and setting. Pools are used for exercise as well as relaxation and this is very important when deciding on the size and look of a pool. Some larger pools incorporate a therapy pool where jets are strategically placed around the sides for the client to be massaged by warm water. The water in the therapy pool may be normal, but quite often it contains mineral-enriched water to increase the benefits. In some spas the pools are the main treatment area, where thermal pools, pools at contrasting temperatures or rich in different minerals/salts/seawater are used to restore health, vitality and alleviate various ailments.

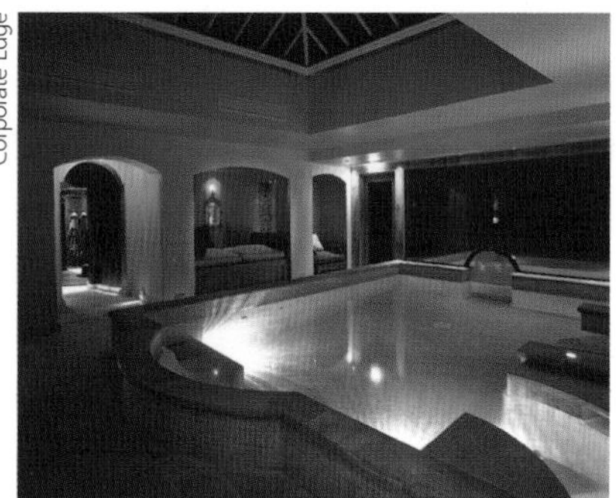

Corporate Edge

Monty's Spa, Charlton House

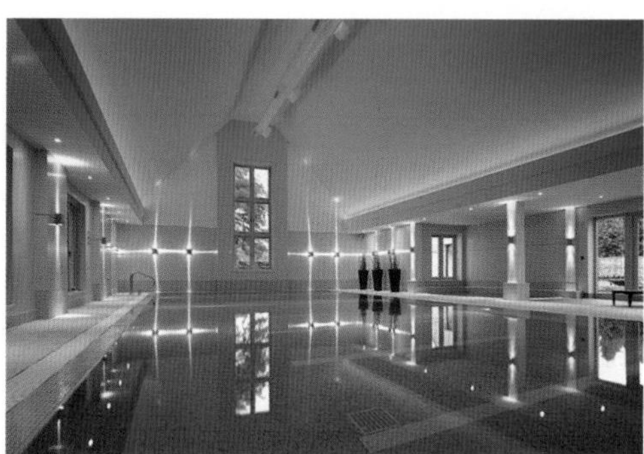

Corporate Edge

Calcot Manor Spa

WATSU

Watsu is based on the synthesis of shiatsu and water as relaxing aquatic bodywork. The emphasis of **water shiatsu** is on stretching the body in warm water, which acts as a support for freeing the joints and muscles and also promotes deep relaxation. The movements are performed by the client being held in the warm water and the practitioner moving the body through gentle stretches and rotations in a slow rhythmic motion in time with the client's breath. The body is allowed to float effortlessly in the warmth, releasing tension, stress and pain and being moved into positions that had previous limitations.

Each watsu session is unique to the client but usually lasts for about 1 hour. As with all spa treatments, a full consultation must be carried out beforehand to ascertain the client's needs and any precautions or contra-indications.

Benefits of watsu include:

- reduces stress and anxiety
- increases energy levels
- increases client's range of motion

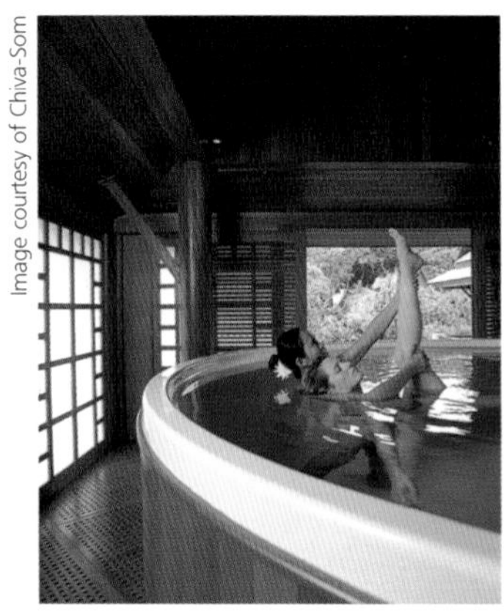

Watsu treatment at Chiva-Som

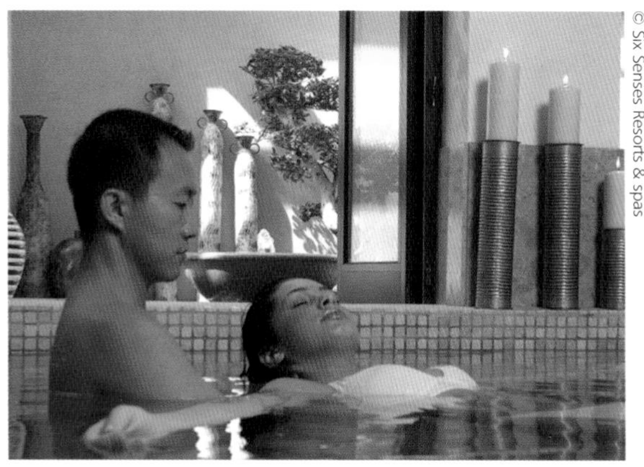

Watsu treatment at Six Senses Spa

SPA TIP

For water-based treatments the products you may be using could include ingredients such as mineral salts (Dead Sea), seaweed, essential oils and algae. These can be used in the bath/shower, body creams, slimming/contouring creams, body masks and in tablets to aid detoxification.

SPA TIP 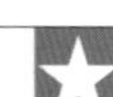

Dry skin brushing is recommended before any body treatment in order to stimulate blood and lymph circulation and remove toxins. The client can also do this very easily at home before they have a bath or shower and it is very good in helping combat cellulite.

- decreases pain, fatigue and muscle tension
- improves breathing patterns
- improves insomnia
- improves body awareness and releases emotional stress.

The water provides elderly, physically handicapped and pregnant clients with a feeling of being lighter, loosens muscles and joints and increase flexibility where mobility was restricted previously.

Psychologically, the client feels safe and nurtured and an intuitive trust develops between the practitioner and the client as the client is held quietly in the water and gently rocked.

Watsu as a treatment in spas is increasing in popularity, with specialized pools being built to carry out the treatments.

POST-TREATMENT ADVICE

After you have completed a spa hydrotherapy treatment, it is always important to give advice to the client on homecare and the products they may use. Record their feedback on the treatment and the further treatments that you recommend. The following guidelines are important:

- The client must drink plenty of water after a treatment and relax until body temperature returns to normal.
- Drinking water, herb teas and natural juices will help rehydrate the client and also aid further detoxification of the body. The client should try to avoid caffeine drinks or alcohol for the next 24 hours so as to gain the most benefit from their treatment.
- The client must not do too much physical exercise for a few hours following treatment as they may still feel dizzy – pilates, yoga or a gentle walk would be OK.

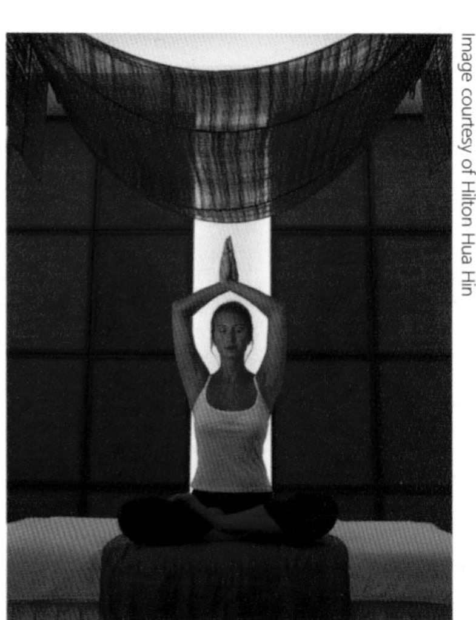

Yoga pose

SIGNATURE TREATMENT S

Champneys Health Resorts

'Thalassotherapy Salt Water Experience: A mineral rich warm pool with hydrotherapy jets to stimulate and tone tired aching muscles. Excellent for treating cellulite, arthritis and general muscular and joint pains.'

- Further treatments may be given after hydrotherapy and may be part of the client's treatment plan, particularly if they are staying at a spa for a few days.
- If the client is losing weight or on a detox plan then they may have received advice from the spa's nutritionist, but, if not, then you may want to recommend healthy eating habits and suitable exercises for them to do at home.
- To maintain and enhance the benefits of any treatment, it is important to recommend products for the client to use at home.

LINKED TREATMENTS

Hydrotherapy

A lot of the water treatments offered at a spa do not involve hands-on contact with the client by the therapist, so other more personal treatments complement hydrotherapy:

- Body/aromatherapy massage – to further enhance relaxation and relieve tension in muscles.
- Rasul – ideal as a pre-treatment as the client has already warmed up their body tissue and started to absorb mineral-rich properties from the mud.
- Crystal healing – assists in balancing the client's energy levels and allows the client to really relax.
- Herbal/seaweed wrap – ideal after a water treatment as it encourages the body to continue detoxing whilst absorbing minerals, etc.
- Exfoliation – good as a pre-treatment to remove dead skin cells.

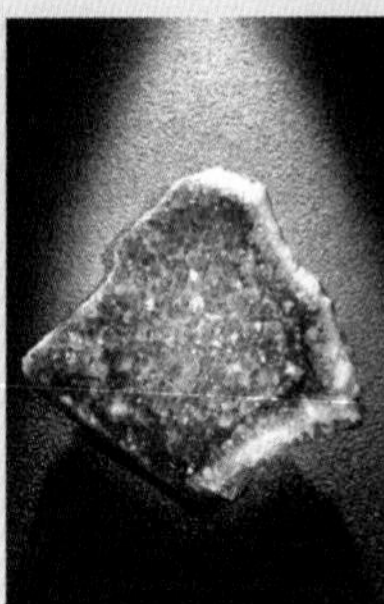

Courtesy of The Spa at Mandarin Oriental

Amethyst Geode in Amethyst Crystal Steam Room, Mandarin Oriental

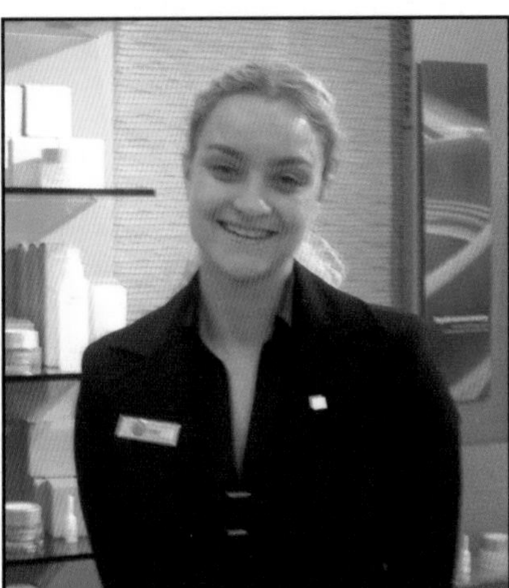

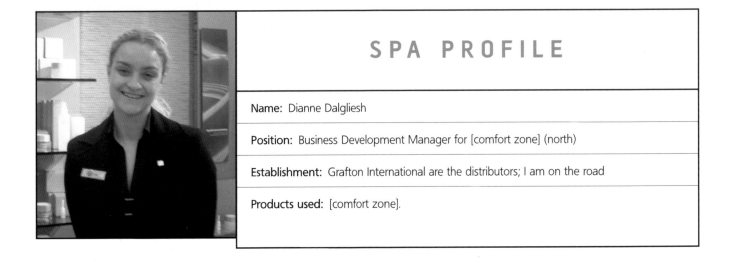

SPA PROFILE

Name: Dianne Dalgliesh

Position: Business Development Manager for [comfort zone] (north)

Establishment: Grafton International are the distributors; I am on the road

Products used: [comfort zone].

Number of staff/roles: Team of 5 people concentrate on [comfort zone] but we are expanding very quickly.

Training/experience: South Trafford College – qualified in Beauty Therapy in 1991; Ragdale Hall health hydro; health and beauty salon; in-flight beauty therapist for Virgin Atlantic; training manager for Kanebo Cosmetics; Group Sales and Membership Co-ordinator for Spa La Manga Club for Hyatt Hotels.

Main responsibilities: Service all existing accounts which stock [comfort zone]; monthly visits to inform of promotions and offers; on-site training for new staff; promotion days to increase sales; source new business.

Best parts of the job: Putting together action plans to help existing accounts improve their business; opening new accounts and watching this exciting brand grow and expand rapidly.

Secrets of a successful spa therapist: This profession is not just a job, it is a vocation. A successful spa therapist will want to give the best treatment to every client with an extremely caring nature. The client should feel confident and safe in their hands. You can have the best products and the best establishment but it is the therapist that makes the difference! A successful spa therapist will be: confident, well groomed, able to give expert advice, professional, caring and able to empathize with the client when needed. Most of all, love what they do!

KEY/CORE SKILLS OPPORTUNITIES

To be an excellent spa therapist you must be able to communicate well, both orally and in writing. To be able to succeed and progress in the spa industry, it is also essential that you have an ability to work with numbers and information technology (IT). Increasingly, employers are looking for spa therapists with these 'key' skills when they recruit staff. NVQ/SVQ unit **BT29** provides you with an opportunity to develop evidence for the following:

KEY SKILLS	CORE SKILLS
Communication Level 2; C2.1a, C2.2	Communication Intermediate 1; Task 1 and 3
Working with others Level 2; WO2.1, WO2.2	Working with others Intermediate 1; Tasks 1, 2 and 3
Improving own learning and performance Level 3; LP3.1, LP3.2	(no parallel unit in core skills)

Assessment of knowledge and understanding

When you have some free time, test your understanding and knowledge by answering the following questions. Do this at regular intervals and it will reinforce your learning and help you retain the knowledge, so you are able to perform better in your assessments.

Consult with the client

1 Name six contra-indications to check for before giving any hydrotherapy treatment.

2 Why is it important to check the client continually when giving a hydrotherapy bath treatment?

3 What considerations must you take into account when devising a treatment plan for a client who is on a detox programme and would like a series of water-based treatments?

4 How would the client be prepared before a spa water treatment?

5 What important instructions must you give to a client before a flotation treatment?

6 What does the Greek word 'thalassotherapy' mean?

7 How would you carry out a skin test to establish whether the client is allergic to a product used in a water treatment.

Prepare for the treatment

1 Name six conditions that benefit from water-based treatments.

2 What types of products can be used in hydrotherapy/spa pool treatments?

3 How would you prepare the treatment room and equipment for the following treatments:
 a. hydrotherapy bath?
 b. flotation tank?
 c. Swiss shower?

4 What is the ideal temperature for the water in a spa pool/hydrotherapy bath?

5 What kind of water can be used in a blitz/Scotch shower?

6 How would you accustom the client to the water temperature in a cold water treatment?

Carry out water therapy treatments

1 How often can the client receive a hydrotherapy bath treatment in a single week?

2 Name five physical effects on the body of water treatments.

3 Name three psychological effects of water-based treatments.

4 What benefits do Dead Sea salts have in a flotation treatment?

5 Why is it important for the client to take a shower after some water treatments?

6 What benefits will the client receive from having a treatment using alternate cold and hot water jets.

7 Give three water-based treatments that would be beneficial for a client with cellulite.

8 What precautions must the client take before bathing in water containing a high concentration of salts?

Provide aftercare advice to the client

1 Name four adverse reactions the client may experience after a water treatment and how you would treat the client for them.

2 Why is it important that the client is advised to rest and drink plenty of water after a treatment?

3 What further spa treatments may be give after hydrotherapy?

4 What type of products could you advise the client to use at home following thalassotherapy-based treatments?

chapter 10

Testing, control and monitoring of spa/water treatments

BT28

Set up, monitor and shut down water, temperature and spa facilities

BT15

Assist with spa treatments

Learning objectives

This chapter covers the skills a spa therapist needs for setting up, monitoring and shutting down water, temperature and spa facilties.

It describes the skills and knowledge necessary to enable you to:

- **prepare, clean and maintain the spa environment**
- **monitor water, temperature and spa treatments and environment**
- **provide aftercare advice**
- **complete shut down of treatment areas and spa environment**

When setting up, monitoring and shutting down water, temperature and spa facilties it is important to use the skills you have learnt in the following core units:

G1 Ensure your own actions reduce risks to health and safety

G6 Promote additional products or services to clients

G11 Contribute to the financial effectiveness of the business

INTRODUCTION

Spa equipment monitoring and maintenance is an important part of the spa therapist's daily routine. As spas are a communal area there are Health and Safety regulations to adhere to in order to make the environment as hygienic as possible and safe for everyone using it. The set up, monitoring and shut down of spa equipment will be slightly different depending on the individual manufacturer but the basic procedures will be the same.

SPA HEALTH AND SAFETY REGULATIONS

There is much legislation in the United Kingdom that relates to the safe maintenance of equipment, the providing of a healthy environment for both clients and employees, the correct storage of equipment and chemicals and monitoring of possible hazards within the spa. It is the responsibility of all employees as well as management to maintain these standards. Management's key function in this respect is to make sure that staff are properly trained and aware of all Health and Safety regulations.

World wide, each country will have its own regulations that must be followed and which will be carefully monitored by the local authorities.

The following Health and Safety regulations are mandatory within the UK spa environment, while further regulations and First Aid requirements are covered in more depth in chapter 5.

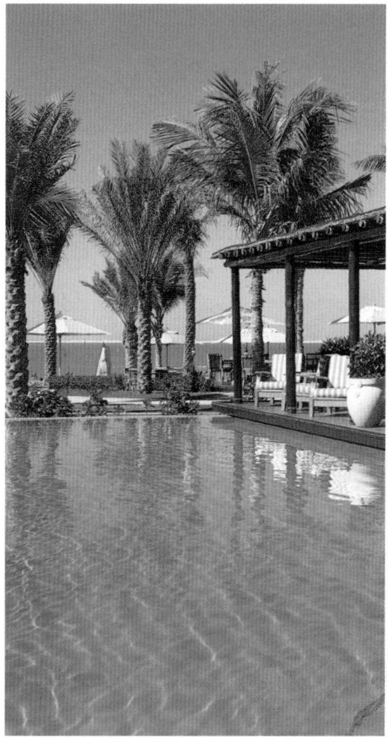

Arabian Court Pool, One&Only Royal Mirage, Dubai

Health and Safety at Work Act 1974

- It is the employer's responsibility to ensure that the workplace is maintained to high standards of Health and Safety for both clients and employees.
- This act must be displayed clearly for employees to see.
- All staff must abide by these regulations and report to management any hazards they notice that could be of potential danger to clients and employees.

Personal Protective Equipment at Work Regulations 1992 (PPE)

Appropriate equipment and clothing must be provided for employees where a risk or hazard in their job/duties has been identified

Control of Substances Hazardous to Health Regulations 1999 (COSHH)

- Substances that are hazardous to health and used in the spa must be clearly identified and stored in the correct place.
- Manufacturers have to provide clear guidelines on how the product should be stored and handled.

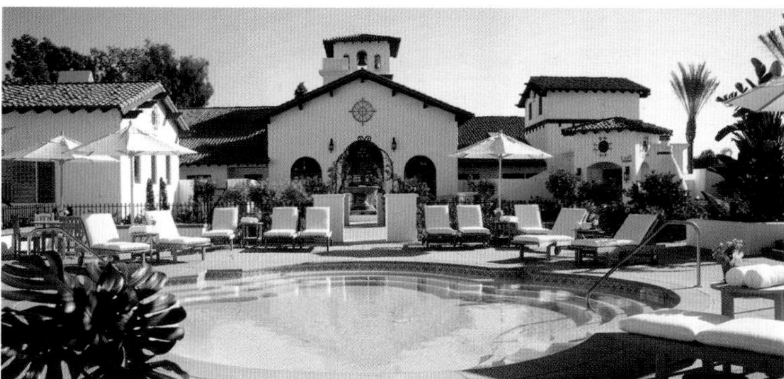

Spa courtyard, La Costa Resort & Spa, California

ACTIVITY

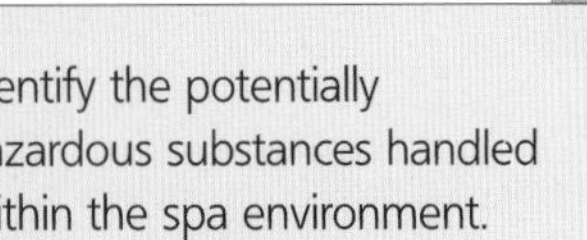

Identify the potentially hazardous substances handled within the spa environment. Is there a need for protective equipment to be made available to the spa therapist?

- Chemicals – such as those used in water testing and maintenance – should be stored securely in a fire-resistant room or cupboard, away from public areas.
- All staff who use hazardous materials should be trained correctly in their use.

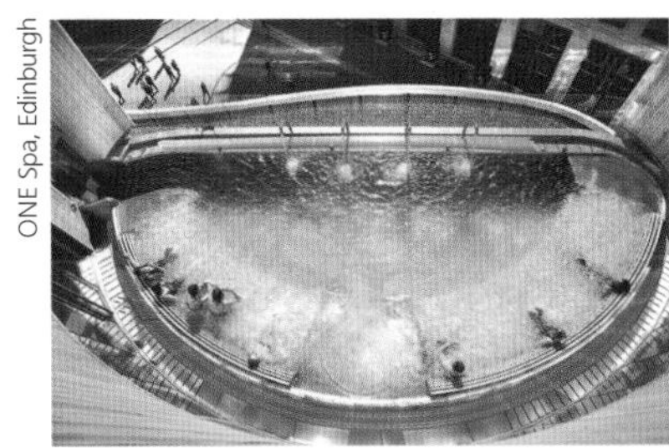

ONE Spa, Edinburgh

Hydropool

Workplace (Health, Safety and Welfare) Regulations 1992

These regulations relate to the basic management of the environment, such as ventilation, lighting, temperature, storage and handling of waste materials, cleanliness, washing, toilet and changing facilities, fresh drinking water and staff areas for resting and eating.

PREPARE, CLEAN AND MAINTAIN THE SPA ENVIRONMENT

SPA TIP

A dirty, untidy spa will not have the clients rushing back for more! This is so important in today's competitive spa market where it is vital that the client receives the best treatment in the most hygienic environment.

It is important that all treatment areas are cleaned and kept at a high standard of health and safety for the benefit of the clients, as well as for the good impression that it makes. Most large spas employ cleaners who will clean the spa at the beginning and end of the working day, but it is the therapist's job to keep their area clean throughout the day between clients and treatments. Work surfaces, floors and equipment should be cleaned and disinfected according to manufacturers' guidelines to prevent the breeding of bacteria.

Managers should inspect the spa area thoroughly on a weekly basis, but on a **daily basis** they should walk through all working areas to ensure they are being maintained to the required standard.

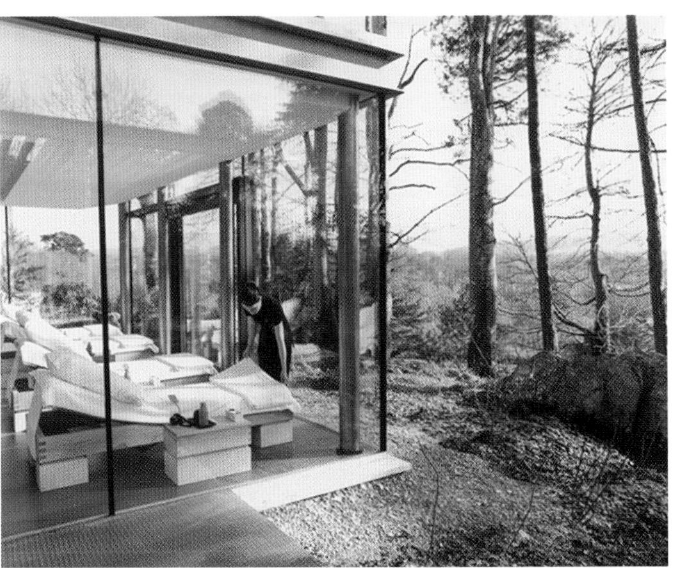

Relaxation area, Sámas

Cleaning of spa areas/equipment

Sauna	*Steam*	*Showers*	*Spa pool*	*Flotation*
• Daily wipe down flooring and surfaces with appropriate disinfectant cleaner • Keep the door open at night when the sauna is switched off to allow in fresh air • Do not allow water to stagnate in a bucket – empty daily!	• Daily wipe down flooring and surfaces with appropriate disinfectant cleaner • Make sure there is no moisture or water left in the room or cabinet as it will start to smell unpleasant	• Clean the shower area with appropriate cleaning products • Make sure any product or its residue are removed from plugholes between clients as it looks unprofessional not to • Swiss/Vichy shower tables should be cleaned with disinfectant between clients as recommended by the manufacturers,	• The water in the pool is regularly maintained by being filtered and chemically treated • In a hydrotherapy bath the water is changed for each client. The bath should be cleaned with appropriate cleaning products and the jets cleaned daily according to manufacturers' instructions • The floor around the pool or bath should be cleaned daily and regularly throughout the day, and any water on the floor wiped up	• The water should be filtered between clients to remove any residue and make it perfectly clear • The bath or tank should be regularly cleaned inside according to manufacturers' instructions • The floor around the bath or tank should be cleaned daily with appropriate cleaner

Water treatment

Correct water treatment ensures that the spa pool water is safe for client treatments and clean to swim and bathe in. As the spa pool or swimming pool are not drained daily, they rely on being continually filtered and chemically treated to achieve safe and sparkling water conditions.

There are numerous chemical products on the market to disinfect, control and balance the water in a spa pool.

HEALTH AND SAFETY !

Clients should be encouraged to take showers before using spa pools, baths, saunas or flotation tanks to prevent cross-infection and their leaving creams or oil residue in the water.

Chlorine

This was one of the most widely used disinfectants for swimming pools and must be regularly measured to control the chlorination process. High levels of chlorine contaminants may make the eyes sting, which used to be a common complaint when people used public swimming baths.

Bromine

Bromine tablets slowly dissolve in water and are used in the disinfection of spa water and other water treatments. As they are in tablet form they can be dispensed into the water using an erosion feeder or brominator. They are less likely to irritate the skin than chlorine and are more suited to the higher temperatures of spa pools. Regular measurement of bromine-treated water is essential, as twice the quantity of bromine is needed to achieve the same results as chlorine.

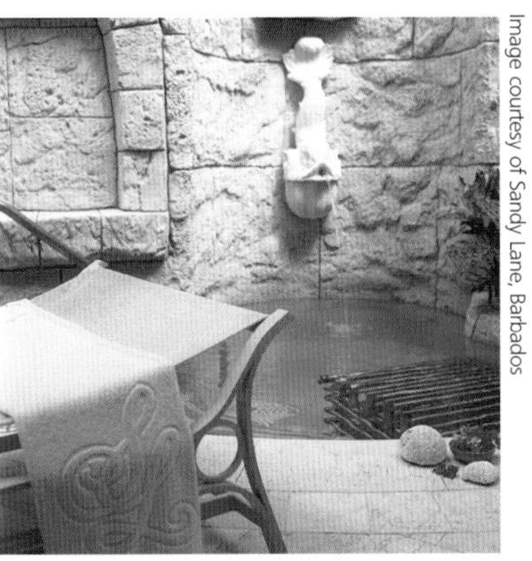

Image courtesy of Sandy Lane, Barbados

Private jet pool

HEALTH AND SAFETY !

Corrosive water will try to saturate itself by dissolving the structure of the pool. Scale, formed by the separation of salts from hard water, causes cloudy water and will eventually come to form a coating on pool components.

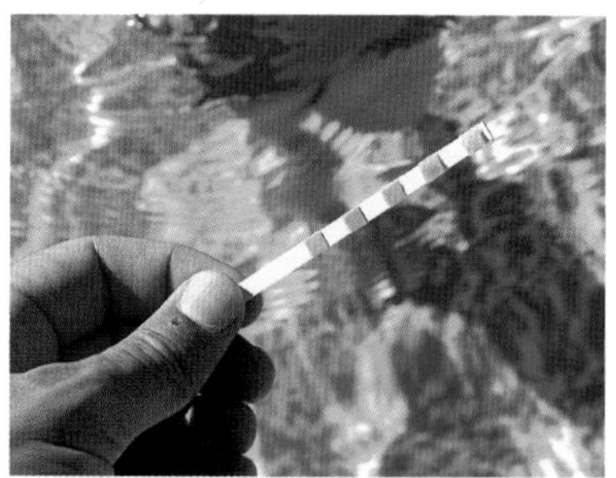

All water testing results should be written down and kept for any local authority inspectors to check when they visit

HEALTH AND SAFETY !

Disinfectants will not work properly if debris has been allowed to build up in the pool and around the filters and fixtures.

HEALTH AND SAFETY !

It is important that the client showers before any water treatment to prevent the spread of waterborne infections.

Ozone

This is a relatively new way of treating spa pool water. An ozone generator destroys bacteria and viruses in the water naturally through ozone. The advantages of this method are that there is no smell and less chance of any irritation to the skin. It is also less corrosive than chlorine, so will not damage the equipment or allow any build-up of scale around the pool and fixtures.

Other chemicals used in the treatment of water are hypochlorous acid, sodium and calcium hypochlorite and chloramine.

Water testing

Water testing is carried out in accordance with the chemicals used to ensure that it is safe and effective and to determine whether the water is corrosive, scale-forming or nicely balanced.

The Langelier Saturation Index is used to calculate:

- Calcium hardness in the water – 75 to 150 mg per litre.
- pH – range of 7.2 to 7.6; this is important as it affects the power of the disinfectant.
- Alkalinity – 100 to 150 mg per litre.
- Temperature – ideally between 27–30 °C in commercial pools and 34–37 °C in spa pools.

These are considered safe operating levels and water samples are measured against this index.

Regular testing of the water, cleaning of pipes and filters, maintaining disinfectant levels and keeping records of all water treatment will help to reduce the risks.

There are various pool tester kits on the market designed for simple pool water disinfection control and pH monitoring. Some are more elaborate than others but they all basically use the worldwide recommended DPD test which is used by all companies to check the chlorine levels in drinking water.

Monitoring and testing water

- Always check the temperature of the pool water regularly using a thermometer.
- Take a sample of water in a sample tube to test pH, alkalinity and chlorine/bromine levels.

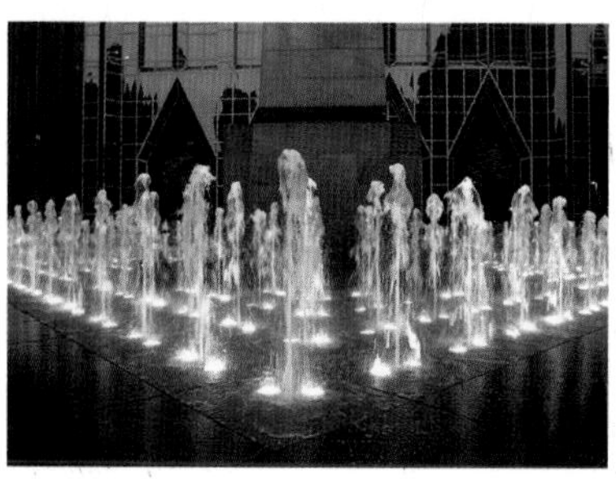

HEALTH AND SAFETY !

Environmental Health Officer (EHO) is employed by the local authority to reinforce the various Health and Safety at work regulations and ensure all businesses are abiding by them. If they find any areas of danger, they give a period of notice in which the problem must be rectified. If this is not complied with, they can then close a business down until such time as they are satisfied there is no longer any risk.

- By adding a DPD 1 tablet to the water to calculate the free chlorine concentration, you will see a colour change which can either be measured against a coloured metric disk or by an instrument into which the sample tube is placed – by simply pressing a button the concentration is immediately displayed on a screen.
- A phenol red tablet can be added to the water sample to measure the pH level in the same way as testing for chlorine.
- Alkalinity, ozone levels and calcium hardness can also be measured using tablet count tests.

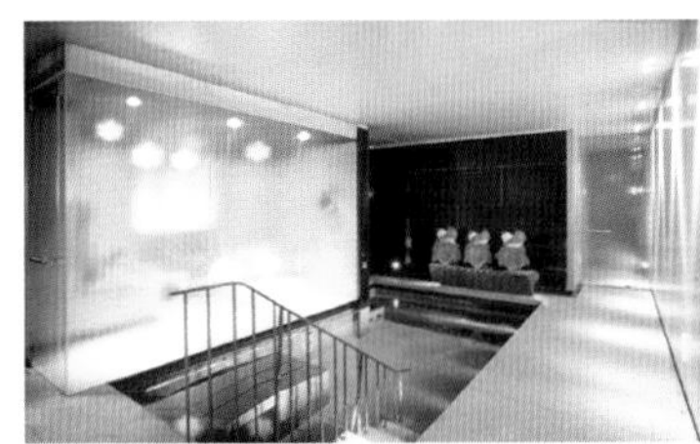
Courtesy of The Spa at Mandarin Oriental

Vitality Pool, Mandarin Oriental

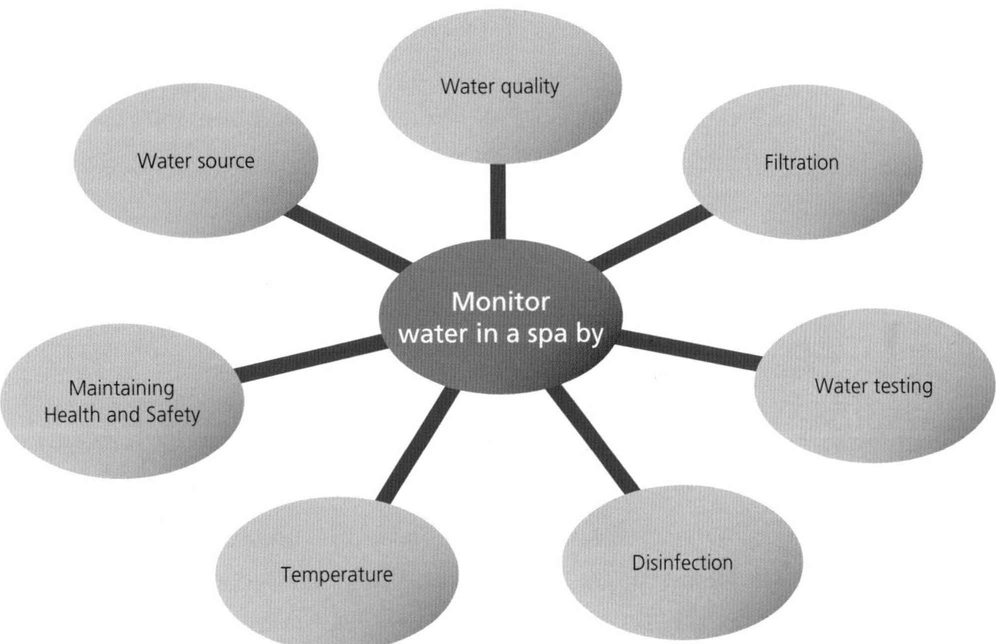

Legionnaires' disease

Recent public scares concerning spa pools have been raised by experts warning that they could be a breeding ground for legionnaires' disease. It is the high temperature of the water in spa pools and its re-circulation that is said to provide an ideal environment for the bacteria. Symptoms of the disease include aching muscles, tiredness, headaches, cough and fever. The infection can be treated with antibiotics but there have been fatalities as a result of the disease.

HEALTH AND SAFETY !

Cloudy pool water can be dangerous as it prevents a person in distress at the bottom of a pool being seen.

Filtration of spa water

Water is pumped through a filter in order to remove any small particles and fine debris, which if left in the water may turn the water cloudy. Inadequate filtration of the water allows the build-up of debris, which means the pool chemicals cannot do their job properly and algae and bacteria may start to take over the water.

Most filters are switched on for at least 10 hours during the day, when the water is being used most, but some pool operators find that it is less expensive to have it running 24 hours with a reduced capacity at night. Weekly

HEALTH AND SAFETY !

To check for high standards of Health and Safety in a swimming pool look for visible notices reminding clients to shower before using the pool. The smell of chlorine in the water should be mild and the water clear, bright and sparkling.

Exclusive Spas Australia. Image Collection – Copyright

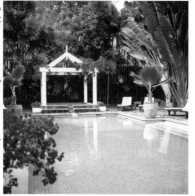

Pergola and pool, Sebel Reef House Palm Cove, Australia

> **SPA TIP** 
>
> Flooring is important in a spa area where water is being used, as potential risks, such as a client slipping on a wet floor, are high. Non-slip tiling is the most suitable floor surface, as it is easy to clean, good looking and can incorporate designs, such as mosaics.

> **FACT** !
>
> The Institute of Sports and Recreation Management has created an award for the management of public swimming pools. This award covers water treatment systems, water treatment plant and heating and ventilation systems. Pools which apply for this and meet the nationally approved specifications will receive a plaque, which they can display. Every 2 years the application is reviewed.

> **HEALTH AND SAFETY** !
>
> The Swimming Pool and Allied Trades Association (SPATA) is the trade association for the swimming pool industry in the United Kingdom. SPATA sets down standards governing the construction and operation of pools, spas, saunas and steam rooms and a list of suitable qualified and approved pool and spa installers is available.

backwash cleaning of the filter is important as loose dirt and debris get caught in the filter; this should only take about 5 minutes. Several times a year it is necessary to chemically clean the filter to remove stubborn debris and oils.

Testing and maintenance of the water is important in water filtration as, if scale is allowed to form, it tends to clog up the filter first, thereby making it incapable of filtering the water adequately.

SPA POOL MAINTENANCE SCHEDULE

Every week a full service should be carried out on spa pool facilities to check the water balancing and filtration systems. This should consist of the following maintenance procedures:

- Water sample to test pH, alkalinity, chemical levels and calcium hardness.
- Drain out the spa water and clean all the equipment, pool and filters with cleaning products appropriate for a spa.
- Check all equipment – filtration, treatment plants, etc. – and equipment settings.
- Check all pool maintenance records and report any areas of concern.
- Re-fill the spa.
- Check chemical levels in the treatment plant and re-supply as necessary.
- Check water temperature.

SHUTTING DOWN SPA EQUIPMENT

At the end of the day all spa equipment needs to be shut down in accordance with manufacturers' instructions and the training that has been given with these.

- All water treatment equipment, apart from the spa pool and swimming pool, should be switched off at the electricity mains and in accordance with the manufacturers' guidelines.
- A switch in the plant room should turn off the spa pool and any other pool facilities. The water filter system may be left on overnight.
- Some spas may test the water again at the end of the working day to ensure water levels are ok for the following morning.

- Any water on the floors should be removed so that they are dry – some spa floors may be cleaned with a high-pressure hose first, depending on what treatments have been carried out in the area.
- All baths, showers and wet table surfaces should be cleaned with the appropriate cleaner.
- Remove and clean floor mats in the shower as they can harbour bacteria.
- Tiled areas should be cleaned with a suitable tile disinfectant.
- Remove any towels from the spa area and place them in laundry baskets to be laundered.
- All rubbish should be removed in a sealed waste bag to an appropriate area – this may be at the back, outside the spa.
- The treatment areas and pool should be left clean, ready for use the following day.

SIGNATURE TREATMENT S

Altira SPA Majorca

'Algotherm Thalasso Bath with underwater shower: With this fundamental and highly effective technique, the guest lies in a bath of warm seawater and receives a whole body massage from a powerful underwater jet. This treatment is a particularly effective method for stimulating the circulation in the lower limbs. It also improves muscle tone and circulation while promoting a sense of relaxation.'

SPA PROFILE

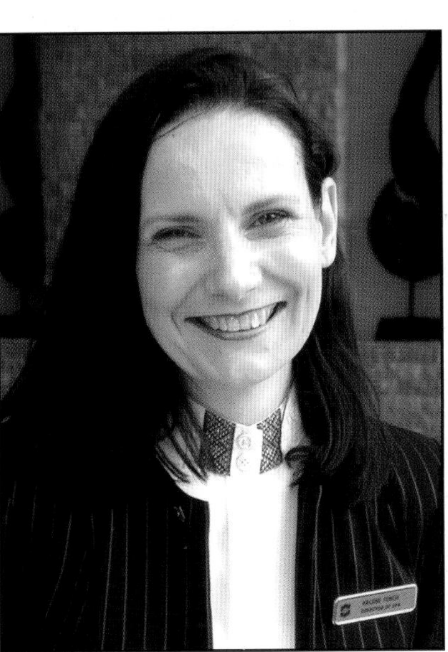

Name: Arlene Finch

Position: Spa Director

Establishment: Chi, The Spa at Shangri-La, Bangkok, Thailand

Products used: 'Chi' spa products.

Number of staff/roles: Spa Director; Assistant Spa Manager; 22 therapists; 10 spa attendants; 5 spa receptionists.

Training/experience: Australia – beauty therapy and remedial therapy training; salon in Sydney, Australia – therapist; cosmetic company – sales, training and state management; Clarins – set-up/operation of 'Gold Salon' programme; Estee Lauder – promotional manager; Jurlique – spa development (Duty Free, department stores and pharmacies); Spa of Siam, Asia – spa development and consultancy (13 spas in Asia); 'Chi' The Spa at Shangri-La, Bangkok – Spa Director since February 2004.

Main responsibilities: Setting up the spa and the day-to-day running of the establishment; revenue generation – targets, budgets, planning; recruitment and selection of staff; marketing and promotion; developing the retail sales area; staff issues: schedules, appraisals, target setting; staff training and development.

Best parts of the job: I enjoy dealing with people from a variety of backgrounds; guests, staff, journalists, etc. The interaction with my team and guests is what makes the role so enjoyable.

Secrets of a successful spa Therapist: Caring and nurturing capacity, a natural instinct for reading the body, adapting and adjusting your treatments to the client's individual needs, you need to really want to look after the client and take care of them, a passion for the industry and the treatments you offer, the passion should come from the heart – it's more than just a job!

SPA PROFILE

Name: Jessica Wadley

Position: COO

Establishment: La Jolla Spa MD, La Jolla, California

Products used and treatments: Spa MD Skin Care Line, Elemis line of body products. Medical procedures include: botox therapy, vein treatments, liposculpture, dermatologic surgery, laser therapy, laser hair removal, plastic surgery, hair transplantation, acupuncture and spa and medical packages.

Number of staff/roles: 76 members of staff, including aestheticians, massage therapists, nurse practitioners, physicians, dermatologists, plastic/cosmetic surgeons. All treatments are available under one roof.

Training/experience: BA in Business Management: 'I started off in a small spa and worked my way up through the industry including working for Steiner Day Spa Division in the States.'

Main responsibilities: 'Managing the finances and driving the revenue of the spa to ensure it runs smoothly and efficiently. Training and developing staff. As one of America's leading medical spas we offer state-of-the-art cosmetic surgery and dermatology combined with spa therapies to give the client the most complete care possible. Due to the calibre of the staff at the spa and it's reputation we also educate and train other physicians and healthcare providers in the latest treatments and our research department is involved in developing the latest technologies in the medical spa industry.'

Best parts of the job: 'Being part of a successful team and working with the calibre and talent of the physicians that work at the spa. Being involved in the latest technology and its research and development in the most advanced medical techniques being offered.'

Secrets of a successful spa therapist: 'A confident therapist who has a passion to address clients' skincare concerns and help to recommend and resolve their skin care issues.' 'When employing cosmetic surgeons it is important that they have double board certification.'

Assessment of knowledge and understanding

When you have some free time, test your understanding and knowledge by answering the following questions. Do this at regular intervals and it will reinforce your learning and help you retain the knowledge, so you are able to perform better in your assessments.

1. State three ways in which cross-infection can be avoided in the spa area.
2. Describe briefly the Health and Safety at Work Act 1974.
3. Give four potentially hazardous substances that may be found within the spa area.
4. Describe briefly the daily maintenance routine for a spa pool.
5. Why should a client take a shower before using the spa?
6. What is chlorine used for?
7. Why is testing of pool water carried out in the spa?
8. What does the Langelier Saturation Index calculate?
9. What is an ideal temperature for a commercial pool?
10. Briefly describe the role of an Environmental Health Officer (EHO).
11. How can legionnaires' disease be prevented in a spa pool?
12. Why is water filtered in a pool?
13. What does the acromyn SPATA stand for?
14. List the key points in monitoring water in a spa.
15. How is the spa area and equipment shut down at the end of a day?

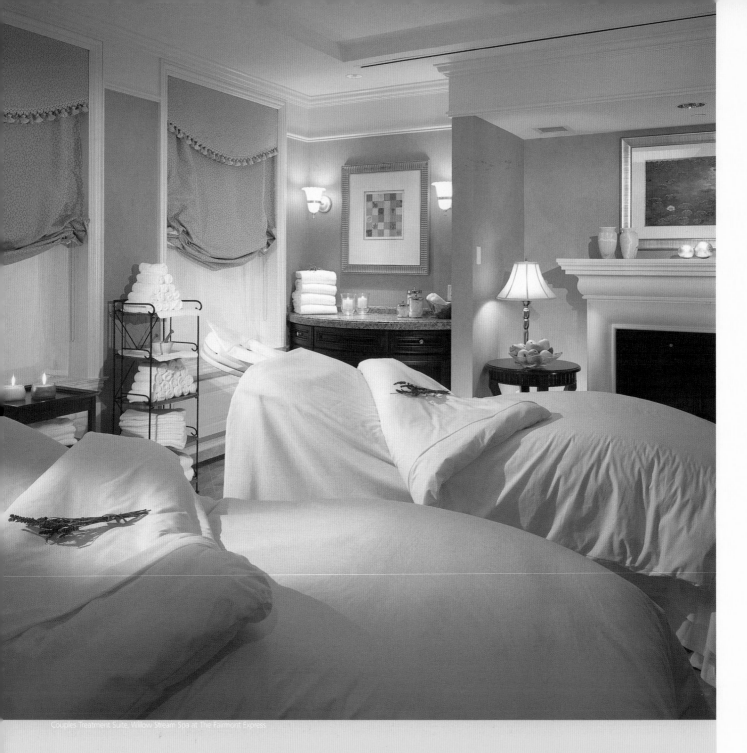

Couples Treatment Suite, Willow Stream Spa at The Fairmont Express

*It's a truly **exciting** time to be part of the spa industry – we have proven that spa is more than just a fad, it is a major player in the hospitality and leisure arena. Spa therapies are increasingly recognized for their benefits to overall wellbeing and, more importantly, our guests are finding inspiration from spas that they are embracing in their everyday lives, from design to fitness to skin care regimes. We are a **passionate** industry that cares about the **wellbeing** and **health** of our guests . . . we are on a **mission** to be a source of **inspiration** and **guidance** to **living** life with abundant **energy**.*

ANNE MCCALL WILSON, GENERAL MANAGER, WILLOW STREAM THE SPAS AT FAIRMONT, FAIRMONT SPAS INC.

6 SOOTHE

It is a very exciting and inspirational time to join the spa industry. There is tremendous diversity and record growth in all segments, from medical spas to companies associated with the spa lifestyle. In addition, there are new career opportunities for individuals who want to bring wellness and health to spa goers all over the world.

SUSIE ELLIS, PRESIDENT, SPA FINDER INC.

It is such an exciting time to be joining the spa industry due to the explosion of quality new spas that are emerging world-wide and the increasing focus on standards. The sheer variety of treatments and therapies now available are tremendous, e.g. Ayurvedic, Complementary – Watsu, Shiatsu, Cranio-Sacral, Reiki. Heat & Hydro experiences – Laconium, Hammam, Bio-Saunas Tepidarium, hydropool. This rapid expansion opens up a wide range of job opportunities, such as Therapists, spa Managers, Lifestyle Consultants, Spa Directors, this in turn gives great opportunities for international travel.

BRIAN HUNTER, SPA GENERAL MANAGER – ONE SPA, SHERATON GRAND HOTEL & SPA, EDINBURGH, SCOTLAND

chapter 11

Body massage

BT17

Provide head and body massage treatments

BT20

Provide Indian head massage treatment

Learning objectives

This chapter covers the skills a spa therapist needs to provide head and body massage treatment. This may be performed **manually**, where the therapist's hands manipulate the client's skin, tissue and muscle, or **mechanically** using a machine.

This chapter describes the skills and knowledge necessary to enable you to:

- **consult with the client**
- **plan the treatment**
- **prepare for the treatment**
- **massage the client's body using suitable massage techniques**
- **perform mechanical massage treatments**
- **complete the treatment**

Courtesy of Ragdale Hall

Manual massage treatment

Refer to chapter 13 for details on head massage.

When providing body massage it is important to use the skills you have learnt in the following core units:

G1 Ensure your own actions reduce risks to health and safety

G6 Promote additional products or services to clients

G11 Contribute to the financial effectiveness of the business

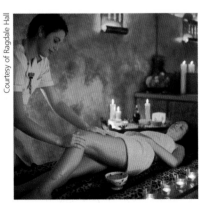

INTRODUCTION

Body massage is often viewed as a core treatment, and can be the foundation for many other skills such as aromatherapy, Indian head massage and sports massage. Many spa routines and packages involve some form of massage, and clients come to view this part of the experience as one of the most relaxing and enjoyable.

HISTORY OF MASSAGE

Massage is a skill that has been passed down through the ages for many thousands of years. In chapter 1 you will find lots of details relating to the history of spas that helped shape 'massage' we know it today.

Massage produces heat in the tissues and can have a relaxing or stimulating effect on the body. It is important to adapt your massage strokes and techniques to suit the client's needs, and there are two ways body massage is performed:

1 **Manual massage** involves the manipulation of the soft body tissues with your hands, to produce benefits to the vascular, muscular and nervous systems. This technique is extremely popular and has many benefits, both physiological and psychological. Clients can be invigorated or relaxed depending on the techniques used.
2 **Mechanical massage** involves using a piece of equipment to simulate a manual massage. The effects are similar to those of manual massage, but with a less personal approach. Mechanical massage can bring a different dimension to the treatment, and for maximum effect can be combined with manual techniques. The two most popular mechanical massage treatments are:
   - **gyratory massage** (e.g. G5) – this equipment involves a hand-held applicator with different massage heads, which simulate the different massage strokes.
   - **audio-sonic** – this smaller piece of equipment uses sound waves to gently vibrate the tissues of the body, without stimulating the surface of the skin.

TERMINOLOGY

Massage thought to be derived from the Arabic word 'to press softly' and the Greek word 'to knead'. Massage can be described as a 'scientific method of manipulating the body tissues'.

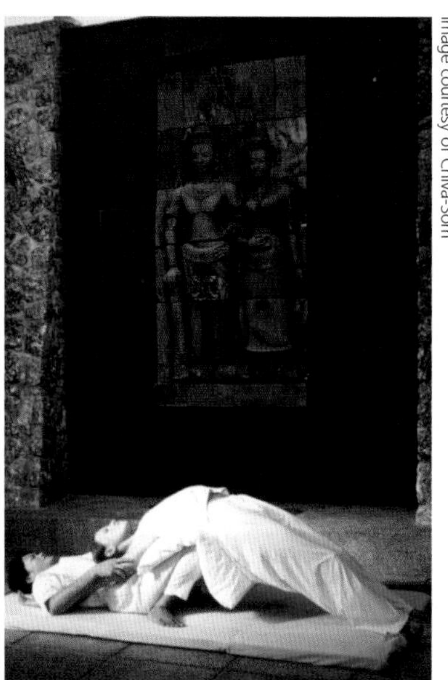
Image courtesy of Chiva-Som

Thai massage

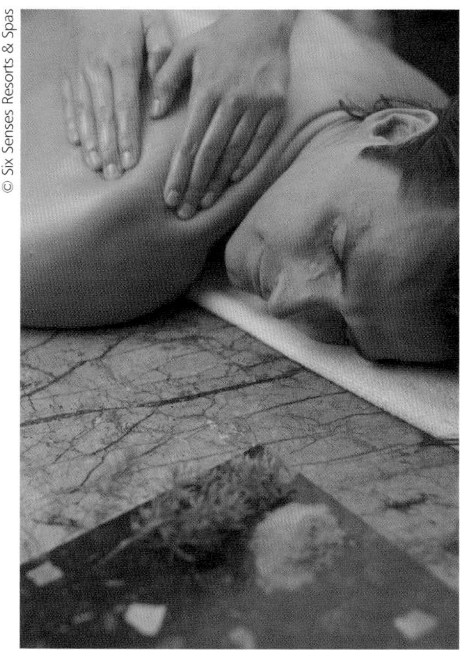
© Six Senses Resorts & Spas

Manual body massage treatment

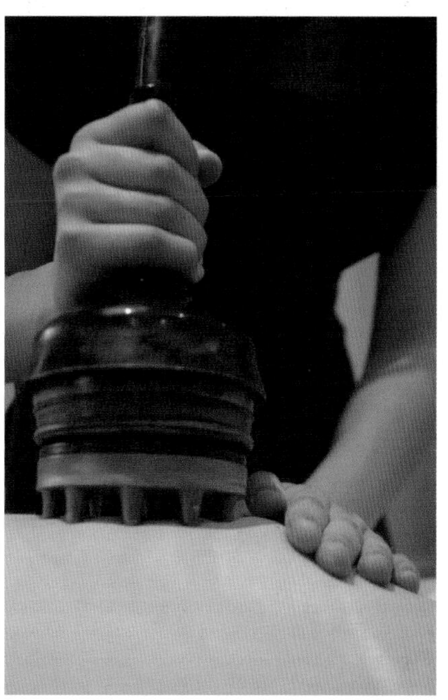

Mechanical body massage treatment

TERMINOLOGY

Desquamation in this context means the removal of dead skin cells in layers or flakes through rubbing or general friction.

EFFECTS OF HEAD AND BODY MASSAGE

Massage has far reaching effects on the body and you need to understand in detail the systems of the body as covered in chapter 6. The systems that are particularly relevant to massage are:

- muscular
- skeletal
- circulatory
- lymphatic
- nervous
- skin
- endocrine
- respiratory
- digestive
- excretory
- olfactory.

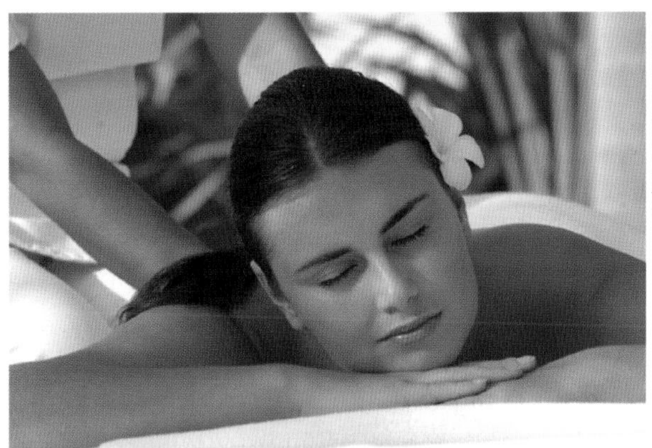

Massage encourages a feeling of wellbeing

GENERAL PHYSIOLOGICAL EFFECTS

The general physiological effects of massage are:

- increase in blood circulation, producing a hyperaemia and providing nourishment to all the cells and tissues of the body
- increase in lymphatic circulation, improving the removal of waste products and toxins
- warms muscles, relaxes tense and tight muscles
- promotes relaxation
- nerve endings are soothed or stimulated, depending on the technique used
- aids desquamation, improving texture of skin
- skin condition is improved due to increased blood flow, improving regeneration of cells and improving elasticity
- increase in sebum produced by the sebaceous glands, helps soften the skin
- softens and 'mobilizes' fatty deposits
- encourages a feeling of 'wellbeing', leaving the client feeling invigorated, rejuvenated, motivated and more focused on health and wellness
- can mobilize scar tissue
- helps reduce non-medical swelling, e.g. gravitational oedema.

HEALTH AND SAFETY !

The difference between hyperaemia and erythaema is:

Hyperaemia usually refers to the instant, short-term reddening effect of a treatment, such as massage, heat treatments, etc.

Erythaema is a deeper-seated, longer-lasting redness produced by ultraviolet exposure or certain allergies. A histamine reaction is usually involved. There are a number of degrees of erythaema, ranging from first degree, which involves a mild pinking, to a fourth degree, with blisters and peeling.

EFFECTS ON SPECIFIC AREAS

Blood and lymphatic systems

- Improves blood circulation, making vessels dilate and producing a reddening of the skin (hyperaemia).
- Increases the removal of waste products and carbon dioxide by the veins.
- Nourishes cell and tissues by improving venous circulation and bringing oxygen and nutrients to the affected area.
- Contracts the surface capillaries, creating a cooling effect on the body.
- Effleurage and kneading movements can accelerate lymph circulation.
- Can reduce swelling in non-medical oedemas and lymph node infections.

Muscular system

- Refreshes muscles by increasing the blood supply which nourishes the muscle and absorbs waste products.
- Improves blood supply making the whole body feel warmer.
- Maintains muscle tone and delays wastage of muscles through disuse (especially during illness).
- Can help correct postural faults.
- Prevents adhesions and increases the mobility of the joint.

Nervous system

- Soothes the nervous system – locally or the entire body.
- Vigorous manipulations can revitalize tired nerves suffering from exhaustion.
- Pressure on nerves can have a deadening effect and will temporarily relieve pain.
- Can have a reflex effect on nerves, making tissues and organs function more efficiently.

Bone and joints

- Pressure against the periosteum of the bone stimulates the blood circulation which nourishes the bone and joints.
- Prevents adhesions and stiffness in joints.
- Can help correct mild postural problems caused by tense muscles that can otherwise unduly influence bone growth and development.

SIGNATURE TREATMENT S

The Spa, Sandy Lane, Barbados

'Bajan Synchronised Massage: Paradise is achieved with a combination of stretching and rolling movements and long deep strokes using oil enriched with fragrant spices. Two therapists work in synchronised harmony to achieve mental and spiritual bliss commencing with a welcoming foot ritual and a complete vital energy point massage of the face, body and scalp. 2 hours'

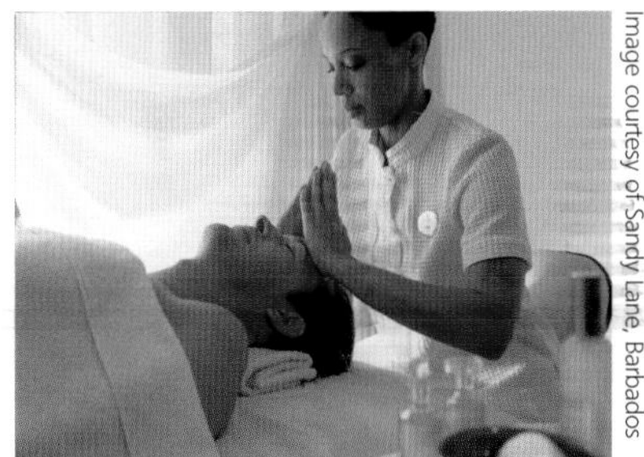

Image courtesy of Sandy Lane, Barbados

TERMINOLOGY

Metabolism the term used to describe how the body converts food and other substances into energy for its own use. If food is not correctly metabolized, certain diseases can occur, such as obesity, gout and diabetes, while a lethargic metabolism can lead to skin problems and an overall sluggish, sallow and dull appearance.

TERMINOLOGY

Adipose tissue the term used to describe the fatty tissue of the body. Massage cannot break down fatty tissue, as this could be very dangerous.

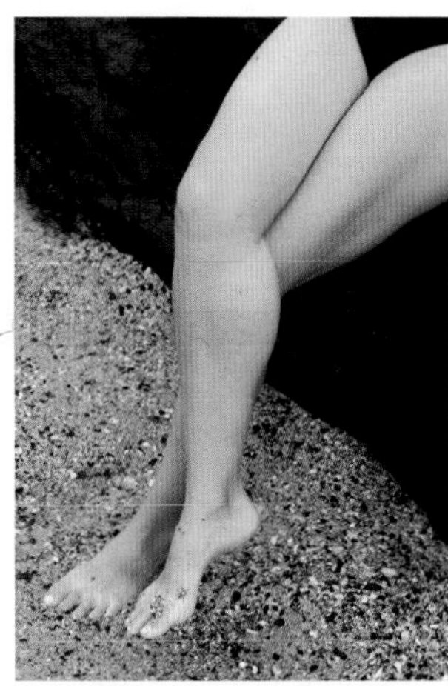

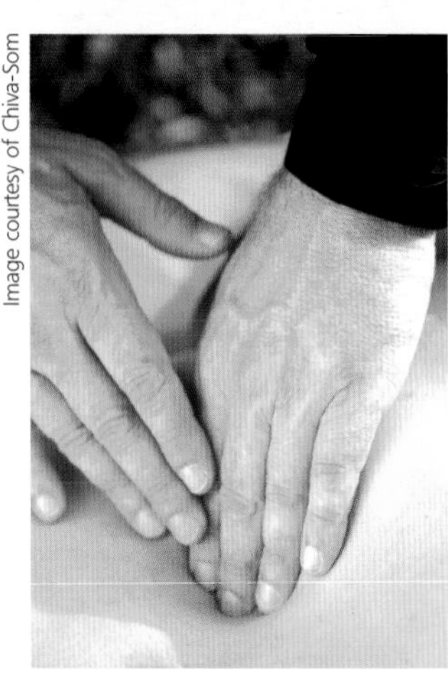

Image courtesy of Chiva-Som

Massage can help increase the vitality and function of the abdominal organs

The skin

- Improves blood circulation, making skin soft, supple and more resistant to infection.
- Simulates sweat glands, making them excrete urea and other waste products.
- Removes dead skin cells, improving the overall condition and appearance of the skin.
- Can soothe or stimulate nerve endings, according to the requirements of the treatment.

The lungs

- Deeper massage movements, such as percussion strokes (e.g. cupping), can increase circulation to the bronchioles of the lungs.
- Improved circulation to the lungs can increase the gaseous exchange, helping replace carbon dioxide with oxygen.

Metabolism

Massage can be very beneficial in correcting the effects of a faulty metabolism, promoting health and wellness throughout the body.

Adipose tissue

- By generating heat within fatty tissues, massage can aid the absorption of fat, and the increased metabolism can help convert this to energy.
- Regular and vigorous treatment can soften areas of firm solid fat and, when combined with a healthy eating plan, aid weight loss.
- Improved circulation helps drain fluid using the lymph glands and increases the conversion of fatty tissues into energy through the body's metabolic process.

Abdominal organs

- Can vitalize abdominal organs and aid digestion.
- Kneading manipulations over the colon can affect the involuntary muscle wall and increase the peristaltic action – aiding peristalsis.
- Vibrations can soothe the nerves of the alimentary tract, relieving spasm and flatulence.

PSYCHOLOGICAL EFFECTS OF MASSAGE

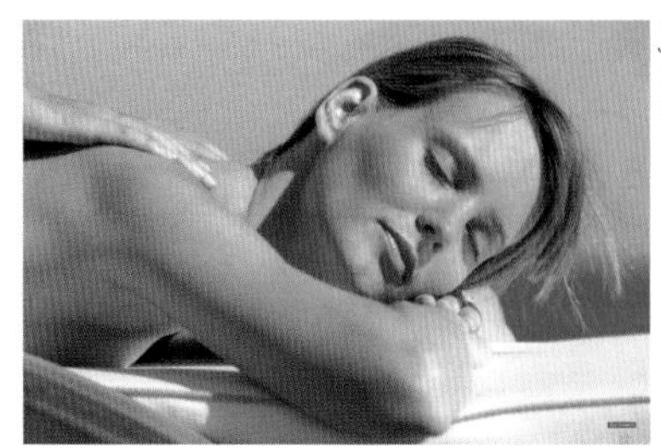
Phytomer

Massage can promote a feeling of health and wellbeing

As part of a thorough consultation with the client, you will assess their psychological needs: Do they want to relax and calm down after a busy period, or are they feeling low and need uplifting? Depending on the strokes and techniques used, a massage can:

- promote a feeling of increased energy and vigour
- promote a feeling of increased health and wellbeing
- increase confidence and positive outlook
- reduce stress levels, relaxing the client and increasing a feeling of contentment and satisfaction
- increase the client's feeling of being cared for, supported and nurtured.

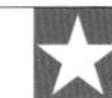

SPA TIP

To improve the psychological effect of massage, consider using pre-blended massage oils. Certain blends contain oils that have an 'uplifting' effect on the body, and can enhance the effect of the massage and help create a feeling of wellbeing. Many spas have their own signature blends.

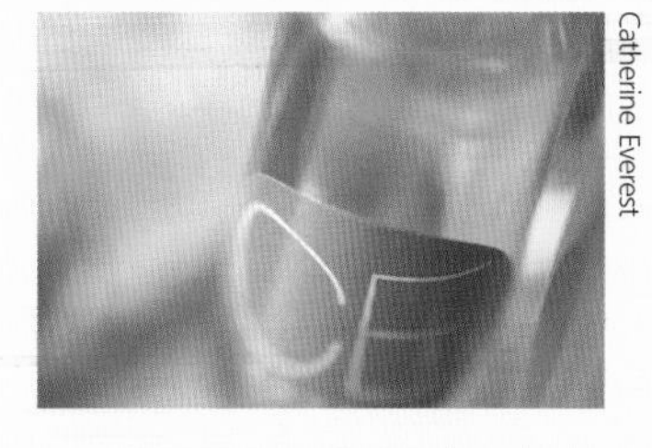
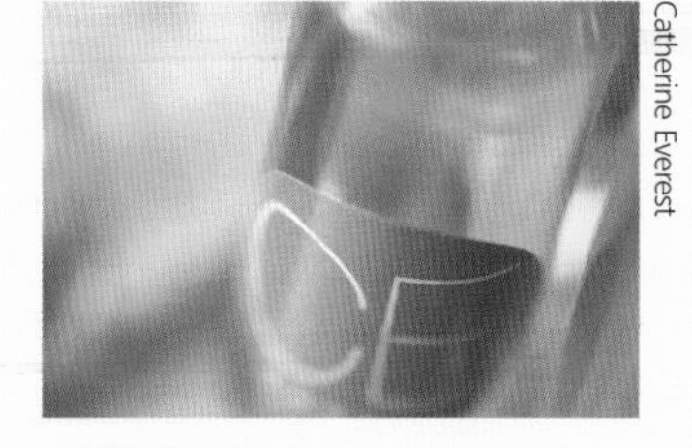
Catherine Everest

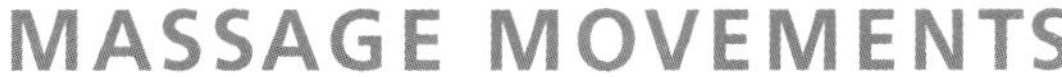

MASSAGE MOVEMENTS

There are four main groups of massage movements, each with a different effect on the body:

1. effleurage
2. petrissage
3. percussion or tapotement
4. vibrations.

Each group is further divided into specific manipulations, as the table below shows.

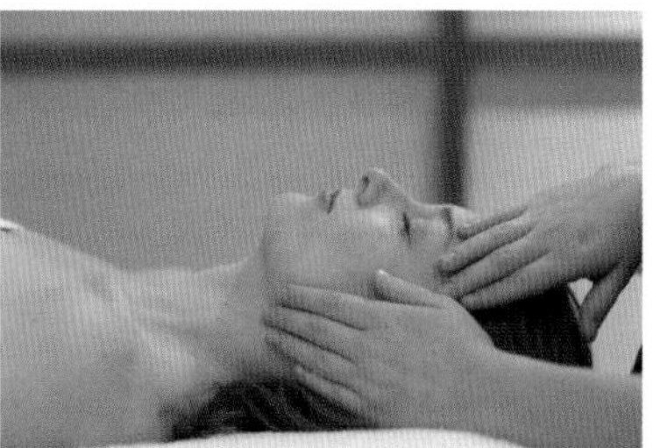
The Forum Health Club and Spa at the Celtic Manor Resort

Effleurage – one of the four main massage movements

Classification of massage

Group	*Manipulation/stroke*
Effleurage	Effleurage Stroking
Petrissage	Kneading Wringing Picking-up Skin rolling Frictions
Percussion/tapotement	Hacking Cupping/clapping Beating Pounding
Vibrations	Vibrations Shaking

TERMINOLOGY

Effleurage a French word meaning 'to skim over'.

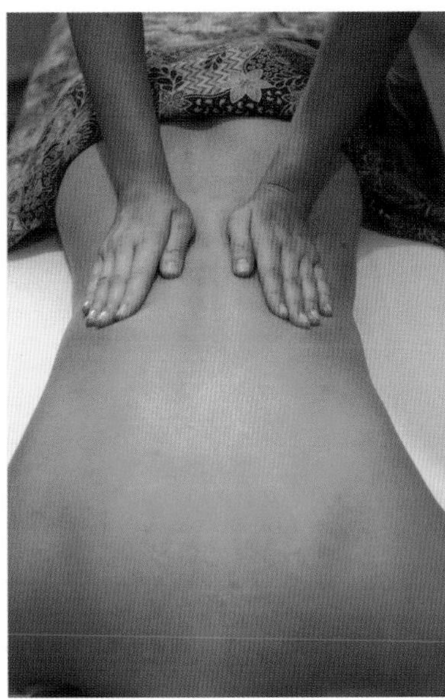

Effleurage to the back

Effleurage group

Effleurage stroke

Effleurage movements are very soothing and relaxing. The whole of the palm is usually employed, although only the fingers are used in certain circumstances. Effleurage can either be superficial or deep; this depends upon the requirements of the client and the effect needed. Whatever depth is applied, effleurage must always be performed in the direction of 'venous return'.

Effects of effleurage

- Increases blood circulation, providing nourishment to all the tissues of the body.
- Increases lymphatic circulation and speeds up the removal of waste products.
- Relaxes muscles and soothes nerve endings to relieve tension.
- Aids desquamation, improving the condition of the skin.
- Helps reduce non-medical oedema.

Uses of effleurage

- To evenly distribute the massage medium, e.g. oil or cream.
- To help the client get used to the therapist's hands, aids relaxation.
- Prepares the body tissues for the deeper movements to follow.
- Helps improve sluggish circulation.
- Helps to prevent swelling/oedema.
- Before exercise, can help warm up muscles.
- After exercise, can help to remove waste products that could lead to stiffness.
- As a link movement, helping to provide a smooth, seamless massage.

Stroking stroke

Stroking is very similar to effleurage, however it differs in three ways:

1. It can be performed in any direction, whereas effleurage always follows 'venous return' and the direction of the lymph glands.
2. The hands can lift off the body on the return stroke, whereas with effleurage it is usual to keep contact with the body on the return stroke.
3. Pressure does not increase at the end of the stroke, if anything it can become lighter. Whereas with effleurage, a slight increase in pressure is applied towards the lymph glands at the end of the stroke.

Stroking can be done in a variety of ways: with one hand, both hands together or alternately with one hand following the path of the other. Stroking can be either 'stimulating' or 'soothing' depending on the depth applied and the result needed.

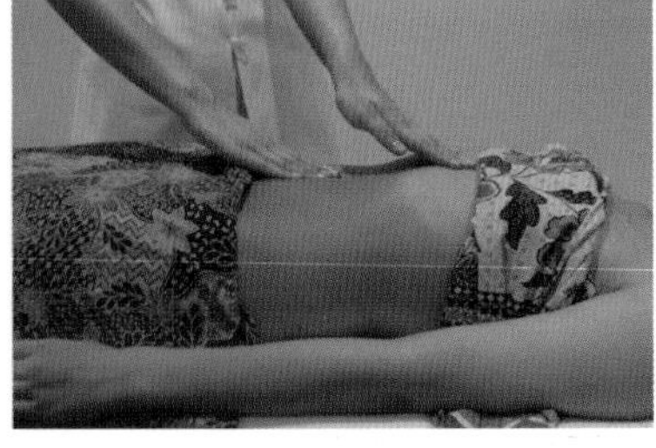

Stroking to the abdomen

Effects of soothing stroking

- Cools down an area by contracting the superficial capillaries.
- Helps relaxation by soothing sensory nerve endings. Deep relaxation can be achieved by prolonged stroking.

Uses of soothing stroking

- To cool down hot, swollen areas (non-medical oedema).
- Relax a nervous, anxious, tense client.
- Help with sleep problems, such as insomnia.

Effects of stimulating stroking

- Dilates superficial capillaries, warms and reddens the area.
- Sensory nerve endings are stimulated, producing a feeling of invigoration.
- Sebaceous glands are stimulated, more sebum is produced, helping to keep skin supple.
- Sudoriferous glands are stimulated, increasing sweat production.
- When performed over the abdomen, can stimulate peristalsis and improve movement in the colon.

Uses of stimulating stroking

- To warm up an area, produces a hyperaemia.
- Invigoration – can stimulate and perk up a tired, lethargic client.
- Helps constipation, or prevent it occuring.
- Improves skin condition by increasing activity of the sebaceous and sudoriferous glands and improving circulation.

Petrissage group

Kneading stroke

Kneading can be performed in a variety of ways, each an adaption of the basic kneading movement. The different types of kneading are:

- Thumb kneading – using only the pads of the thumb.
- Finger kneading – usually the index, middle and ring fingers are used.
- Palmar kneading – using the palmar surface of the hand. Variations of palmar kneading exist:
  - single-handed palmar kneading: one hand supports the tissue while the other hand performs the kneading movement, e.g. on the biceps
  - alternate palmar kneading: hands work alternately in a rhythmical movement, e.g. on each side of the spine
  - reinforced kneading/ironing: one hand is placed directly on top of the other to reinforce the effect. This is a very deep manipulation used on the large muscle groups, e.g. the back.

TERMINOLOGY

Petrissage a french word derived from the verb 'petrir', which means 'to knead'.

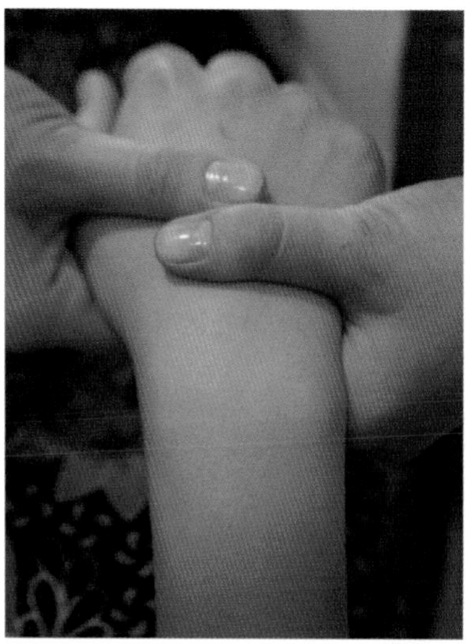

Thumb kneading on the back of the hand

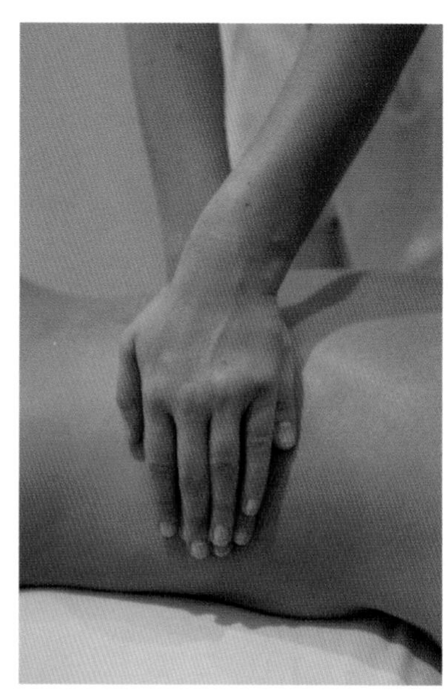

Petrissage movement to the abdomen (reinforced kneading/ironing)

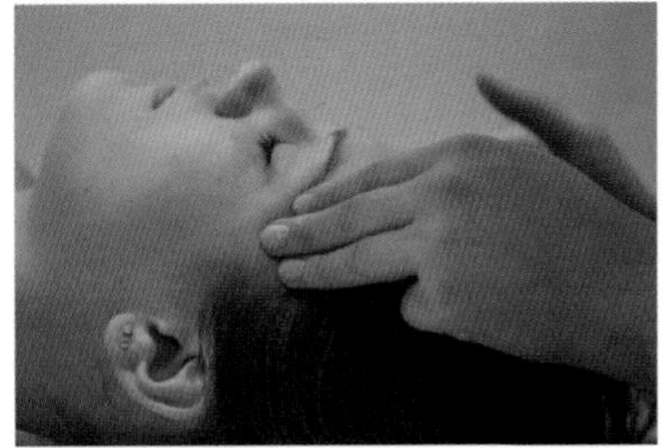

Finger kneading to the temples

Effects of kneading

- Increases blood circulation throughout the body, nourishing tissues, muscle fibres and bone tissue.
- Increases lymphatic circulation, improving the removal of waste products.
- Mobilizes tight fascia, and loosens adhesions.
- Improves skin condition by increasing activity of the sebaceous and sudoriferous glands and enhances blood circulation –; desquamation and the massage cream or oil medium used provide extra nourishment.

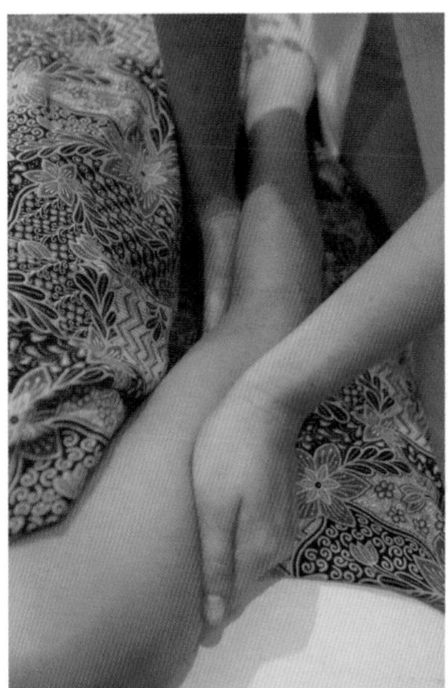

Single-handed palmar kneading to the triceps

Uses of kneading

- Improves muscle relaxation.
- Mobilizes and loosens adhesions and tight fascia and tissues.
- Before exercise, to warm up muscles and prevent injury.
- After exercise, to prevent muscle stiffness.
- Maintain muscle tone and elasticity.
- Improves lymphatic circulation, prevents non-medical swelling.
- Improves blood circulation, prevents varicose veins.

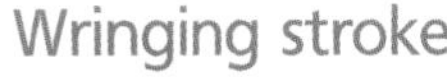

Wringing stroke

The tissues are lifted away from the underlying bone, and twisted between the fingers and thumb in a 'wringing' movement. The manipulation works methodically along the length of the muscle.

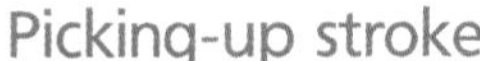

Picking-up stroke

The tissues are lifted away from the underlying bone, squeezed, then released. The stroke can be performed with one hand or by both hands, either alternately or reinforcing one another.

SPA TIP

Four-hands massage is increasingly popular in some spas. Each establishment devises its own unique treatment technique. The two therapists required need to be of a similar build so that the pressures they exert are equal. The technique takes a long time to perfect as it involves the two therapists working in harmony with synchronized movements. The hypnotic rhythm of the strokes has a deeply relaxing effect on the body.

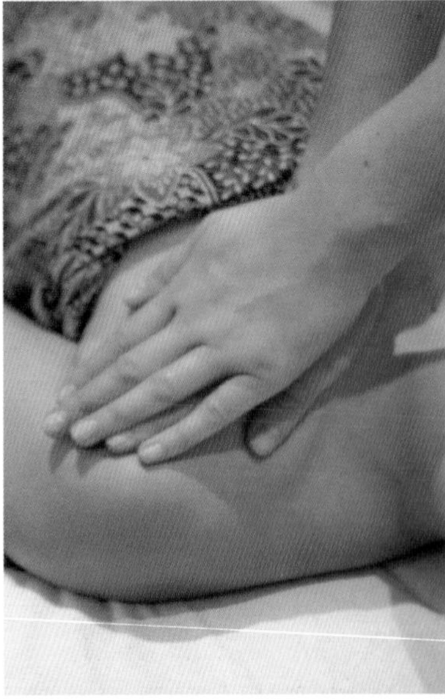

Reinforced kneading/ironing to the chest

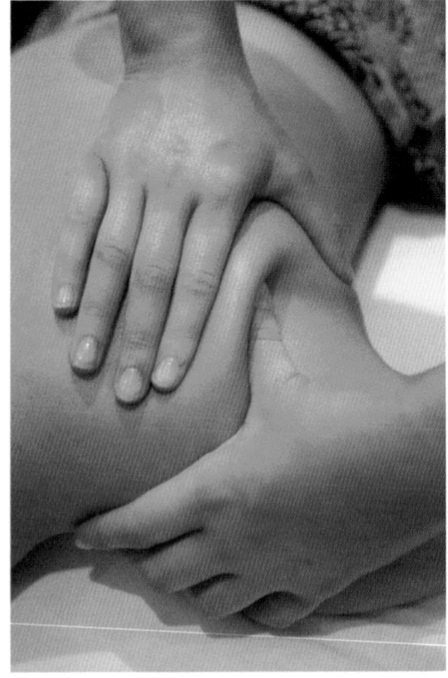

Wringing to the back

Effects of wringing and picking up

- Increases blood circulation, raises temperature slightly, increases metabolism and improves nutrition to the treated area.
- Increases lymphatic circulation because of the squeezing movement.
- Softens and mobilizes adipose tissue.
- Stimulates or soothes nerve endings, depending on how the stroke is performed.
- Improves elasticity of muscles and can help stretch tight muscles and fascia.

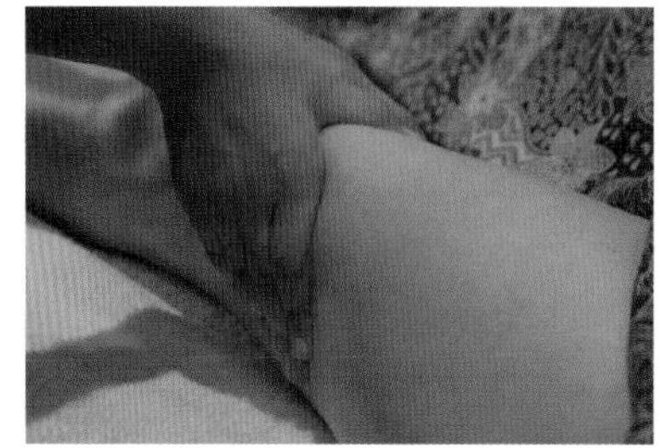

Double-handed picking-up to the thigh

Uses of wringing and picking up

- Relaxation, if performed slowly.
- Invigoration, if performed briskly.
- Warms muscles –; useful before exercise.
- Relieves tense and tight muscles –; useful after exercise.
- Improves blood circulation and warmth is produced.
- Softens and mobilizes adipose tissue.
- Mobilizes and improves elasticity of skin and muscles.

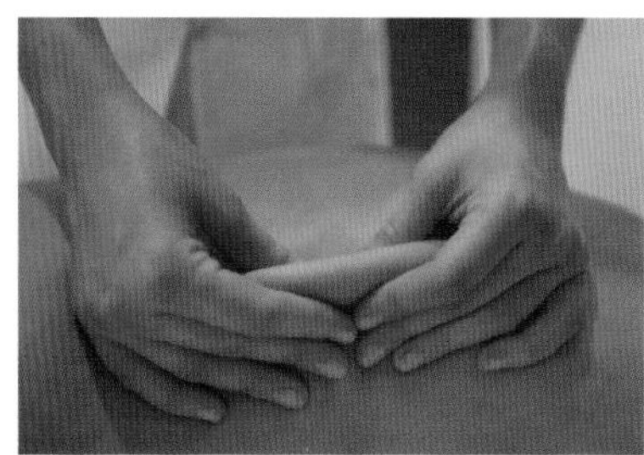

Skin rolling to the back

Skin rolling stroke

The tissue is lifted away from the underlying bone and rolled between the fingers and thumb. Requires a bony surface on which to manipulate the tissues.

Effects of skin rolling

- Increased blood circulation, producing a hyperaemia.
- Stimulates and mobilizes adipose tissue.
- Stimulates sebaceous glands – more sebum produced.
- Stimulates sudoriferous glands – more sweat produced.
- Improves elasticity and suppleness of skin, softening old scar tissue.

Uses of skin rolling

- Relaxation, if performed slowly, or invigoration, if performed briskly.
- Softens and mobilizes adipose tissue and old scar tissue, and increases skin elasticity.

Frictions stroke

These are deep, localized movements performed by the thumb or fingers. They can be applied in a circular movement or transversely across the muscle fibres. The pressure can be constant or get slowly deeper. This pressure must be released at the end of the stroke, before moving slowly along the body to repeat the movement. Frictions differ from finger kneading, which involves an upward pressure as part of a circular movement.

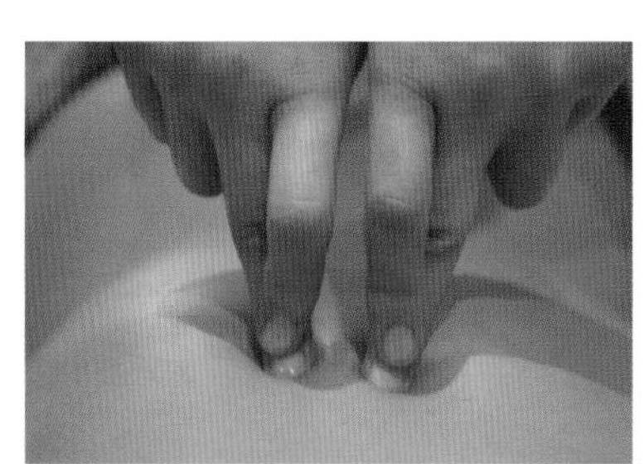

Frictions to each side of the spine

Effects of frictions

- Increases blood circulation, causing a hyperaemia.
- Increases blood flow, resulting in improved nourishment to ligaments and joints, helping to improve mobility.
- Improves mobility and helps loosen scar tissue.
- Stimulates and invigorates spinal nerves when performed on either side of the spine.
- Can mobilize adhesions, fibrous nodules and fibrositic conditions.

Uses of frictions

- Improves joint mobility.
- Improves blood circulation and helps tissue healing.
- Mobilizes and loosens old scar tissue.
- Tired and lethargic clients can be invigorated.
- Helps improve tension nodules and adhesions in muscles, e.g. the trapezius.

Percussion/tapotement group

Hacking strokes

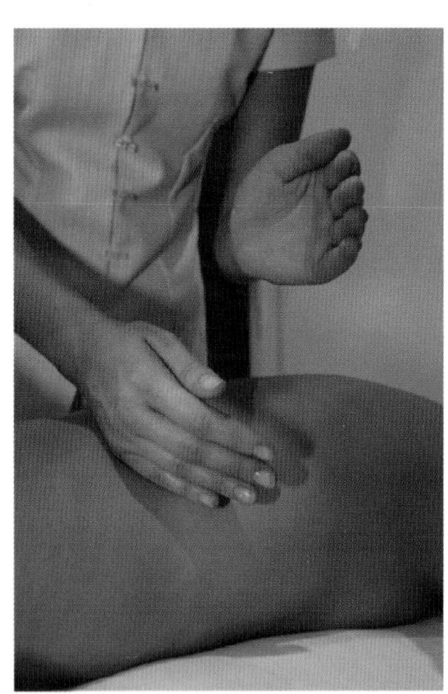

Hacking to the back

The ulnar border of the hand and the middle, ring and little finger strike the body. The forearm rotates, and the fingers alternately strike in a rapid and springy manner. The fingers should be relaxed, giving a light, stimulating movement, rather than a heavy-handed banging of the tissues. It can be a difficult stroke to perfect. To begin with you can practice on the bed or pillow, varying depth until a prolonged period of hacking can be mastered.

Effects of hacking

- Increases blood circulation, producing a hyperaemia.
- Raises metabolic rate.
- Stimulates and mobilizes adipose tissue.
- Stimulates spinal nerves when performed either side of the spine.
- The briskness of the stroke increases muscle tone by stimulating the reflex action of the muscle fibres.

Uses of hacking

- To stimulate poor muscle tone – can revitalize tired muscles.
- To increase blood circulation and warm an area of the body.
- Provides a feeling of invigoration and wellbeing.
- Can mobilize and soften adipose tissue.

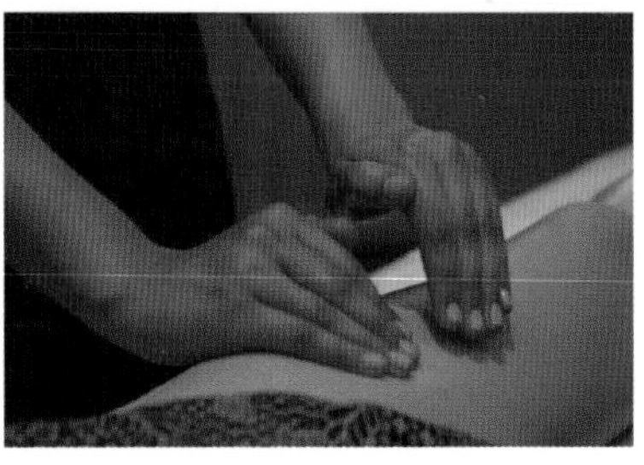

Cupping to the thigh

Cupping/clapping strokes

The hand is cupped in a pyramid shape, and each hand alternately strikes the body in a brisk manner. A hollow cupping sound is produced, similar to horses' hooves.

No 'slapping' sounds should be produced; this would be uncomfortable and mean the hand is not held in a sufficiently hollow shape.

Effects of cupping/clapping

- Increases blood circulation, producing a hyperaemia.
- Warms the area and raises the metabolic rate.
- Stimulates and mobilizes adipose tissue.

Uses of cupping/clapping

- To increase blood circulation and warm an area of the body.
- Provides a feeling of invigoration and wellbeing.
- Can mobilize and soften adipose tissue.

Beating strokes

A heavy percussion manipulation, often used on solid areas of adipose tissue, such as the buttocks. A loosely clenched fist strikes the body, alternately using the heel of the hand and back of the fingers. Wrists flex and extend similarly to cupping, but hands fall heavier on the body.

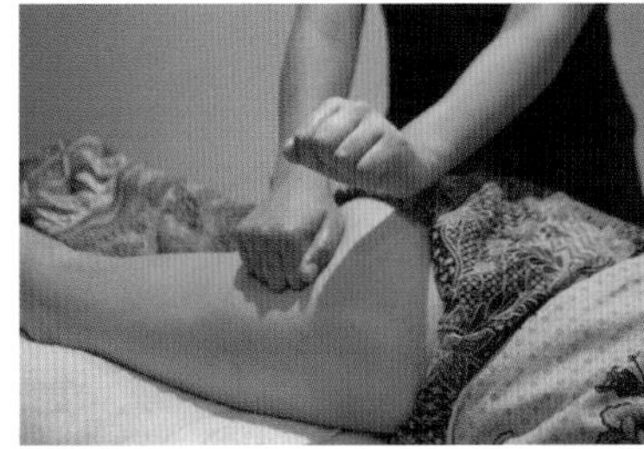

Beating to the glutteals

Pounding strokes

This is a very heavy movement using the ulnar border of a loosely clenched fist to alternately strike the body. Elbows are abducted from the body, and the wrists rotate similarly to hacking.

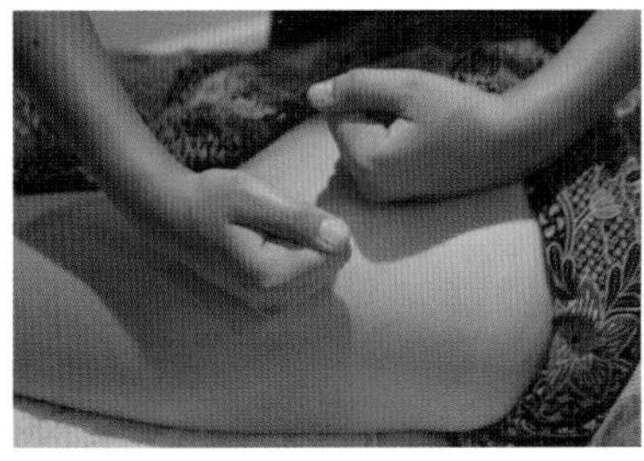

Pounding to the glutteals

Effects and uses of beating and pounding

- Increases blood flow and warms up an area of the body.
- Stimulates, softens and 'mobilizes' stubborn fatty tissue.
- Stimulates muscles, to improve poor tone.
- Creates an invigorating and glowing feeling, and promotes a sense of wellbeing.

Vibrations group

Vibrations strokes

Normally performed by one hand, but both hands can be used over larger areas. The hand can be moved up and down or from side to side to produce a tremor-like movement that vibrates the tissues.

Effects of vibrations

- Soothes nerve endings and promotes relaxation.
- Can promote absorption of tissue fluid.
- When used over the colon, can improve peristalis and help relieve flatulence.

Uses of vibrations

- Relaxes muscles and relieves tension in the back and neck area.
- Invigorates and improves sluggish, puffy areas.
- Relieves flatulence.

Shaking strokes

Both hands can work together, or one hand supports the area whilst the other grasps and shakes the muscle. This movement is beneficial when carried out over the chest as it can loosen secretions and mucous.

Effects of Shaking

- Aids muscle relaxation.
- Helps reduce pain and stiffness in muscles.

Uses of shaking

- To relieve pain and stiffness in muscles.
- Very effective after overexertion or exercise.

SPA TIP

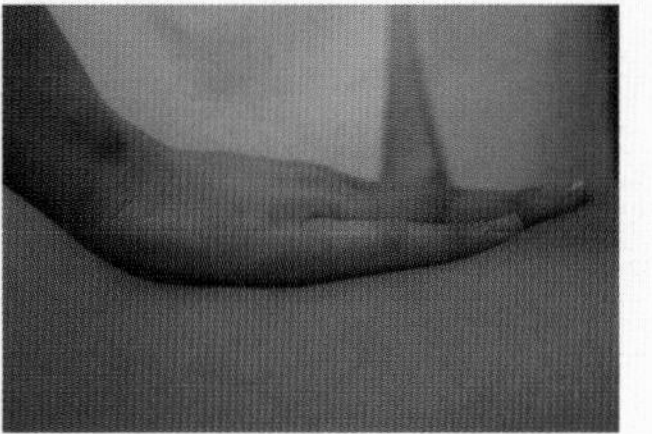

Hands should be warm and moulded to the part of the body you are treating

Your hands should be clean, soft, with short, well-manicured (unpolished) nails because:

- Rough, calloused hands can cause discomfort to the client. In some cases, rough cuticles with 'hangnails' can scratch a client.
- Dirty hands are unhygienic and can spread infection.
- Nail enamel can cause allergies in some clients, plus it can harbour germs and hide dirty nails.
- It looks professional to have well-cared-for immaculate hands.

QUALITIES OF A MASSAGE THERAPIST

Well-trained hands

This is probably the most important requirement for massage and your sense of touch will develop gradually as your understanding of underlying structures and musculature increases.

Flexible hands can be developed by practising massage movements, while regular exercising of the hands encourages suppleness and can avoid injuries.

Rate of movement

This is the speed or rate at which the massage is carried out – usually it is at a moderately slow speed, but this depends upon the effect that is required:

- slower speed – for a more relaxing massage
- faster speed – for an invigorating/stimulating massage.

Rhythm and flow

Good technique will depend upon how you make use of 'rhythm and flow' throughout the massage. All movements should 'flow' into one another with no interruptions. Where possible, your hands should not leave the body; use effleurage strokes to link manipulations together. As in music, 'rhythm' is the 'beat' or pulse of the massage; it should be even, continuous and consistent. Rhythm is produced by a swaying motion, backwards and forwards from the ankles, knees and hips.

Stance

This is important for you to obtain a good rhythm and freedom of movement. Good stance is very closely linked with good posture. As a spa therapist you must maintain good posture because:

- It enables you to carry out a much better massage, with the correct pressure, rhythm and flow.
- It prevents tiredness, backache, sore muscles and medical problems from developing.
- It looks professional and correct. As a therapist working with clients you must practise what you preach with regard to health, posture, etc. Never lean on the couch or the client.

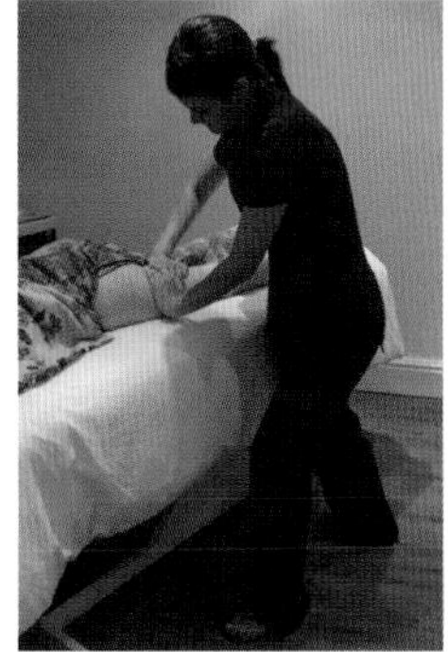
Walk standing: for working along the length of the body

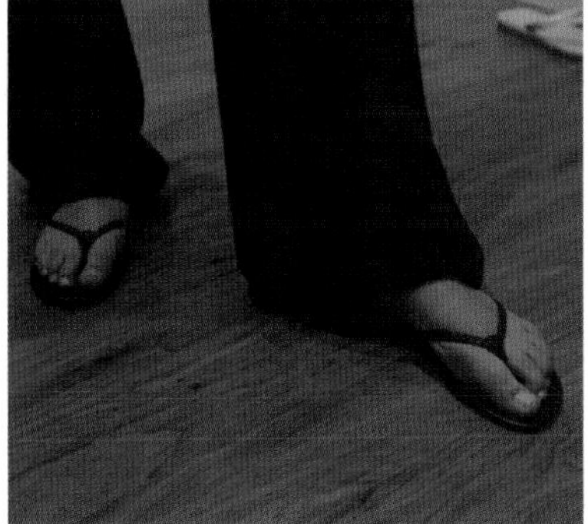
Walk standing: position of the feet

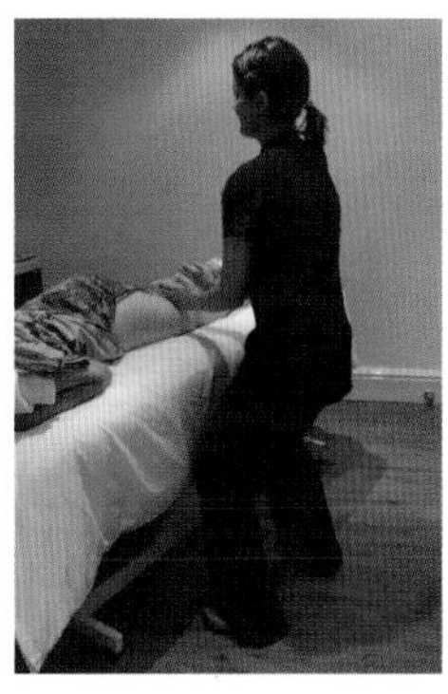
Stride standing: for working across the body

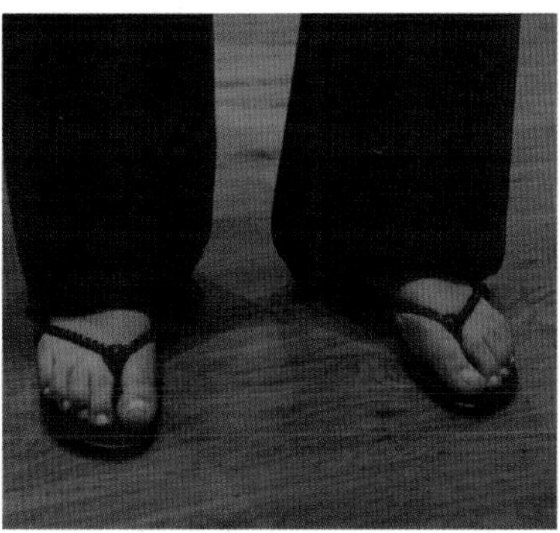
Stride standing: position of the feet

There are two main standing positions:

1 Walk standing – used when you are working longitudinally along the length of the body or limb, e.g. effleurage of the leg. When performing the stroke, one foot is in front of the other (as in walking) and you simply transfer your body weight from your back foot to your front foot. This stance allows the massage stroke to benefit from your body weight, enabling you to give a deep treatment.
2 Stride standing – used when you are working transversely across the body, e.g. ironing on the back. When performing the stroke, both feet are side by side but hip-distance apart, your back is straight and knees are slightly bent.

Depth of pressure

The depth of pressure depends upon the body area being treated and the sensitivity of the tissues. Depth of pressure is obtained by correct use of body weight transferred through the arms and into the hands. Not, as some inexperienced therapists think, by pushing harder into the body, squeezing tighter or massaging quicker. Generally, the back and lower limbs require a deeper pressure than that for the neck, chest, abdomen and upper limbs.

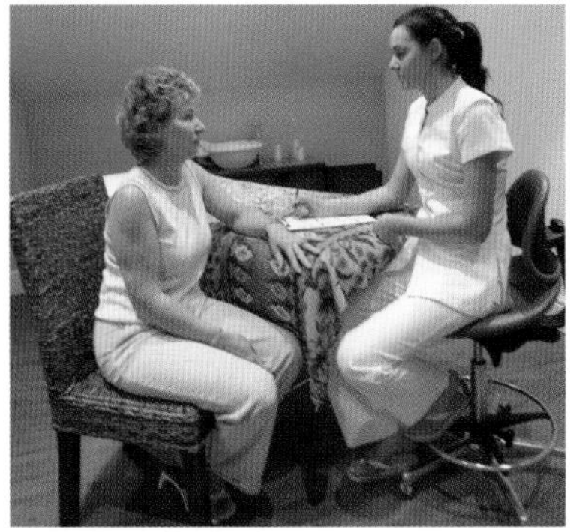

Consultation for massage

- Lighter pressure – can be more relaxing, inducing sleep, etc. (but be careful it is not tickly and irritating).
- Deeper pressure – can be more stimulating and invigorating, but can also be deeply relaxing, e.g. ironing.

PREPARE, CONSULT AND PLAN FOR TREATMENT

As outlined in chapter 15, preparation is critical for successful spa treatment, and when preparing your treatment area for body massage you should consider every stage of the **Prepare for treatment** checklist.

PREPARE FOR TREATMENT CHECKLIST

Body massage

- correct environment
- health and safety/hygiene
- professional appearance
- equipment/products/consummables
- record card
- private changing facilities
- bathrobe
- help client onto massage couch
- correct client positioning
- client warm, relaxed and comfortable
- wash hands, cleanse skin
- select massage medium

CONSULTATION

As outlined in chapter 15, a full consultation should be carried out to ensure the treatment is safe and effective and every stage of the consultation checklist should be cleared prior to treatment.

CONSULTATION CHECKLIST

Body massage

- quiet private area, client privacy
- plenty of time
- client comfortable and at ease
- aims of treatment/outcome/treatment plan
- postural check
- fill in record card, client signs
- check contra-indications/explain contra-actions
- client questions

CONTRA-INDICATIONS TO BODY MASSAGE

The therapist must be aware of all the contra-indications to massage, so that the treatment is carried out with full regard for the client's safety and wellbeing. Each client is assessed so that the treatment can be adapted to meet their individual needs. If there is any concern about the client's health, the therapist should advise them to seek medical advice.

Contra-indications to massage can be divided into three categories:

1. General – contra-indications that affect the entire body, e.g. diabetes. Massage could not be carried out whilst these conditions exist.
2. Local – contra-indications that only involve a local area of the body, e.g. scar tissue. Massage could be carried out as long as the area is avoided.
3. Temporary – contra-indications that do not last very long, e.g. bruising. Massage is temporarily stopped, but can be carried out once the condition clears up.

TERMINOLOGY

Contra-indication a condition of the body that prevents the treatment from being carried out.

Contra-indications to massage are listed in the table below.

General	*Temporary*	*Local*
Heart disease/conditions	Pregnancy	Skin disorders
Circulatory disorders	Allergies	Skin diseases
High or low blood pressure	Heavy bruising	Psoriasis
Cancer	Medication	Eczema
Lung disease	Skin abrasions	Recent scar tissue
Deep vein thrombosis/ embolism	During chemotherapy/ radiotherapy	Recent operations
Phlebitis	Skin disorders	Recent fractures
Epilepsy	Skin diseases	Varicose veins
Diabetes	High temperature/fever	Painful/swollen joints
Rheumatism	Spastic/contracted muscles	Cuts/abrasions
Haemophilia	Under influence of alcohol or drugs	Local bruising
Recent haemorrhage	Medical oedema	Large or inflamed moles
Neuritis (inflammed nerves)		Warts/skin tags
Disorders of nervous system		Metal pins or plates
Certain medication		Sunburn/windburn
Loss of skin sensation		
Postural deformities		
Undiagnosed lumps, bumps and swellings		
Very thin, bony frame		

HEALTH AND SAFETY !

If massage is contra-indicated, its important that you do not alarm or upset the client. Gently and diplomatically explain that it is for their own wellbeing, and that there may be a risk of worsening the condition. Explain that you can continue treatment when the condition has cleared up or when they have sought medical consent.

HEALTH AND SAFETY !

Older clients may have thin, overstretched, crepey skin. Gentle massage can be given, but the pressure should be very light, avoiding percussion strokes altogether. Be sure to apply plenty of lubricant to avoid overstretching the skin.

SELECTING THE MASSAGE MEDIUM

When massaging a client, the choice of 'massage medium' depends upon the desired effect and the client's own preference.

Before applying the massage medium ensure the client's skin is clean, with no other products on it. The client can either have a shower before the treatment, or you must clean each area of the body with either witch hazel or eau de cologne, applied with clean cotton wool.

Once the medium has been selected, apply it to your own hands first and not directly onto the client. Apply with effleurage strokes. Never apply oil or talc directly from the bottle, or cream via a spatula straight on to the skin.

HEALTH AND SAFETY !

To enable massage to take place safely, the therapist can cover certain local contra-indications, such as warts, skin tags, abrasions, cuts, bites, etc., with a small sticking plaster.

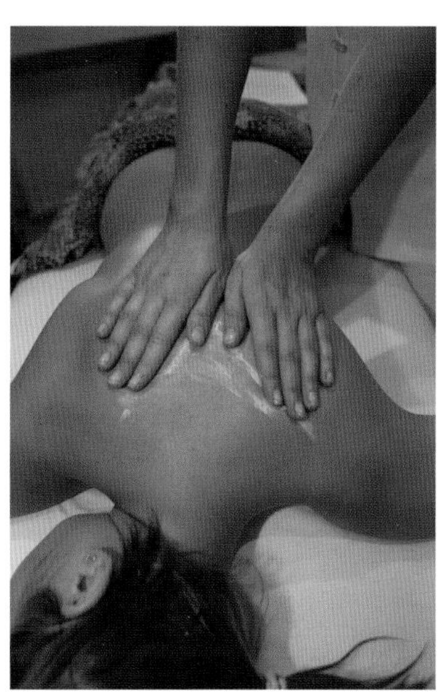

Apply the massage medium with effleurage strokes

Spa tip

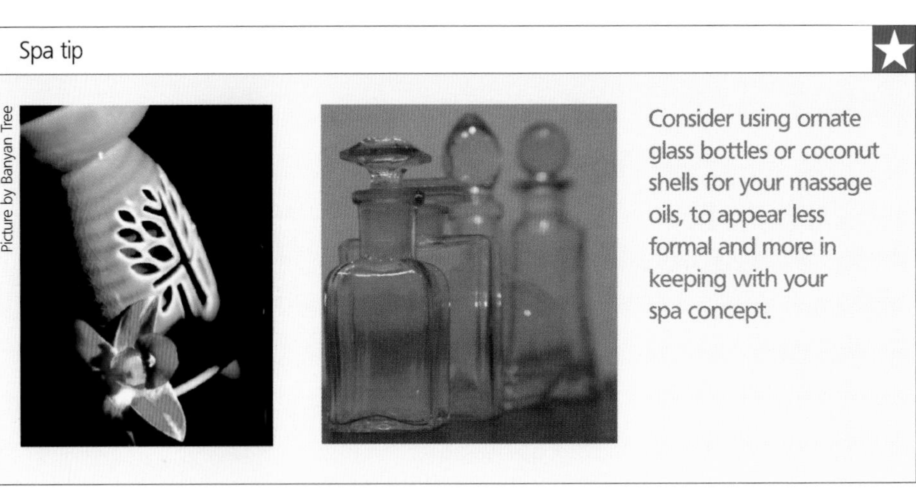

Picture by Banyan Tree

Consider using ornate glass bottles or coconut shells for your massage oils, to appear less formal and more in keeping with your spa concept.

Selecting the massage medium

Medium	*Description*
Massage oil	Usually a good quality vegetable/plant oil such as almond (see chapter 12 for usage details). Very beneficial for normal to dry skin types as it softens and nourishes while providing plenty of 'slip', enabling a deep massage to be given. Avoid using too much, as it will be unpleasant and difficult to massage
Cream	Preferred by some therapists over oil as its increased thickness and viscosity helps their technique. Very nourishing for normal to dry skin and can be more comfortable on hairy areas
Emulsion	A combination of oil and water which is not as rich as oil or cream, so may be better for normal skin types. Easily absorbed by the skin and needs re-applying to avoid discomfort from dragging the skin
Gel	Commercially available massage gels are often light and readily absorbed. Depending on the ingredients, they can be better than oil or creams for normal to oily skin
Talcum powder	Allows the therapist's hands to slide easily over the body and beneficial for oily and combination skin as it can absorb excess sebum. Never use on dry, dehydrated skin as it could irritate, and use the finest available powder, preferably unperfumed

TREATMENT PLAN

Plan the treatment carefully, so you do not waste time and maximize the effectiveness of your massage:

- check client record card – complete, signed
- check equipment is in working order
- follow manufacturer's instructions, and health and safety procedures

SPA TIP 

Courtesy of Aromatherapy Associates

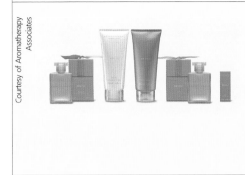

Clients enjoy the additional benefits of the massage medium. It can enhance the relaxing qualities of the massage. The texture and fragrance of the medium used can make them feel the massage has added value, and that they are getting something extra. The product used can be available to purchase and use at home, to recreate the 'spa experience' between visits.

EQUIPMENT LIST

You will need to prepare the following for a **body massage** treatment:

- room lighting, warmth, music, etc.
- massage couch
- bed linen
- disposable paper bedroll
- trolley/table
- massage chair/stool
- towels
- bathrobe/bath towel
- witch hazel or eau de Cologne
- make-up cleanser
- massage oil
- massage cream
- massage gel
- massage emulsion
- purified talc
- cotton wool
- tissues
- spatulas
- metal or plastic bowls
- petroleum jelly
- record card
- eye mask
- burner/candles

Optional

- infra-red lamp
- gyratory massage equipment
- audio-sonic machine

- confirm outcome/aim of treatment
- confirm areas of body to focus on
- confirm treatment, timing, etc.
- select massage medium
- select massage technique, e.g. manual or mechanical.

AFTERCARE AND TREATMENT ADVICE

On completion of the massage routine, check to see if there is any excess massage medium on the skin. Usually most of the lubricant has been absorbed by the skin while any that remains can be left on to provide ongoing nourishment, but be sure to ask your client if they want you to remove any excess. This can be done by using:

- a warm dry towel
- strong large tissues
- hot damp towels, heated either by a purpose-built steam cabinet or by simply placing them in hot water and then wringing each towel out well. Be careful to check that the towels are not too hot for the clients and apply carefully
- cotton wool pads with eau de cologne or witch hazel.

At the end of the massage treatment, it is important that the client does not quickly get up and start getting dressed. Cover the client and keep them warm. Explain that they need to rest for at least 5 minutes, as, after lying for an hour, the body needs to rise slowly in order to get used to being in an upright position again. If they are too quick and rush, they may feel faint and dizzy, as the blood rushes from their head.

Whilst the client is resting, you have an opportunity to go through the aftercare and treatment advice listed below. Offer the client a glass of water, and advise them to drink plenty of water during the next few hours. Furthermore, to ensure they maximize the effectiveness of the treatment, advise the client to take it easy for a few hours after treatment, and avoid eating a heavy meal or drinking alcohol.

SPA HYGIENE

Manual massage

- clean couch with hot soapy water, and wipe with disinfectant
- clean, fresh bed linen and towels
- use disposable paper bedroll
- wipe trolley with disinfectant
- plastic spatulas are washed and sanitized in an ultraviolet cabinet.

Aghadoe Heights, Ireland

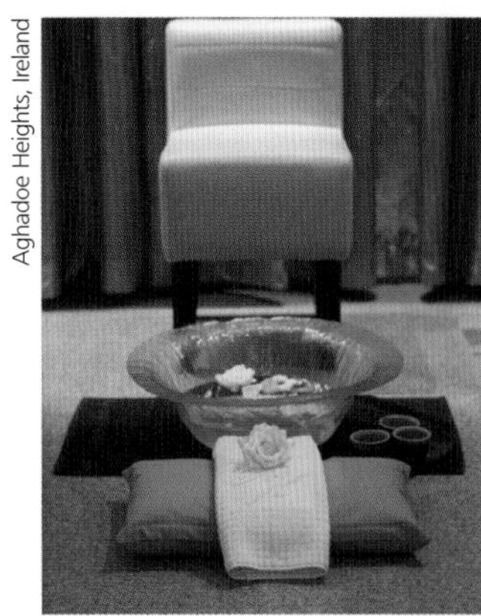

Every aspect of your treatment must be prepared in advance

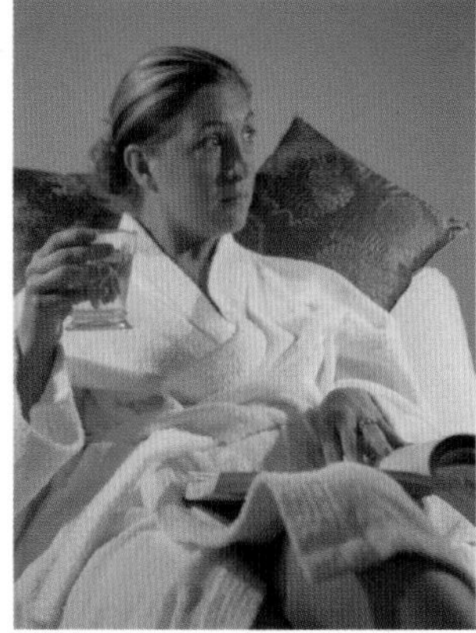

The client must relax after the treatment

Como Shambala

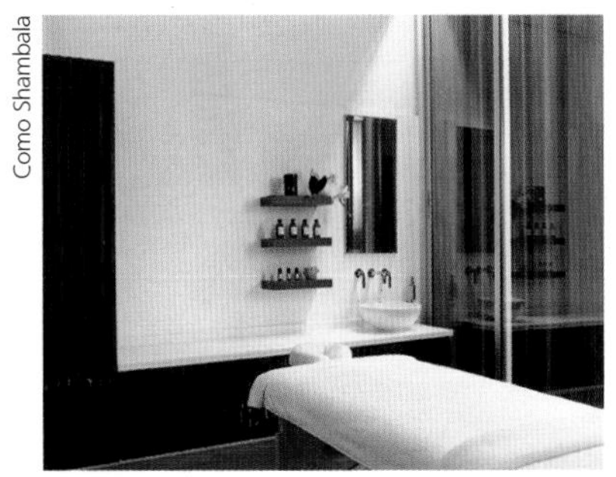

Ensure your treatment area, equipment and materials are totally safe and hygienic

AFTERCARE AND TREATMENT ADVICE

After-treatment advice	✔ Rest period ✔ Monitor reactions ✔ Water/refreshment ✔ Avoidance of stimulants
Products used in the treatment	✔ Explain details of products ✔ Homecare recommendation ✔ How to use the products ✔ Written prescription ✔ Additions – candles, body brush, eye mask, etc.
Contra-actions	✔ Explain possible reactions ✔ Advise on recommended action
Posture	✔ Posture awareness ✔ Postural advice
Lifestyle pattern	✔ Dietary and fluid intake ✔ Exercise habits ✔ Smoking habits ✔ Sleep patterns ✔ Hobbies/interests ✔ Means of relaxation
Further massage treatment	✔ Benefits of continuing treatments ✔ Courses/financial incentives
Linked treatments	✔ Benefits of combining with other treatments, e.g. heat, electrical
Frequency of treatments	✔ Recommended frequency and time intervals

MASSAGE TREATMENT ROUTINES AND ADAPTIONS

In a spa, clients can select either a full body massage or a shorter treatment concentrating on a specific area of the body, e.g. back massage. Also, massage may be combined with other treatments as part of a package or client 'journey'. Usually the treatment menu will give the details of all the different treatments available, so that the client can read these before booking an appointment.

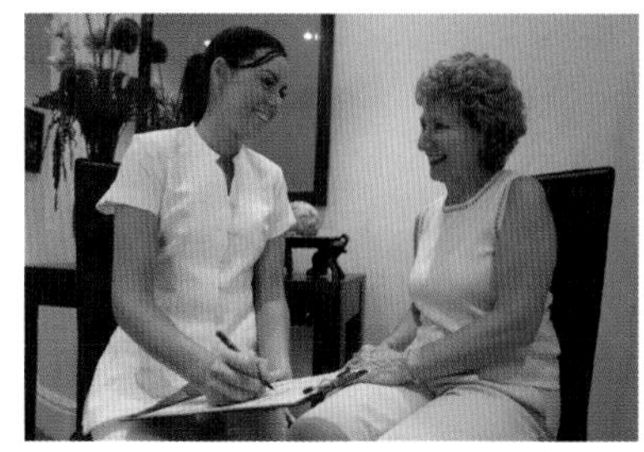

Always confirm the detail of the treatment with the client

Timings of treatments are unique to each spa, and are set when the treatments are formulated and developed. Treatment service times can vary dramatically according to client needs, treatment requirements and service delivery. However, the following standard service times can be used as a guide:

Full body massage	1 hour
Full body and head massage	1 hour and 15 minutes
Back massage	30 minutes
Neck/shoulder massage	30 minutes

SPA TIP 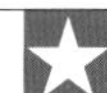

Some clients will ask the receptionist for advice before deciding on the best treatment. It is very important that the receptionist confirms the details of the appointment with the client, so that the correct amount of time is booked. This avoids confusion and disappointment later.

Within the overall time available, you will adapt the timings for each part of the body to suit the individual requirements of the client. It is therefore difficult to be prescriptive about the exact number of minutes spent on each area. Below is a guide for a standard body and head massage routine lasting 1 hour 15 minutes:

BODY AND HEAD MASSAGE TREATMENT PROCEDURES

It is important to have a smooth methodical approach to a full body massage. The therapist should work smoothly around the couch, not back and forwards in an erratic manner. This approach is efficient, effective and professional, and allows the maximum treatment time with no time wasting.

TERMINOLOGY

Supine lying means face up.

Prone lying means face down.

A common sequence for a full body and head massage is:

- **Client lying face upwards (supine)**
  - right arm
  - right leg (front)
  - left leg (front)
  - left arm
  - neck and chest
  - abdomen
  - head.
- **Client lying face downwards (prone)**
  - back of right leg (including buttocks)
  - back of left leg (including buttocks)
  - back.

Body area and order of massage	*Timing (minutes)*
Client lying face up (supine)	
Right arm	5
Front of right leg	5
Front of left leg	5
Left arm	5
Neck/chest	5
Abdomen	5
Head	10
Client lying face down (prone)	
Back of right leg (including buttocks)	10
Back of left leg (including buttocks)	10
Back	15

TREATMENT APPLICATION

Each training establishment will have its own massage routine. The following pages present, step-by-step, a standard routine for a full body and head massage. The details of each type of massage manipulation are covered earlier in this chapter.

STEP-BY-STEP: Arm massage routine (approximately 5 minutes each arm)

1 Effleurage
   - 3 times to the posterior surface of the arm
   - 3 times to the anterior surface of the arm.
2 Palmar kneading to the deltoid, with both hands.
3 Single-handed palmar kneading to the triceps.
4 Single-handed palmar kneading to the biceps.
5 Alternate palmar kneading to the biceps and triceps.
6 Wringing to the triceps.
7 Wringing to the biceps.
8 Double-handed picking-up to the deltoid.
9 Picking-up to triceps.
10 Picking-up to biceps.
11 Finger kneading around the elbow.
12 Alternate palmar kneading to the flexors and extensors of the forearm.

TERMINOLOGY

Flexor muscles cause a 'flexion' movement, which is a bending or folding action at a joint, e.g. bending the elbow.

TERMINOLOGY

Anterior means front.

Posterior means back.

13 Picking-up to flexors.

14 Picking-up to extensors.

15 Thumb kneading to the interosseous groove of the forearm.

16 Thumb kneading on back of hand, wrist and palm.

17 Hacking
   – softer on anterior surface
   – deeper on posterior surface.

18 Effleurage
   – 3 times on anterior surface
   – 3 times on posterior surface.

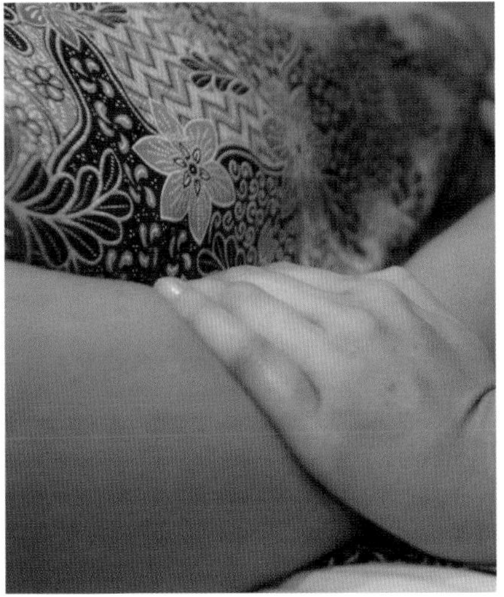

Effleurage to the arm

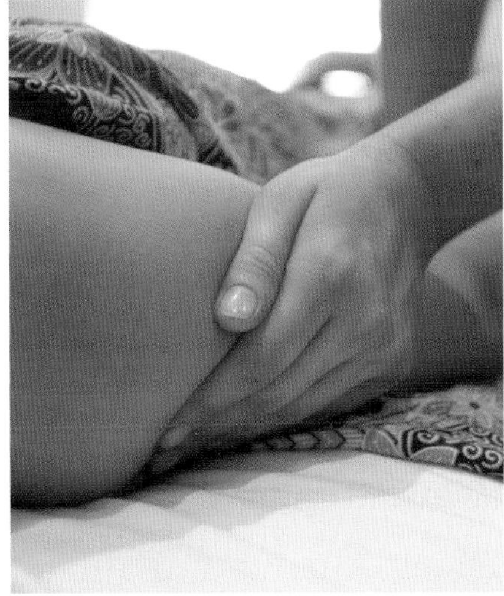

Single-handed kneading to the triceps

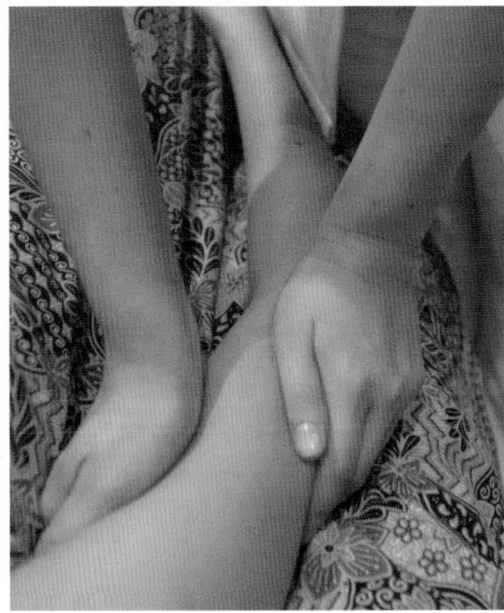

Alternate palmar kneading to the triceps and biceps

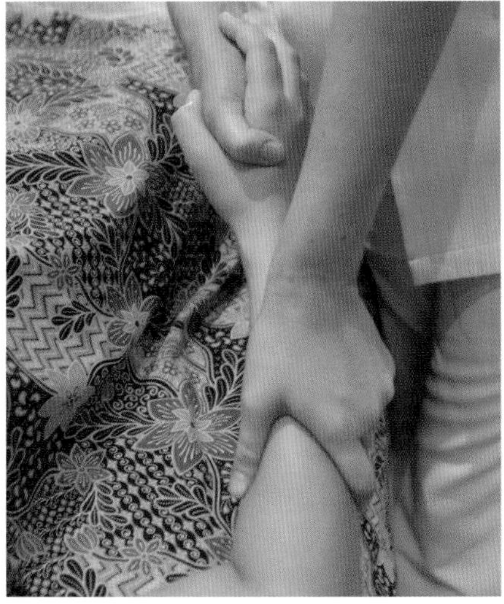

Picking-up to the extensors of the forearm

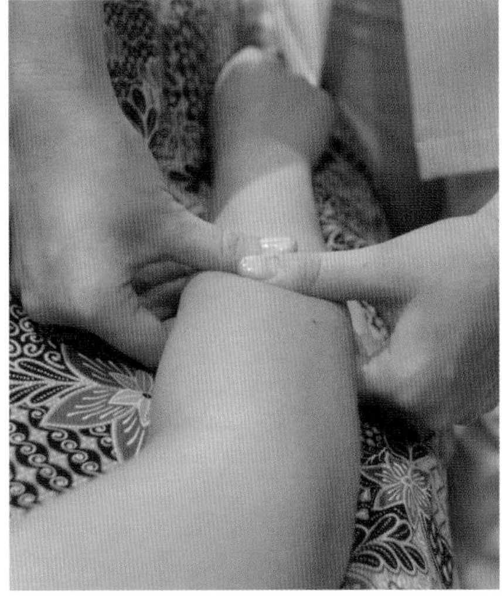

Thumb kneading to the interosseous groove

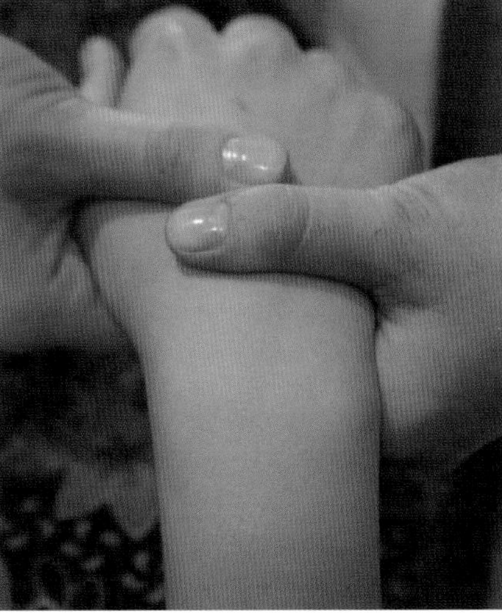

Thumb kneading to the back of the hand

SPA TIP 

If the client suffers from gravitational oedema support the leg with pillows, ensuring that the ankle is elevated. This helps drain excess fluid from the leg.

TERMINOLOGY

Medial the correct term for inner surface.

Lateral means outer surface.

FACT

The **interosseous groove** is literally the groove between two bones: the tibia and fibula bones in the leg and the ulna and radius bones in the arm. Fluid can often stagnate in these areas. Thumb kneading can help relieve the sensation of tired and heavy limbs.

STEP-BY-STEP: Leg massage routine – anterior/front surface (approximately 5 minutes each leg)

1. Effleurage
   - 3 times on anterior surface
   - 3 times on lateral/medial surface.
2. Single-handed kneading to the abductors of the thigh.
3. Single-handed kneading to the adductors of the thigh.
4. Alternate kneading to the abductors and adductors.
5. Reinforced double-handed kneading to the quadriceps.
6. Wringing to the whole of the thigh.
7. Double-handed picking-up to the quadriceps.
8. Picking-up to the abductors.
9. Picking-up to the adductors.
10. Hacking to the whole of the thigh.
11. Cupping to the whole of the thigh.
12. Effleurage to the knee.
13. Finger-kneading around the knee joint.
14. Effleurage to the knee.
15. Thumb kneading to the interosseous groove.
16. Effleurage to the ankle and foot.
17. Finger kneading around the ankle joint.
18. Thumb kneading to the top of the foot.
19. Effleurage
    - 3 times on the medial/lateral surfaces
    - 3 times on the anterior surface.

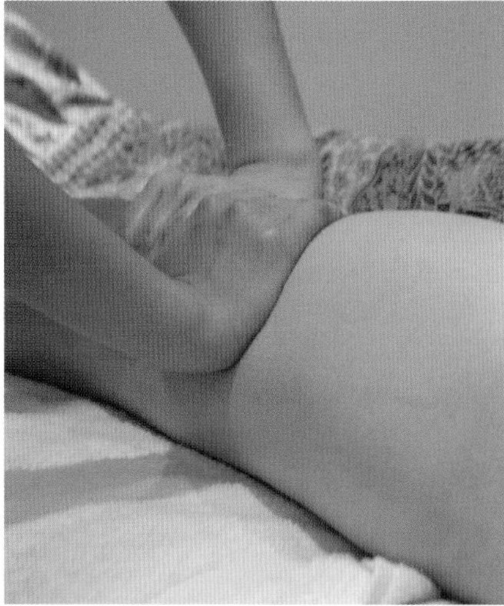

Effleurage to the thigh

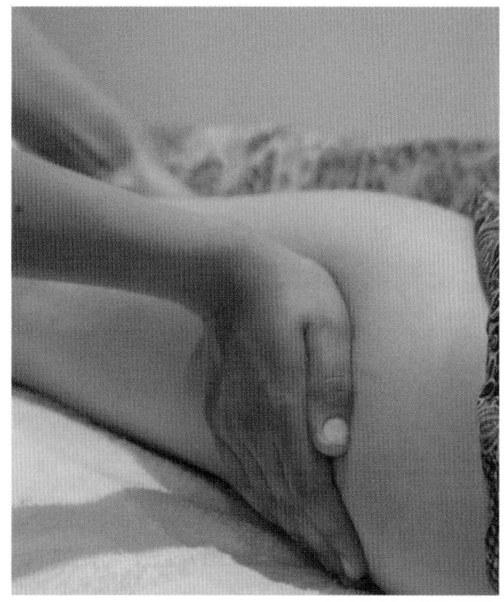

Single-handed kneading to the abductors of the thigh

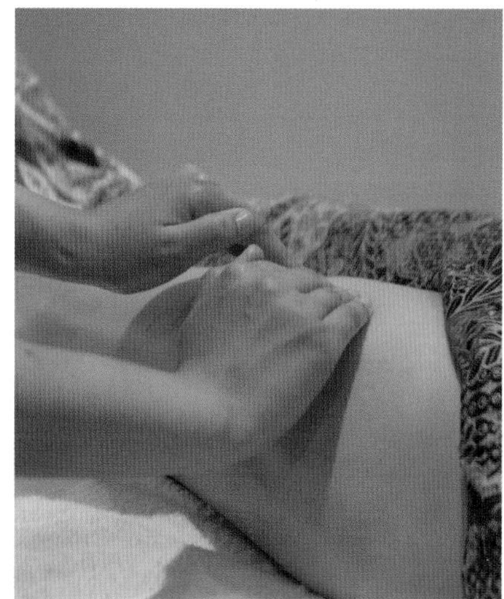

Cupping to the thigh

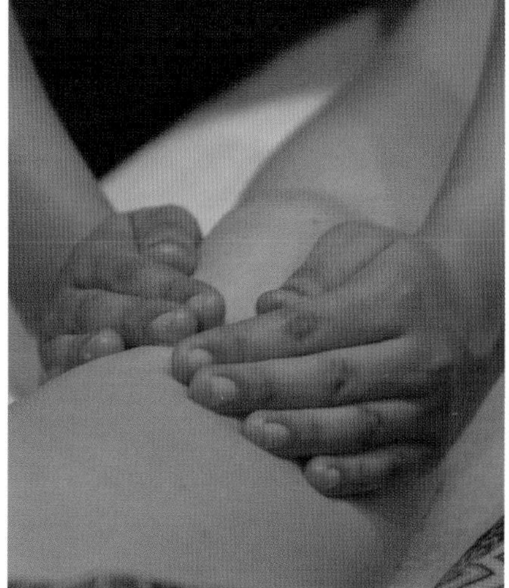

Effleurage to the knee

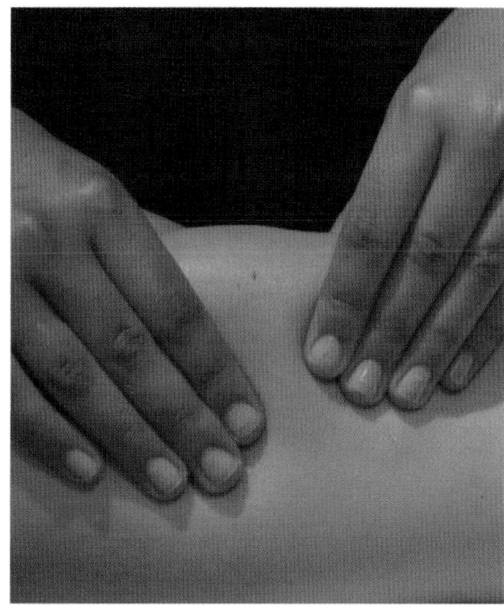

Finger kneading around the knee joint

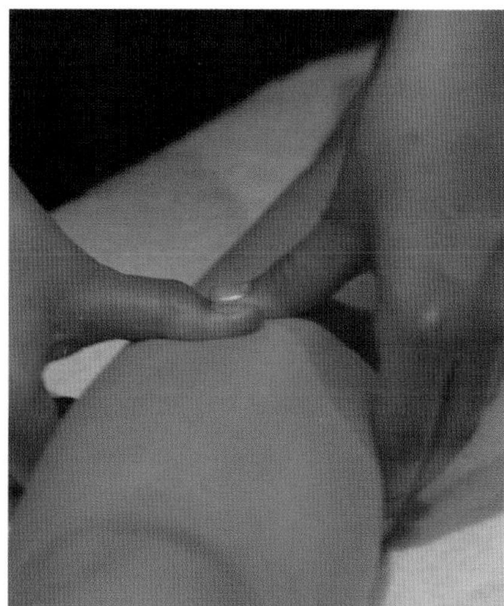

Thumb kneading to the interosseous groove

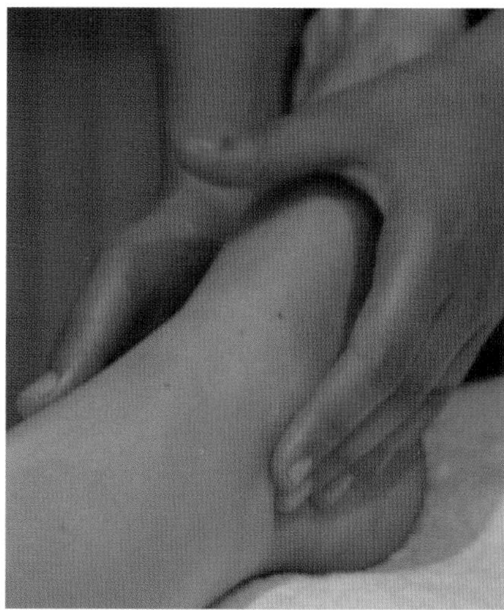

Finger kneading around the ankle joint

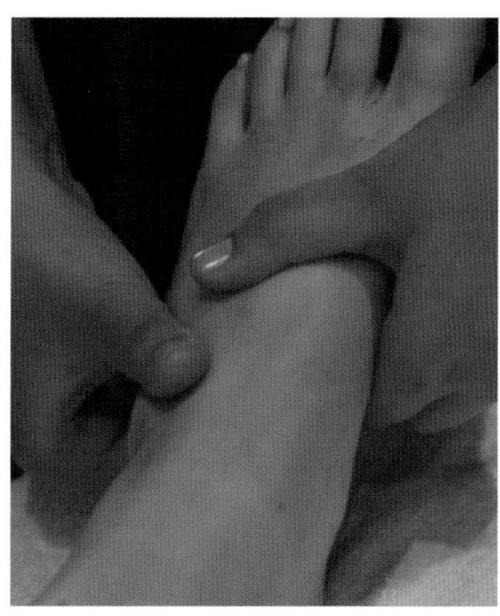

Thumb kneading to the top of the foot

TERMINOLOGY

Clavicle the correct name for the collar-bone.

Sternum the name for the breastbone.

SPA TIP

Before starting the abdomen massage, some spa therapists 'connect' with the client's energy over the solar plexus. Breathing techniques used in yoga can encourage the client to relax.

STEP-BY-STEP: Neck/chest massage routine (approximately 5 minutes)

Standing behind the client:

1. Effleurage around the shoulders, using both hands.
2. Thumb kneading to the trapezius.
3. Effleurage around the shoulders using both hands, standing at the side of the client.
4. Effleurage to the chest, using both hands alternately.
5. Reinforced double-handed kneading (ironing) to the chest.
6. Finger kneading around the clavicles, using both hands.
7. Vibrations across the chest.
8. Very light hacking to the chest.
9. Effleurage to the chest, using both hands alternately.
10. Soothing stroking.

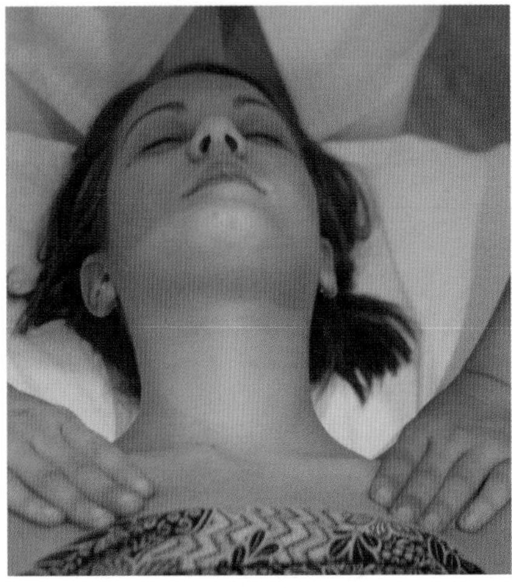

Effleurage around the shoulders (standing behind the client)

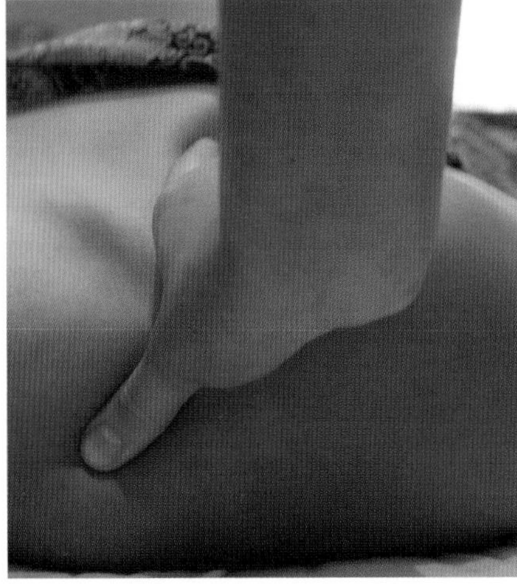

Thumb kneading to the trapezius (standing behind the client)

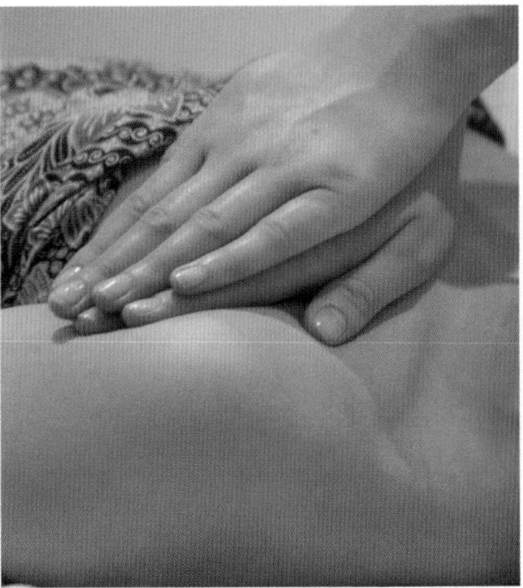

Reinforced double-handed kneading (ironing) to the chest

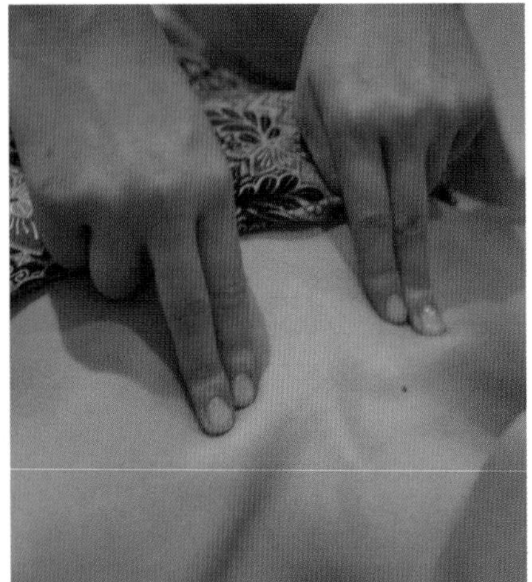

Finger kneading around the clavicles, using both hands

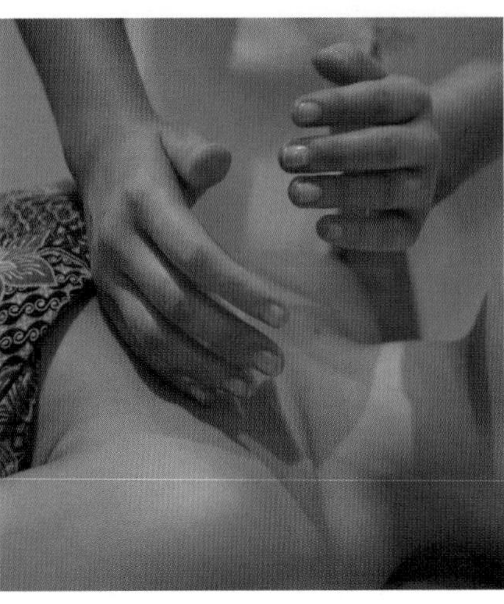

Very light hacking to the chest

STEP-BY-STEP: Abdomen massage routine (approximately 5 minutes)

1 Effleurage from waist towards the groin, using both hands.
2 Palmar kneading from waist towards the groin, using both hands together.
3 Palmar kneading from waist towards groin, using hands alternately.
4 Reinforced double-handed kneading (ironing) to the abdomen.
5 Wringing to the abdomen.
6 Picking-up to the abdomen.
7 If required, extra work on the colon: kneading, ironing and effleurage.
8 Vibrations across the abdomen.
9 Effleurage from waist towards the groin, using both hands.
10 Soothing stroking.

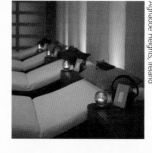

SPA TIP

After treatment, allow the client to spend time in a relaxation room, with reclining couches, fresh fruit, water and books and magazines to read.

Aghadoe Heights, Ireland

Relaxation room

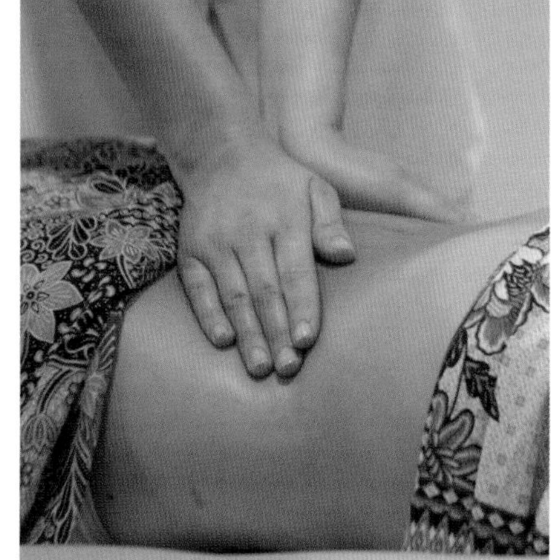

Effleurage from the waist towards the groin

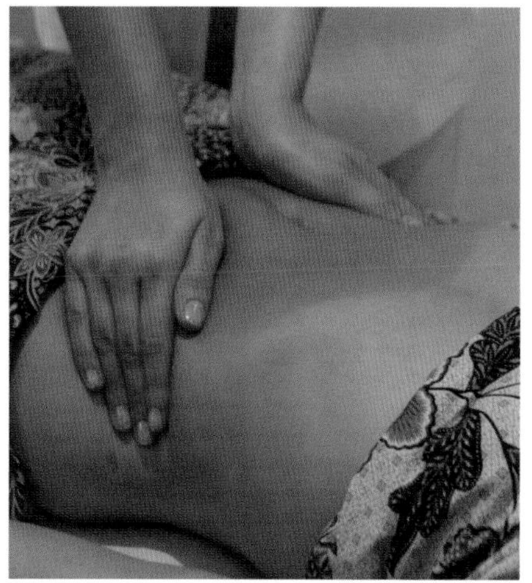

Palmar kneading from the waist towards the groin, using both hands together

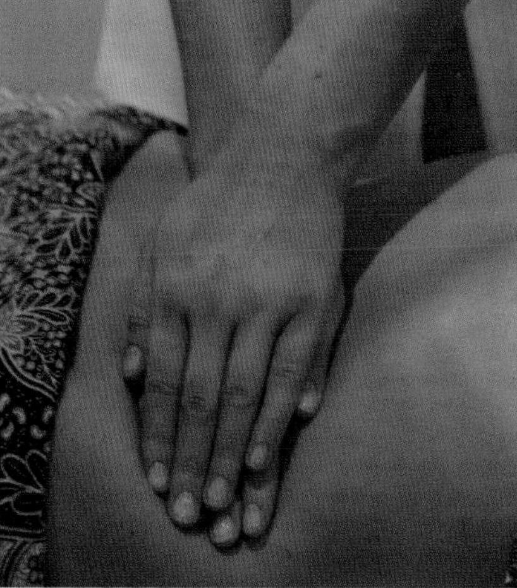

Reinforced double-handed kneading (ironing) to the abdomen

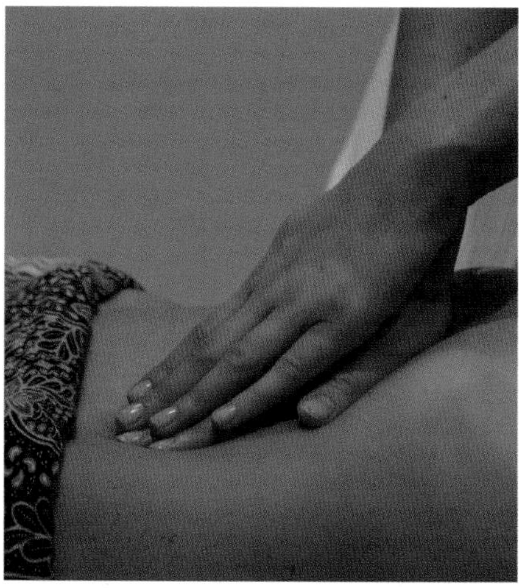

Reinforced double-handed kneading (ironing) to the colon

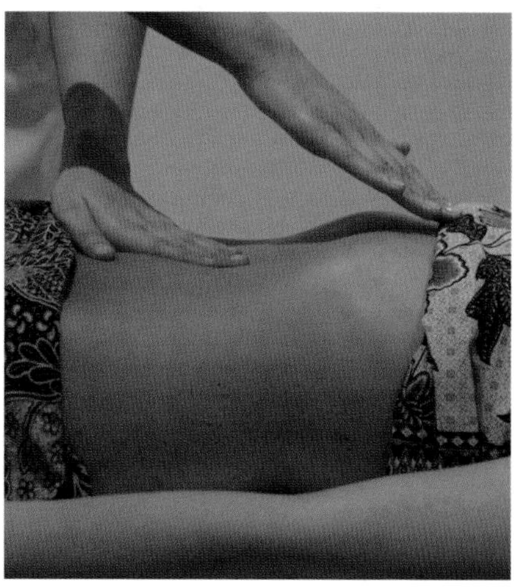

Soothing stroking to the abdomen

SPA TIP

When a client is lying face down for a back massage, their view through the hole in the couch to the floor below is not an attractive one. Excellent spas think of every detail, and some place an attractive bowl of fragranced water (e.g. lime blossom) with floating real flower heads below the couch. Others may instead choose to position a large ornament, such as a spiritual elephant, for the client to focus on. Some international spas are designed so that the treatment couches are directly over the ocean, so the view from the couch is of the sea, or even below the sea – bliss!

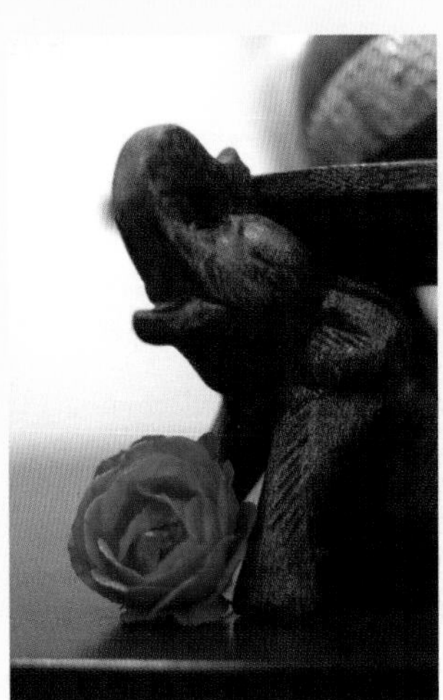

The client can focus on an object placed on the floor under the breathing hole in the couch

STEP-BY-STEP: Leg massage routine – posterior/back surface (approximately 10 minutes each leg)

1. Effleurage – 3 strokes to the posterior surface and onto the glutteal.
2. Single-handed kneading to the glutteals and onto the hamstrings.
3. Reinforced double-handed kneading (ironing) to the glutteals and hamstrings.
4. Wringing to the area.
5. Picking-up to the area.
6. Hacking to the area.
7. Beating to the glutteals.
8. Pounding to the glutteals.
9. Effleurage to the calf area.
10. Single-handed kneading to the inner/medial surface of the gastrocnemius.
11. Single-handed kneading to the outer/lateral surface of the gastrocnemius.
12. Kneading to both medial and lateral surfaces of the gastrocnemius, with both hands alternately.
13. Wringing to the gastrocnemius, and entire calf area.
14. Double-handed picking-up to the gastrocnemius.
15. Light hacking to the calf area.
16. Effleurage to the calf area.
17. Finger kneading around the Achilles tendon and ankle joint.
18. Thumb kneading to the sole of the foot.
19. Effleurage – 3 strokes to the posterior surface and onto the glutteals.

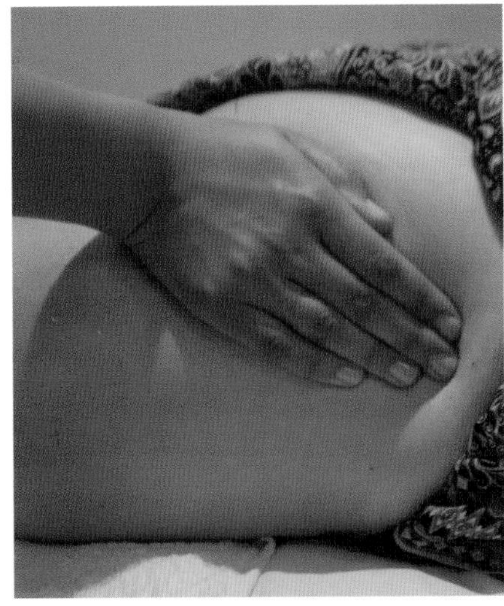
Single-handed kneading to the glutteals

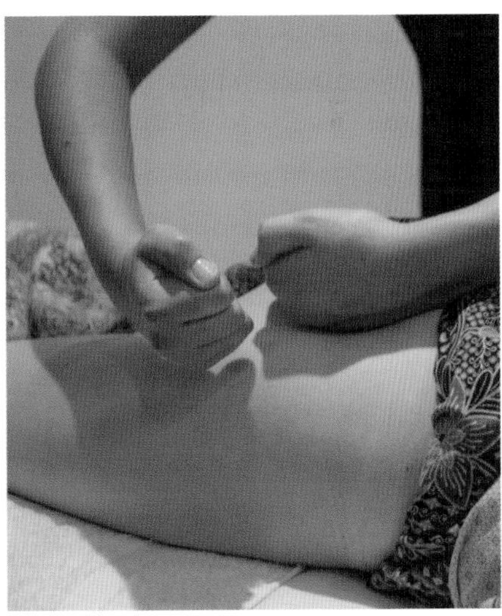
Pounding to the glutteals

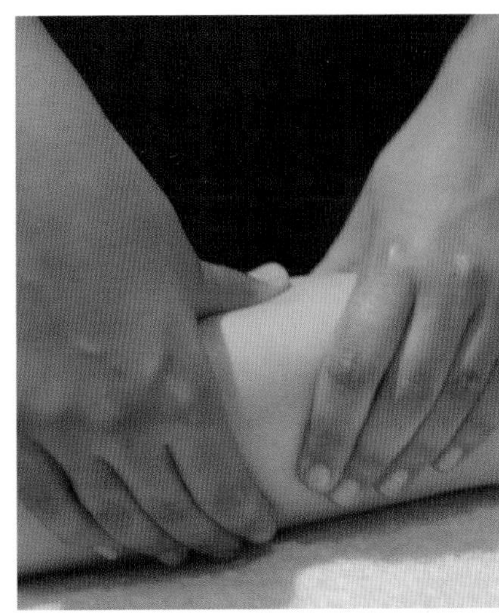
Wringing to the gastrocnemius

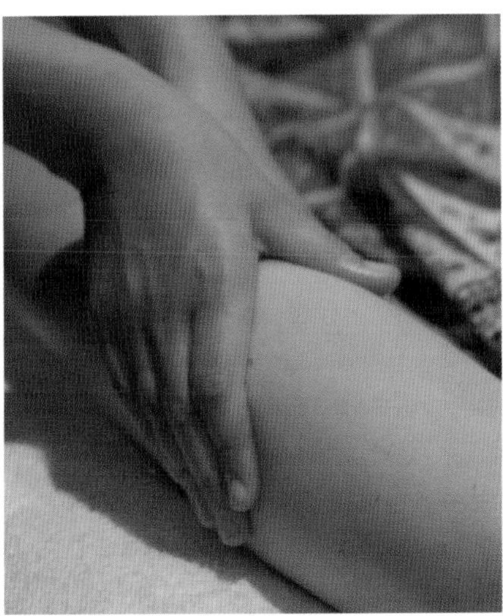
Double-handed picking-up to the gastrocnemius

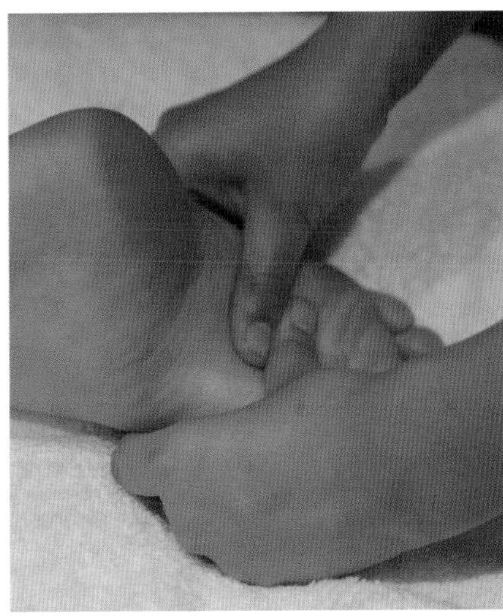
Thumb kneading to the sole of the foot

SPA TIP 

Ask the client if there is an area of the back they want you to concentrate on. Spend more time on this area. Focus on lots of kneading movements, interspersed with effleurage.

SPA TIP 

Some spas use feng shui small bells to signal the end of the treatment.

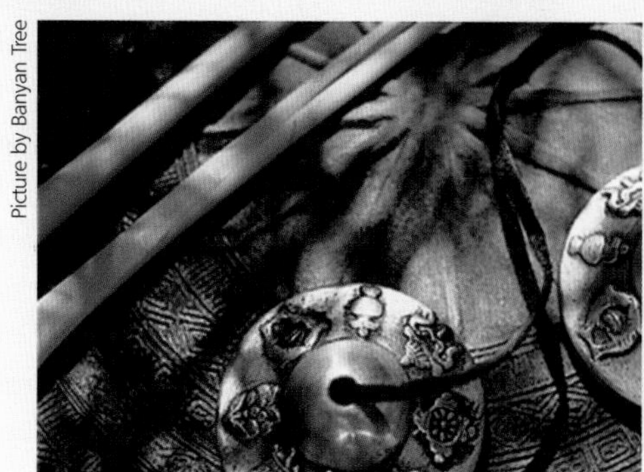

Picture by Banyan Tree

Tibetan bells can signal the end of the treatment

STEP-BY-STEP: Back massage routine (approximately 15–20 minutes)

1 Effleurage
   – 3 strokes towards the neck
   – 3 strokes towards the axillary area
   – 3 strokes towards the waist.
2 Palmar kneading, using both hands together.
3 Palmar kneading, using both hands alternately.
4 Reinforced double-handed kneading (ironing).
5 Wringing to the whole of the back.
6 Picking-up to the whole of the back.
7 Finger kneading around the border of the scapula.
8 If required, smoothly move to the top of the couch and work on the trapezius: effleurage, thumb kneading, effleurage.
9 Frictions down either side of the spine.
10 Skin rolling.
11 Hacking.
12 Cupping.
13 Effleurage
   – 3 strokes towards the neck
   – 3 strokes towards the axillary area
   – 3 strokes towards the waist.
14 Soothing stroking.

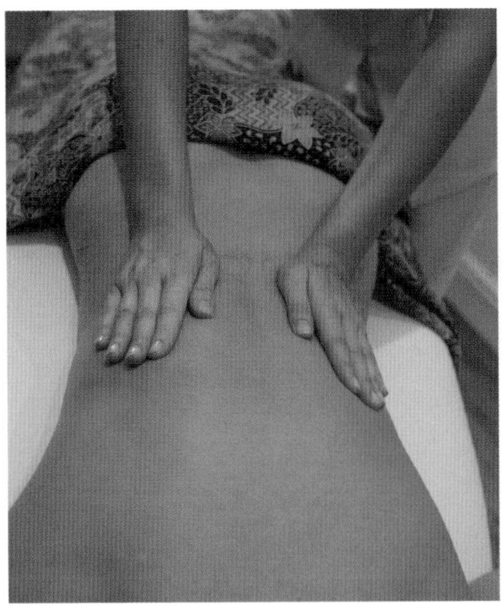
Effleurage to the back

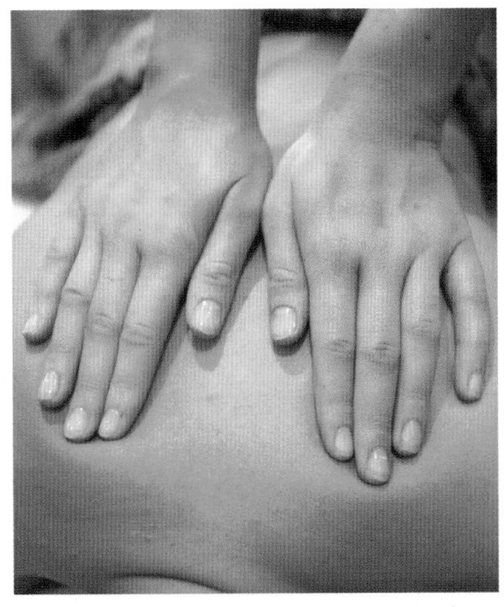
Palmar kneading, using both hands together

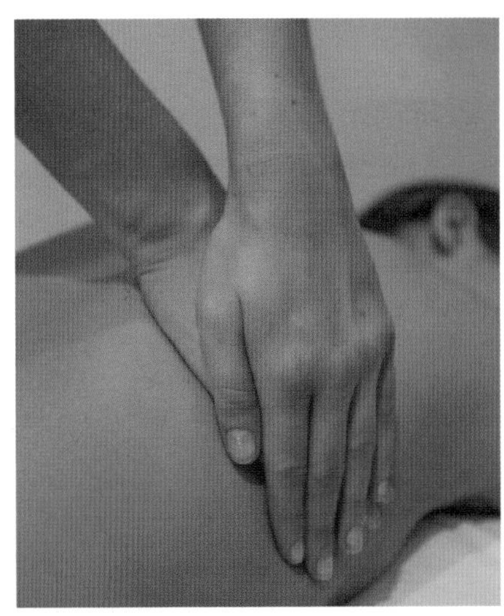
Reinforced double-handed kneading (ironing)

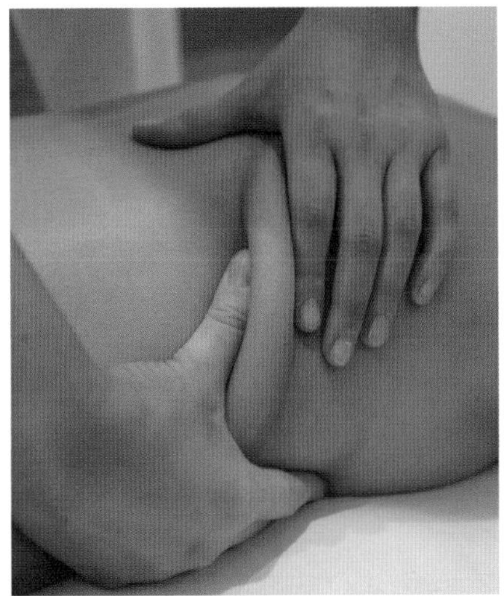
Wringing to the back

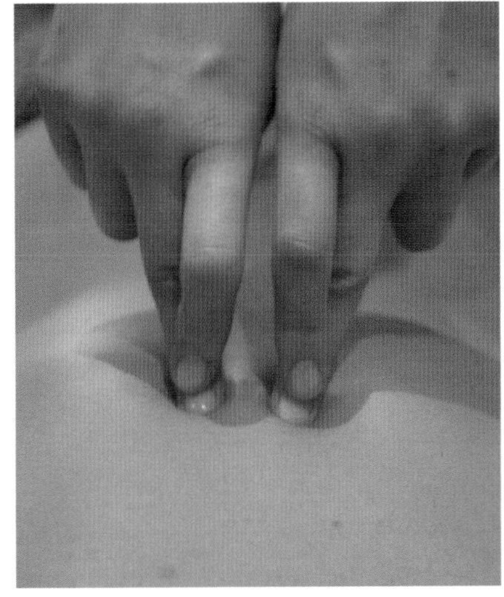
Frictions down either side of the spine

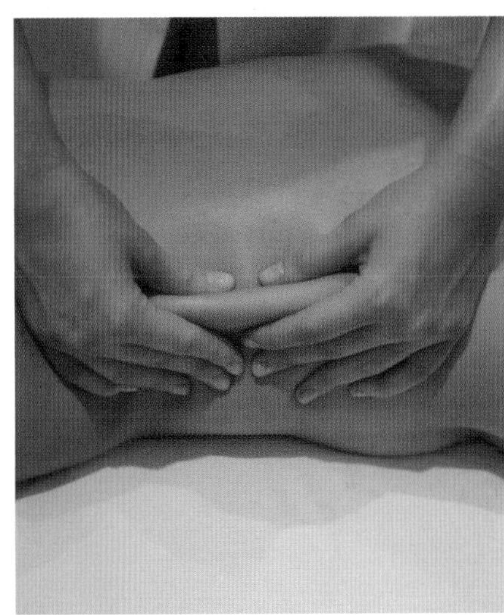
Skin rolling

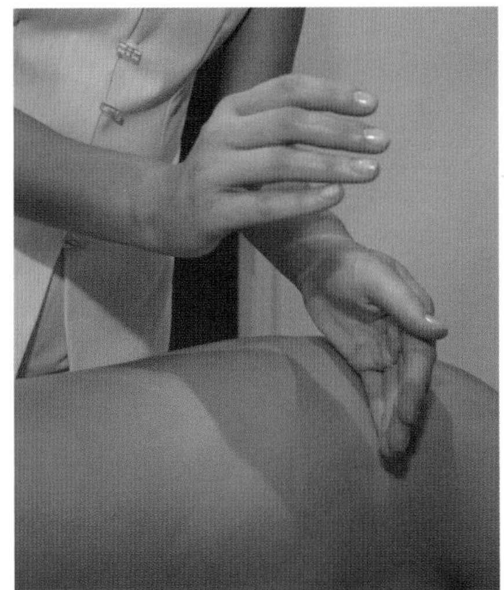
Hacking

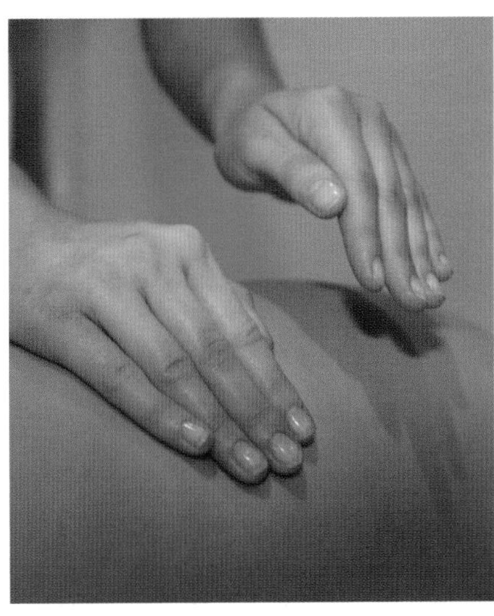
Cupping

FACT

Head massage
Head massage can be included with a body massage to increase the overall relaxing effect. Usually the head can be massaged whilst the client is lying face up, just before they turn over to have the backs of their legs and back massaged. Often the head massage is carried out 'dry', but a treatment oil can be used to nourish the scalp and hair. If possible, the oil should be left on for the rest of the day, as it will continue to feed and nourish the skin and hair.

For full details of head massage, refer to chapter 13.

COMMON FAULTS WITH MASSAGE

A massage is a very individual treatment, and the client will have unique needs and expectations. Failure to go through a very detailed consultation, and take the time to find out the client's requirements will typically result in the following faults:

- incorrect use of lubricant – either too much or too little
- inappropriate pressure – either too light or too heavy
- inconsistent flow and rhythm – makes the massage irritating, and not relaxing
- uncomfortable position on the couch – lack of supporting pillows, etc.
- temperature – either too hot or too cold; both can be irritating
- communication – either too much chatting by the therapist and the client can't relax, or too little and the therapist may come over as unfriendly and uncaring. It is a fine balance, but an experienced therapist should be able to gauge each client and the level of communication needed.

CONTRA-ACTIONS FROM MASSAGE TREATMENT

TERMINOLOGY

Contra-actions are unwanted reactions to the treatment.

- Bruising – caused by poor technique or too much pressure, such as with tapotement strokes, e.g. cupping.
- Skin reaction – could be a heat reaction, or an allergy to the product used, e.g. cream.
- Light-headedness and fainting – could be an effect of the increased blood flow and changed blood pressure. Also, the client may feel dizzy if they get up too quickly after lying down for the massage.
- Nausea, sickness or headache – could be a result of the increased circulation encouraging more waste products to be eliminated, similar to the headaches clients get when they are following a 'de-tox' programme.

Should a client suffer from an adverse reaction to massage, they must be allowed to relax and recover before leaving the spa. It is suggested that the therapist:

- provides a room for relaxation that is well ventilated
- ensures the client's gown or clothing is not too tight, and that they can breathe freely and easily
- provides a glass of water or other refreshment
- applies a cold compress or soothing lotion to any irritated skin condition
- advise the client to seek medical assistance if symptoms persist.

On completion of the treatment, make a full note on the client's record card of any adverse reactions, so that future treatments can be adapted. If appropriate, you can contact the client during the following few days to enquire about their health and wellbeing.

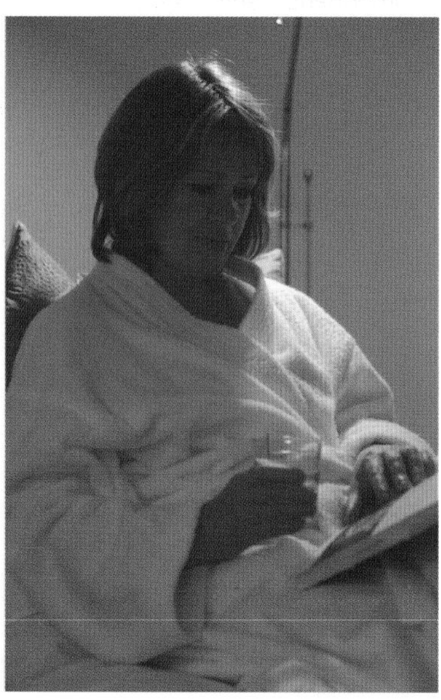

Allow the client to relax after the massage

ADAPTION OF MASSAGE FOR SPECIFIC CONDITIONS

Stress and tension

- A pre-'heat' treatment can increase the effectiveness of the treatment by warming the muscles and generally relaxing the client.
- The rhythm of the massage must be slow, constant and of a medium depth.
- Concentrate on the effleurage and petrissage/kneading movements.
- Soothing stroking can be used more, especially on the back.
- Avoid tapotement movements, as they are too stimulating.
- Concentrate on specific areas of tension, such as the shoulders/neck, lower back and large muscle groups, e.g. thighs.

Provide homecare advice (e.g. relaxation techniques) to help the client learn how to cope with stress in their day-to-day lives.

SPA TIP 

Stress can affect people in different ways, some of the more common problems include headaches, disturbed sleep, high blood pressure and lack of energy. It is vital that the treatment is given in a calm and relaxing environment.

Tight and contracted muscles

- A pre-heat treatment can increase the effectiveness of the treatment by warming the muscles and generally relaxing the client.
- The rhythm of the massage must be slow, constant and of a medium depth.
- As muscles warm and relax, the pressure can get deeper.
- Concentrate on the effleurage and petrissage/kneading movements, as they help warm, relax and stretch the muscles.

SPA TIP 

Very tight muscles are often caused by poor posture or a postural problem (e.g. scoliosis) or can be found in very sporty and athletic clients who have been overdoing it or having insufficient rest between activity.

Avoid tapotement movements, as they are too stimulating and could further tighten the muscles, causing discomfort and pain.

Slack muscles

- Start with a medium depth, increasing the pressure slowly as the muscles respond and become more toned.
- To stimulate the muscles, concentrate on deep petrissage/kneading and tapotement movements. The increased blood supply will increase the nourishment to the muscles.

SPA TIP 

Slack muscles can occur after an operation, pregnancy, quick weight loss, periods of illness, especially if confined to bed, or during the normal ageing process.

Homecare advice is very important. Gentle exercise should be taken to slowly and safely improve the strength and tone of the muscles.

Stiffness of joints

- A pre-heat treatment can increase the effectiveness of the treatment by warming the muscles and generally relaxing the client.
- The rhythm is constant, brisk and of a medium depth.
- A heat treatment may be beneficial prior to the massage, e.g. heat lamp, sauna or paraffin wax.
- Localized finger kneading and frictions around the joint can help relieve stiffness, and increase blood circulation and nourishment to the joint area.

SPA TIP 

Stiffness of joints can be a temporary condition after excessive exercise or activity, but if the stiffness persists, it is recommended that the client consults their doctor to obtain their permission before you treat them.

Homecare advice is very important. Gentle, passive and mobility exercise can be carried out to help joint stiffness and maintain long-term joint stability.

SPA TIP 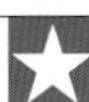

It is important to identify if muscular aches/pains are a result of overexertion (e.g. too much gardening) or if the client has an injury. If there is any possibility that it might be a medical condition, this would contra-indicate the treatment and a doctor's consultation is required.

SIGNATURE TREATMENT S

The Refinery, London

'Turbo Boost (2 hrs 30 mins)

Running on reserve?

Then refuel with our power-up combination.

Guaranteed to leave you feeling super-charged, invigorated and refreshed.

SALT SCRUB

HYDRATING BODY WRAP

DEEP TISSUE MASSAGE'

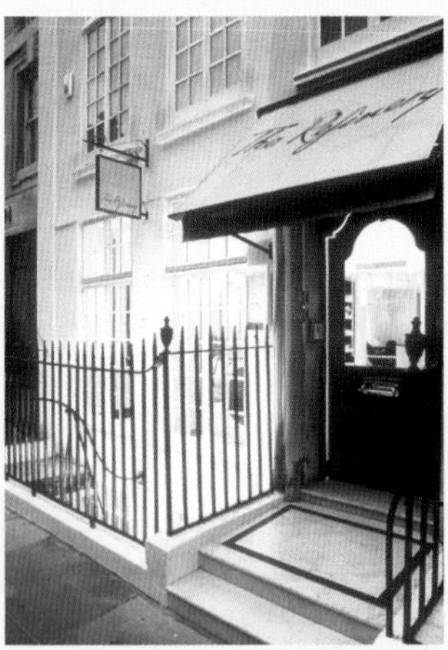

The Refinery, London

SPA TIP 

Massage is not a miracle cure for weight loss. It can, however, be effective when part of a treatment package, combined with exercise and healthy eating, and can also improve the overall appearance and condition of the skin.

Massage improves blood and lymphatic circulation. It is therefore ideal for reducing oedema and can also help prevent it from occuring.

Concentrate on the effleurage, stroking, squeezing kneading and vibration type massage movements.

- All muscles attached to the joint must be massaged as part of a thorough treatment.
- Combine localized finger kneading with lots of effleurage strokes to help increase lymphatic drainage.

General muscular aches, pains and stiffness

- A pre-heat treatment may be beneficial, e.g. sauna, as it can increase the effectiveness of the treatment by warming the muscles and generally relaxing the client.
- Ensure that the area to be massaged is supported well – if not, the client could develop more aches and pains.
- Ask the client to identify problem areas, and allocate more time to the affected areas.
- Intersperse all the massage movements with lots of effleurage and stroking, as this will help stiffness by dispersing waste products, e.g. lactic acid.
- The therapist can concentrate on petrissage movements, with plenty of deep kneading, wringing, picking-up, finger/thumb kneading and frictions.

Weight problems and cellulite

- Very deep massage movement should be applied to a long-standing cellulite condition.
- Kneading, picking-up, skin rolling and wringing can be used on areas of adipose tissue and cellulite.
- Hacking, cupping, beating and pounding are beneficial on very heavy, dense adipose tissue.
- Intersperse all massage movements with firm effleurage strokes, to encourage lymphatic drainage and removal of waste products.

TERMINOLOGY

Oedema refers to a swelling, usually associated with a build up of tissue fluid which the lymphatic vessels have failed to drain. Typical causes include standing for long periods of time, injury, lack of muscle activity or lymphatic system disruption, e.g. infection.

SPA TIP 

Gravitational oedema can occur after standing for long periods. The lack of muscle contraction and effect of gravity means that the lymphatic drainage of the leg slows down. The legs swell, especially around the ankles, which can feel very uncomfortable as the skin becomes tight. A good leg massage can help reduce this type of oedema, and can improve the tired and heavy sensation in the legs.

HEALTH AND SAFETY 

Swelling is a contra-indication to massage treatment. If in any doubt, always recommend that the client seeks medical attention. Their doctor can decide whether massage would benefit the condition.

Oedema

- Elevate the massage area, so gravity can help drain the fluid.
- To avoid skin damage, great care should be taken with swollen areas, as the skin can become stretched, thin and shiny.
- It is advisable to start massage strokes nearest the lymph nodes, and work gradually further and further away. This is so that a 'draining' effect occurs and clears the vessels closest to the nodes, avoiding the area becoming jammed or 'engorged'.
- Follow the direction of the lymphatic flow, applying a squeezing type of kneading (petrissage) movement.
- Intersperse all kneading movements with lots of effleurage and stroking to drain the area, therefore reducing the swelling.

Hormonal problems

- If a client is underweight and bony, avoid tapotement movements.
- If the client is stressed and tense, use more effleurage and petrissage strokes, avoiding the tapotement movements.
- Areas of excess fat can usually tolerate increased depth and pressure.
- On heavy areas, concentrate on stimulating movements, such as petrissage (kneading, wringing, picking-up, skin rolling) and tapotment (hacking, clapping, beating and pounding).

Skin conditions

- Very dry, sensitive skin – check with the client for any allergies, to avoid a reaction to the massage medium. Use a high-quality oil or cream that can be absorbed readily by the body. Be careful with deep pressure or a lengthy treatment, as the skin can become overstimulated, red and irritated.
- Skin that lacks elasticity – apply plenty of massage medium, and avoid overstretching the skin by omitting stretching movements, such as wringing, picking-up and skin rolling.
- Oily skin type – massage could overstimulate a very oily skin. Acne vulgaris can often affect the back and chest area, and the massage would

SPA TIP 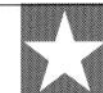

Hormonal imbalance can be responsible for a whole host of body conditions, such as an over- or under-active thyroid and menopause. The client needs to consult their doctor to ensure that the appropriate medication is in place, and that they give their permission for treatments to go ahead.

Homecare advice is very important. Massage is best combined with exercise and nutritional advice to benefit the individual condition.

Massage has many beneficial effects on the skin. However, certain skin conditions need an adapted massage technique to ensure you do not make the situation worse.

Older clients should be treated extra cautiously, and a thorough consultation is necessary to check all aspects, such as medication, recent operations, medical treatment, etc.

need to be adapted. If there are papules and pustules present, it is best to avoid the area until they have healed, as it could be uncomfortable and spread any infection present. Talc is often the best massage medium for oily skin, although many companies produce specialist creams for oily skin conditions.

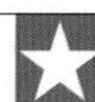

SPA TIP

Increasingly, men are becoming more aware of the benefits of looking after their skin, bodies and health. A huge industry is growing up around male skin care and the specialist products developed to meet the needs of these clients. Many spas are capitalizing on this new client group and are tailoring treatment packages or journeys for the male market.

Older clients

- Ensure the client is well supported on the treatment couch, so no aches or pains develop during the treatment.
- Check that the client is ok to lie flat on the couch – it may be necessary for them to lie in a semi-reclining position to avoid dizziness.
- To prevent dizziness, be extra careful when the client gets up after the treatment.
- Avoid excess pressure – start lightly and increase the pressure, if the client can tolerate a medium depth.
- Avoid overstretching the skin.
- If appropriate avoid deep and stimulating percussion movements.

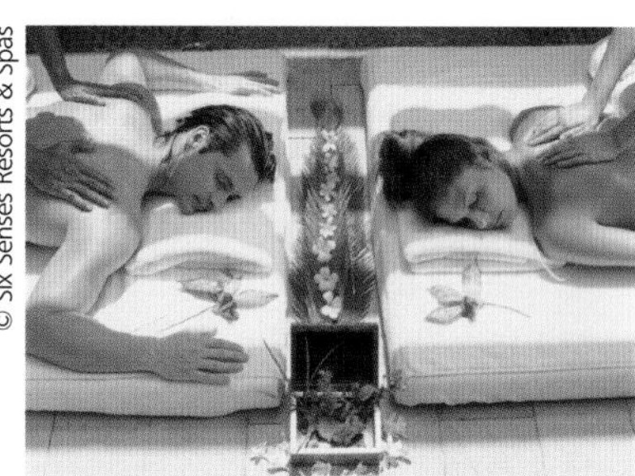

Spa treatments are very popular with men, Six Senses Spa

Male clients

- With excess body hair, be very careful, as the massage could become uncomfortable if not enough medium is used and, in extreme cases, an excessively hairy area may need to be avoided.
- If the client has strong, toned and bulky muscles, then the massage needs to be much deeper than usual.
- Stroking does not need to follow the direction of 'venous return', instead it can be performed – with plenty of oil/cream – in the direction of hair growth.
- The therapist can concentrate on petrissage movements, with plenty of deep kneading, wringing, picking up and skin rolling.
- Extra percussion movements can be performed, concentrating on hacking, cupping, beating and pounding.

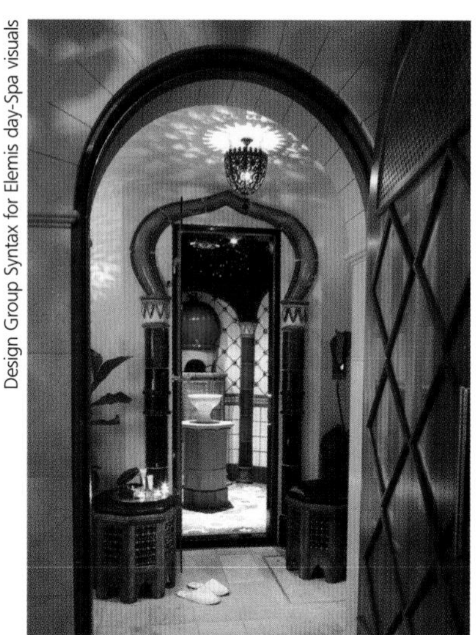

A rasul treatment links well with a massage

LINKED TREATMENTS

Body massage

Massage is a fantastic treatment, and can readily be combined with a huge range of other treatments. The following treatments can 'link' with massage:

- heat treatments, e.g. sauna, steam, rasul, dry float, herbal bath, etc.
- water treatments, e.g. spa pool, jet massage, flotation
- other massage treatments, e.g. Indian head massage, pre-blended oils massage, Thai massage, Balinese massage, remedial massage
- body envelopments, wraps, scrubs, exfoliation
- relaxation, e.g. sound therapy, tepidarium.

SPA TIP 

Indonesian massage is a very intuitive technique, often using a scented massage oil. It involves long sensual strokes, rolling skin between thumb and forefinger to stimulate blood and nerve endings, and pressure point work on the feet and hand reflexes.

Thai massage has an ability to heal, relax and re-align the body. Using the stretching techniques of Indian Ayurveda, plus pressure points, Thai massage is a very deep treatment. The feet, scalp, face and ears are very important areas in Thai massage.

GYRATORY MASSAGE

This type of equipment works on two planes – vertical and horizontal – in an attempt to simulate manual massage. The applicator 'heads' move up and down, as well as in a circular direction. With the various types of 'heads', the machine can simulate the main massage strokes: effleurage, petrissage and percussion. The various gyratory massage machines are usually floor-standing on a pedestal, although there are also hand-held models. This treatment is often referred to as **G5**, as this was the original model from France, which is still in use today.

Effects of a gyratory vibrator

- Increases blood circulation, nourishing the cells and improving skin colour.
- Increases lymphatic circulation, improving the removal of waste materials and toxins.
- Relaxes tight, tense muscles and helps ease muscular pain.
- Increases desquamation, improves skin texture and colour.
- Mobilizes adipose tissue, particularly hard, stubborn deposits. Can help to motivate clients and encourage them to keep to a healthy, balanced eating plan.
- Stimulates sensory nerve endings.
- Stimulates sebaceous glands.

Uses of gyratory vibrator

- For very deep massage, when manual massage is insufficient (useful for male clients).
- Spot reduction – provides deep strong massage on problem fatty areas.
- Less tiring than manual massage, especially when heavy deep massage is needed.
- To help mobilize cellulite.
- Improves poor blood circulation.
- Increases a sluggish lymphatic system.
- Improves dry skin by increasing desquamation and stimulating sebaceous glands.

EQUIPMENT LIST

You will need to prepare the following for a gyratory massage treatment:

towels/bathrobe

witch hazel or eau de cologne

make-up cleanser, purified talc

cotton wool/tissues, spatulas

metal or plastic bowls

gyratory vibration machine

applicator heads

record card

Gyratory massage heads

Name	*Use*	*Picture*
Round sponge	General use to simulate effleurage. Starts and finishes the treatment. Useful for the 'trunk' and large areas	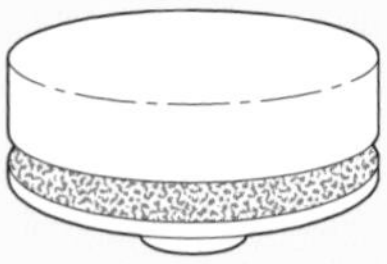
Curved sponge	As above, but is a curved shape to mould to the contours of the arms and legs	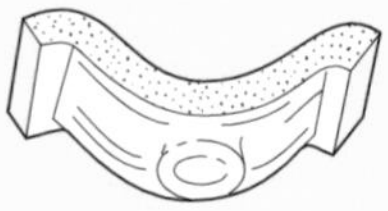
Round, smooth rubber	Simulates effleurage and petrissage, for clients with sensitive skin who cannot tolerate the sponge heads	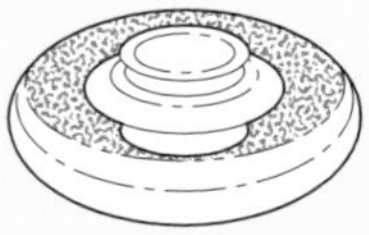
Round, smooth water-filled head	Simulates effleurage and petrissage. Can be filled with: – cold water to create an invigorating and stimulating effect – hot water to soothe and encourage relaxation	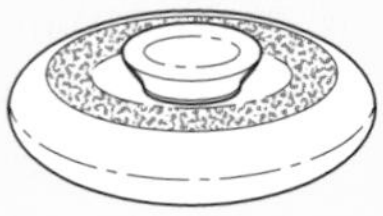
Eggbox	Simulates petrissage. Is useful for heavy areas of adipose tissue, such as the glutteals and thighs	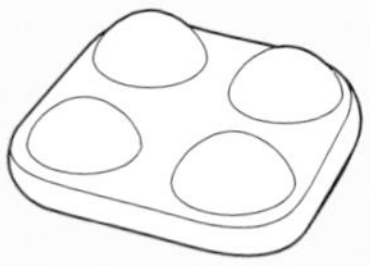
Heavy prong	Simulates petrissage. Also useful on heavy areas of adipose tissue, such as the glutteals and thighs	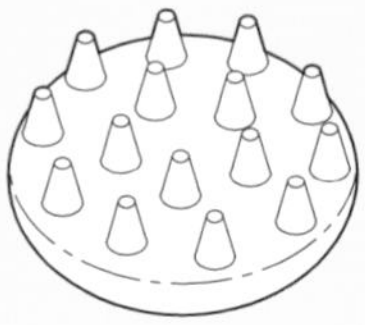
Football	Simulates petrissage. Used on flabby areas of adipose tissue, such as the the trunk. Also can be used for colonic kneading as it can help peristalsis	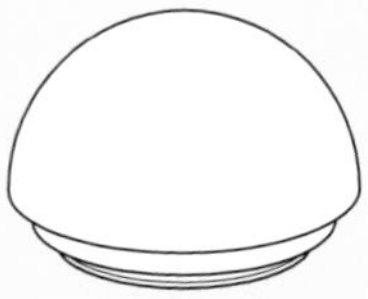
Spiky/ pin-cushion	Simulates percussion. It stimulates the surface of the skin very quickly, causing an immediate hyperaemia (do not use on very sensitive skin). It improves skin texture and condition as it aids desquamation	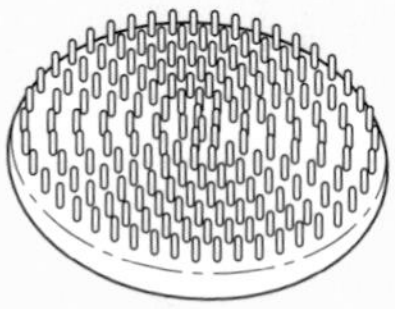
Lighthouse/ pepper-pot	Simulates frictions. Can be used to treat nodules of tension in muscles, and down either side of the spine, and around joints. Could also be used alongside the 'football' head for colonic kneading	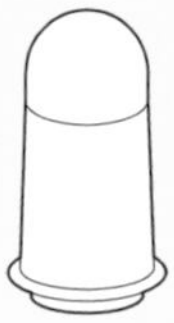

Contra-indications to gyratory massage

- Heart or circulatory conditions.
- Thrombosis.
- Varicose veins.
- Very vascular, sensitive skin.
- Excessively hairy areas.
- Broken skin/bruising.
- Recent fractures, painful joints.
- Skin diseases or disorders.
- Swelling (medical).
- Thin, bony or elderly clients.
- Skin tags, moles, raised skin conditions.
- Loose folds of skin/very old senile skin.
- Scar tissue.
- Skin inflammation.

PREPARE FOR TREATMENT CHECKLIST
Gyratory massage treatment

- ✔ correct environment
- ✔ health and safety
- ✔ hygiene
- ✔ professional appearance
- ✔ equipment/products/consumables
- ✔ record card
- ✔ private changing facilities/bathrobe
- ✔ help client onto massage couch
- ✔ correct client positioning
- ✔ client warm, relaxed and comfortable
- ✔ wash hands
- ✔ explain treatment/sensation
- ✔ remove jewellery
- ✔ cleanse and dry the skin
- ✔ select applicator heads
- ✔ sterilize applicator heads
- ✔ apply unperfumed talc to the area

SPA HYGIENE

Gyratory massage treatment

- after use wash all attachments/heads in warm soapy water
- dry thoroughly
- sanitize heads in an ultraviolet cabinet
- sponge applicators can be covered by a plastic cover, which can then be sanitized
- disposable covers can be used over applicator heads
- store in a clean, dry, safe place.

HEALTH AND SAFETY !

To avoid bruising the client, make sure you do not:

- over-treat (too long)
- apply too much pressure
- use the wrong applicator heads
- use too little talc.

STEP-BY-STEP: Gyratory massage treatment procedure

1. Prepare the client.
2. Select and attach the appropriate applicator head firmly.
3. For a full body treatment, the order follows that of a manual massage, with the client starting face upwards and then turning over for the back of the legs and back to be treated.
4. Start with the effleurage applicators (sponge) and use smooth straight strokes in the direction of the blood and lymph flow. Your free hand can lead or follow the applicator head for continuity and it feels more soothing.
5. Follow the stroke pattern in the diagram opposite.
6. Switch off the machine and change the head to a petrissage one. Perform circular motions, with your free hand lifting the tissue towards the applicator head. Start at the upper part of the area and, in circular motions, work slowly down the body.
7. The pressure and emphasis of the stroke must always be upwards and in the direction of the blood and lymph flow.
8. Change to the head that simulates frictions (lighthouse/pepper-pot) and make small movements around the joint or over tension nodules.
9. Next, change to the spiky/pin-cushion head to simulate percussion. This head can be used either in flowing straight lines or in a circular motion.
10. Always use the effleurage (sponge) heads at the end of the treatment (as with manual massage) to sooth and relax the client.
11. Remove any excess talc, and continue with the next treatment, e.g. manual massage.
12. Complete the record card, giving details of the treatment.

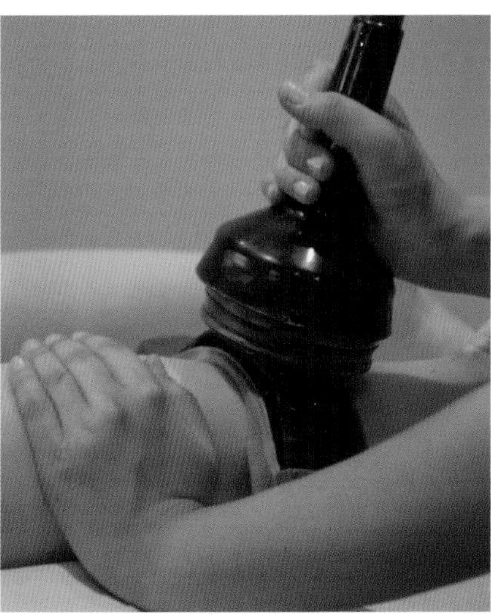

Treatment to the thigh using the 'curved sponge' applicator head

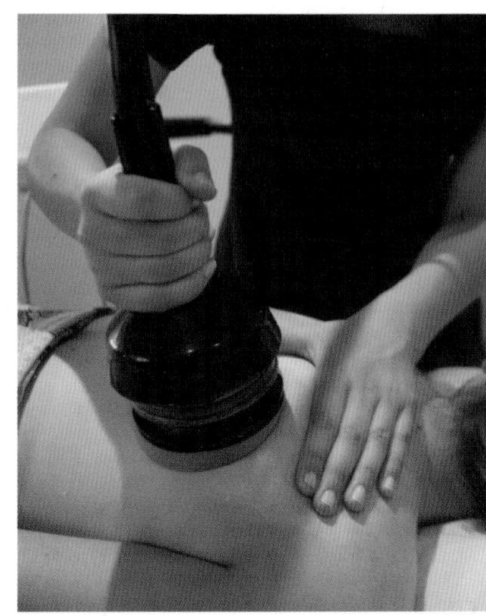

Treatment to the back using the 'round sponge' applicator head

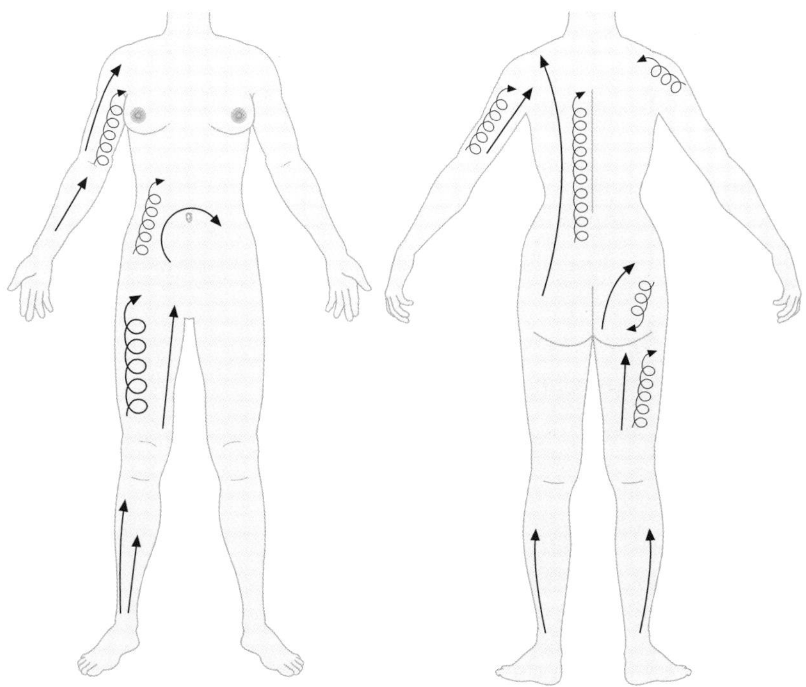

Gliding strokes towards the venous return lymphatic nodes

Rotary movements along muscle length or localised area

Round smooth sponge applicator

Round smooth massage head

Curved sponge applicator

Spiky rubber applicator

Round smooth applicator

Eggbox rubber applicator

Pronged rubber applicator

Football rubber applicator

Lighthouse rubber applicator (used on upper fibres of trapezius muscle)

Application of gyratory vibrator treatment. The straight arrows show the direction of 'effleurage' applicator heads. The circular arrows show the direction for the 'petrissage' applicator heads

AUDIO-SONIC MASSAGE

This is a small hand-held piece of equipment that uses sound waves to produce a vibratory effect. The sound waves vibrate into the skin to a depth of approximately 5–6 cm. Audio-sonic is often chosen for sensitive skin, as the tissues can be massaged without any surface friction or stimulation.

Audio-sonic attachment heads

- Disc or flat plate – used for larger areas of the body and face.
- Round ball-shape – used for smaller areas, for deep body effects, such as to treat tension nodules in muscles.

HEALTH AND SAFETY !

Be careful in case the client experiences a contra-action, which could include:

- excessive redness due to a treatment that was too long
- irritated skin because pressure was applied (no need to apply pressure)
- discomfort due to insufficient lubricant
- sensitivity because the frequency was incorrect over bony areas.

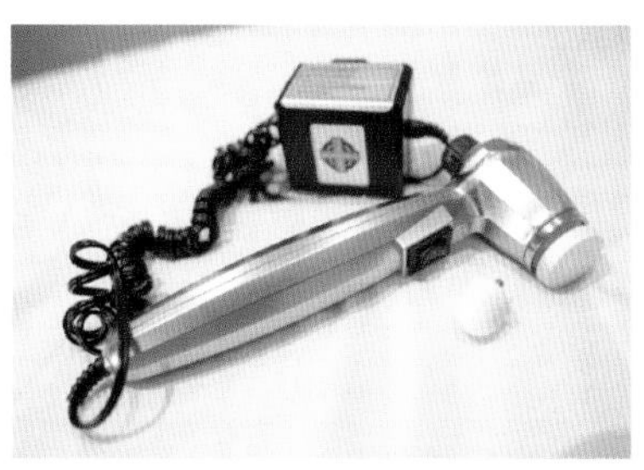

Audio-sonic equipment

EQUIPMENT LIST

You will need to prepare the following for an audio-sonic treatment:

- towels
- cotton wool and tissues
- metal or plastic bowls
- record card
- audio-sonic machine
- 2 attachment heads (disc and ball)
- skin cleanser
- lubricant – talc/oil/cream
- surgical spirit

SPA HYGIENE 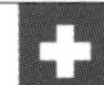

Audio-sonic treatment

- after use, wash attachment heads in warm soapy water
- wipe over individual heads with spirit-based cleaner
- sanitize heads in ultraviolet cabinet, or soaked in a disinfectant solution
- store in a clean, dry, safe place.

Effects of audio-sonic vibrator

- The sound waves shake and vibrate the tissues, cells are compressed and decompressed.
- Blood circulation is increased, which provides more nourishment and oxygen to the cells and the skin colour is improved.
- Stimulates lymph circulation. This improves the removal of waste products and toxins.
- Tissues are warmed.
- Relaxes muscles and helps relieve tension nodules.
- Mobilizes soft adipose tissue.

Uses of audio-sonic vibrator

Body

- To generally relieve tension in tight, contracted muscles.
- To relieve nodules of tension, e.g. in trapezius muscle.
- To mobilize cellulite.
- Use when the gyratory vibrator is contra-indicated because it may irritate and make the area too sensitive.

Face

- Mature skin – to brighten, tone, stimulate and increase the nourishment to cells.
- Sensitive skin or vascular areas.

Contra-indications to audio-sonic massage

- Very bony areas or clients
- varicose veins
- metal pins or plates
- recent scar tissue
- recent fractures
- very vascular skin, e.g. large network of dilated capillaries
- skin disorders/diseases, e.g. psoriasis, impetigo
- skin inflammation, or sensitivity, e.g. sunburn, rash
- broken skin
- bruising
- painful, swollen joints
- eye area
- pregnancy
- pacemaker fitted.

PREPARE FOR TREATMENT CHECKLIST
Audio-sonic treatment

✔ correct environment	✔ correct client positioning
✔ health and safety	✔ client warm, relaxed and comfortable
✔ hygiene	✔ wash hands
✔ professional appearance	✔ explain treatment/sensation
✔ equipment/products/consumables	✔ remove jewellery
✔ record card	✔ cleanse and dry the skin
✔ private changing facilities/bathrobe	✔ select attachment heads
✔ help client onto massage couch	✔ apply lubricant to the skin

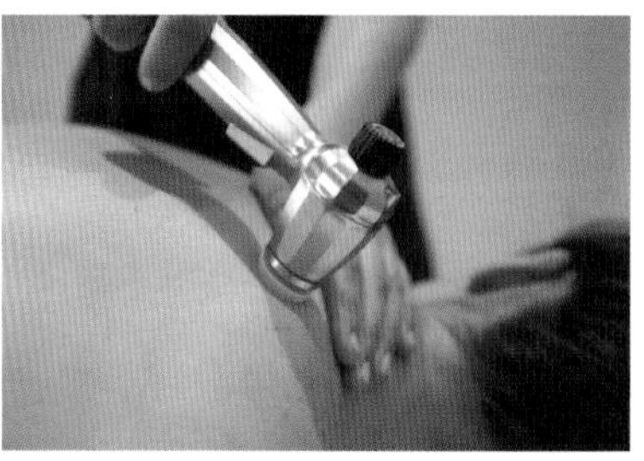

Audio-sonic treatment on the back

HEALTH AND SAFETY 

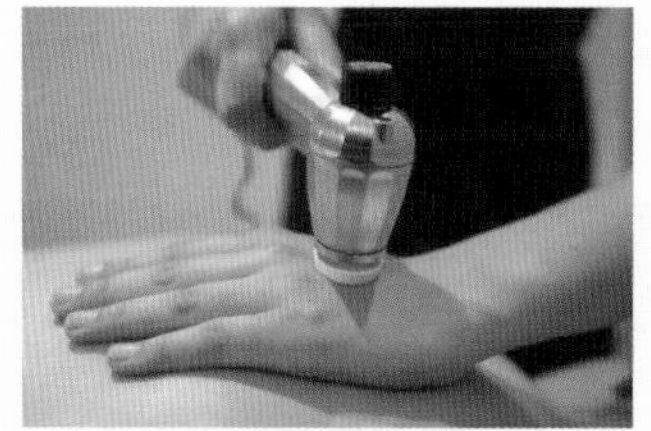

Be careful over bony areas, such as the scapula. Where appropriate, place your hand over the area and apply the audio-sonic to your own hand. The vibrations will travel into the client, but will be much gentler.

SPA TIP 

After the audio-sonic treatment, go through your usual aftercare and homecare advice. Advise the client on skin and body products that will suit them and that are available to buy in the spa. If stress or poor posture is involved, recommend some relaxation techniques and postural exercises.

Audio-sonic treatment procedure

1. Prepare the client.
2. Select the appropriate head for the treatment.
3. Attach the head firmly.
4. Switch machine on at the electricity mains, test the intensity, then clean the head with surgical spirit.
5. Usually small, localized areas of the body are treated, but if a full body treatment is required start on the feet, work up the legs, arms, trunk then the back.
6. Work in straight lines, and circular movements along the length of muscles, in the direction of the heart. Always keep the head moving.
7. Adapt the treatment to different areas by adjusting the frequency control, which regulates the depth of the vibrations.
8. To change heads, always switch off the machine.
9. At the end of the treatment, switch off and unplug the machine.
10. Remove the massage medium and continue with the next treatment, e.g. manual massage.
11. Complete the record card, giving details of the treatment.

HEAT TREATMENTS

On many occasions, a pre-'heat' treatment can be carried out before the massage. This helps increase the effects of the treatment, and is particularly beneficial if the client is in need of deep relaxation. The additional effects of the heat are to increase blood circulation, soothe nerve endings and relax muscles.

> **HEALTH AND SAFETY** !
>
> Always carry out a **thermal skin sensitivity test** before a client has a heat treatment. If they have a reduced sensitivity to heat, this could cause a burn, so the treatment would be contra-indicated.

There is a wide range of pre-heat treatments (many are covered in chapter 7):

- sauna bath
- steam bath
- rasul
- paraffin wax
- dry float.

INFRA-RED LAMP TREATMENT

Whereas many of the heat treatments affect the entire body, infrared treatment is more localized. This is ideal if you only want to treat a specific area, such as the back, or the client does not want (or hasn't the time) to go through the bathing routine involved with other heat treatments.

The lamp used produces infra-red rays which heat the body.

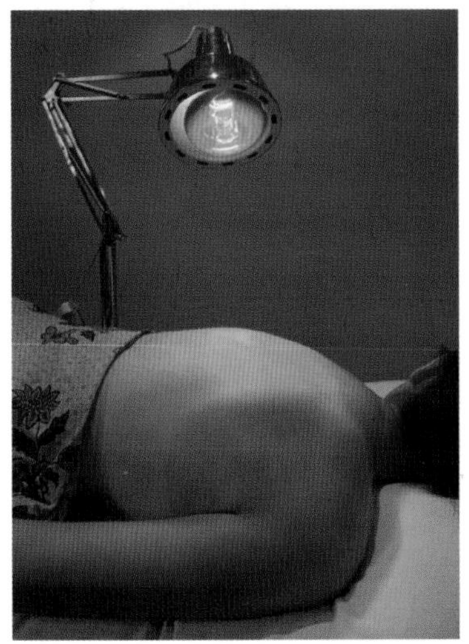
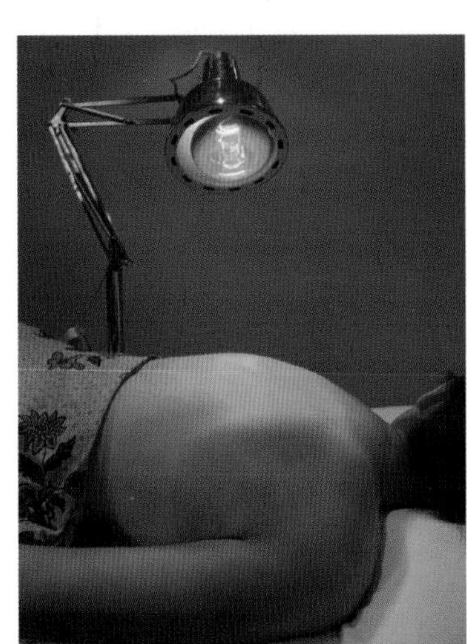

Infra-red lamp treatment to the back

Effects of infra-red heat lamps

- Increase body temperature and stimulate sweat glands.
- Wamth produced in the tissues, hyperaemia develops.
- Increase in blood circulation – improves nourishment to the cells and speeds up removal of waste products.
- Relaxation of muscles.
- Pain relief – the sensory nerve endings are soothed by mild heat.

Uses of infra-red heat lamps

- Preparation of the body – relaxing muscles and allowing oils and creams to be absorbed more readily.
- Relax tight muscles and soothe muscle tension.
- Relax clients who are nervous and tense.
- As an alternative to the 'wet' heat treatments, for clients who haven't the time or do not want the 'bathing' experience.
- Pain relief for sore joints or muscular aches.

> **HEALTH AND SAFETY** !
>
> When conducting an infra-red treatment make sure the client does not:
>
> - touch the hot lamp
> - overheat
> - look directly at the infra-red lamp
> - wear jewellery during treatment
> - have body lotion or oil on their skin
> - trip over the flex of the lamp
> - try to move the lamp during treatment.

Contra-indications to infra-red heat lamps

- Loss of skin sensation
- diabetes
- sunburn or other burn
- high or low blood pressure
- metal pins or plates
- heart conditions

- circulatory problems
- skin diseases or disorders
- very sensitive, vascular skin.

Infra-red treatment procedure

1. Ensure the tactile and thermal skin sensitivity tests have been carried out, and that the client's sensitivity is normal.
2. Check contra-indications.
3. Heat the lamp away from the client in a safe place.
4. Clean the skin (shower or wipe).
5. Position the lamp between 40–60 cm from the body, with the rays striking the body at 90 degrees.
6. Follow manufacturer's instructions.
7. Stay with the client throughout treatment.
8. Check regularly that the client is not too hot or uncomfortable.

Treatment lasts between 5 and 15 minutes, depending on the client and the reason for treatment.

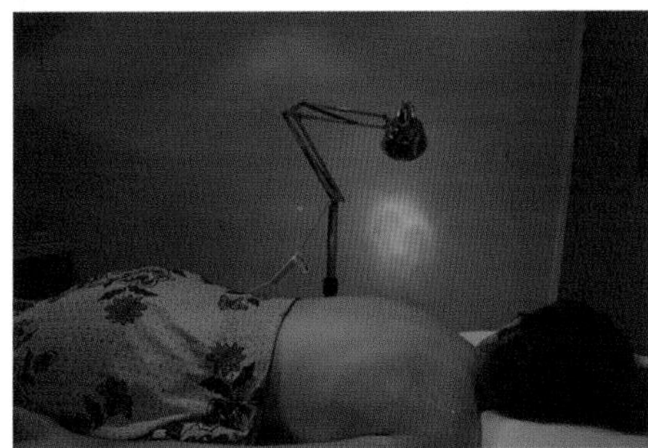

Always heat the lamp away from the client, and out of harm's way

HEALTH AND SAFETY !

The rays of the infra-red lamp must strike the body at 90 degrees to ensure maximum penetration and avoid burning due to 'hot-spots'.

HEALTH AND SAFETY !

Check:

- the lamp is in good working order
- you have followed the manufacturer's instructions
- the bulb is firmly screwed in
- the plug and flex are not worn or damaged
- the reflector of the lamp is clean and has no dents
- no one can trip over the flex to the lamp
- no one can bump into the lamp when it is heating up
- the joint on the arm of the lamp can be tightened sufficiently.

SPA PROFILE

Name: Gemma Stewart

Position: Spa Manager

Establishment: Cowshed, The Scotsman Hotel, Edinburgh

Products used: 'Cowshed' Products.

Number of staff/roles: Spa Manager. 5 full-time spa therapists; 1 part-time therapist; 1 part-time massage therapist.

Training/experience: Perth College – HND Beauty Therapy; Crieff Hydro Hotel – Therapist; Escape at The Scotsman Hotel – Senior Therapist; Cowshed at The Scotsman Hotel – Spa Manager since August 2004.

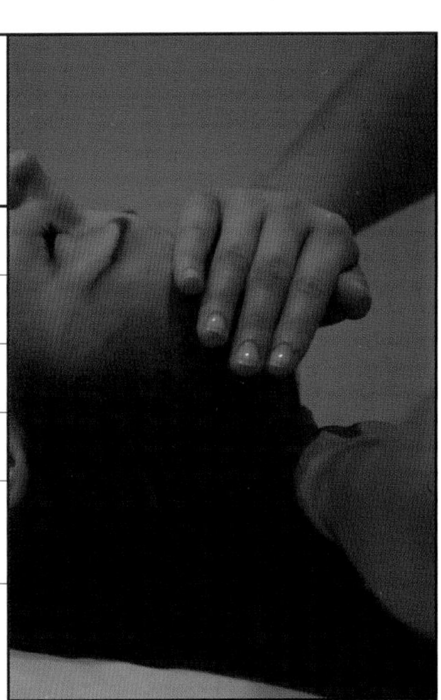

Main responsibilities: Recruitment and selection; training and development; promotions/marketing; stock – ordering, checks; human resources – staff problems, issues; treatments; co-ordinating groups/corporate bookings.

Best parts of the job:
Interaction with different types of guests

Meeting people

I have a great team, we work really well together, with very low staff turnover

I love the 'hands on' part of the job, and still do treatments on guests

I like the uniqueness of the 'Cowshed' philosophy, the treatments and the products.

Secrets of a successful spa therapist:
Commitment is very important

Strong personal interest in therapies, products and treatments

Good people skills

Exceptionally high professional standards

Good understanding of the industry

Very high standard of treatment.

KEY/CORE SKILLS OPPORTUNITIES

To be an excellent spa therapist you must be able to communicate well, both orally and in writing. To be able to succeed and progress in the spa industry, it is also essential that you have an ability to work with numbers and information technology (IT). Increasingly, employers are looking for spa therapists with these 'key' skills when they recruit staff. NVQ/SVQ unit **BT17** provides you with an opportunity to develop evidence for the following:

KEY SKILLS	CORE SKILLS
Communication Level 3; C3.1a, C3.2	Communication Intermediate 2; Task 1 and 3
Working with others Level 2; WO2.1, WO2.2, WO2.3	Working with others Intermediate 1; Tasks 1, 2 and 3
Improving own learning and performance Level 3; LP3.1, LP3.2	(no parallel unit in CORE SKILLS)
Problem solving Level 2; PS2.1, PS2.2, PS2.3	Problem solving Intermediate Level 1; Tasks 1, 2 and 3

Assessment of knowledge and understanding

When you have some free time, test your understanding and knowledge by answering the following questions. Do this at regular intervals and it will reinforce your learning and help you retain the knowledge, so you are able to perform better in your assessments.

Organizational and legal requirements

1 What does the abbreviation COSHH mean?

2 When performing a massage treatment, what are your responsibilities under the Health and Safety at Work Act 1974?

3 When performing a mechanical gyratory massage treatment, what are your responsibilities under the Electricity at Work Regulations 1989?

4 Why is it important when performing body massage treatments to have clean, soft, well-manicured hands and nails?

5 What precautions will you take to ensure your massage treatment is hygienic and avoids cross-infection?

6 Why is the spa therapist's posture important when performing a massage treatment?

7 Why is it important to keep up-to-date records of client treatments?

8 When keeping client record cards what are your responsibilities in relation to the Data Protection Act 1998?

9 Why should treatments be completed in the given time? And what are the commercially acceptable timings for the following treatments?:
   a. full body and head massage
   b. full body massage
   c. back massage.

Client consultation

1 During the consultation why should you allow sufficient time and encourage clients to ask questions?

2 Why would you encourage a client with a contra-indication to seek advice from their doctor?

3 Why would you ask the client to sign the record card during the consultation?

4 What beneficial effects can result from a client changing their lifestyle pattern?

5 Describe three postural conditions that the client could suffer from?

Preparation for treatment

1 Describe the ideal environment for a relaxing massage treatment?

2 Which areas of the body would need cleansing before massage treatment?

3 Describe the following skin types:
   a. sensitive
   b. mature
   c. oily.

4 Which would be the ideal massage medium for the following skin types?:
 a. oily
 b. normal
 c. dry/mature.

5 What are the benefits of a pre-heat treatment before performing a massage?

Contra-indications

1 List four 'general' contra-indications that prevent body massage treatment.

2 List four 'temporary' contra-indications that prevent massage treatment.

3 List four 'local' contra-indications that would restrict massage to particular areas of the body.

4 Why should the client consult their doctor if a contra-indication is identified?

Equipment and materials

1 How would you sanitize the following equipment?:
 a. plastic spatulas
 b. trolley/table
 c. gyrator massage applicator heads.

2 How would you ensure the treatment couch is in a clean and hygienic condition for each client?

Treatment specific knowledge

1 What is a contra-action? Describe possible contra-actions to massage treatment.

2 Which skin types may be aggravated or irritated by the following massage mediums?:
 a. purified talc
 b. massage oil.

3 What effect does body massage treatment have on the following?:
 a. muscles
 b. blood system
 c. lymph system
 d. skin
 e. nerves.

4 What are the psychological effects of massage?

5 Why is it important to complete stretching exercises prior to performing massage?

6 What are the uses of the following massage manipulations?:
 a. effleurage
 b. palmar kneading
 c. hacking
 d. finger kneading.

7 What precautions should you take to avoid discomfort when performing a gyratory massage treatment?

8 Why is it important to evaluate how effective the body massage treatment has been?

Treatment advice

1 What advice regarding fluid intake should you give the client after the massage?

2 Why is it important to record all treatment details, including contra-actions, on the record card?

3 How often would you recommend the client has a body massage treatment? And what would be the benefits of regular treatments?

4 Which treatments could easily be combined or 'linked' to body massage?

5 What products, linked to body massage, could you recommend for the client to buy and use at home?

6 What nutritional and lifestyle advice could you give to a client who is hoping to lose weight and tone up their body?

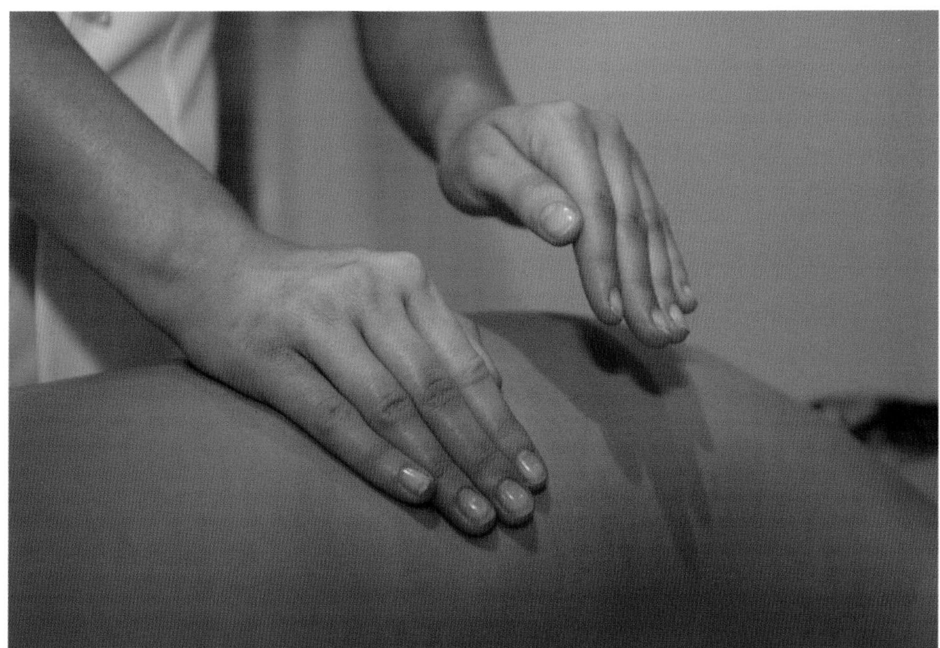

chapter 12

Massage with pre-blended oils

BT21

Provide massage using pre-blended aromatherapy oils

Learning objectives

This chapter covers the skills spa therapists need for preparing clients for, and delivering, massage using pre-blended aromatherapy oils.

It describes the skills and knowledge necessary to enable you to:

- **consult with the client**
- **plan the treatment**
- **prepare for the treatment**
- **massage client's head and body using suitable massage techniques**
- **complete the treatment**

FACT

The use of aromatic plants for medicinal and cosmetic purposes has been traced back to the Egyptians as early as 3000 BC, who famously used frankincense in the embalming process to help preserve mummies.

When providing massage using pre-blended aromatherapy oils it is important to use the skills you have learnt in the following core units:

G1 Ensure your own actions reduce risks to Health and Safety

G6 Promote additional products or services to clients

G11 Contribute to the financial effectiveness of the business

INTRODUCTION

Aromatherapy has been used for thousands of years, but it is the resurgence of aromatherapy over the past 10 years that has made it one of the most popular alternative treatments offered in spas today.

Aromatherapy is what the name implies, a therapy using aroma (or smells). It uses essential oils extracted from plants, trees and fruits, and their individual properties are known to benefit physical and psychological problems.

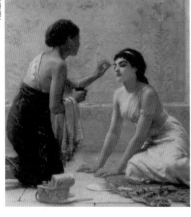

Kurland

Ancient practice of aromatherapy

USES OF AROMATHERAPY

Many people are turning to alternative therapies to cope with the pressures faced in today's world. Aromatherapy can be used as a preventative treatment to help maintain optimum health.

Essential oils can be applied through several methods other than massage – baths, burners, inhalation, creams and lotions – but massage is seen as the most effective way of introducing essential oils to the body.

Aromatherapy can be used to treat clients on a psychological level as well as a physical level:

Physical

- penetrates the skin
- strongly antiseptic
- stimulates and soothes the nervous system
- promotes healthy cell growth.

Psychological

- sedative
- euphoriant
- stimulating/uplifting
- aphrodisiac.

SPA TIP 

As a therapist recognize your limitations in your therapy, do not give too many aromatherapy treatments, and it may be necessary to refer a client to their GP if you are not happy with their progress.

SIGNATURE TREATMENT S

Willow Stream Spa at the Fairmont Empress, Victoria, Canada

'Island Senses – 120 minutes Rejuvenate in the coastal wonders and mystical harmony of the elements found on Vancouver Island. Begin your island experience with your arrival by ocean – an invigorating "salts of the sea" body scrub for exfoliation. Follow your ocean journey by a refreshing walk in the forests with an aromatic pine hydrotherapy bath. Experience the invigorating walking and hiking trails through the earth aroma of a detoxifying mud wrap. Draw from the gentle fields of Victoria abundant with lavender, and take pleasure in a restoring and healthy massage of lavender. Your senses delight as energy is restored.'

ESSENTIAL OILS

Essential oils are the highly aromatic, natural oils found in plants. The essential oil is present within the root, stem, flower, fruit, leaf or bark and the percentage of oil in the plant depends upon the part the oil is extracted from.

The natural molecular structure of essential oils is very complex, but they are largely made up of the three elements – carbon, hydrogen and oxygen. It is their complex state which stops them from being replicated by scientists, as their structure is naturally occurring and depends on external factors, such as the weather, time of harvesting the plant and environmental conditions.

The molecules of essential oils are very small which allows them to penetrate through the skin easily and pass into the bloodstream. Even though each essential oil has a different chemical structure and effect, they basically have the same physical properties:

- are highly volatile
- do not feel greasy
- have no lubricating properties
- mix with alcohol
- mix with vegetable oils
- do not mix with water
- have an odour.

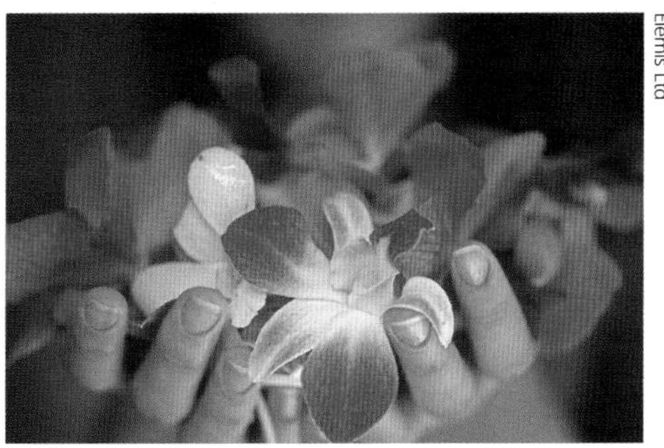

Elemis Ltd

Storage of essential oils

Essential oils are highly volatile (evaporate easily) and need to be stored in dark glass bottles, in a dark cool place away from sunlight. The top of the essential oil bottle should be fitted with a dropper top to stop oxygen getting in and the bottle labelled clearly.

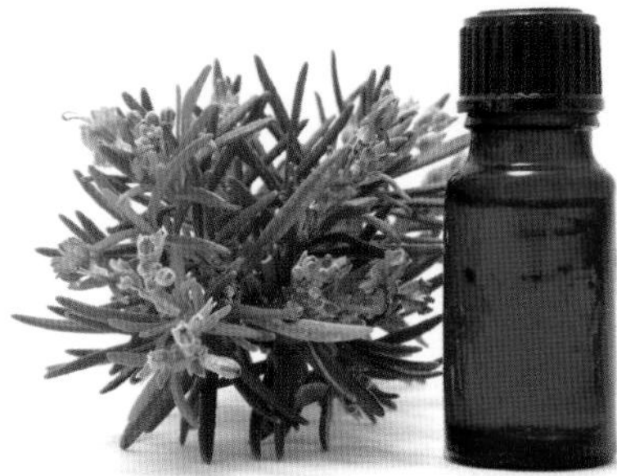

Rosemary herb and oil

> **HEALTH AND SAFETY !**
>
> The volatility of essential oils makes them catch fire easily, so care should be taken when near a naked flame, e.g. in a burner. Make sure that any burner you purchase has been properly sealed to stop oil leaking through onto the candle.

> **HEALTH AND SAFETY !**
>
> Essential oil bottles become sticky after constant use so always wipe the outsides with surgical spirit.

Picture by Banyan Tree

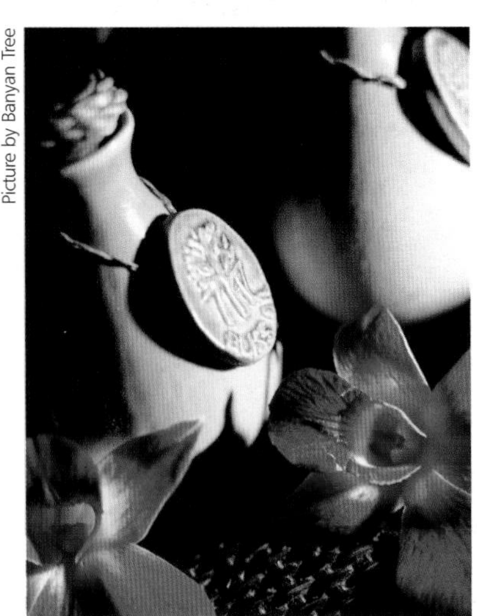

Evaporation of essential oils

The rates at which individual essential oils evaporate have been put into three catagories.

Top note	*Middle note*	*Base note*
Evaporate quickly	Evaporate moderately quickly	Evaporate slowly
Lasts approximately 24 hours	Lasts for 2–3 days	Lasts for about 1 week
Absorbed quickly into the body	Absorbed moderately quickly into the body	Absorbed slowly into the body
Have a sharp aroma	Generally have physical therapeutic effects	Heavy aroma with relaxing and soothing properties
Have a stimulating/ uplifting effect	Produced from flowers and herbs such as lavender, geranium, chamomile and rosemary	Are known as fixatives as they prolong the life of a blend
Examples are citrus oils such as orange, lemon, grapefruit and herb oils such as peppermint		Produced from woods and resins generally, for example sandalwood, rosewood, myrrh and ylang-ylang

Classifications of essential oils in plants

Essential oils are yielded from different parts of the plant.

Flowers	Jasmine, neroli, rose, ylang-ylang
Leaves	Citronella, lemongrass, petitgrain, palmarosa
Bark	Cinnamon
Wood	Cedarwood, sandalwood, rosewood
Roots	Ginger, vetiver
Entire plant	Geranium, lavender, rosemary, spike lavender
Fruit peel	Bergamot, lemon, lime, bitter and sweet orange, tangerine, mandarin

Methods of extracting essential oils from plants

Steam distillation

Distillation is the most common method used in extracting essential oil molecules from plant material. Plant material is prepared by drying, crushing or breaking in order to break up the glands that contain the essence of the

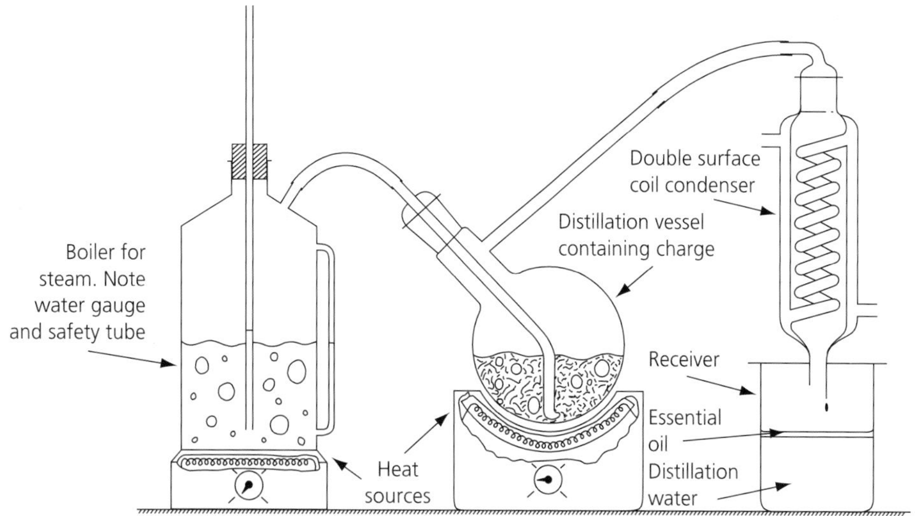

Water and steam distillation processes

Steam distillation

plant, then put into a large closed container, known as a vat, which steam is forced through. The heat and pressure cause the release of the tiny droplets of essential oil from the plant material, which then rise with the steam out through a spiral tube. This cools the steam, condensing it into liquid. As oil and water do not mix, you are left with the oil floating on top of the water, which is then removed.

> **FACT**
>
> **Hydrolats** or **flower water** is the water solution left at the end of distillation once the essential oil has been removed. This can be used to make skincare products or used as a toner/facial spray on the skin. Peppermint flower water is very good for cooling down the skin when on the beach or as a pick-me-up when travelling.

Enfleurage

Enfleurage is the old-fashioned method of extracting the scent from thick-petalled flowers, such as rose, jasmine and ylang-ylang. A thin layer of pure, odourless fat is spread onto a glass frame and the fresh flowers are put in layers on top of this. After about 30 hours the essential oil from the flowers will have become absorbed in the fat. This process is repeated several times with fresh flowers until the fat is completely saturated with scent. The fat is then scraped off the glass, placed in a clean glass container and alcohol is added. Over a few weeks the alcohol absorbs the essential oil. The alcohol is then gently separated from the fat under vacuum, leaving pure essential oil.

Expression

This is used on the rinds of citrus fruit to obtain essential oils such as lemon, lime and orange. A machine squeezes the rinds of the fruit until the oil glands burst releasing the essential oil, which is then collected.

Solvent extraction

Mainly used on flowers. The flowers are covered with a solvent (usually petrol ether), which extracts the essential oil. The solvent is then evaporated off, leaving the essential oil in the container. Essential oils, which use this method, are known as **absolutes**.

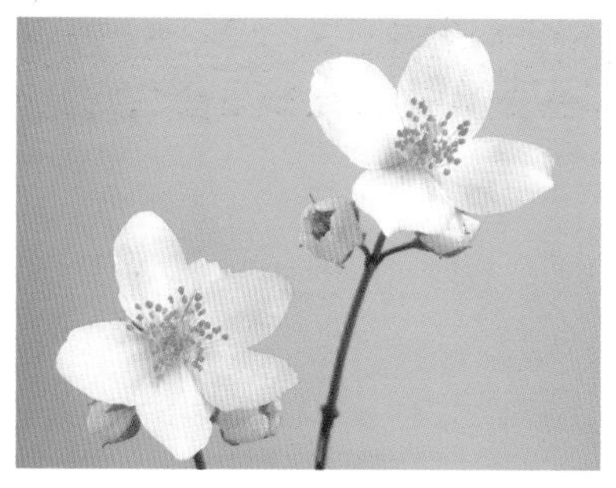
Jasmine

FACT

There are over 15 different species of lavender, with one species, English lavender, having over 40 named varieties with different shades of flowers.

SPA TIP 

To make chamomile tea put a tablespoon of dried flower heads (can be obtained at a good health shop) in a mug, pour boiling water over and cover for 10–15 minutes. Add honey and strain the flowers before drinking. This tea will calm you down, help sleep and ease stomach cramps.

HEALTH AND SAFETY

There have been a number of reports lately of skin irritation due to the prolonged use or overuse of tea tree oil neat on the skin. The oil can be applied neat onto spots or boils, but not onto larger areas of skin. It should always be diluted before use, for most other purposes.

Sources and uses of essential oils

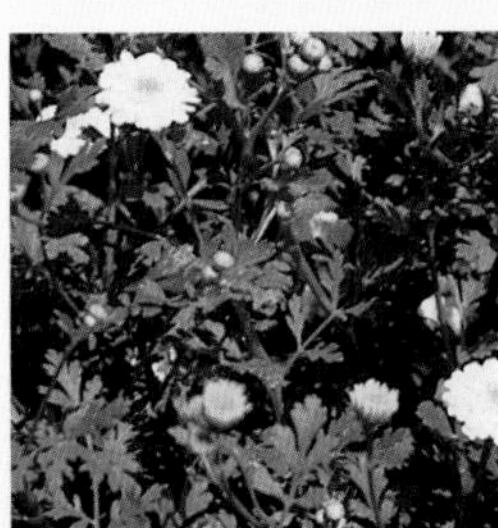

Chamomile Roman
Latin name – *Anthemis nobilis.*
Steam distilled from the dried flowers of the chamomile plant.
Is a middle note.
Country of origin – Eastern Europe, France, Morocco.
Uses – menstrual problems, headaches, nausea, sensitive skin conditions, inflammation, insomnia, headaches, calming, aches and pains, very useful for children.
Precautions – none.

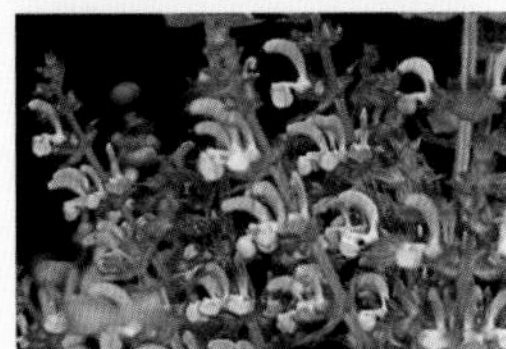

Clary sage
Latin name – *Salvia sclarea.*
Steam distilled from the flowering tops and leaves.
Is a top note.
Country of origin – Russia, Morocco and southern Europe.
Uses – balancing menstrual problems, painful periods, muscular aches and pains, depressions (including post-natal), lowers high blood pressure.
Precautions – do not use during pregnancy and avoid using the oil shortly before or after drinking alcohol as it can exaggerate drunkenness.

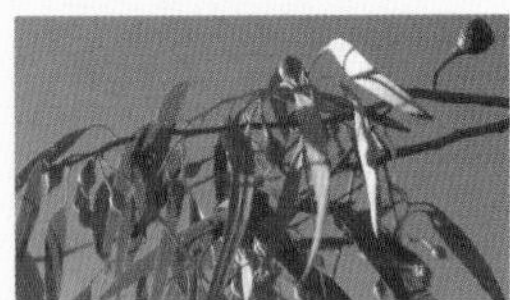

Eucalyptus
Latin name – *Eucalyptus globulus* or *Eucalyptus radiata* – depending on the species of plant the oil comes from.
Steam distilled from the leaves.
Is a top note.
Country of origin – native to Australia and Tasmania. Today most of the oil is produced in Spain, Portugal, Brazil and California.
Uses – respiratory system, colds and flu, muscular aches, fungal infections, burns, cuts, open wounds.
Precautions – always use well diluted, do not use eucalyptus globules for babies or young children, not compatible with homeopathic treatments.

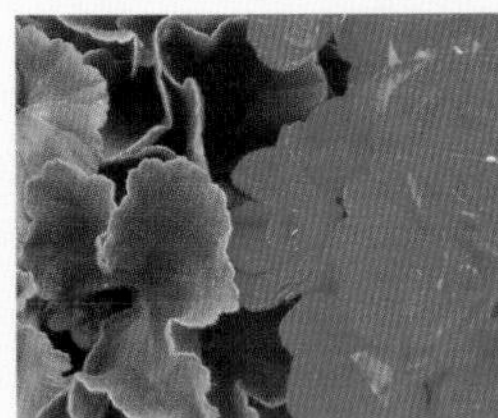

Geranium
Latin name – *Pelargonium graveolens.*
Steam distilled from both the flowers and flowering tops.
Is a middle note.
Country of origin – South Africa, Egypt, Russia, southern Europe.
Uses – anxiety, depression, menopausal symptoms, fluid retention, skincare for dry and oily skin as it balances.
Precautions – may cause irritation in hypersensitive skin.

Grapefruit
Latin name – *Citrus paradisi.*
Expressed from the peel of the fruit.
Is a top note.
Country of origin – Florida, California, Brazil, Israel.
Uses – depression, uplifting, cellulite, fluid retention, oily skin.
Precautions – avoid direct exposure to sunlight or ultraviolet rays for 12 hours after using the oil.

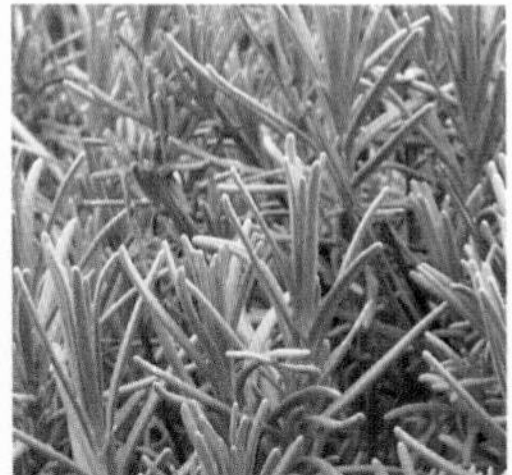

Lavender
Latin name – *Lavendula angustifolia.*
Steam distilled from the flowering tops.
Is a middle note.
Country of origin – France, southern Europe, north-west Africa
Uses – relaxation, insomnia, healing burns, calming skin conditions, aches and pains, lowers high blood pressure and is generally a very versatile oil.
Precautions – none.

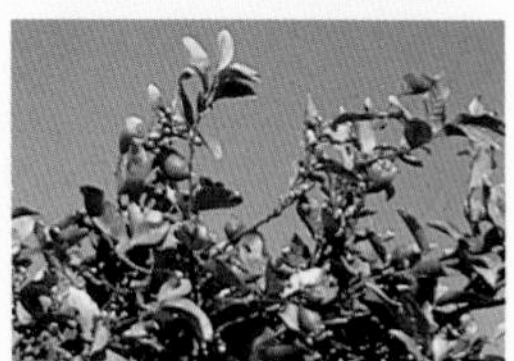

Lemon
Latin name – *Citrus limonium.*
Expressed from the peel of the fruit.
Is a top note.
Country of origin – Spain, Italy, California, northern India.
Uses – loss of appetite, digestive problems, uplifting, asthma, cellulite, oily skin, bites and stings.
Precautions – can cause skin irritation and avoid exposure to direct sunlight for 12 hours after using the oil.

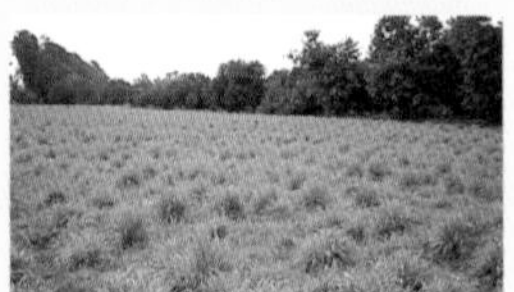

Lemongrass
Latin name – *Cymbopogon citrates.*
Steam distilled from the fresh or partially dried grass.
Is a top note.
Country of origin – southern India, Sri Lanka, West Indies.
Uses – uplifting, cooling for feverish conditions, digestive problems, indigestion, stress, fungal infections, muscular aches and pains, insect repellent, antiseptic.
Precautions – strong aroma, use with care on sensitive skins.

Marjoram
Latin name – *Origanum marjorana.*
Steam distilled from the flowering tops.
Is a middle note.
Country of origin – north Africa, Mediterranean, Egypt, Morocco.
Uses – insomnia, grief, muscular aches, respiratory problems, menstrual pain, overactive sex drive.
Precautions – do not use during pregnancy.

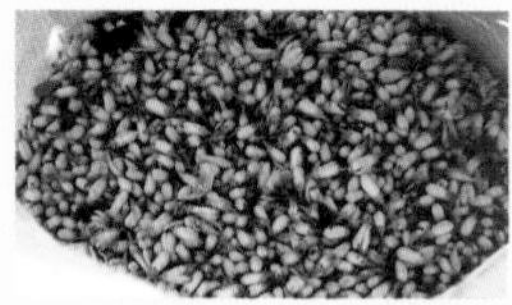

Neroli
Latin name – *Citrus aurantium.*
Steam distilled from the blossom/flowers of the bitter orange tree.
Is a base note.
Country of origin – south of France, Tunisia, Morocco, Egypt.
Uses – stress, depression, calming, sedating, PMT, heart palpitations, stretch marks, poor circulation.
Precautions – none.

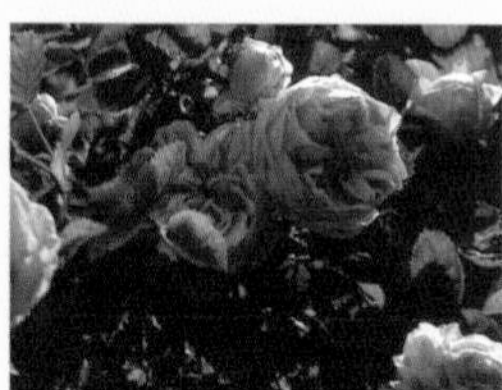

Rose Bulgar
Latin name – *Rosa damascena.*
Steam distilled from the petals.
Is a base note.
Country of origin – Syria, Bulgaria, Turkey, Morocco, Tunisia, France.
Uses – depression, dry/ageing skin, broken capillaries, impotence, menstrual problems, palpitations, stress, meditation.
Precautions – none.

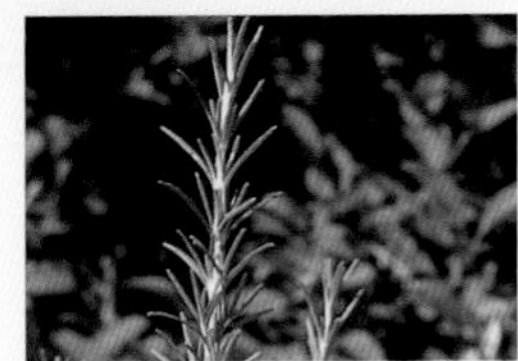

Rosemary
Latin name – *Rosmarinus officinalis.*
Steam distilled from the tops, leaves and smaller twigs.
Is a middle note.
Country of origin – south of France, Spain, Hungary, Italy, Greece, Tunisia, Morocco, Corsica.
Uses – stimulates the mind, uplifting, asthma, coughs, aches and pains, arthritis, improves circulation, cleansing, antiseptic, oily skin, dandruff.
Precautions – avoid if you are pregnant, have high blood pressure or epilepsy.

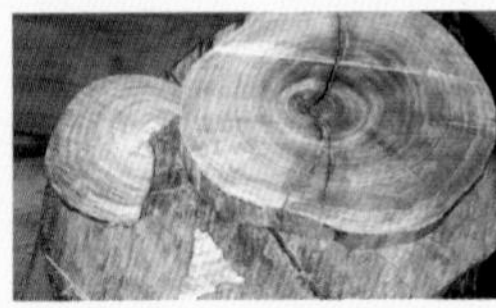

Sandalwood
Latin name – *Santalum album.*
Steam distilled from the coarsely powdered wood and roots.
Is a base note.
Country of origin – the best oil comes from the Mysore region of India.
Uses – depression, anxiety, respiratory ailments, cystitis, skincare, aphrodisiac, meditation, moth repellent.
Precautions – none.

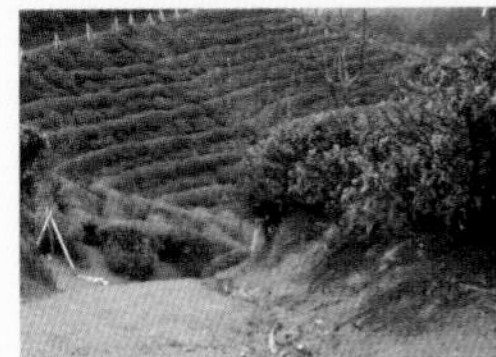

Tea Tree
Latin name – *Melaleuca alternifolia.*
Steam distillation of the leaves twigs.
Is a top note.
Country of origin – Australia.
Uses – strong antiseptic, fungal infections, burns, cuts, deep wounds, insect bites, thrush, athletes foot, spots, head lice, acne, coughs, colds, sinus congestion, low immune system.
Precautions – do not use neat or in high concentration on very sensitive skin.

Ylang-Ylang
Latin name – *Cananga odorata.*
Steam distilled from the flowers.
Is a base note.
Country of origin – Madagascar, Reunion, south-east Asia.
Uses – aphrodisiac, malaria, fevers, insomnia, anxiety, stress, lowers high blood pressure, palpitations, PMT, low self-esteem, skincare, perfume.
Precautions – heavy scent may cause headaches or nausea in some individuals if used in high concentration.

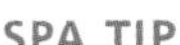

SPA TIP

Lavender and marjoram essential oils are good blended together if you have trouble sleeping. Lavender and chamomile essential oils are more effective in calming down inflamed skin when they are used together.

FACT

In Indonesia it is customary to spread ylang-ylang flowers on the bed of a couple on their wedding night. The aroma is believed to calm the nerves and lessen inhibition.

Risk assessment of essential oil safety

Toxic if ingested	Drink large quantities of full-fat milk (absorbs essential oils) Contact the nearest Accident & Emergency department
Over inhalation of essential oils	Go outside and breathe in deeply plenty of fresh air
Irritation on the skin	Wash off immediately
Oil in the eye	Wipe the eye with vegetable oil or full-fat milk then wash out thoroughly

HEALTH AND SAFETY !

Unsafe oils

The following essential oils should be avoided for use in aromatherapy:

Bitter almond
Calamus
Camphor
Costus
Horseradish
Mugwort
Mustard
Pennyroyal
Rue
Sassafras
Savin
Tansy
Thuja
Wintergreen
Wormseed
Wormwood

Chemotypes

A chemotype is a plant that has been cloned and which has the same characteristics as the mother plant but produces different quantities of chemical constituents in their essential oils. This is important when purchasing essential oils, as the differences in the composition of the oil will affect the therapeutic properties of the oil. The Latin name of the essential oil means you can identify the exact plant from which the oil has been extracted.

ABSORPTION OF ESSENTIAL OILS INTO THE BODY

Essential oils can be taken into the body in different ways. They absorb through the skin by massage, creams, touch or lying in a bath and into the lungs and nose through the vapour being inhaled into the body. Once applied to the skin, essential oils are absorbed by muscle tissue and blood vessels. The circulatory system distributes the small essential oil molecules throughout the body where they affect all aspects of it – joints, digestive system, all internal organs – and they are eventually excreted via the skin, kidneys, lungs and bladder (small amounts of essential oil have been found in urine!).

Olfactory system

When we inhale essential oils, the aroma molecules pass through the olfactory system, which is found high up inside the nose. The nerves in the olfactory system then relay messages to the limbic system in the brain, where a chain of chemical and physiological reactions take place. The limbic system in the brain is a complex structure and is responsible for:

- anger and emotion
- learning and memory
- relaying messages to the hypothalamus.

This is why when we sometimes smell a certain aroma it reminds us of a particular experience, emotion or person. The hypothalamus releases chemical

TERMINOLOGY

Toxicity is what we call poisonousness and may become fatal. In aromatherapy this depends upon whether the oil has been taken orally or absorbed through the skin.

Phototoxic refers to some essential oils that make the skin more sensitive to sunlight.

ACTIVITY 

On a piece of tissue put a drop of cinnamon oil and a drop of orange and see what occasion it reminds you of.

messages into the bloodstream stimulating: the autonomic nervous system, which can make the heart beat faster; the motor response, as in picking something up; and the pituitary gland, which has a hormonal reaction – one of the reasons why scent can be an aphrodisiac.

The brain and the olfactory nerves work together to recognize a smell and start to identify it.

SPA TIP 

Buying essential oils

- Always buy from a reputable supplier.
- The essential oil bottle should be clearly labelled with the Latin name of the oil, the use by date and the part of the plant the oil came from (if relevant).
- Not all essential oils are the same price – expect to pay a lot more for essential oils such as rose, sandalwood and jasmine and less for citrus oils.
- Remember, certain essential oils have a longer shelf life than others – top notes tend to lose their properties much more quickly than base notes.

PHYSIOLOGICAL EFFECTS OF ESSENTIAL OILS ON THE BODY

Cardiovascular system Circulation can be stimulated by essential oils – black pepper, rosemary and eucalyptus. Oils such as ginger can raise body temperature and black pepper and peppermint can take it down. Blood pressure can be decreased by chamomile and ylang-ylang.

Lymphatic system Thyme and lemon can have an antibacterial effect on the immune system.

Respiratory system Fennel, peppermint and rose prevent spasms of the bronchial tubes. Eucalyptus, lemon and benzoin act as expectorants.

Urinary system Juniper, fennel and rosemary are good diuretics.

Reproductive system Jasmine, ylang-ylang and rose are aphrodisiacs.

Endocrine system Lemongrass is similar to the male hormone testosterone. Clary sage and fennel are similar to the female hormone oestrogen.

Digestive system Marjoram, ginger and rosemary act as laxatives.

CARRIER OILS

SPA TIP 

When you have blended essential oils with a carrier oil, try and use your blend within 6 months as carrier oils have a relatively short life.

Essential oils are too strong to be applied neat to the skin and need diluting in a suitable carrier or base oil. In massage, cold pressed vegetable oils such as grapeseed or sweet almond are commonly used. Vegetable based oils penetrate the skin aiding the absorption of essential oils into the bloodstream. Carrier oils are also ideal bases in massage, as they act as a lubricant and have little or no aroma and don't interfere with the essential oil. Vegetable carrier oils have the following physical properties:

- little or no aroma
- non-volatile – do not evaporate

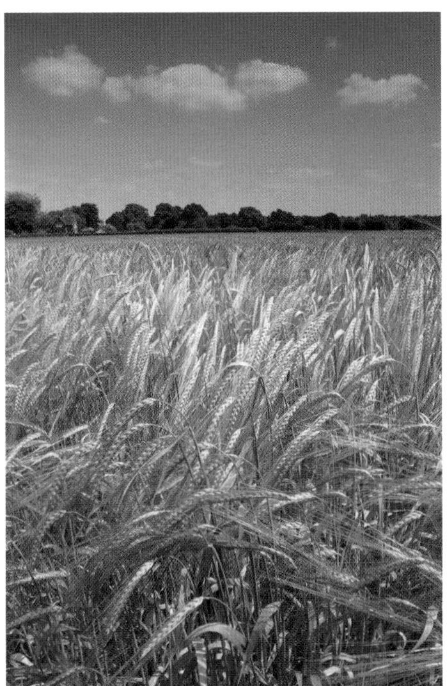

Wheatfield

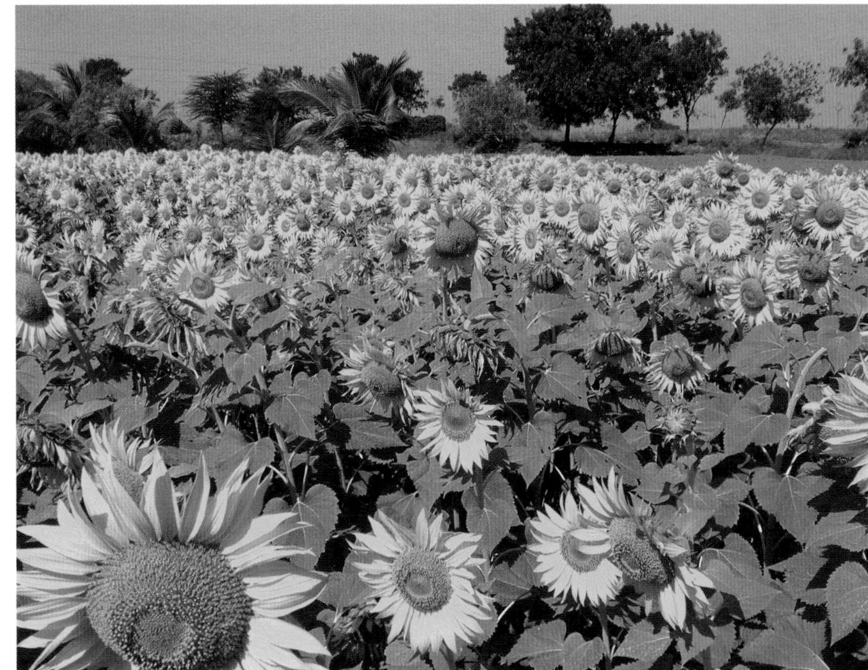

Sunflower

- lubricating quality
- oily
- pale in colour
- do not mix with alcohol.

The quality of the carrier oil is as important as the quality of an essential oil, as carrier oils have their own therapeutic values to the therapist. Two or more carrier oils can be blended together to get a particular effect and this is often used in face oils as they have important skin nourishing nutrients. The quality of the carrier oil can be affected by:

- time of harvesting
- storage conditions
- method of extraction.

> **FACT**
>
> Mineral oil is not a suitable carrier for essential oils as it is very oily and greasy and tends to clog the pores. It also acts more as a barrier on the skin so it is used in baby oil, helping to reduce the risk of nappy rash.

Vegetable oils are derived from the following:

Vegetable	Carrot, corn
Nuts	Sweet almond, peach kernel, apricot kernel, jojoba, hazelnut, macadamia, walnut, peanut
Seeds	Wheatgerm, soya, sunflower, grapeseed, evening primrose, camellia, safflower
Fruit	Olive, avocado, coconut

SPA TIP 

Buy only as much carrier oils as you will use within a few months, particularly the heavier oils such as avocado

HEALTH AND SAFETY 

Avoid using nut oils on children and clients with nut allergies. Also avoid using wheatgerm oil on clients with wheat allergies.

Methods of extraction

Cold pressing

A certain amount of heat is used, but nothing higher than 60 °C. The raw material such as seeds, nuts or kernels are simply pressed with a hydraulic press and the oil is squeezed out. The first pressing of oil is known as 'virgin oil' (as in the virgin olive oil available in supermarkets), and after pressing the oil is filtered through cotton cloths and finally through a paper filter.

Maceration

This method is used to obtain additional properties to normal vegetable oils. Particular parts of certain plants are chopped up and put into a vat of a vegetable oil and agitated for several days before being left in the sun for a few more days. The therapeutic properties from the plant are absorbed into the vegetable oil, which is then filtered to remove any remaining plant material before being bottled.

Storage of carrier oils

Carrier oils contain no preservatives and have a shorter shelf life than essential oils (a carrier oil with essential oils in it will last slightly longer than

Carrier oils

Oil	Description
Sweet almond *Prunus amygdalis*	A very light oil, odourless, colourless to pale golden yellow, it is ideally suited to body massage as it blends well with all other oils. Rich in proteins and vitamins it is nourishing for dry, irritated skin and is safe to use on children and babies.
Grapeseed oil *Vitis vinifera*	Has a slight smell and is a pale greenish-yellow colour, it is a very light oil and is easily absorbed in the skin. Can be used on all skin types and is inexpensive, so is an ideal base for massage.
Apricot kernel *Prunus armenica*	Suitable for all skin types, but especially skincare as it is very light and well absorbed. The oil is odourless and is colourless to pale yellow.
Hazelnut *Corylus avellana*	It has a slightly heavy texture, and is obtained from the kernel. Pale yellow in colour, it can be stimulating to the circulation and is good for oily skin.
Macademia *Macadamia ternifolia*	Suitable for dry, ageing skin conditions due to its profile resembling human sebum. Oil is obtained from the kernel and is a yellow, fine textured oil.
Jojoba *Simmondsia chinesis*	Has a slight smell, pale to golden yellow in colour with a fine wax-like texture. It is one of the best carrier oils to use, but is slightly expensive. It is suitable for all skin conditions and blends well with other carrier oils.
Avocado *Persea americana*	Cold pressed from the dried and sliced flesh of the fruit, when refined it is always pale yellow and lacks the rich green colour of the cold pressed oil. Slightly expensive, the unrefined oil has a shorter shelf life and is best blended with another carrier oil. As it is slightly heavy in texture it is good for dry skin and eczema.
Wheatgerm *Triticum vulgare*	Strong odour which can dominate a blend, it is yellow to orange in colour and has a high vitamin E content which makes it a good antioxidant and suitable to add into another carrier oil to lengthen the shelf life. Suitable for dry mature skin, eczema, stretch marks and scar tissue.

one without). Bulk quantities should be stored in stainless steel containers in a cool, dark place. Carrier oils with a high vitamin E content or oils that have been blended with one that has, such as wheatgerm, will last longer as it acts as an antioxidant and helps prevent the oil going rancid. Once a blend has been made with essential oils use it as quickly as possible – never make up too large a bottle.

SPA TIP

As well as using carrier oils to blend with essential oils there are many other natural bases available on the market, such as creams/lotions, that sometimes may be more suitable for particular clients.

BLENDING ESSENTIAL OILS

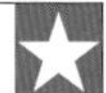
SPA TIP

If you have not got a burner and want to create an aroma in a room, put a few drops of essential oil onto a cotton wool ball and place behind a warm radiator to release the scent.

There are a number of things to consider when prescribing and blending essential oils: the client's condition and personal preference, the client's skin type and condition, the carrier oil being used, the treatment objectives, and the area being treated. The most important aspect of aromatherapy is that the essential oils work **synergistically** together, meaning that they work together in harmony, e.g. chamomile and lavender together increase their healing effects. It is also important to consider whether the oils are top, middle or base notes, as this still forms the basis of most blends. The main blending guidelines are:

- For full body massage you should use 25 ml of carrier oil with 7–12 drops of essential oil.
- For a child's massage use 10 ml carrier oil with 1 drop of essential oil.
- If you are using a burner/vaporizer add 5–15 drops of essential oil into the dish of water, which is placed over a burner.
- If you are using essential oil in a bath add the essential oil to a capful of full-fat milk to make sure it is dispersed into the water – 4–6 drops for an adult bath, 1–3 for a young child and 1 drop for a baby.

AROMATHERAPY MASSAGE TREATMENT

Aromatherapy massage is one of the most popular treatments in spas. It is available throughout the world and will slightly differ depending on the country, traditions and the therapist's training and background. Through the massage movements, essential oils penetrate into the skin and are absorbed into the body's organs to help alleviate any ailments, whilst the massage activates and soothes nerve endings, helping the client to relax. The basic movements used in an aromatherapy massage are:

- Swedish massage – using mainly effleurage and kneading strokes.
- Neuromuscular – much firmer pressure than Swedish. The overall effect is the stimulation and balancing of the nervous system.
- Lymphatic massage – a lot of lymphatic drainage techniques are used in aromatherapy massage.
- Acupressure massage and shiatsu – an oriental massage technique focusing on energy fields of the body along the meridians and tsubo points. Firm pressure using the thumbs or fingers is applied to these points to release blocked energy.

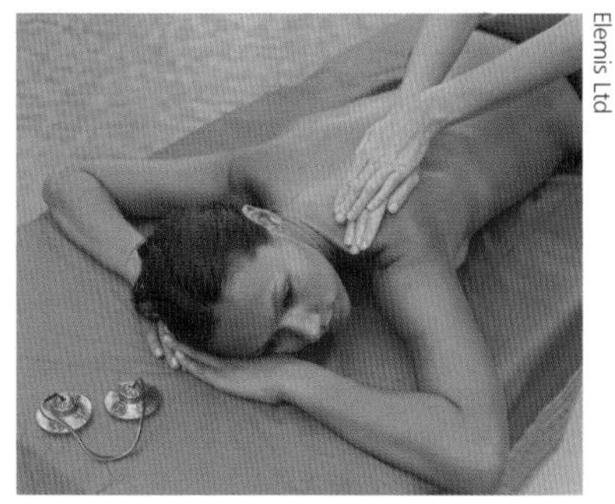
Elemis Ltd

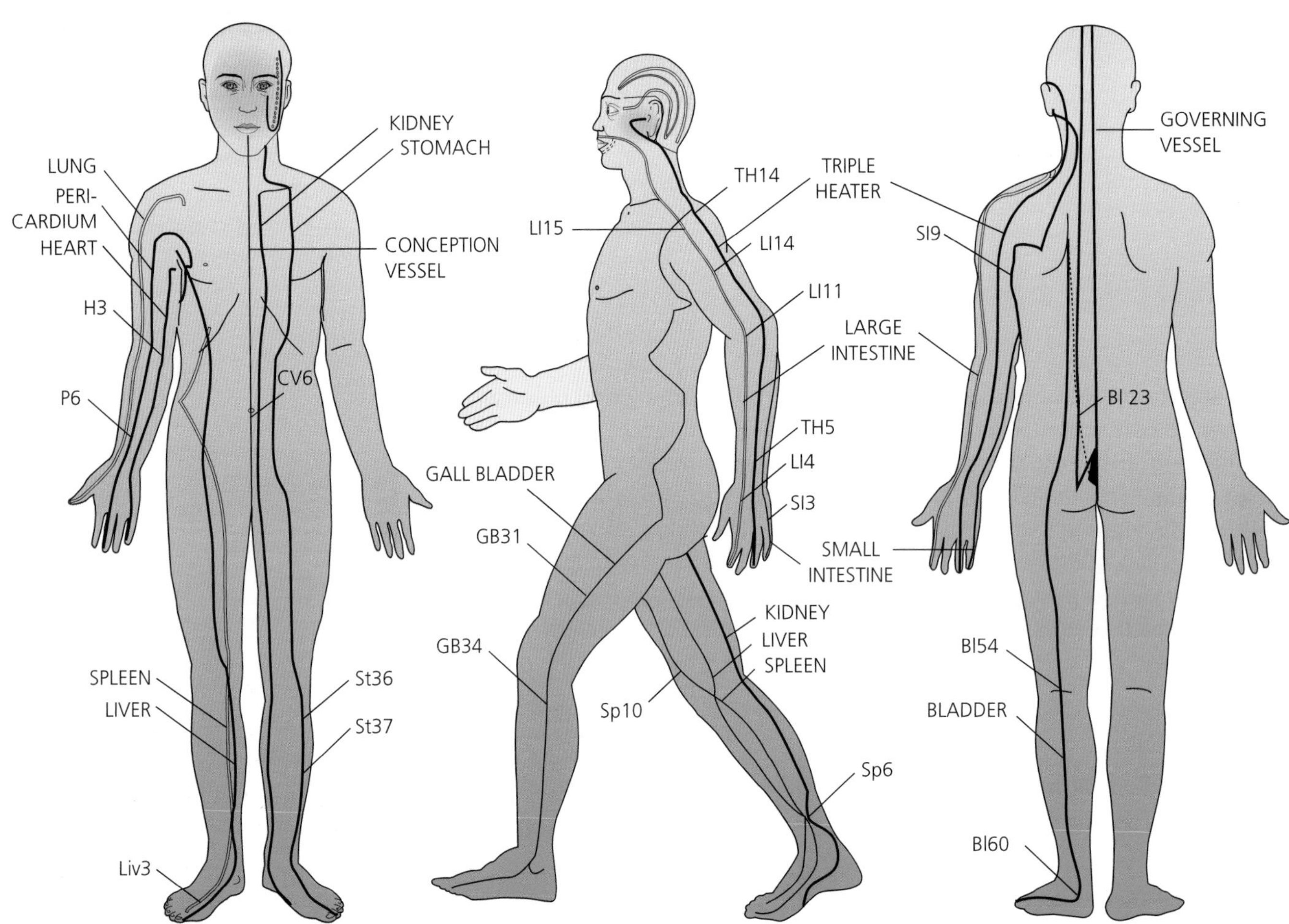

Shiatsu points and meridians

Contra-indications to aromatherapy massage treatment	*Contra-indications which may restrict aromatherapy massage*
Infectious or contagious diseases	Pregnancy – be careful with the essential oils that you use, and you will have to adapt the client's positioning as the baby grows
High temperature	Recent scar tissue – avoid massaging on that area for up to 6 months
Heart condition – seek doctor's permission	Severe bruising – avoid the area
Epilepsy	Varicose veins – if severe avoid massaging the legs, if they are quite faint use gentle effleurage strokes over the area
Cancer – seek doctor's permission	Cuts and abrasions – avoid the area
Diabetes – seek doctor's permission	Fractures – avoid the area for up to 3 months
Recent inoculations – wait at least 24 hours	Asthma – be careful with your selection of oils and position the client so that they have a clear airway to breathe
If the client has recently drunk a lot of alcohol	High and low blood pressure – be careful with your selection of oils, if you are unsure about the severity of the client's condition always get the doctor's approval first
Straight after a heavy meal	First 2 days of menstruation – avoid heavy massage movements over the abdomen area
Immediately after a hot bath/sauna/steam – wait an hour	
Strong medication – seek doctor's permission	

CONSULTATION

As explained in chapter 15, a record card must be filled in for all spa treatments, but in aromatherapy it is very important that we ascertain as much information as we can about the client's lifestyle and emotional and physical state so that we can select the appropriate blended massage oils.

Ideally a client should follow their treatment plan, attend regularly and follow all your aftercare advice, but most clients do not fall into this category and your treatment plan will need to be adapted to suit the client's individual needs.

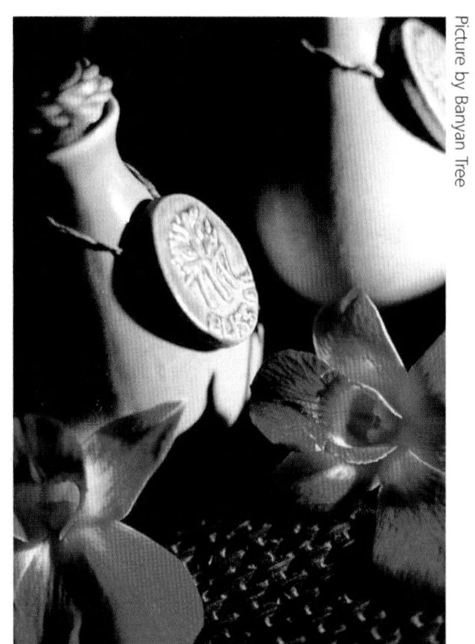

Picture by Banyan Tree

Patch test

If your client has a sensitive skin or thinks they may be allergic to an essential or carrier oil, then a patch test should be carried out 24 hours prior to treatment. A 2 per cent blend, e.g. 2 drops of essential oil in 2 mls carrier oil, is applied in the crease of the client's elbow. The client should be advised to keep the area clean for 24 hours. If the client has a positive reaction they may show signs of redness, itching or swelling in the area. If this occurs they should clean the area immediately and inform the spa, so that they can be booked in for an alternative treatment or an alternative product used.

Clinical aromatherapist

In this unit aromatherapy massage incorporates using pre-blended oils for the client's treatment, with the main objectives of the treatment being for relaxation, sense of wellbeing or uplifting. If your client presents quite a few medical conditions or is looking for more therapeutic benefits from aromatherapy, then you need to be able to refer them on to a clinical aromatherapist who has been trained in mixing and blending essential oils. A clinical aromatherapist will have studied for 2 years part-time or completed a private course that is recognized by one of the professional aromatherapy organizations. It is important for them to be a member of such an organization and abide by that organization's code of practice, for example, the International Federation of Aromatherapists or the AC (Aromatherapy Consortium).

Preparation of the treatment room

The treatment room should be warm, quiet and well-ventilated, and have a nice aroma, soft lighting and subtle music playing. The working area should be kept clean at all times, including all surfaces and floors – it is important not only to prevent cross-infection, but also to give a professional image to the client.

The ambience created in a treatment room is individual to the spa's style and the individual therapist's interpretation of this, e.g. the couch may be set up with Balinese sheets on it and rose petals scattered over. A good spa manager will make sure that all rooms follow a similar theme and are of the highest professional standard so that the client receives the same level of service

EQUIPMENT LIST

Aromatherapy massage

- treatment couch – ideally with a face hole
- clean towels – small hand and large bath sheets
- Balinese wraps/sheets – may be appropriate for your spa
- heated base blanket – some spas use to keep the client warm
- small support pillow – may be used for supporting knee when massaging
- blanket or quilt – may be used if client feels cold
- facial products on the trolley – to cleanse face before facial massage
- lavender eye pillow – can be used at the end of the treatment, whilst the client is relaxing
- selection of essential oils and carrier oils or pre-blended bottles of aromatherapy massage oil
- glass rod and glass measuring jar – to blend essential oils
- aromatherapy burner – the room should have a nice aroma when the client enters
- candles – may be scented to create aroma or used for subtle lighting

SPA HYGIENE

- All towels and bed linen should be washed in very hot, soapy water in order to remove any oil.
- All work surfaces should be cleaned with surgical spirit. In particular the trolley where the oil bottles are kept should be done after each client, and daily with a disinfectant spray.
- All floors should be cleaned daily.
- Use fresh towels/gowns for each client.
- All empty bottles, measuring jars, etc., should be washed in warm soapy water and any pre-blended massage oil bottles should be wiped over after each client.

whichever room or therapist they have for their treatments. Health and Safety legislation applies and must be adhered to, particularly the Health and Safety at Work Act 1974 and COSHH 1992 (as discussed in chapter 5).

TREATMENT PROCEDURE

Once the consultation and treatment plan have been completed you need to select a suitable pre-blended aromatherapy massage oil. The following table contains some ideas of blends suitable for particular outcomes but once you are confident in using essential oils you may want to create your own blends. For a full body massage you will need approximately 25 ml of carrier oil and 10–12 drops of essential oil. Remember not to blend more than 3–4 essential oils in one blend and ideally use a top, middle and base note oil and check the properties of the essential oils, ensuring they are suitable for your client.

This is just a sample of blends that you could choose. You may be working in a spa where they use a well-known beauty company's products such as Elemis, Espa, Pevonia, Aromatherapy Associates, etc., and they will have their own ready-blended massage oils to use.

Relaxation	*Uplifting*	*Sense of wellbeing*
Lavender, chamomile & geranium	Eucalyptus, rosemary & grapefruit	Clary sage, lemon & ylang-ylang
Lavender, marjoram & chamomile	Rosemary, clary sage & lemon	Neroli & sandalwood
Clary sage, rose & sandalwood	Lemongrass & eucalyptus	Lemon, geranium & sandalwood
Geranium, lavender & marjoram	Lemon, grapefruit & tea tree	Rose, geranium & grapefruit
Ylang-ylang & clary sage		Rosemary, chamomile & lavender

PREPARING THE CLIENT

- Once you have chosen the blend of oils for the client, massage a little bit of the oil onto the back of the client's hand to make sure that they like the aroma.
- If the client hasn't already undressed and put on a gown allow them to do so now privately – if possible offer the client a warm shower before they have a massage.
- Help the client onto the couch, lying face down and make sure that they are covered with the appropriate bedding and that they feel warm – there is nothing worse than having a massage and lying there feeling cold.

SPA TIP

The spa at Jimbaran, Four Seasons Resort uses a blend of sandalwood, ylang-ylang and a touch of citrus oils in their massage blend for calming and grounding. The Mandara Spa's signature blend is a mix of sandalwood and patchouli oil for romance and dry skin conditions.

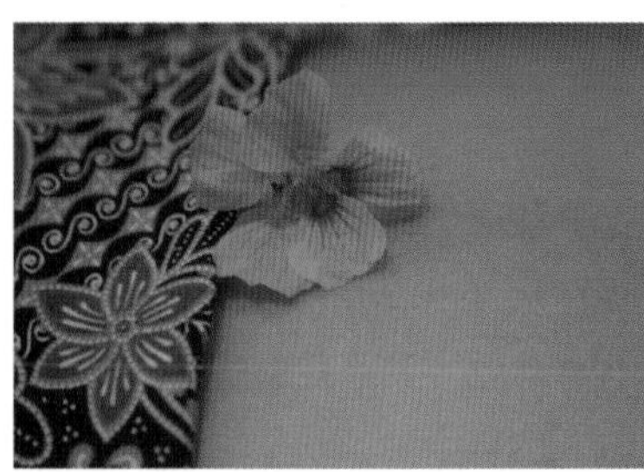

- Explain to the client the treatment procedure and answer any questions they may have now so that whilst you are carrying out the massage the client relaxes thoroughly.
- Wash your hands in view of the client before you apply massage oil and make sure that you are not disturbed in the room – some salons/spas have little signs or symbols to put on the treatment room door handles to signal that a treatment is taking place.
- An aromatherapy massage should last approximately one and a half hours.

SPA TIP 

The client throughout the aromatherapy massage should carry out the abdominal breathing technique as it helps in relaxing the client and brings in more oxygen to the body. This technique is often used in yoga and other meditation practices.

PREPARE FOR TREATMENT CHECKLIST Aromatherapy

✔ Correct environment	✔ Bathrobe
✔ Health and safety	✔ Help client onto massage couch
✔ Hygiene	✔ Correct client positioning
✔ Professional appearance	✔ Client warm, relaxed and comfortable
✔ Equipment/products/consumables	✔ Wash hands
✔ Record card	✔ Cleanse skin
✔ Private changing facilities	✔ Select massage oils

Picture by Banyan Tree

Order of aromatherapy massage

As you gain in confidence and experience you will develop and alter your massage routine. The following sequence starts with the back as this is a good area to start relaxing the client and most people suffer at some time with back pain:

1. back
2. back of legs
3. front of legs and feet
4. abdomen
5. arms and hands
6. neck and chest
7. face
8. scalp.

Before giving a face and scalp massage, cleanse the client's face with appropriate cleansing products.

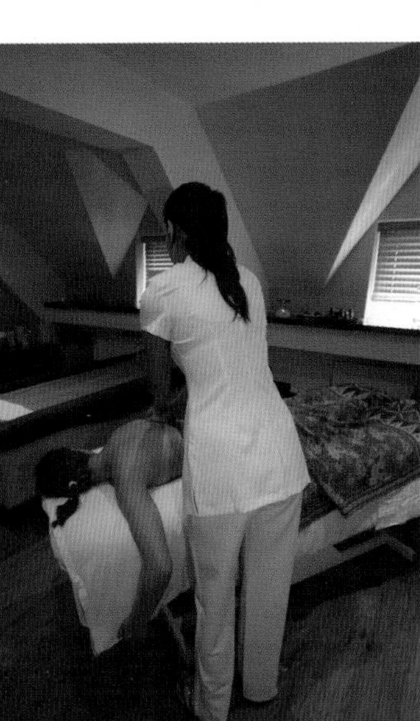

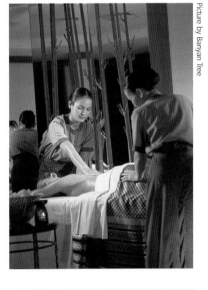

Therapist's posture

It is important for the therapist to maintain a good posture throughout an aromatherapy massage – follow the same guidelines as you would when giving a massage as discussed in chapter 11. If you have poor posture you are more likely to tire easily and suffer from aches and pains, and in some spas and salons you may be carrying out massage treatments all day.

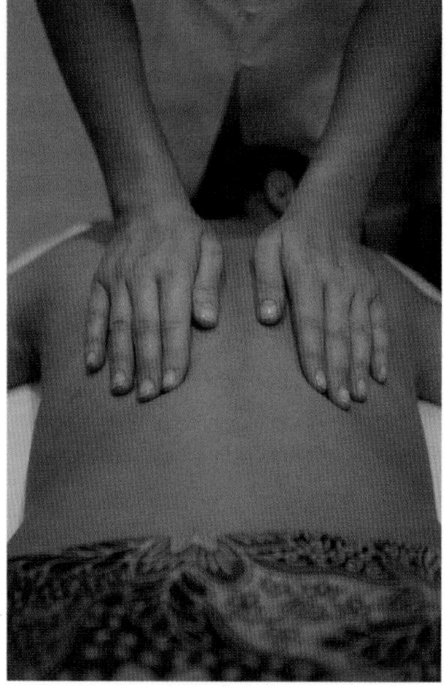
Reverse effleurage on the back

LINKED TREATMENTS

- Manicure/pedicure – essential oils can be added into the water and massage creams (tea tree oil is very good for fungal infections!).
- Sauna/steam bath – essential oil can be added into the water or directly onto the hot stones to help decongestion.
- Hydrotherapy/spa bath – only use essential oils which will be dispersed constantly in the water.
- Floral bath – using essential oils and flowers such as jasmine, gardenia, rose petals, hibiscus placed onto the water.
- Milk bath – essential oils and milk mix very well and this is excellent for softening the skin.
- Reflexology – essential oils absorb very quickly into the body through the feet and this is an excellent way of relaxing the client.
- Indian head massage – ideal for client who cannot lie down on a couch, and more exotic oils can be used following Ayurvedic principles.
- Hot stone massage – the use of hot stones can be incorporated into an aromatherapy massage to warm the body and relax the muscles.

ADAPTING MASSAGE TECHNIQUES

For aromatherapy massage you will have learnt a standard routine – either at college or one specifically designed by the spa or the beauty company whose products you are using. Depending on the condition you are treating your client for, you may have to adapt your massage movements.

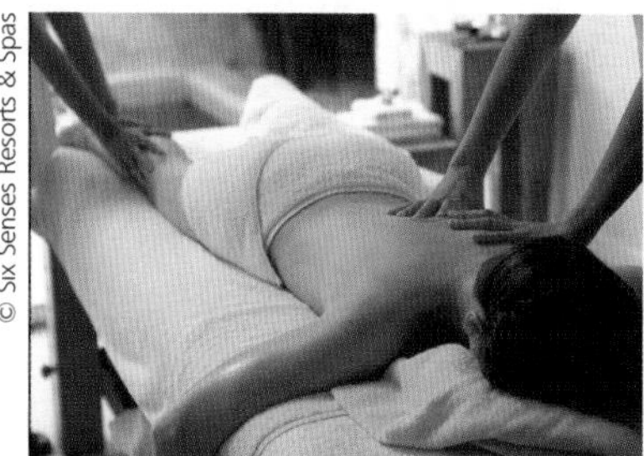
© Six Senses Resorts & Spas

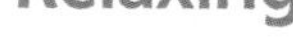

Relaxing

- Increase the amount of effleurage and stroking movements used.
- Encourage the client's abdominal breathing throughout the treatment.
- Keep all movements at a slow and even pace.
- Spend a bit more time on the back, neck, shoulders and scalp – as these areas hold a lot of tension.

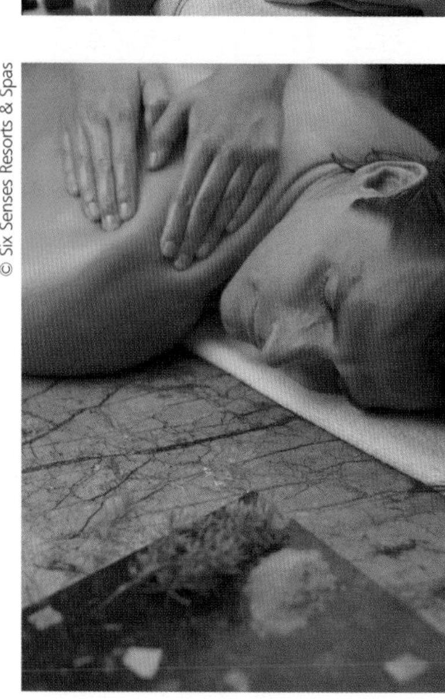
© Six Senses Resorts & Spas

Uplifting

- Apply deeper and stronger movements.
- Increase the amount of neuromuscular, acupressure and shiatsu movements.
- Reduce effleurage strokes.
- Make all movements quicker and more invigorating.

Wellbeing

- Do plenty of effleurage, lymphatic drainage and pressure point movements.
- Spend a bit longer on the abdomen area, particularly the solar plexus, and the feet – if you know any reflexology movements, you could include a few here.
- Encourage the client's abdominal breathing.

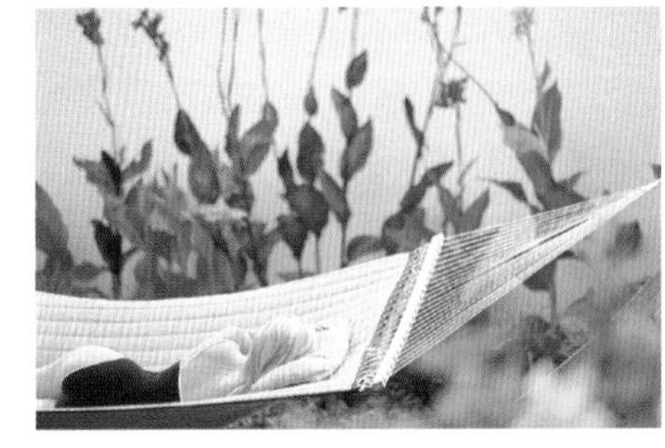

Client relaxing in the spa's courtyard, La Costa Resort & Spa, California

EFFECTIVENESS OF THE AROMATHERAPY MASSAGE

This should be judged continually throughout the treatment by looking at the client's body language, how well they relax, if they fall asleep, if they fidget, any comments that are made during the treatment and by asking the client verbally at the end of the treatment how they felt, and if the massage needs to be adapted in any way for their next treatment. Any comments and feedback should be recorded on the client's record card.

SPA TIP 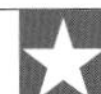

When you have completed an aromatherapy massage, cover the client with a warm towel and use warm mitts to remove any excess oil from the face.

POST-TREATMENT ADVICE

After you have completed the aromatherapy massage allow the client to relax for 5 minutes and offer them a glass of water. Whilst the client is relaxing write down on their record card the aromatherapy oils used, quantity, any reactions the client had and start to think about any recommendations you are going to add to their treatment plan.

It is important that at the end of each treatment you explain to the client any reactions they may experience and most importantly give homecare advice to enhance the effects of their treatment. The following advice must be given:

- Avoid a bath or shower for the next 6–8 hours to allow the oils to carry on penetrating into the body.
- Drink plenty of water or herb teas and try to avoid caffeine drinks such as tea or coffee and alcohol for the next 24 hours, as the body will continue to de-tox from the treatment.
- Don't do too much physical exercise for a few hours, and allow the body to continue relaxing.

If the client is having a treatment in a hotel spa, then they can be advised to go back to their room to relax for the next hour, or if there is a relaxation area in the spa, they could spend some quiet time with a book or magazine. Any form of relaxation afterwards will enhance the benefits of the treatment.

To continue the therapeutic effects of aromatherapy for the client, it is important that they incorporate the use of essential oils into their

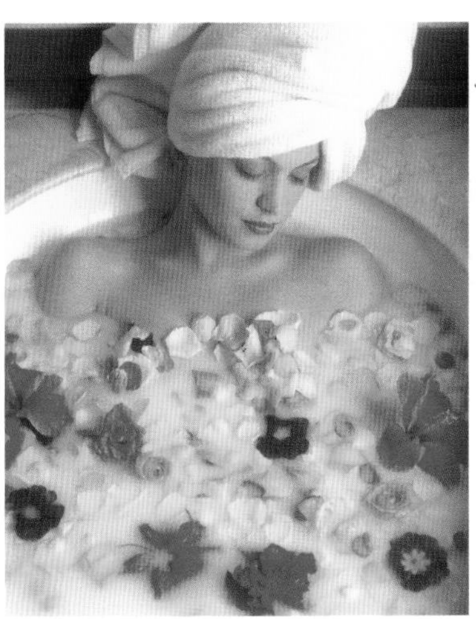

Courtesy of Chiva-Som

Floral bath, Chiva-Som

LINKED PRODUCTS 

Burner/aromastone – both methods require essential oils to be dropped onto a small amount of water and heated. This is ideal for the client who is having trouble sleeping, is suffering from stress and needs to relax at home or needs uplifting/invigorating during the day

LINKED PRODUCTS 

Bathing
If you are working with a beauty or spa company's products, then they will have their own aromatherapy bath oil products to retail to clients, which can be a safe way for the client to use essential oils at home as they are already blended for them.

LINKED PRODUCTS 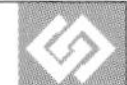

Aromatherapy candles – these are a good way of creating a mood-enhancing ambience at home, but you must make sure that they are from a reputable beauty/aromatherapy company as those available from a supermarket are perfumed with synthetic fragrances.

SIGNATURE TREATMENT 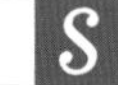

C-Side, Cowely Manor Hotel
'Cloud 9: The ultimate. A deeply relaxing and rebalancing treatment, which effortlessly combines aromatherapy, Qi energy balancing, reflexology and acupressure. This is the signature C-Side treatment. You are taken to Cloud 9 during this extensive all-over massage that covers the whole body as well as the face and head. It is, quite simply, unique.'

homecare routine. Quite a lot of the top spas/hotels have created their own aromatherapy scented blends of massage/bath oils for the clients to use at home. These enhance the various treatments that the client can have and can be an easy way of the therapist retailing to the client.

CONTRA-ACTIONS FROM AROMATHERAPY MASSAGE

As the essential oils work through the body and the client relaxes, they may suffer from some of the following reactions to the treatment:

- Erythaema – this is a reddening of the skin caused by stimulation of the circulation through the massage movements and is a normal reaction to the treatment, which should disappear within an hour.
- Headache/dizziness – this is just part of nature's reaction to the release of some toxins into the body and should disappear within a few hours. If this occurs the client should drink a lot of water, sit down and relax immediately after the treatment and avoid tea/coffee and alcohol for the next 24 hours.
- Excessive urination – the client may feel they need to visit the toilet a lot after treatment as the excretory system is stimulated and toxins are removed. Drinking plenty of water and herb teas will help replenish the body.
- Allergic skin reaction – this would appear as a red swollen area of skin, blisters may appear and the skin would feel very itchy. This may take a few days to disappear, and if it hasn't disappeared within 2–3 days then the client may need to see their doctor. If it appears straight after the treatment, remove all the oil from the area with water and note down on the client's record card the reaction.

Always record any reaction/comments the client has on their record card for future reference.

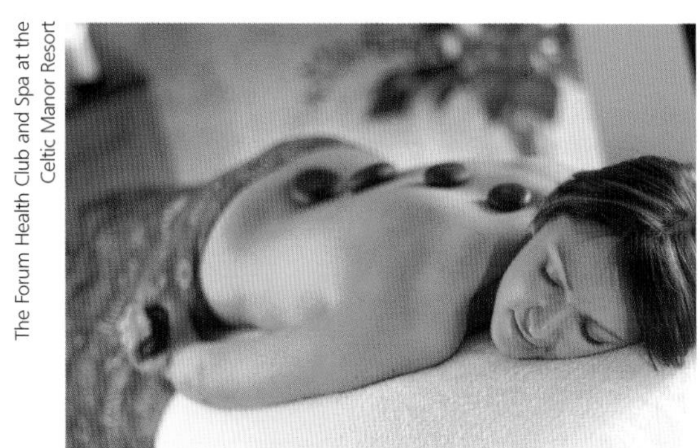

The Forum Health Club and Spa at the Celtic Manor Resort

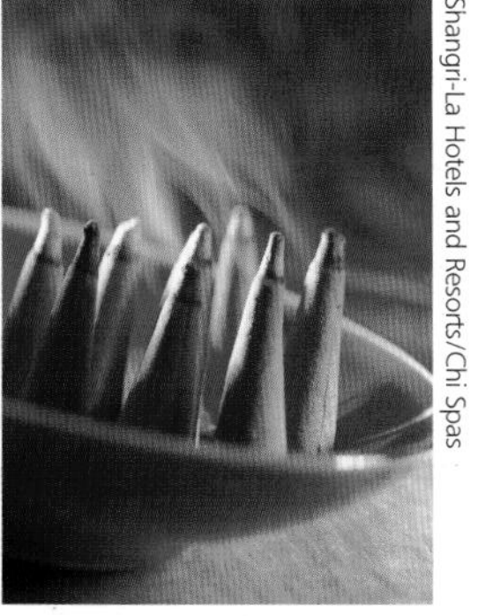

Shangri-La Hotels and Resorts/Chi Spas

The essence of Chi, Shangri-La

SPA PROFILE

Name: Helen Norman

Position: Spa Manager

Establishment: The Spa at Mandarin Oriental, London

Products used: Mandarin Oriental signature products, clothing and tea, E'SPA.

Number of staff/roles: 36 staff, including: Spa Manager; Assistant Spa Manager – Treatments; Assistant Spa Manager – Operations; Senior Spa Concierge; Head Therapist Trainer; Spa Concierge; therapists; spa attendants.

Training/experience: Therapist: 18 month training plan – treatments; ongoing weekly training plan – treatments; customer care; Legendary Quality Experiences training.

Main responsibilities: Strategic planning; finance and budgeting; training and development.

Best parts of the job:
Working with amazing and inspiring individuals.

Watching the development and growth of my team.

Researching new ideas and practices as well as sourcing the quality products we use and sell.

And the best bit really is seeing the expression on our guests' faces and watching their body language as they leave our spa, rejuvenated and invigorated!

Secrets of a successful spa therapist: To achieve the standards of excellence essential in delivering these specialized treatments requires a therapist to be grounded as an individual, professionally qualified and caring as a guardian of their guests.

KEY/CORE SKILLS OPPORTUNITIES

To be an excellent spa therapist you must be able to communicate well, both orally and in writing. To be able to succeed and progress in the spa industry, it is also essential that you have an ability to work with numbers and information technology (IT). Increasingly, employers are looking for spa therapists with these 'key' skills when they recruit staff. NVQ/SVQ unit **BT21** provides you with an opportunity to develop evidence for the following:

KEY SKILLS	CORE SKILLS
Communication Level 2; C2.1a, C2.2	Communication Intermediate 1; Task 1 and 3
Working with others Level 2; WO2.1, WO2.2, WO2.3	Working with others Intermediate 1; Tasks 1, 2 and 3
Improving own learning and performance Level 3; LP3.1, LP3.2	(no parallel unit in CORE SKILLS)
Problem solving Level 2; PS2.1, PS2.2	Problem solving Intermediate Level 1; Tasks 1, 2 and 3

Assessment of knowledge and understanding

When you have some free time, test your understanding and knowledge by answering the following questions. Do this at regular intervals and it will reinforce your learning and help you retain the knowledge, so you are able to perform better in your assessments.

Consult with the client

1 Give four points to consider when preparing the client for a treatment.

2 Why is it important to keep client record cards?

3 Name three conditions that may restrict an aromatherapy treatment.

4 How would you carry out a patch test?

5 Why is the client's signature very important on a record card?

6 List four contra-indications to an aromatherapy massage treatment.

7 What information do you need to keep updating on an aromatherapy record card?

8 If a client is allergic to an essential oil, what reaction would you expect?

Plan the treatment

1 Name two points you need to consider with your client whilst formulating their treatment plan.

2 What limitations may the client have in coming for a series of aromatherapy massages?

3 What two pieces of Health and Safety legislation particularly apply to aromatherapy?

Prepare for the treatment

1 How should essential oils be stored?

2 How many drops of essential oil would you use in 25 ml of carrier oil?

3 How long should an aromatherapy massage take?

4 What precautions must you consider when using essential oils?

5 How would you create an ambience in your treatment room appropriate for an aromatherapy massage treatment?

6 How should you prepare the client for an aromatherapy treatment?

7 Give an appropriate blend of essential oils for the following outcomes:
a. relaxing
b. uplifting
c. sense of wellbeing.

8 Name two carrier oils that are suitable to use on their own for an aromatherapy massage?

9 List four ways in which the therapist can ensure that the equipment and treatment room are properly sterilized?

10 Give five essential oils that are unsafe to use in aromatherapy?

Massage the body using pre-blended aromatherapy oils

1 List four psychological effects essential oils have?

2 From which part of the plant do we obtain the following essential oils?:
   a. jasmine
   b. lemongrass
   c. cinnamon
   d. sandalwood
   e. petitgrain.

3 How do essential oils affect the cardiovascular system?

4 How are essential oils absorbed into the body?

5 Give four basic massage movements used in an aromatherapy massage.

6 What four contra-actions may occur to the client after an aromatherapy treatment?

7 How would you adapt your massage if the client wanted relaxation?

8 Why is posture important for the therapist when giving a massage?

9 Where in the body is the olfactory system and how do aroma molecules affect it?

10 What action would you take if you got essential oil into someone's eye?

Complete the treatment

1 Give three pieces of advice that must be given to a client following an aromatherapy treatment?

2 Name three ways in which the client may use aromatherapy at home?

3 What should be recorded onto the client's record card after an aromatherapy treatment?

4 Devise a de-stress plan for a client to use at home – to include suitable essential oils.

5 How could aromatherapy be incorporated with other spa treatments?

chapter 13

Indian head massage

BT20

Provide Indian head massage treatment

Learning objectives

This chapter covers the skills a spa therapist needs to provide Indian head massage treatment. It describes the skills and knowledge necessary to enable you to:

- **consult with the client**
- **plan the treatment**
- **prepare for the treatment**
- **carry out the procedure for Indian head massage**
- **provide aftercare advice**

When providing Indian head massage it is important to use the skills you have learnt in the following core units:

G1 Ensure your own actions reduce risks to Health and Safety

G6 Promote additional products or services to clients

G11 Contribute to the financial effectiveness of the business

INTRODUCTION

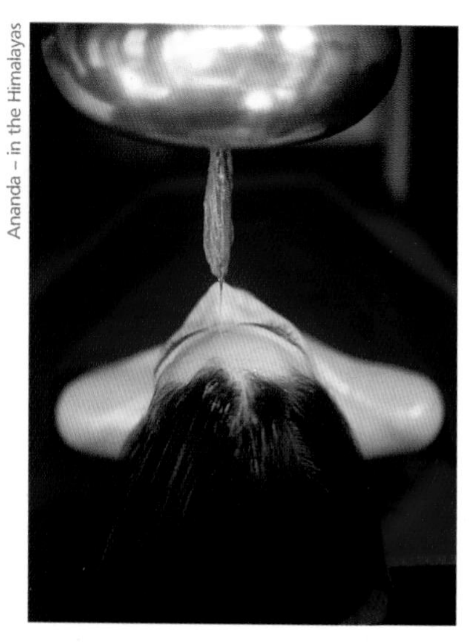

Ananda – in the Himalayas

Shirodhara, Ananda Spa Resort

Indian head massage is an Ayurvedic therapy in which medicated oils are used in a vigorous head and scalp massage. With the rising interest in therapies from Asia, Indian head massage courses have grown in popularity over the past few years. The head is the centre of your nervous system and the seat of your intelligence – if your head feels good, you feel good.

HISTORY, ORIGIN AND TRADITIONS OF INDIAN HEAD MASSAGE

The tradition of massage in India dates back thousands of years and plays a central role in the life of the family. Indian women, who believed it would keep their hair healthy, traditionally used the art of head massage. The technique would be passed down to their children, who would actively be encouraged to massage other family members.

In India, massage is still seen as a family occasion where weekly everyone will give and receive a treatment. If you visit a masseur or barber in India, head massage is given as an integral part of the treatment – even on the beaches and in market squares you will find head massages being given. Oils, such as coconut, sesame, almond or olive, have always been used.

Indian head massage is often classed as an Ayurvedic therapy, the world's most ancient medical tradition. The Ayurvedic concept is that there are three governing forces (doshas) at work inside us:

- vata (air) – artistic, nervous, highly strung temperament
- pitta (fire) – aggressive, driven, hot tempered
- kapha (water) – charitable, loving and prone to weight.

Most people are considered to be a blend of the three doshas, but there is usually one dosha that is predominant. A healthy balance of all three is believed to be integral to wellbeing, while any imbalance results in disease and distress.

FACT

Ayurvedic massage may be performed by one or more therapists, using herbal oils to suit your body type, and is aimed at loosening excess energy towards the organs of elimination.

FACT

'Chavutti pizchil', is a specialized form of Ayurvedic massage where a therapist suspends himself by a string/rope from the ceiling to apply extra pressure with his feet.

The relationship of the seven chakras within Indian head massage

Indian head massage works on the subtle levels of the body as well as the physical. These subtle levels are known as **energy centres** or **chakras** and are important points of focus throughout the treatment. Chakra comes from the ancient Sanskrit word meaning 'wheel', and they are seen as spinning energy centres situated an inch away from the body and are connected to the body via energy channels or **meridians**. A dysfunction in any one of the chakras can build up and cause an imbalance affecting them all and can lead to the client feeling stressed and tense.

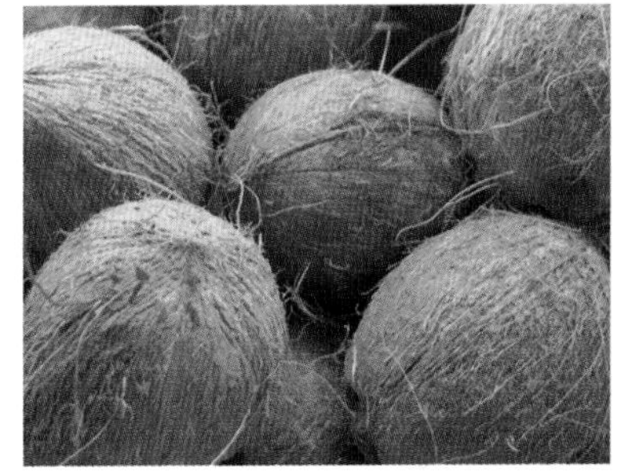

During an Indian head massage treatment, the therapist concentrates mainly on the three higher chakras – the crown, third eye and throat – which has a powerful effect in releasing stagnant energy, balancing the chakras and helping the body to feel more balanced.

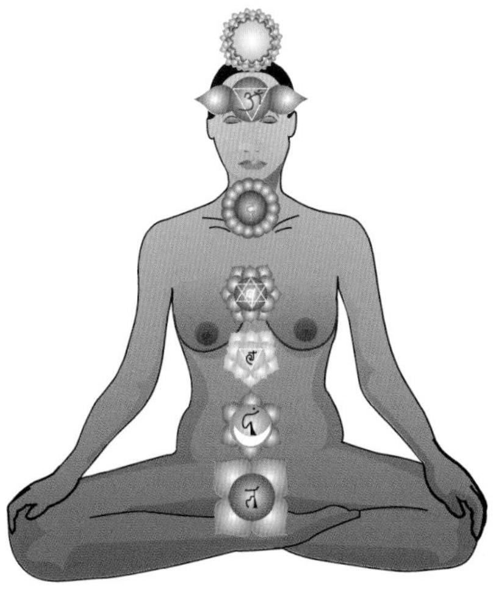

Seven major chakras

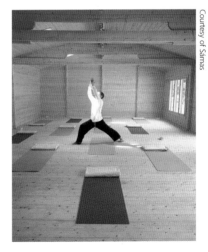

Courtesy of Sámas

Yoga position, Sámas

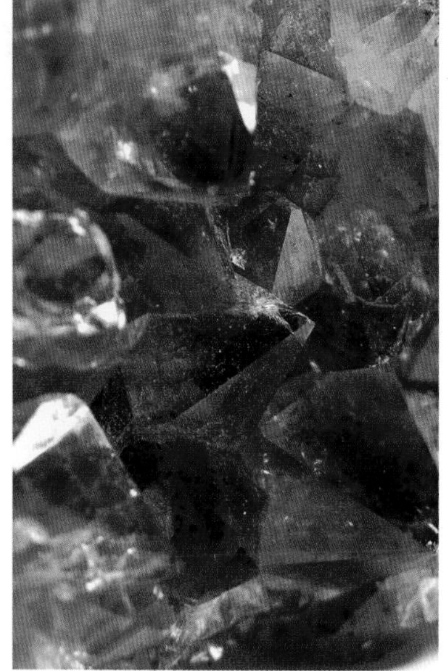

Amethyst crystal

SPA TIP 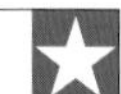

The therapist always begins each head massage treatment, by placing the hands over the crown chakra to open up the chakras and energy field. At the end of the treatment the therapist will do the same to restore balance, energy and a feeling of wellbeing.

The seven chakras are often associated with colours, gemstones and elements:

Chakra	*Element*	*Gemstone*	*Colour*	*Associated with*
Base – root (Muladhara)	Earth	Ruby Red garnet	Red	Relates to earth and keeps you grounded, vitality and sexuality
Sacral – abdomen (Svadisthana)	Water	Tiger's eye	Orange	Emotions, health and energy
Solar plexus – stomach (Manipura)	Fire	Citrine	Yellow	Memory, expressing oneself, energy
Heart – chest (Anahata)	Air	Emerald Rose quartz	Green	Physical and emotional balance
Throat – thyroid (Vishuddha)	Ether	Blue sapphire	Blue	Communication and creativity
Third eye – brow (Ajna)	Mind	Lapis Amethyst	Indigo	Intuition and spiritualism
Crown – top of the head (Sahasrara)	Spirit	Amethyst Clear quartz	Purple	Imagination and thought, cosmic consciousness

Unique advantages of Indian head massage are

- Clothes can be kept on – good for nervous clients, or where a treatment is being given in a working area
- Oils do not always have to be used – the client will gain more therapeutic benefits from using oil but they may be going back to work, shopping or going out and so not want greasy hair
- Versatile – can be carried out in most places where there is a low back chair or couch to lean against, such as the office, shopping mall, client's home, etc.
- Suitable for most people – can be carried out on children, elderly, disabled, pregnant women – where other massages are sometimes difficult to carry out
- Cost effective – a full treatment takes about 30 minutes, and quick treatment at an office desk can be given in 10 minutes

The head, neck and shoulders are all energy centres where tension is most likely to accumulate. As these areas are gently but firmly massaged, the pressures begin to release and generally create a feeling of wellbeing.

Elemis Ltd

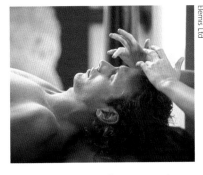

Tension commonly accumulates around the head, neck and shoulders

EFFECTS OF INDIAN HEAD MASSAGE

All the usual benefits of massage apply to an Indian head treatment along with lots of unique physical and psychological effects.

Physical effects

- Relaxation of the muscles.
- Circulation is improved, increasing the oxygen supply to the brain.
- Relief of neck and shoulder stiffness.
- Improvement in the circulation of the lymphatic system, helping to disperse toxins from tense muscles.
- Improved joint mobility in the neck and shoulder area.
- Loosening of the scalp.
- Facial massage movements help to relieve headaches, nasal congestion and eye strain.
- Energy levels can be increased as tension spots are released.
- Massage of the scalp can stimulate hair growth, by increasing the blood supply to hair follicles.
- By using oils in the massage the condition of the scalp and hair can be improved.

Psychological effects

- Relaxation.
- Improved sleep patterns, particularly if the client is suffering with insomnia.
- Stress relief – which is one of the reasons why Indian head massage has become a popular treatment in the workplace.
- Stimulation of the mind – can make the client feel more alert.
- Relief of tension headaches and eye strain.
- Chakra balancing.

SIGNATURE TREATMENT S

Vida Wellness Spa at The Fairmont Chateau, Whistler

'Ayurvedic Swedana: This treatment begins with an Ayurvedic Massage. Following your massage, you will be placed in a handcrafted, West Coast cedar steam cabinet customized with herbs based on your dosha. The steam and herb combination will detoxify and cleanse your system. This is followed by a dry flower brushing of your entire body to further exfoliate the skin and prevent the re-entry of toxins.'

FACT !

Conditions that benefit from Indian head massage are:

alopecia, asthma, arthritis, backache, dandruff, eye strain, headaches, insomnia, muscular tension, poor hair condition, stress, sinusitis.

OILS USED IN INDIAN HEAD MASSAGE

Indian head massage can be given as a treatment without the use of oils and this should be discussed in the consultation. Ideally if oil is being used then it should be warm, but not too hot, as this will aid its penetration into the skin and also be very soothing to the client.

SPA TIP 

As the body relaxes during a treatment, the client may start to talk about their problems and may even get tearful. As a therapist, be a good listener but do not offer advice as a counsellor. Always know when to refer clients to a professional in this field.

FACT

In Ayurvedic treatments the oils are cooked with traditional herbs for their hair strengthening and growth promoting properties.

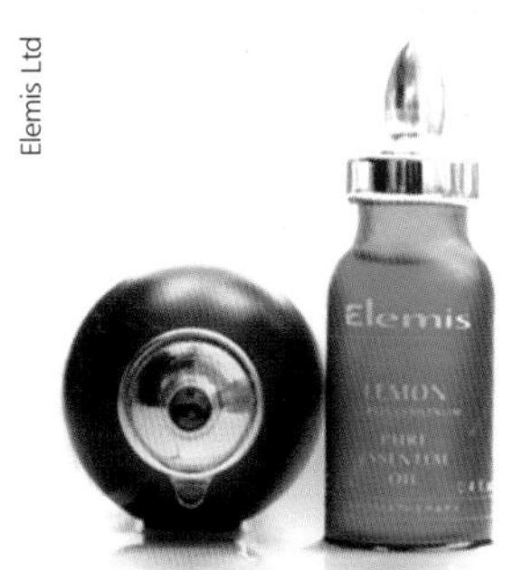

Elemis Ltd

HEALTH AND SAFETY

Remember that if the client is allergic to nuts then do not use any carrier oils obtained from them. If you think the client may be allergic to an oil then always carry out a patch test first (as in an aromatherapy treatment).

HEALTH AND SAFETY 

When using essential oils do not use them neat on the skin, always dilute in a carrier oil.

Traditionally oils such as coconut, sesame, almond or olive have been used in head massage. Organic vegetable carrier oils are the best to use as they are easily absorbed through the skin and have internal and external effects. As well as improving the hair and scalp conditions, oil massage can promote and slow down hair growth. Essential oils can be added to the carrier oils to treat specific hair conditions.

Alternative oils

Other oils that can be used include: jasmine oil, evening primrose, calendula, grapeseed, apricot kernel, sunflower, hazelnut oil, jojoba, macadamia nut oil, St John's wort.

If you were treating a client according to their dosha then you could use the following herbal oils:

- vata – almond, olive, sesame, wheatgerm
- pitta – almond, coconut, sunflower
- kapha – mustard, almond.

Traditional oils

Sesame oil	A traditional Indian favourite, it has a strong odour and is particularly used during the summer. It is said to reduce swelling and muscular aches and pains and delay greying of the hair. It is a good balancing oil. Has been known to cause skin irritation.
Mustard oil	Popular in northern India due to its warming properties. Due to the muscles being warmed it is effective in relieving muscular aches and pains and is good for clients with arthritis. Not suitable for clients with sensitive skin as it may cause irritation.
Olive oil	A thick heavy oil – commonly used in cooking – that can be used to treat very dry skin and hair. In India it is particularly used during the summer as an alternative to sesame oil.
Almond oil	This is one of the most popular carrier oils in the West and is widely used as a base for Swedish and aromatherapy massage. It is a very light oil and is a good alternative to olive oil. Can be used on normal to dry skin and hair.
Coconut oil	Unrefined coconut oil is solid at room temperature and will need gently warming, but has a beautiful aroma and has a good consistency to massage with. This is one of the traditional oils used in the Far East for women's hair treatments.

Or, if you want to blend essential oils with your base oils, then you could use the following recommendations:

- dry hair – geranium, sandalwood, lavender
- damaged hair – sandalwood, lavender, frankincense
- blond hair – lemon, chamomile
- hair loss – juniper, rosemary, lavender
- dandruff – rosemary, cedarwood, tea tree.

If essential oils have been used, then ideally you should blend only 2–3 drops in 10 ml of carrier/base oil.

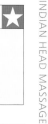

SPA TIP

Hot macadamia oil mixed with your choice of essential oils is used at a spa in Bali.

FACT

Hot coconut milk has been traditionally used in the Far East, passed down through generations of women, for washing and conditioning the hair.

INDIAN HEAD MASSAGE TREATMENT

You will find the anatomy associated with an Indian head treatment in chapter 6. The massage movements used in a treatment follow the same classifications as for Swedish massage (chapter 11) but have had slight adaptations to them to incorporate the traditional Indian techniques. Depending on the technique, the massage movements can either have a stimulating or relaxing effect. The basic movements are:

- Effleurage.
- Tapotement – the movements used in Indian head massage are hacking, tapping and champissage.
- Petrissage.
- Frictions.

TERMINOLOGY

Champissage the traditional term used in India for head massage. It originates from the Hindu word 'champi' which means head massage. In the West this term has been used to describe a hacking technique associated with Indian head massage.

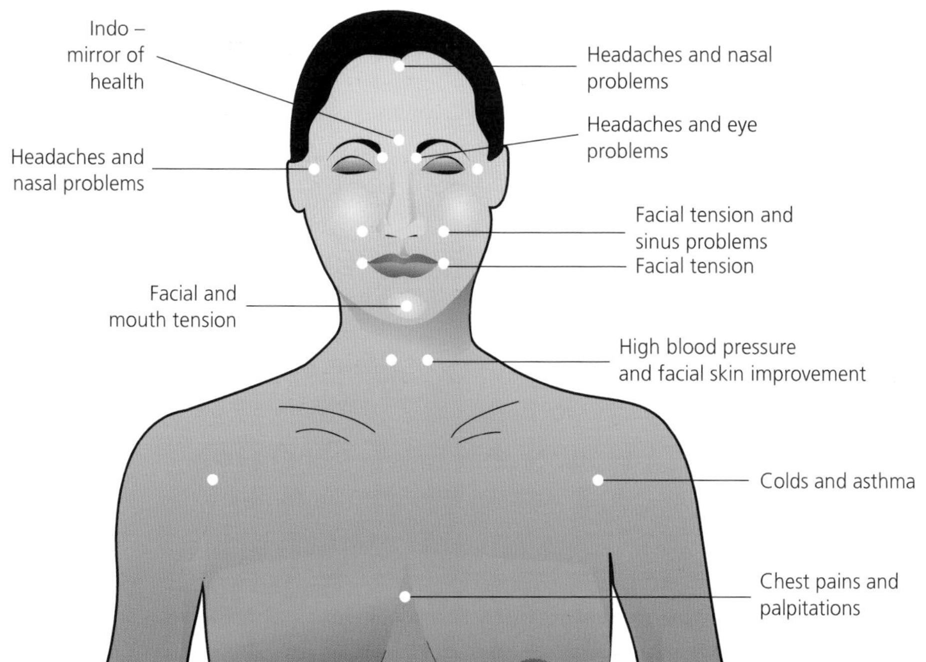

Shiatsu pressure points of the face

> **SPA TIP**
>
> Regular hand exercises will prevent the therapist from straining the wrists and damaging any ligaments in the hand.

- Pressure points – these are used in an Indian head massage treatment to improve energy levels and induce relaxation. The pressure points follow the traditional Ayurvedic marma point massage, which focuses on the face, neck, scalp and shoulders. Massaging the points using either the thumb or index finger relieves anxiety, aids hearing and improves vision.

CONTRA-INDICATIONS TO INDIAN HEAD MASSAGE

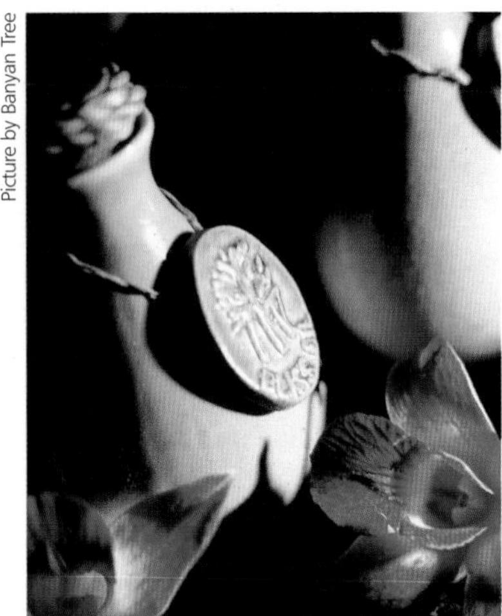
Picture by Banyan Tree

As with massage and aromatherapy, there are some ailments that are total contra-indications, some for which you need to seek medical approval and others which are localized and just restrict a full treatment.

If you are in any doubt about giving a treatment, then always consult a doctor first.

Total contra-indications	*With medical approval*	*Localized*
Contagious or infectious diseases	Pregnancy	Cuts
Fever	Heart conditions	Bruises
Under the influence of drugs or alcohol	Cancer	Scar tissue (avoid for 6 months)
Client suffering from food poisoning	Medical oedema	Sunburn
Head or neck injury	Epilepsy	Recent injury/operation
Migraine	Diabetes	Undiagnosed lumps and bumps
	Asthma	Thrombosis
	Acute rheumatism	
	Severe problems of the nervous system	
	High or low blood pressure	

CONTRA-ACTIONS FROM INDIAN HEAD MASSAGE

As toxins are removed from the body some clients experience a 'healing crisis'. This can differ between clients depending on how much cleansing the body has done and may include some of the following reactions:

- Weepiness.
- Headache/dizziness – this is just part of nature's reaction to the release of some toxins into the body and should disappear within a few hours. If this occurs the client should drink a lot of water, sit down and relax immediately after the treatment and avoid tea/coffee and alcohol for the next 24 hours.
- Tiredness.
- Flu-like symptoms.
- Aching muscles – caused by the release of toxins.

Always record any reactions or any comments the client has on their record card for future reference.

MARMA PRESSURE POINT MASSAGE

Marma points are essentially vital energy points in the body, of which there are 107. Traditionally the massage is practised in southern India but it has been adapted for use in modern spa treatments. A marma point massage is done with the thumb or index finger. Beginning with small circular clockwise movements, the therapist will gradually increase the circular movement and pressure used. The marma point will feel uncomfortable to the client if it is blocked or out of balance. Herbal oils were traditionally used in the massage but in spa treatments essential oils can be used. During an Indian head massage treatment we work on these pressure points on the face and scalp.

CONSULTATION

As with all spa treatments it is important that a thorough consultation and lifestyle analysis is done before an Indian head massage treatment. It is important to ascertain as much information as possible about the client's lifestyle and emotional and physical state as this will help in selecting the appropriate blend of oils to use during the treatment (if the client is having oils used). Refer to chapter 15 on consultation techniques for more detail.

If an Indian head massage treatment will be carried out on-site, e.g. in an office setting, then the consultation may have to be a bit briefer, but it is still important to get the client's details, check for any contra-indications and ascertain their reasons for having the treatment.

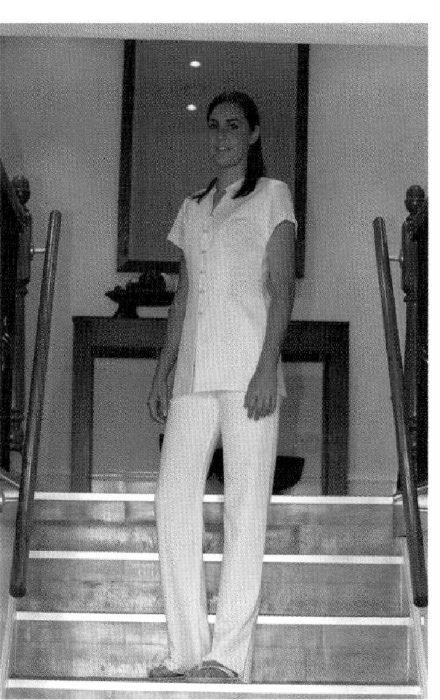

Spa therapist

ACTIVITY

Research the different head massage chairs that are available to buy for use in a spa.

EQUIPMENT LIST

Indian head massage

- low backed chair – preferably a professional head massage chair
- clean towels – small hand and large bath sheets
- Balinese wraps/sheets – may be appropriate for your spa to put around the client
- natural wood comb – you may need to comb the client's hair first if it is long and also after the treatment
- clips – if it is very long the client's hair may need to be clipped up whilst you do the back massage
- facial products on the trolley – to cleanse face before facial massage
- selection of organic carrier oils or bottles of pre-blended massage oil
- small bowl to pour oil into
- aromatherapy burner – the room should have a nice aroma when the client enters
- candles – may be scented to create aroma or used for subtle lighting
- crystals – some therapists like to put crystals in the room when they are working on the chakras

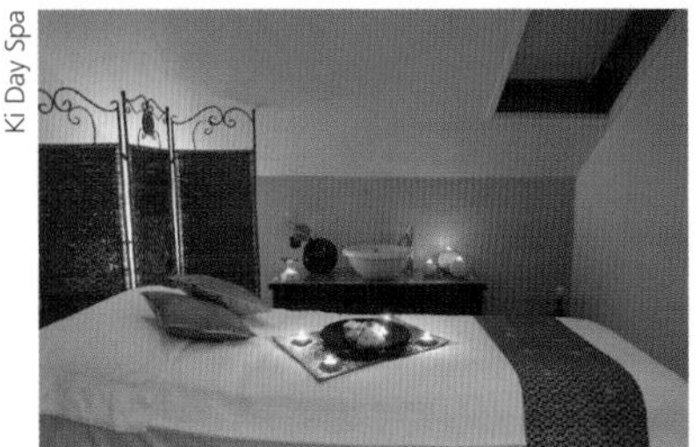

Ki Day Spa

Spa treatment room

PRE-TREATMENT BREATHING

Breathing exercises should be recommended for particularly stressed clients and conducted after the consultation and immediately prior to treatment. A popular exercise involves the client standing relaxed and focusing on their normal breathing pattern while gradually increasing the depth of each breath. The client should maintain these deep breaths for a few moments before gradually reversing the pattern until they are breathing normally again and, if necessary, repeat the entire exercise until they are suitably relaxed.

PREPARATION OF THE TREATMENT ROOM

If using a professional head massage chair it should be positioned where the therapist has got plenty of room to walk around – in some spas this may be outside near the beach, facing a window overlooking the water or on a balcony overlooking rice fields. If the spa has not got a professional chair then use a low backed chair that is a good height for the therapist but comfortable for the client, and allow the client to rest against a few pillows piled up on the treatment couch. Remember that traditionally in India the client could be sat on the beach or in the middle of a market square!

TREATMENT PROCEDURE

Once the consultation and treatment plan have been done, if your client is having a treatment using oils then you will need to select a suitable oil or blend of oils to use. In most spas, Indian head massage treatments nearly always use oil, unlike a salon treatment or a therapist working

SPA HYGIENE 

- Fresh towels/linen/gowns for each client
- All towels, linen should be washed in very hot, soapy water in order to remove any oil
- All work surfaces should be cleaned with surgical spirit, particularly the trolley where the oil bottles are kept, which should be done after each client and daily with a disinfectant spray
- If using a professional chair wipe over with a disinfectant spray after each client, particularly around the head piece
- All floors should be cleaned daily
- All massage bottles should be wiped over after each client, making sure they don't get too oily and look grubby

on-site in an office. You may choose to use carrier oil on its own – the benefits of this were discussed earlier. If you would like to add some essential oils or mix carrier oils, then the table below gives some suggested blends for the particular outcomes. For a full treatment you will need approximately 10 ml of carrier oil and if you are using essential oils do not add more than 2 drops to the blend. If using essential oils, always check the properties of the oil to ensure they are suitable for the client.

This is just a sample of blends that you can use. The spa where you are working may use their own blends of oils or a well-known beauty company's products, such as Elemis and Aromatherapy Associates.

SPA TIP 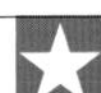

If you are qualified in aromatherapy then you may want to use the following oils in your treatment – for hair loss ginger/rosemary and peppermint, and if the client has head lice then blend thyme, rosemary, eucalyptus and tea tree to use at home.

Relaxation	*Wellbeing*	*Improve condition of scalp and hair*
Almond – rose & sandalwood	Coconut – rose & rosewood	Jojoba, olive & wheatgerm together
Coconut – lavender & chamomile	Coconut – lime & grapefruit	Jojoba – geranium & lavender
Almond & mustard together	Almond – lemon & lime	Sesame – rosemary & sandalwood
	Sesame & almond	

PREPARING THE CLIENT

If the client is having a treatment with oils then you need them to undress, remove any jewellery and put on a gown – if possible, offer the client a warm shower before their treatment. They need to be comfortable in the treatment chair, with legs uncrossed and feet on the floor, and

SPA TIP 

Fresh lemon and grapefruit juice is very good as a rinse for oily hair.

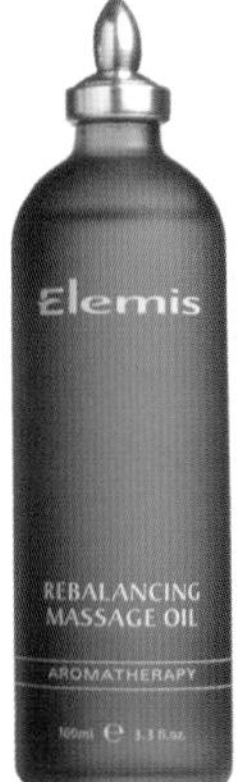

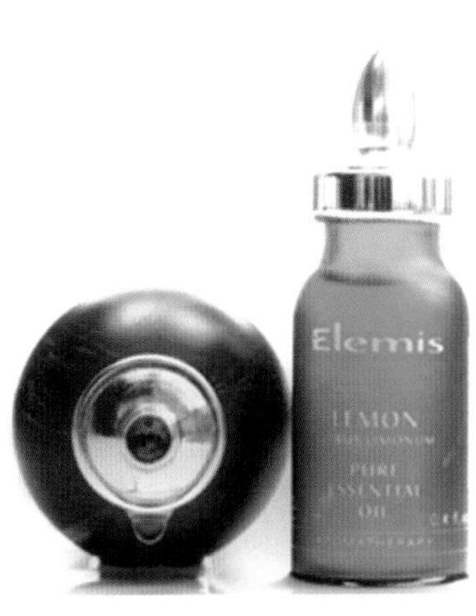

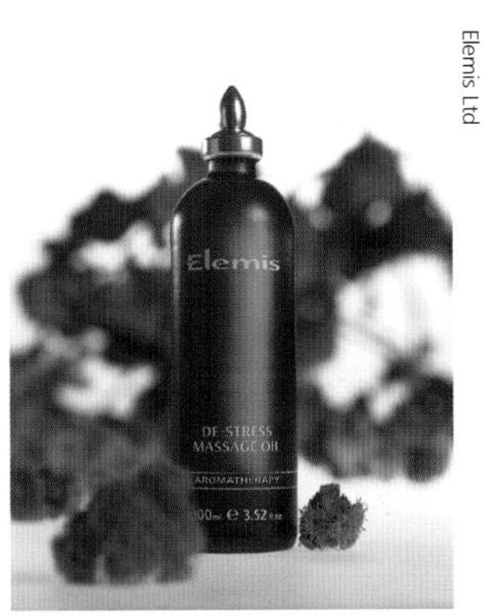

Elemis Ltd

make sure they are appropriately covered. If you have selected the oils then massage a little bit of the oil onto the back of the client's hand to make sure they like the aroma. Explain to the client the treatment procedure and make sure that you wash your hands in view of the client before applying the massage oil. An Indian head massage treatment should last 30 minutes – some spas may allow longer if it is a signature treatment.

PREPARE FOR TREATMENT CHECKLIST
Indian head massage

✔ Correct environment	✔ Bathrobe
✔ Health and safety	✔ Help client onto massage chair
✔ Hygiene	✔ Correct client positioning
✔ Professional appearance	✔ Client warm, relaxed and comfortable
✔ Equipment/products/consumables	✔ Wash hands
✔ Record card	✔ Cleanse skin
✔ Private changing facilities	✔ Select massage medium

TREATMENT APPLICATION

There is no right or wrong way for an Indian head massage and the sequence of movements will vary from one therapist to another. The following step-by-step sequence starts with the shoulder and back and finishes with the face. It is important that the therapist connects with the client before a treatment and becomes grounded, freeing the mind of any negative thoughts, and concentrating your energies into the treatment.

SPA TIP 

Abdominal breathing should be carried out throughout the treatment by the client, as it helps in relaxation and bringing more oxygen into the body. They should breathe in slowly through the nose and out through the mouth.

SPA TIP 

It is important for a therapist to maintain good posture throughout a treatment and follow the same guidelines as you would for body massage. As the client is sitting it is usually easier for the therapist to stand in the stride standing position for comfort and to protect their back. Remember if you have poor posture you are more likely to tire easily and suffer from aches and pains.

STEP-BY-STEP: Preparation or grounding

1 Place the hands gently on the head (crown) and ask the client to close their eyes, and to slowly breathe in through the nose and out through the mouth.
2 Follow the client's breathing with your own breath, helping you to relax and connect with the client.
3 Slowly rest the forearms onto the shoulders and apply gentle pressure on the clients out breath.
4 Then place one hand to the forehead and one to the occipital and hold for 2 minutes.

At this point oil can be applied to the head by parting the hair and pouring a little oil here, massaging in with small circular movements. Remember oil absorbs easily when warm and it will also feel relaxing for the client.

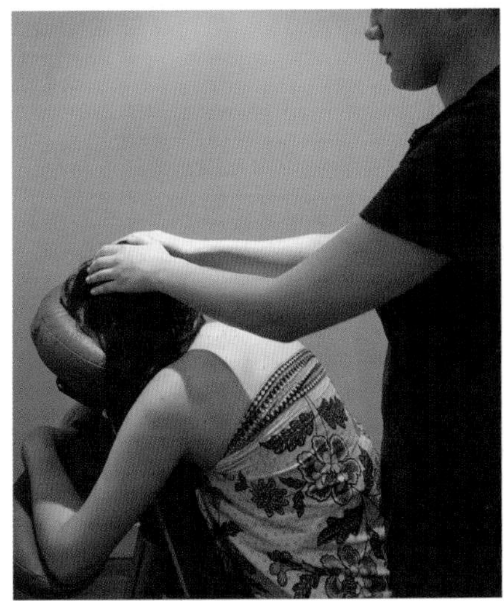

Hands placed on crown chakra

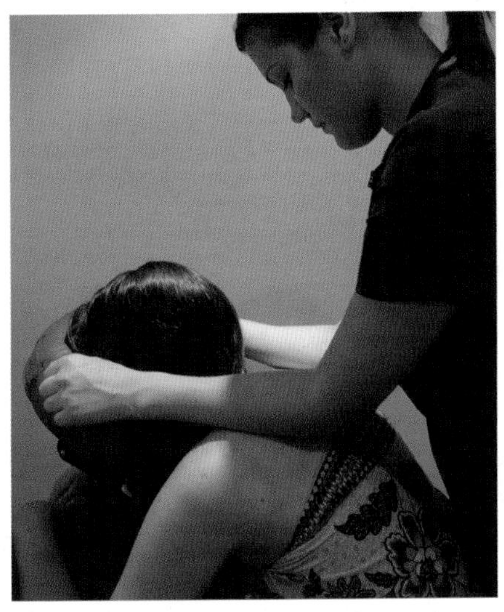

Rest forearms onto shoulders

STEP-BY-STEP: Shoulder and back

1 Ask the client to put their head forward onto the support pillows if you are not using a professional chair.
2 Effleurage oil onto the client's back (if applicable).
3 Re-apply forearm pressure onto the shoulders.
4 Apply frictions using the thumbs to the trapezius in small circular movements.
5 Using the heal of the hand, knead across the shoulder and down the back.
6 Pick up the trapezius muscle by squeezing between the thumb and fingers.
7 Hacking is applied down the sides of the spine and across the shoulders.

8 With both hands iron down the back in circular movements.

9 Using the knuckles apply pressure down the sides of the spine from the shoulder area to the base of the spine using the therapists body weight for the pressure.

10 Repeat the same movement using the thumbs to apply pressure – remember to check the client is well supported.

11 Using the heal of the hand, knead across the shoulder and down the back.

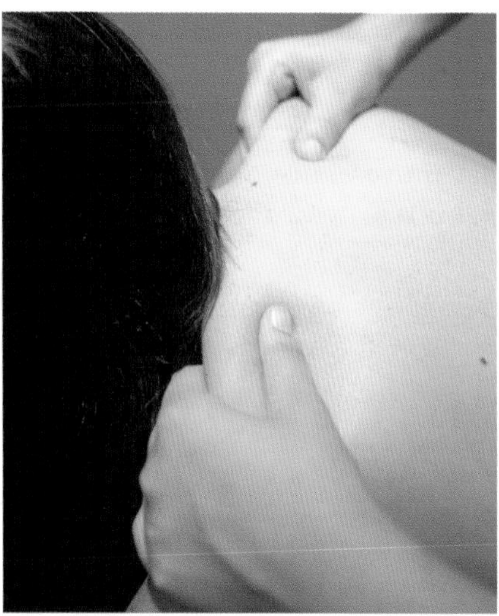

Picking-up trapezius muscles

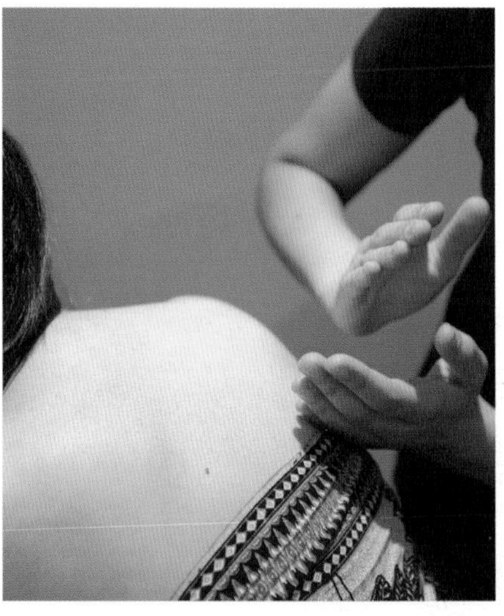

Hacking down the sides of spine

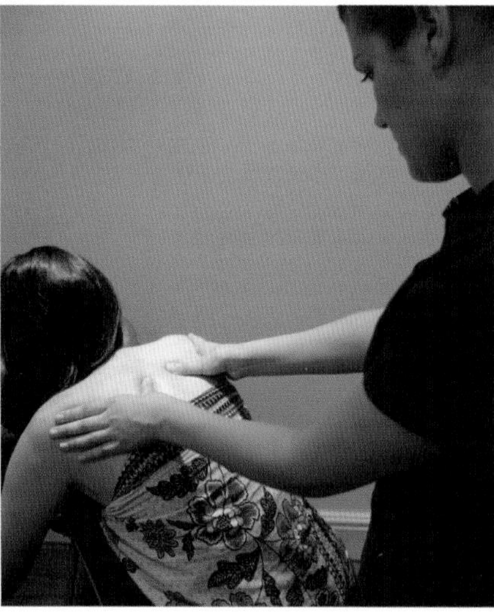

Thumb pressures down sides of spine

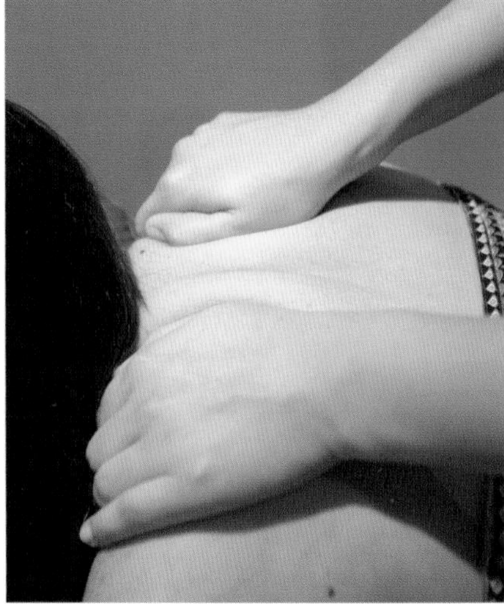

Kneading across shoulders

Neck

1 Knuckle rub down each side of the neck.
2 Pick up the trapezius at the back of the neck between the thumb and fingers – supporting the client's head with the other hand on the forehead.
3 Apply frictions using the thumbs under the occiput in a circular direction.
4 Using the heel of the hand under the occiput, massage in a kneading movement.
5 Using both thumbs apply pressure to points at the base of the skull.
6 Knuckle rub down each side of the neck.

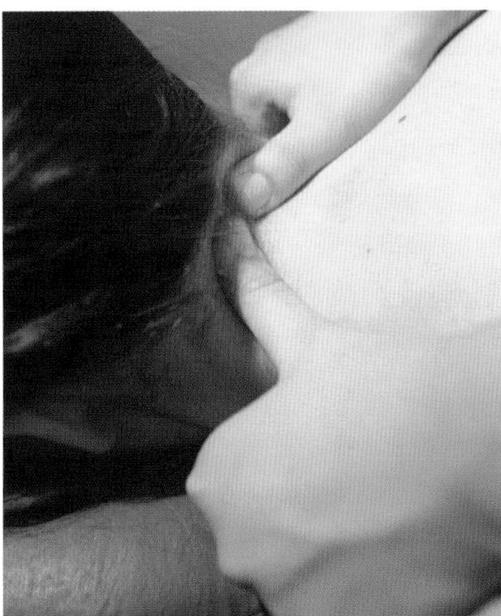

Frictions under the occiput

Arms

1 Ask the client to lift up their head.
2 Using the heel of the hand, quickly roll down the arm, flicking off at the hands.
3 Knead the upper arm by squeezing the deltoid muscle between the fingers and thumb.
4 With the client's arms folded, hold the forearms just below the elbow. As the client breathes in lift the arms upwards and as the client breathes out let them drop slowly.
5 Drain down from the shoulder into the axilla using the thumbs.
6 Hack (champissage) down the side of each arm.
7 Using the heel of the hand, quickly roll down the arm, flicking off at the hands.

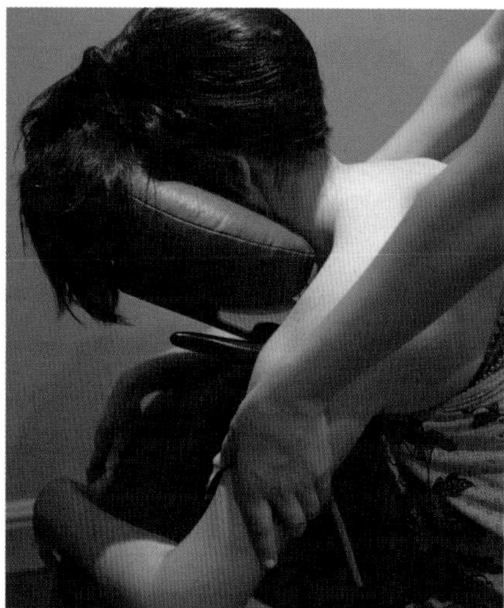

Roll down the arms

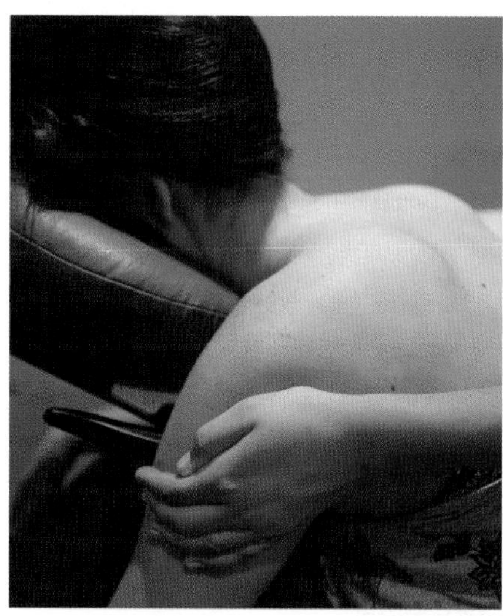

Knead upper arms

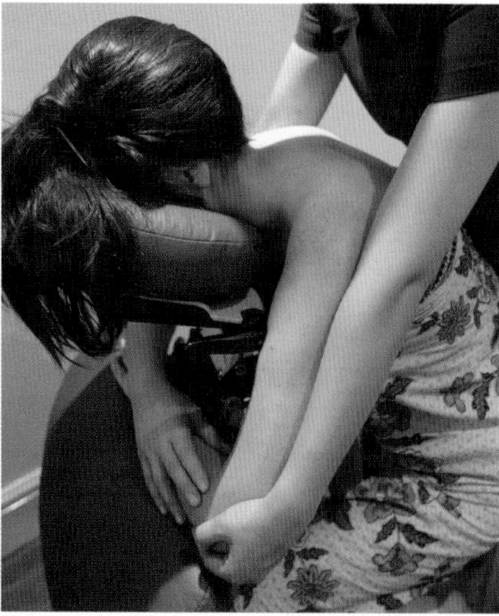

Lift up client's folded arms

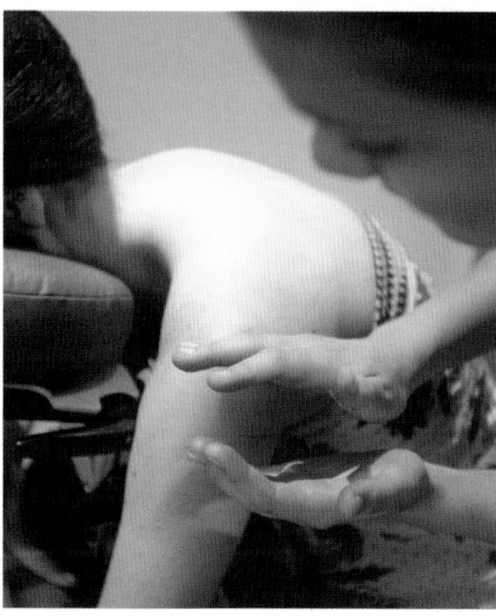

Hacking to the arm

Scalp

1. Effleurage (stroke) through the client's hair alternately with each hand.
2. With the heels of the hands on each temple, apply a short, quick wiping movement on the area.
3. Using the pads of the fingers apply frictions movements all over the scalp (like shampooing).
4. Using the pads of the fingers ruffle the hair.
5. Effleurage (stroke) through the client's hair alternately with each hand.
6. Gently tug the client's hair alternately with each hand.
7. Hack (champissage) over both sides of the head.
8. Interlock the fingers of both hands, and using the heels of the hands squeeze and lift the scalp in a slow circular movement.
9. Using the thumbs apply pressure down the governing vessel and then the bladder meridians starting at the hairline.
10. Effleurage (stroke) through the client's hair alternately with each hand.

Wash your hands after massaging the scalp.

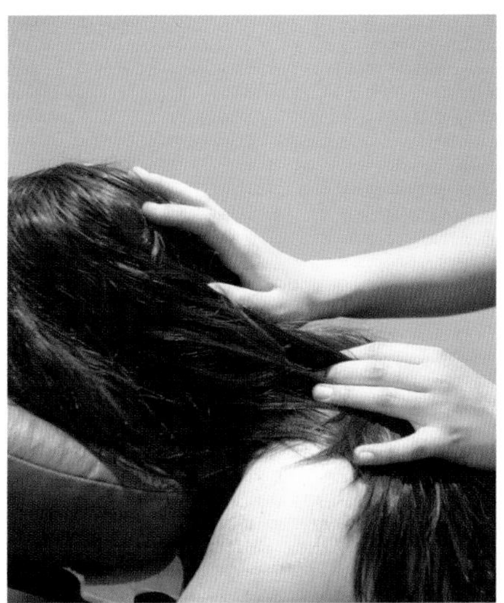

Stroke through the hair

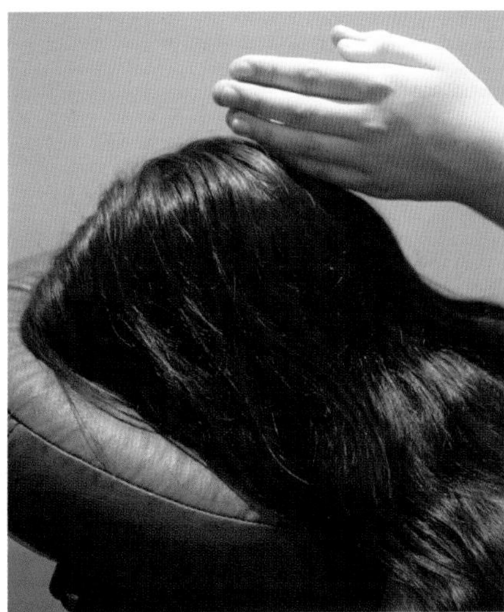

Hacking on the scalp

LINKED TREATMENTS

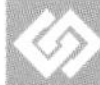

There are other Ayurvedic treatments available in spas that would complement a head massage treatment as well as some of the traditional Western therapies:

- Herbal oil massage – the oils are selected according to the client's doshas and it may be performed by more than one therapist.
- Shirodhara – sometimes referred to as massage of the third eye, a steady stream of herbal oil is directed onto the forehead to alleviate headaches and tension.
- Specialist hair treatments – using natural herbs and mashed fruits as masks for the hair and scalp.
- Body exfoliation – using natural shredded coconut or the traditional Balinese boreh, which is a simple herb and spice mix used in Bali for its heating properties as well as for softening the skin.

Face

1. Ask the client to lean their head into your body.
2. Apply pressure points on the governing vessel – from the top of the nose to the hairline – stroke over afterwards with the middle finger.
3. Stroke over the forehead with alternate hands.
4. Using the middle and ring fingers apply pressure points over the zygomatic (cheek) bone – stroke over afterwards with the middle finger.
5. Gently pinch across the eyebrows using the index finger and thumb.
6. Gently pinch across the jaw line using the index finger and thumb.

7 Using the pads of the fingers and thumb massage the ear lobe in small circular movements then gently pinch around the edges of the ear.

8 Use a gently tapping movement over the face using the pads of the fingers.

9 Apply very slow circular movements to the temples using the index and middle fingers.

10 Slowly rest the forearms onto the shoulders and apply gentle pressure on the client's out breath.

11 Then place one hand to the forehead and one to the occipital and hold for 2 minutes.

12 Give the client a glass of water and let them sit quietly for a few minutes.

13 Wash your hands quietly.

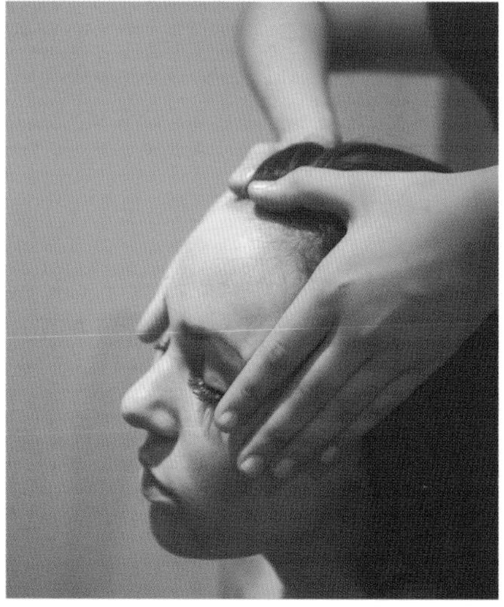

Pressure points to the governing vessel

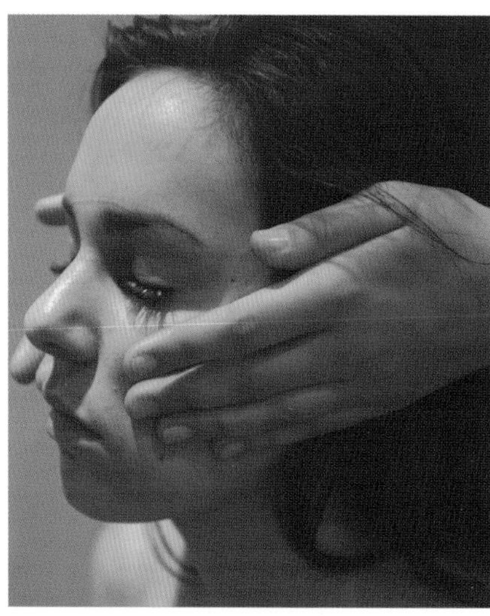

Apply pressure points along the cheek bones

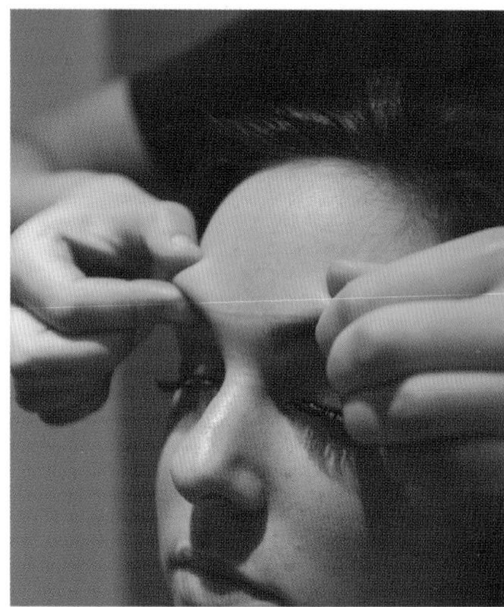

Pinch the eyebrows

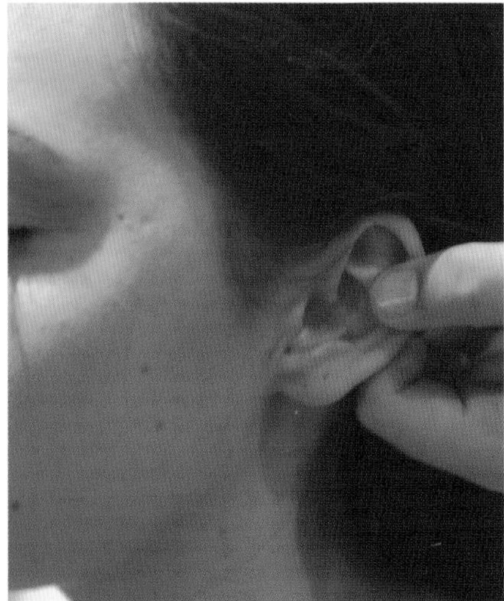

Massage the earlobe

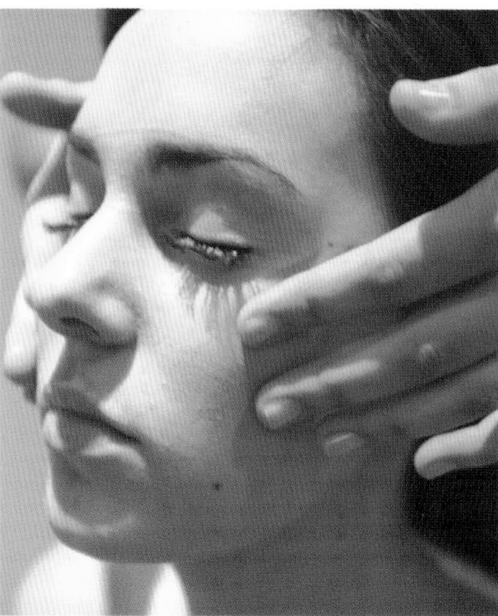

Tapping movement over the face

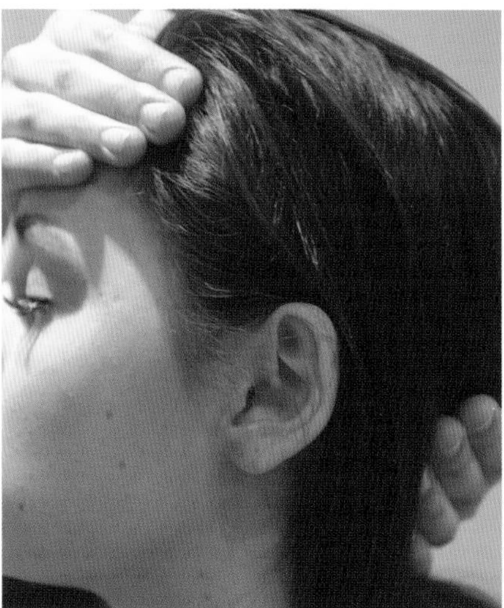

One hand to the forehead and one to the occipital bone and hold

ADAPTING MASSAGE TECHNIQUES

Depending on the condition you are treating your client for, you may have to adapt your massage movements.

Relaxing	You can increase the amount of effleurage and stroking movements used Keep all movements at a slow and even pace Add a few more kneading movements to the neck and shoulders – as these areas hold a lot of tension Omit the hacking movements from the massage
Uplifting	Make all movements quicker and more invigorating Increase the amount of pressure point, hacking movements Increase the pressure applied during kneading movements
Wellbeing	Encourage the clients abdominal breathing Spend longer on the pressure points of the scalp and face Do plenty of effleurage and lymphatic drainage movements Make the massage movements firmer

LINKED TREATMENTS

To continue the therapeutic effects of the treatment for the client, it is important to give them advice on:

- What oils have been used during the treatment and how the client could use them at home – the spa may sell these already blended which are easier to retail to the client
- Advice on products that would be suitable for hair and scalp care
- Advice on changes they may need to make to their lifestyle, e.g. changing their diet, taking more exercise, practising their breathing techniques, spending more quality time at home away from work, etc.
- How often they need an Indian head massage treatment and the benefits of regular massage

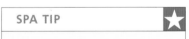

EFFECTIVENESS OF THE INDIAN HEAD MASSAGE

This should be judged continually throughout the treatment by looking at the client's body language, how well they relaxed, did they fidget, any comments that are made during the treatment, and by asking the client at the end of the treatment how they felt and if the massage could be adapted in any way for their next treatment. Any comments and feedback should be recorded on the client's record card.

SPA TIP

A warm towel can be placed over the client's shoulders at the end of the treatment and any excess oil on the face can be removed using warm mitts.

POST-TREATMENT ADVICE

Encourage the client to relax and after their glass of water they could have a herb tea or fruit drink. It is important for the client not to rush as they may feel slightly dizzy after a head massage. At the end of each treatment you need to explain to the client any reactions they may experience and most importantly homecare advice to enhance the effects of their treatment. The following advice must be given:

- Try and relax for the rest of the day, do not do too much physical exercise as the body needs to remain in a stress-free state.

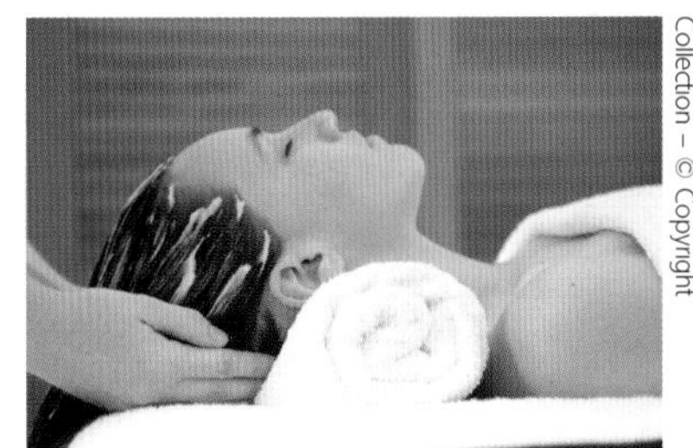

Scalp treatment

SPA TIP

To maintain ongoing relaxation, clients should be encouraged to undertake regular breathing exercises as part of their aftercare advice.

ACTIVITY

Devise a signature treatment for a spa incorporating a Indian head massage treatment. Details of the treatment, time allowed and price should be included.

SPA TIP

If the client is in a spa in a hotel they could be advised to go back to their room and relax or if there is a relaxation area in the spa then they could spend some time there. If they follow this advice then they can expect a good night's sleep and the body to feel more alert.

FACT

The **pizhichil** is a form of Ayurvedic massage carried out at the Ananda Spa in India, where a team of four masseurs work on relaxing the body.

- Drink plenty of water or herb teas and try to avoid caffeine drinks such as tea and coffee and alcohol for the next 24 hours, as the body will continue to de-tox from the treatment.
- If you have used oils try to leave them on for 6–8 hours to gain the maximum benefit from their therapeutic qualities.

SPA PROFILE

Name: Diana Turk

Position: Manager of Massage Department

Establishment: Golden Door Spa, Escondido, California

Products used: Golden Door skin care products.

Number of staff/roles: 32 part time and full time therapists, and 22 fitness staff.

Training/experience: Mueller College of Holistic Studies in San Diego; Certified Massage Therapist (trained in many different techniques); has worked at the Golden Door for 15 years.

Main responsibilities: 'Recruiting new massage staff. Overseeing continuing education and performance of staff to maintain the highest quality of services offered to guests. Creating signature treatments for Golden Door. Scheduling guest massage appointments during their stay.'

Best parts of the job: 'Creating new treatments and researching different massage techniques to enhance the guest experience. Being part of a team of therapists that is aware of Golden Door's world class reputation and is dedicated to exceeding our guests' expectations by giving only the highest quality of service.'

'The Golden Door is a soul-searching respite in a stress-filled world where guests are encouraged to do as much or as little as they wish'. (*Zagat US Hotel, Resort and Spa Guide*)

Secrets of a successful spa therapist: 'A successful therapist is one who is motivated to be the best they can be by taking opportunities for continuing education and training whenever possible. As they consistently nurture and give to others it is also of paramount importance that they nurture themselves, both physically and mentally.'

SPA PROFILE

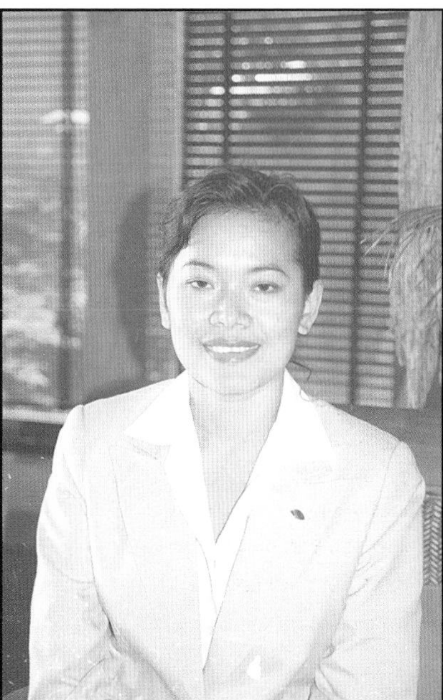

Name: Nongnapat Chaiyawan

Position: Spa Manager

Establishment: The Oriental Spa, Bangkok, Thailand

Products used: Oriental Spa products, Aromatherapy Associates, Valmont.

Number of staff/roles: Spa Manager; Supervisor/Trainer; 22 therapists and 5 receptionists.

Training/experience: Banyon Tree, Phuket – PA to Director of Operations/Asst. Admin. & Support Manager; Angsana Spa, Cairns and Sydney – Assistant Spa Manager; Angsana Spa, Sri Lanka – Spa Manager; Mandara Spa, Bangkok – Assistant Operations Manager (five establishments); Arahmas Resort and Spa, Phuket – Spa Manager; Oriental Spa, Bangkok – Spa Manager since February 2005.

Main responsibilities: Treatment development; marketing and promotions; planning/scheduling staff training and development; staff issues, day to day management; sourcing new therapists/recruitment and selection.

Best parts of the job:
Managing a spa with such a fantastic reputation – I'm very proud to be part of a 'worldclass' spa.

Working closely with the team of staff, everyone is so proud to be part of the 'Oriental Hotel' culture, with a shared vision and values that deliver excellence in guest service.

I love developing new ways of creating more revenue/income and exceeding targets.

Looking at different ways that I can maximize the time of the therapists for the benefit of the guests.

Secrets of a successful spa therapist:
Highly skilled, deliver fantastic treatments.

High standard of guest/client care, they must make them feel very special each time. We are here to make the client feel happy, and then they will return.

The individual needs to have a gentle, kind, caring and respectful nature, but then the training we do with them perfects and polishes their manner so they become the best therapists.

KEY/CORE SKILLS OPPORTUNITIES

To be an excellent spa therapist you must be able to communicate well, both orally and in writing. To be able to succeed and progress in the spa industry, it is also essential that you have an ability to work with numbers and information technology (IT). Increasingly, employers are looking for spa therapists with these 'key' skills when they recruit staff. NVQ/SVQ unit **BT20** provides you with an opportunity to develop evidence for the following:

KEY SKILLS	CORE SKILLS
Communication Level 3; C3.1a, C3.1b, C3.2, C3.3	Communication Intermediate 2; Task 1, 2 and 3
Working with others Level 2; WO2.1, WO2.2, WO2.3	Working with others Intermediate 2; Tasks 1, 2, 3 and 4
Improving own learning and performance Level 3; LP3.1, LP3.2, LP3.3	(no parallel unit in CORE SKILLS)
Problem solving Level 2; PS2.1, PS2.2, PS2.3	Problem solving Intermediate Level 1; Tasks 1, 2 and 3

Assessment of knowledge and understanding

When you have some free time, test your understanding and knowledge by answering the following questions. Do this at regular intervals and it will reinforce your learning and help you retain the knowledge, so you are able to perform better in your assessments.

Consult with the client

1 Why is it important that the client receives a professional consultation from the spa therapist?

2 Give four pieces of information you need from a client for an Indian head massage treatment.

3 Why do you need to know about the client's occupation for a treatment?

4 Name four contra-indications that would prevent a head massage treatment.

5 Name four contra-indications that would restrict a treatment.

6 Give five conditions that would benefit from an Indian head massage.

7 Give four psychological benefits from a treatment.

8 List three unique advantages of an Indian head massage treatment.

Plan the treatment

1 What information would you find on a treatment plan?

2 How long should a treatment take in a spa?

3 What benefits will the client have from a series of treatments?

4 Name two benefits of using oil in a treatment?

Prepare for the treatment

1 How would you create the right ambience in a treatment room for a head massage treatment?

2 What hygiene practices should a spa therapist follow, before and after a treatment?

3 Name and describe three carrier oils that are traditionally used in Indian head massage.

4 How should the client be prepared for the treatment?

Carry out Indian head massage treatment

1 How much carrier oil should be used for a treatment?

2 Name the basic massage movements used in Indian head massage and their benefits.

3 Name the three main chakras the therapist concentrates on during the treatment and list their associations.

4 Why is it important for the therapist to maintain a good posture during treatment?

5 How does the therapist prepare themselves and the client at the beginning of a treatment?

6 How is oil applied to the scalp?

7 How would you adapt your massage movements for the following:
   a. relaxation?
   b. uplifting?

8 Why should the client rest immediately after the treatment has finished?

Provide aftercare advice to the client

1 How can the therapist judge the effectiveness of the treatment?

2 What contra-actions may the client experience after an Indian head massage?

3 Give four important pieces of aftercare advice for the client.

4 What products could a spa therapist retail to a client after an Indian head massage?

chapter 14

Envelopments and exfoliation

BT29

Provide specialist spa treatments

BT15

Assist with spa treatments

Learning objectives

This unit covers the skills a spa therapist needs to provide envelopment and exfoliation treatments. It describes the skills and knowledge necessary to enable you to:

- **consult with and prepare the client for treatment**
- **perform exfoliation treatment**
- **perform envelopment treatments**
- **have an awareness of other associated treatments**

When providing envelopment and exfoliation treatments it is important to use the skills you have learnt in the following core units:

G1 Ensure your own actions reduce risks to health and safety

G6 Promote additional products or services to clients

G11 Contribute to the financial effectiveness of the business

EXFOLIATION

Exfoliation refers to a treatment used to remove dead skin cells from the skin's surface. This has a stimulating, brightening and cleansing effect. On the face there are many different types of exfoliating treatments, such as cleansing brushes, grains and microdermabrasion. On the body, it is more usual to use products such as loofah rubs or body brushes.

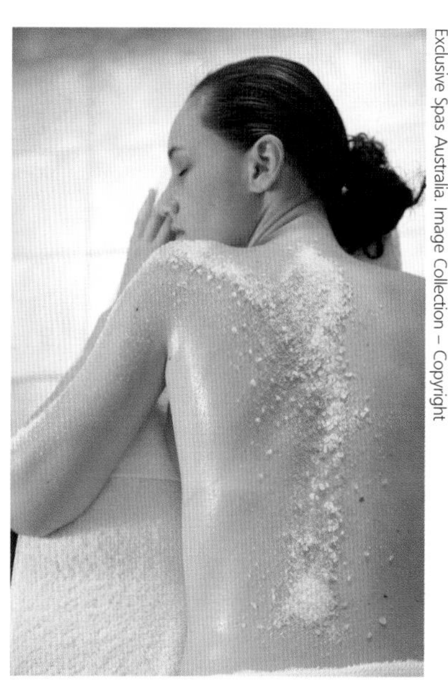

Spa scrub treatment

Uses and effects of exfoliating treatments

- Removes dead skin cells – desquamation.
- Cleanses the skin.
- Stimulates blood circulation, increases cell regeneration.
- Skin colour is improved – the skin appears brighter and more radiant.
- Skin texture is improved – feels smoother, softer and silky.
- Moisturiser can more readily be absorbed after an exfoliation treatment.

FACT

The Devarana Spa in Thailand offers a different scrub each month to suit the time of year, such as Rose Petal (February), Cool Breeze (March) and a special Christmas scrub.

SPA TIP

At the Mandara Spa in Thailand they offer an **Aloe Poultice** to soothe sunburned skin. Natural aloe vera gel is applied, followed by a cooling compress of mint and black tea leaves.

- Excellent for sun-damaged skin.
- Very good treatment before a 'self-tanning' application, as it ensures a more even absorption of the product.

Contra-indications to exfoliation

- Skin diseases.
- Sensitive skin.
- Dilated capillaries.
- Eczema.
- Psoriasis.
- Bruising.
- Recent scar tissue.
- Skin diseases.
- Blood/circulation conditions.

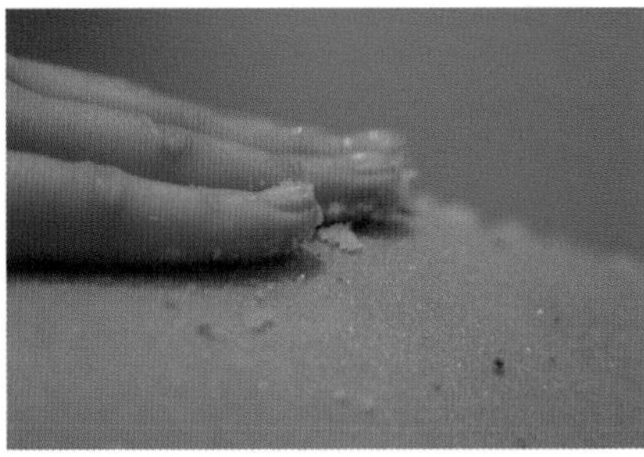

A scrub encourages desquamation and leaves the skin smooth and glowing

CONSULTATION

As outlined in chapter 15, a full consultation should be carried out to make sure the treatment is safe and effective. Every stage of the consultation checklist should be cleared prior to treatment.

CONSULTATION CHECKLIST Envelopments/exfoliation	
✔ quiet private area	✔ fill in record card
✔ client privacy	✔ client signed record card
✔ plenty of time	✔ check contra-indications
✔ client comfortable and at ease	✔ skin/sensitivity test
✔ aims of treatment/outcome	✔ explain contra-actions
✔ treatment plan	✔ client questions
✔ postural check	

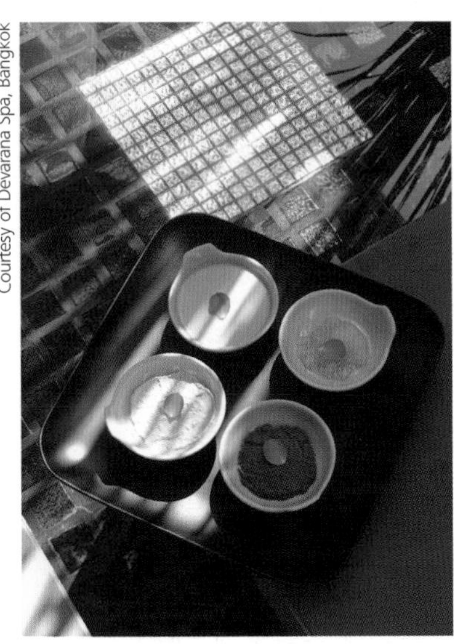

Courtesy of Devarana Spa, Bangkok

Body scrub ingredients

MAIN EXFOLIATING TREATMENTS

Body scrub

There are many products that can be used to 'scrub' the body. It may be a simple combination of sea salt and oil, or a more fragrant exotic blend, e.g. papaya body scrub, coconut body scrub or honey and seed scrub.

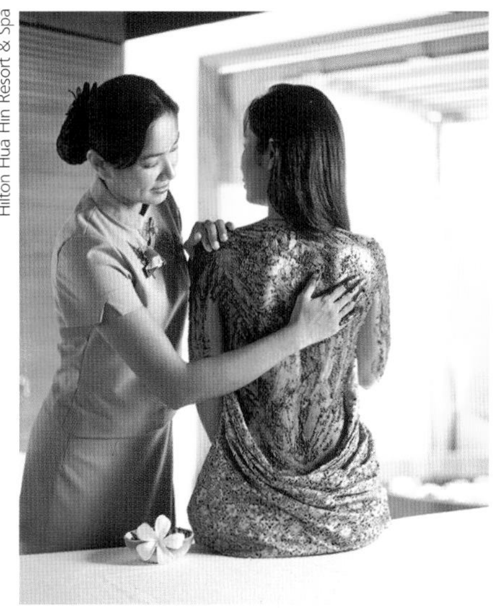

Hilton Hua Hin Resort & Spa

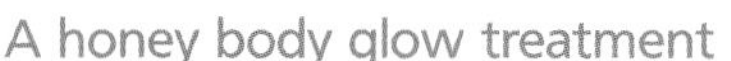

A honey body glow treatment

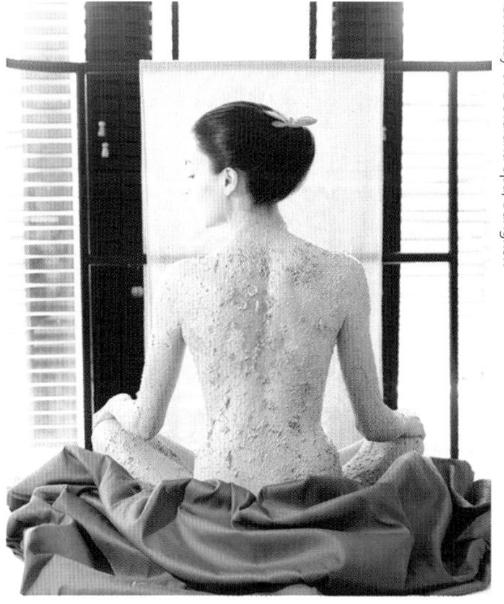

Courtesy of Devarana Spa, Bangkok

An exfoliation treatment

SPA TIP

In Thailand they use the tamarind fruit in their body scrubs, combined with rice, yoghurt and honey. The effect is to whiten, exfoliate, polish and nourish the skin.

Body brushing

In many spas, a loofah or dry body brush is used before treatment to gently exfoliate the skin, preparing it for further treatment. By stimulating blood and lymphatic circulation, body brushing warms the skin and helps remove waste products and toxins.

Each spa will have a set procedure, but make sure that you:

- Ensure the brush is hygienic before the treatment, various companies provide sprays for this purpose.
- Always explain to the client that at first it may feel slightly uncomfortable because of the firm bristles.

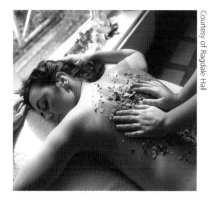

Courtesy of Ragdale Hall

A chocolate body scrub

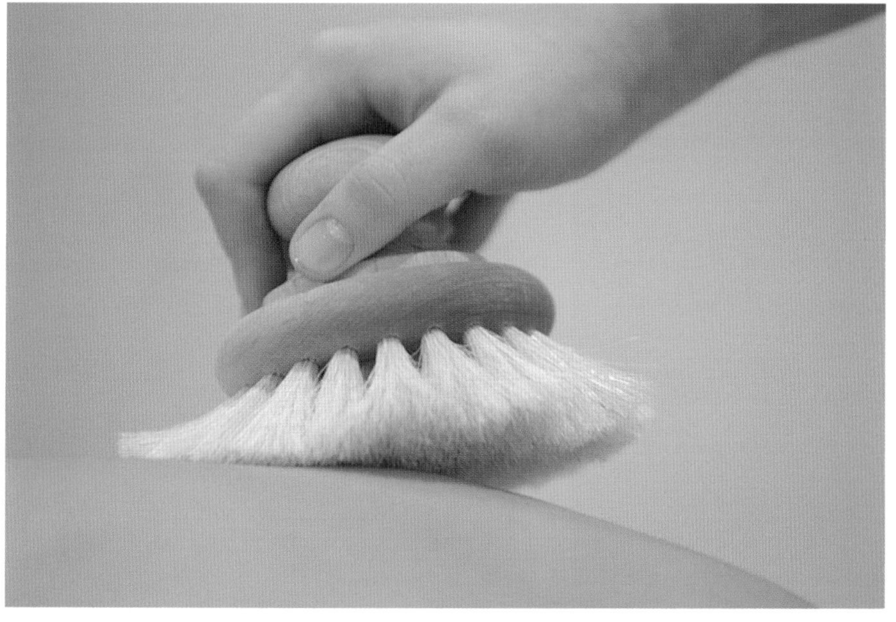

A body brush

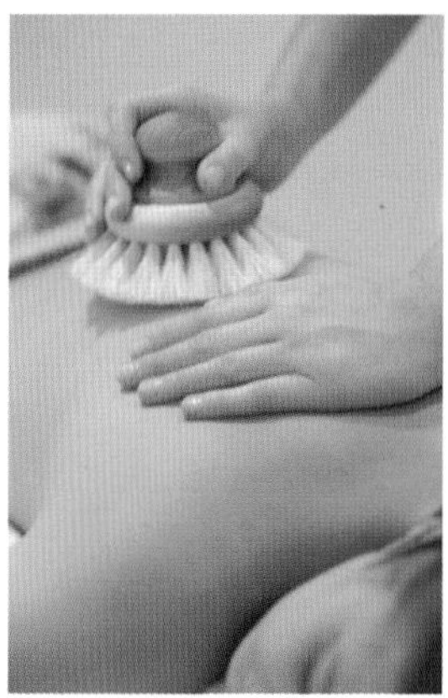

Body brushing to the back

- Always follow the direction of the lymphatic circulation.
- Always use your hand alternately with the brush, this makes it feel much more comfortable.
- Explain to the client the benefits of daily 'body brushing' at home, and if possible provide brushes to retail to the client.

Other types of exfoliating treatments

Javanese lulur

This treatment is often referred to as the 'Queen of Treatments' and has been practised for centuries in Java for the purpose of exfoliation and body polishing. 'Lulur' literally means to 'coat the skin', typically with a mixture of yoghurt and spices, and often combines a massage, spice-wrap and yoghurt coated scrub, and a blossom-filled bath.

The ingredients usually include: turmeric, sandalwood, rice powder, body oil, jasmine oil, natural yoghurt and, water. Each spa has its own unique recipe and a procedure that must be followed carefully. A usual procedure is:

1 Massage the client with an appropriate fragranced oil.
2 Mix the spice ingredients with a small amount of water to form a brown rough paste.
3 The client then showers.
4 Coat the entire body with the yoghurt, covering all areas. The yoghurt moisturizes the skin and restores the acid mantle.
5 Client showers again, meanwhile the bath is prepared with flowers and petals.
6 Client soaks in the warm flower-filled bath for 20 minutes.

Picture by Banyan Tree

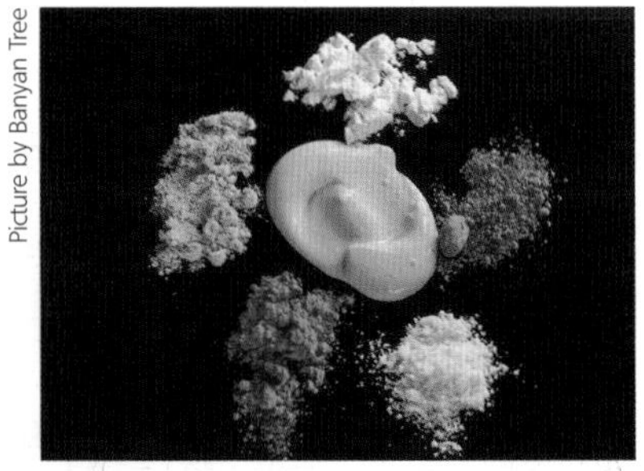
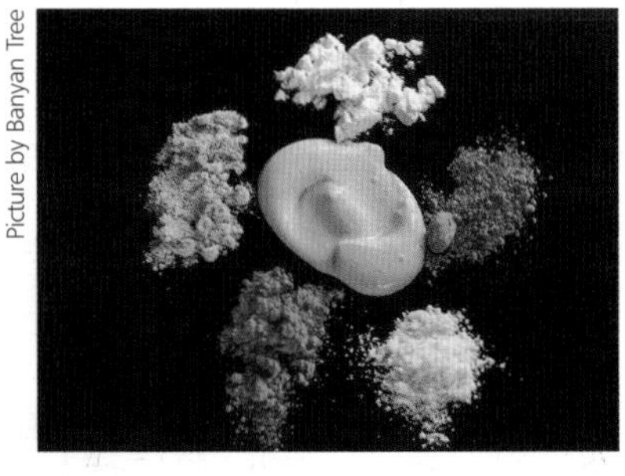

Ingredients for a lulur treatment

SIGNATURE TREATMENT S

Mandara Spa, Thailand
'Ritual of Javanese Lulur
1 Floral foot bath
2 Floral oil massage
3 Lulur scrub
4 Yoghurt splash
5 Mandi susu
6 Refreshment'
(2 hours)

FACT !

The Javanese believe that a bride should be clean, pampered and beautiful on her wedding day, so they have a lulur treatment every day in the week leading up to the wedding.

Picture by Banyan Tree

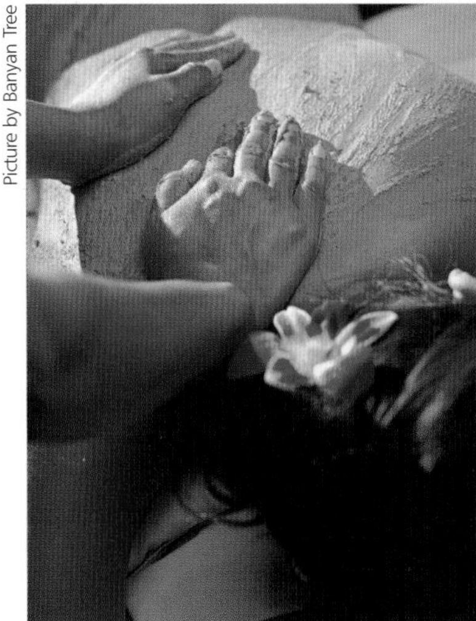

A lulur treatment

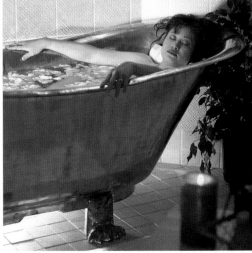

Canyon Ranch

The lulur king's bath treatment

Balinese boreh

This envelopment treatment using a spicy body mask is prepared from a mixture of herbs and spices that warms the body, giving a very deep heat effect. The heat created increases blood circulation and induces perspiration while the rice and cloves act as exfoliators to soften the skin.

The ingredients are usually: cinnamon, ginger, cloves, sandalwood, coriander seeds, turmeric, nutmeg and rice powder. These are mixed together with water to form a paste. The usual procedure is:

1 Combine the ingredients into a thick paste.
2 Cover the entire body with the paste, leave for 10 minutes.
3 Rub the skin vigorously so that the mixture flakes off the body.
4 Grated carrot can then be gently rubbed into the skin, to help replace any moisture lost.
5 The guest then showers and applies moisturizer.

FACT

Balinese boreh is an ancient treatment developed in Bali and used for centuries for headaches, fever, chills, arthritis, and muscular aches and pains.

SPA TIP 

To lessen the heat effect of a boreh treatment, a higher proportion of rice powder can be added.

Brossage

This is a spa treatment using brushes and a fine grained body polish using a salicylic salt. The result is a warm glowing skin, that feels very soft and silky.

Brush and tone

Some envelopment treatments include a pre-stage where body brushes are used. If carried out as a treatment on its own, the brushing should be followed by an application of moisturizing body cream or massage oil.

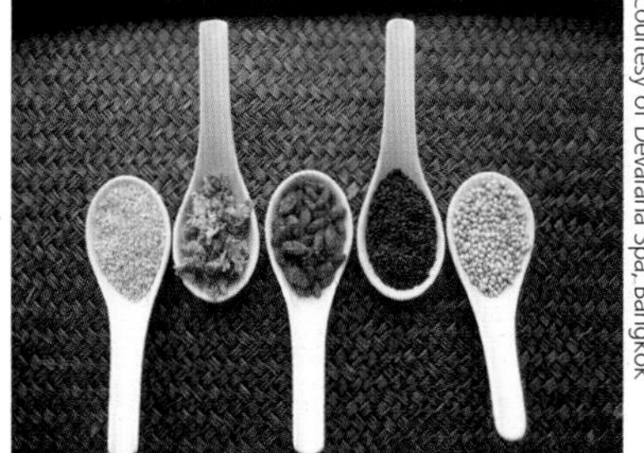
Courtesy of Devarana Spa, Bangkok

Prepare all the ingredients carefully for a boreh treatment

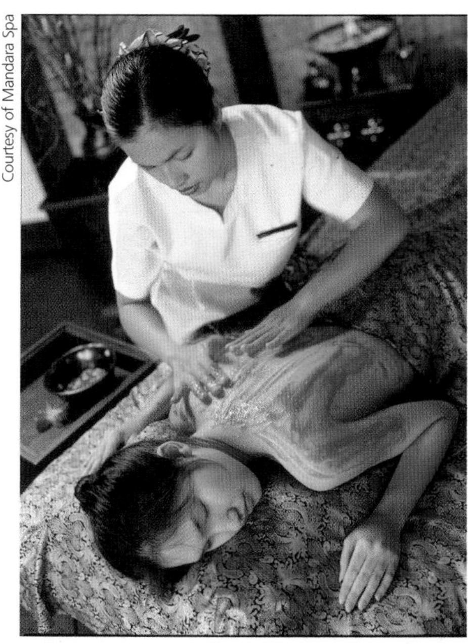
Courtesy of Mandara Spa

A boreh treatment

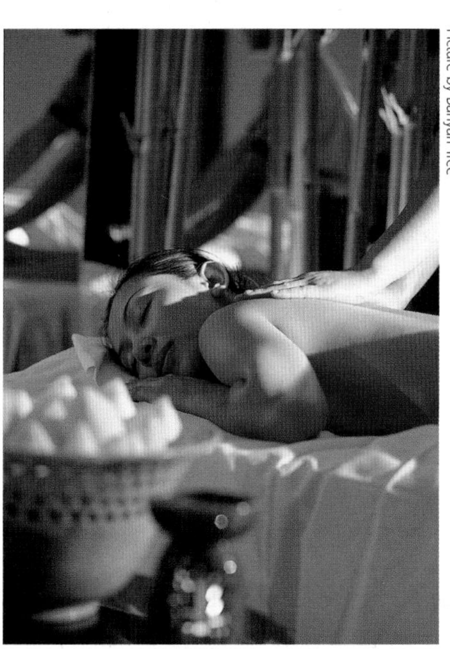
Picture by Banyan Tree

A brush and tone is a great way to prepare the skin before a massage

LINKED TREATMENTS

Exfoliation is a very popular spa treatment as it is so beneficial when carried out before other body treatments, particularly:

- massage
- envelopments
- pedicures
- self-tanning.

the wet plinth room, ONE Spa Edinburgh

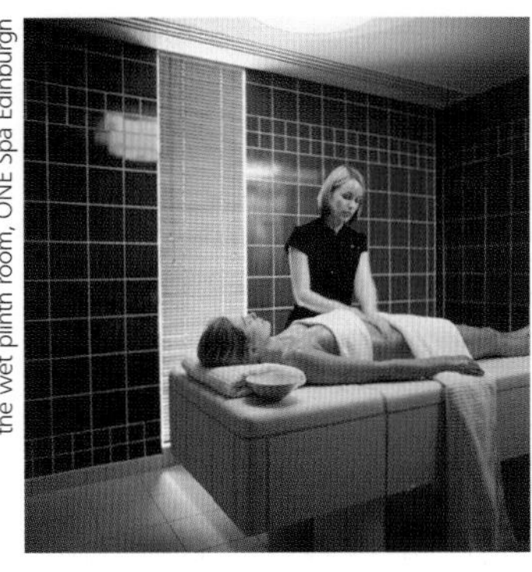

A salt rub/glow treatment

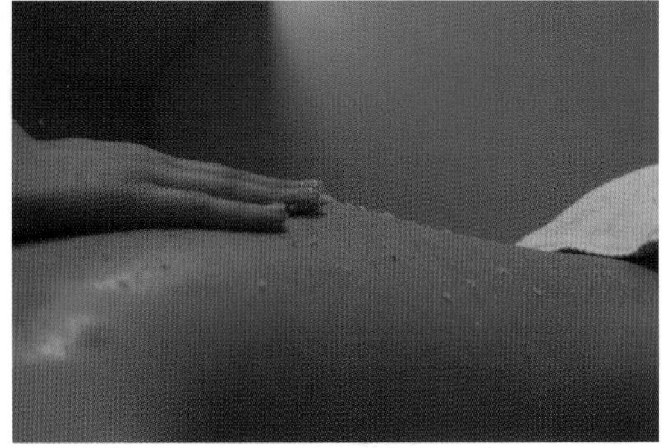

A salt rub leaves the skin 'glowing'

Salt rub/salt glow

A combination of sea salt, essential oil and water is used. The mixture is rubbed all over the body, paying particular attention to areas of rough skin (knees, elbows, etc.). Be careful to check that the client doesn't have any cuts or abrasions as the salt would sting. The client then showers and hydrating body cream or oil is applied. This treatment literally leaves the client 'glowing'.

Dulse scrub

A body scrub using dulse seaweed. The effect is to leave the skin very clean, soft, smooth and re-mineralized.

Picture by Banyan Tree

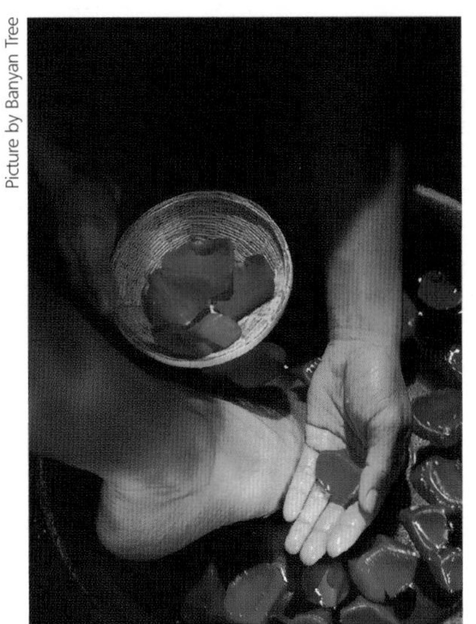

BODY ENVELOPMENTS (WRAPS)

There are a variety of envelopment and wrap treatments available, each with specific products and active ingredients. Some procedures involve applying the product directly onto the skin, then wrapping the client. Others instruct the therapist to soak bandages in the product, then wrap the client with the damp material. Depending on the product and technique used, the 'wrapping' could be with linen bandages, plastic sheeting, foil or blankets, while a variety of products are used on the skin, commonly using clay, seaweed or essential oils as active ingredients. Most systems suggest body brushing at the start of the treatment, and involve covering the client up snugly to keep them warm and maintain the heat within the 'wrap'.

LINKED PRODUCTS

Exfoliation

Products that should be available for the client to purchase in the spa:

- body wash/foam
- body scrub
- body brush
- loofah mitt
- body oil/cream
- available from reception: bathrobes, slippers, towels, eye masks, toilet bags, oil burners, candles, vitamins, etc.

General uses of envelopments

- Temporary inch loss, due to physical pressure from the bandages.
- Relaxation.
- To improve skin appearance – active ingredients are absorbed.

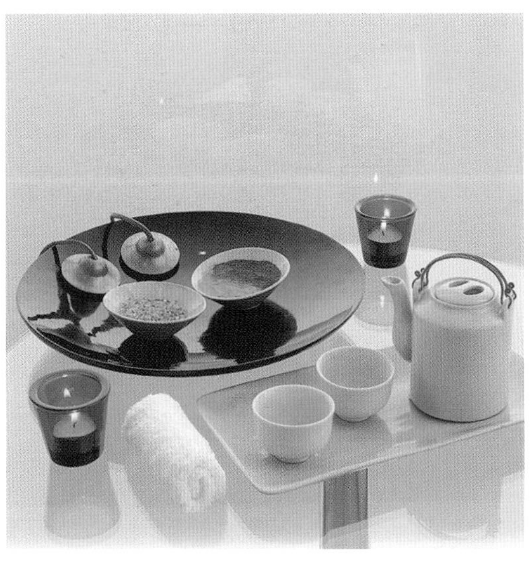

Ensure you have everything prepared before you start the treatment

TERMINOLOGY

Envelopment usually refers to a treatment where the body is wrapped fully – the limbs are not individually wrapped, but together with the body. This is usually carried out for de-toxifying, and skin conditioning purposes.

Wrap usually refers to a treatment where each limb is tightly wrapped or bandaged seperately. The purpose is usually for inch loss and fluid reduction.

- For non-medical swelling (oedema) such as that caused by gravity.
- As part of a cellulite programme.
- Re-mineralize the body– active ingredients are absorbed into a warm moist skin.

General effects of envelopment treatments

- Rise in body temperature.
- Increase in perspiration – cleansing effect.
- Increase in blood circulation – improves nourishment to the cells of the body.
- Increase in lymphatic circulation – excess fluid, waste products and toxins are removed.
- Increase in pulse rate.
- Increase in circulation to the skin – improves function and appearance of the skin.
- A warm skin more readily absorbs active ingredients.
- The warmth created helps muscles to relax.

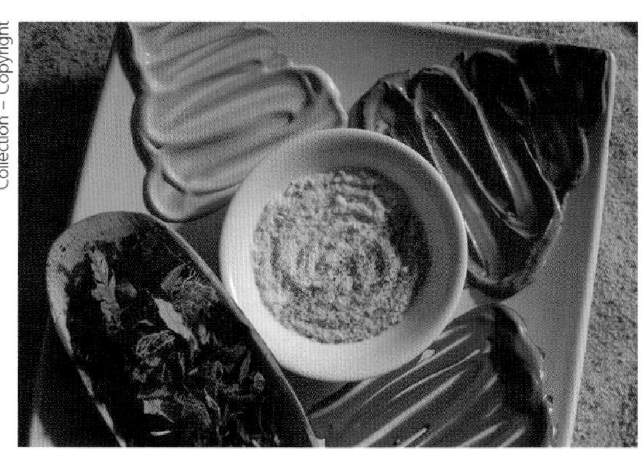

A variety of muds may be used in envelopment treatments

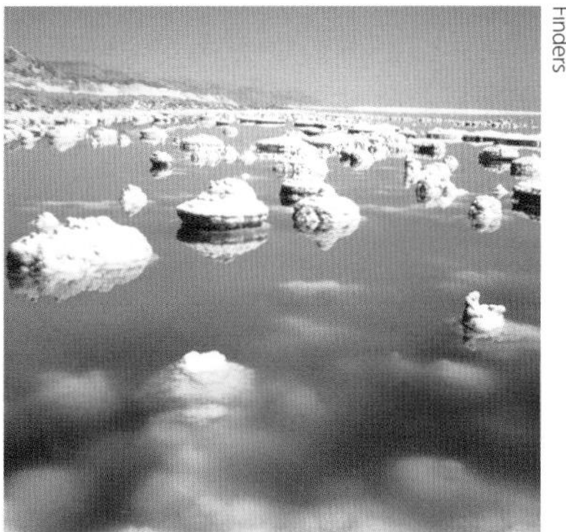

Dead Sea mud can be used as an active ingredient in envelopment treatments

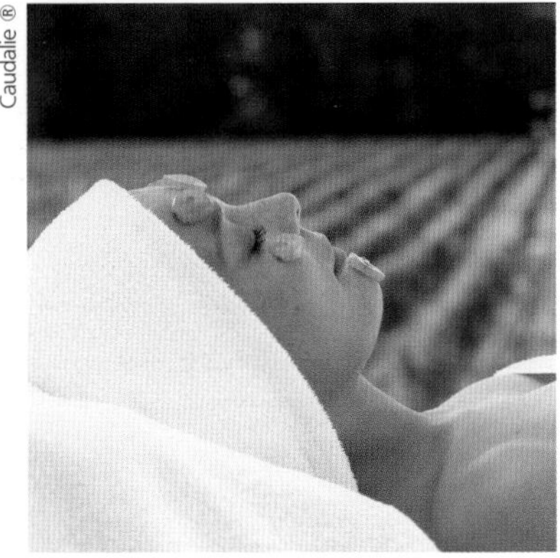

The range of active ingredients and products used for envelopment/wraps:

Active ingredient	*Use/benefit*
Chalk	Finer than mud, and very absorbing, making it ideal for oilier skins
Silt	Inland lakes provide silt that is rich in salts and minerals, especially beneficial for skin conditions, e.g. psoriasis
Peat	Very high in amino acids, stimulates autonomic nervous system and regenerates the skin
Dead Sea mud	Mineral content increases energy, improves gland functions and detoxifies and relaxes the body
Fango mud	High mineral, vitamin and trace element content. Nourishing, healing and detoxifying
Algae/seaweed	Deep cleaning and detoxifying
Herbs and flowers	Revitalizing and soothing
Hay	Cleansing, and gently stimulates blood circulation. Benefits rheumatic conditions, improves immune system
Wine	Grape polyphenols counteract free radicals, stimulating circulation and improving the immune system
Coconut	Rich in vitamins, very cleansing and moisturizing. Ideal ingredient to combine with fragrant oils, flowers and herbs
Milk products	Very rich in vitamins, and contains calcium, magnesium, potassium and sodium. Can improve sensitive, dry and stressed skins.

FACT

Seaweed is often categorized into the following groups:

- red (rhodophyta)
- green (chlorophyta)
- brown (phaeophyta)
- blue (cyanophyta).

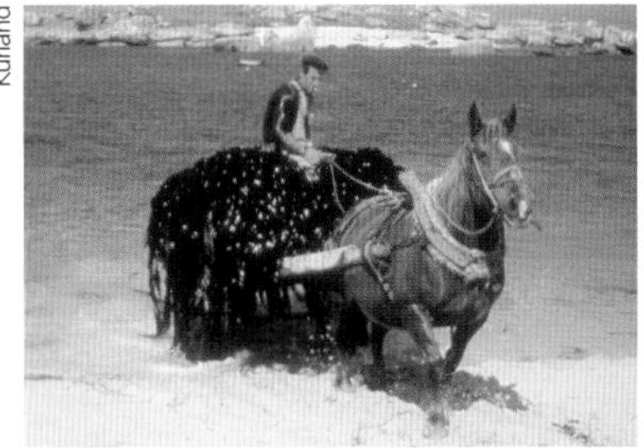

Seaweed is used in a range of different body treatments, including envelopments

FACT

Seaweed is often used as a nutritional supplement. Spirulina is found in the salt lakes of North America and often referred to as a 'super food' because of its high nutritional content.

Seaweed

The sea is a rich source of nutrients that have a beneficial effect on the body. There are over 20 000 different types of seaweed, most contain proteins, minerals and trace elements that can be used in a variety of treatments. The seaweed releases the active ingredients into the water or product and this in turn is absorbed by the body. Seaweed can be used in a range of treatments such as specialized body treatments, bath soaks and envelopment/wrap treatments.

Many products use the following ingredients for specific effects:

- Sea fennel – to cleanse the colon and help constipation.
- Sea buckthorn – to detox and help improve cellulite conditions.
- Bladderwrack sea kelp – to improve fluid retention.
- Fucus – detoxifies, helps eliminate toxins and improves fluid retention.
- Laminaria algae – aids fat absorption and moisturizes/protects the skin.

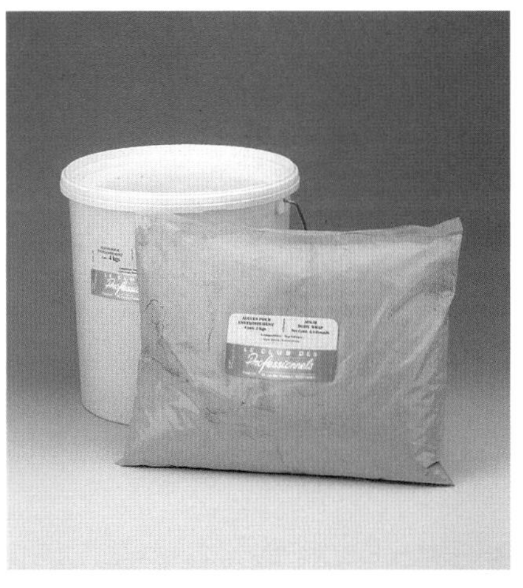

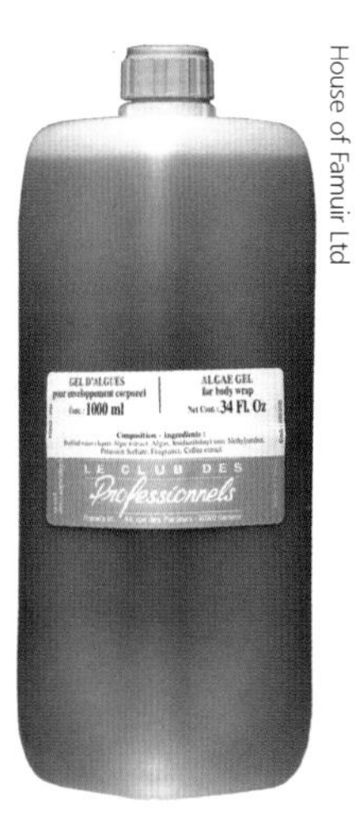

House of Famuir Ltd

There are a variety of products available that use seaweed as the active ingredient

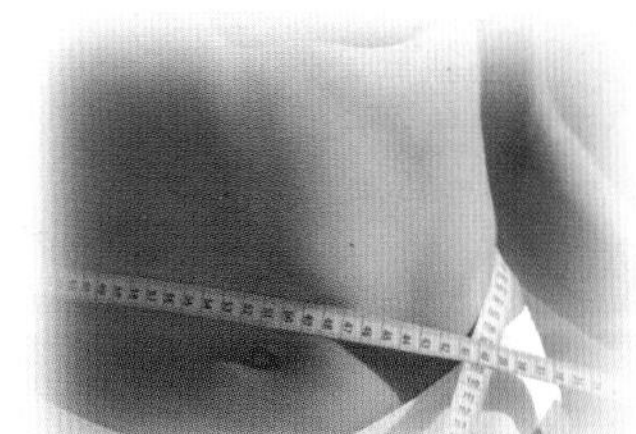

House of Famuir Ltd

A 'wrap' treatment is often used for inch loss

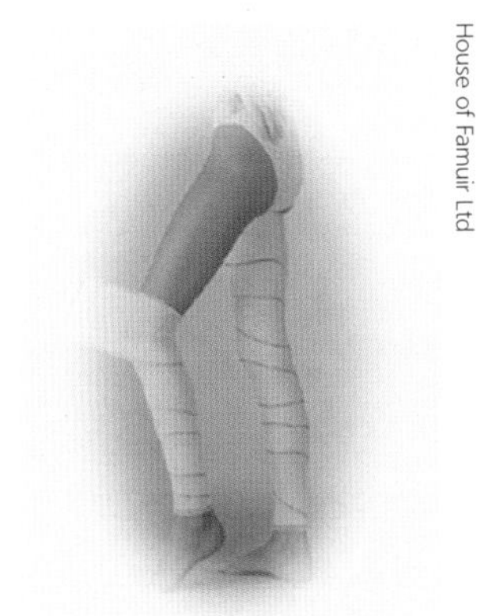

House of Famuir Ltd

Wraps can involve fabric bandages or . . .

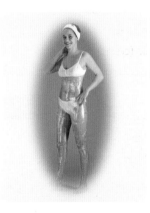

House of Famuir Ltd

. . . cellophane bandages

RECEPTION

A client can have body envelopment treatments up to 3 times each week, if part of a course of treatments. Courses are often designed as part of a slimming or re-contouring programme, and may include 10 treatments over 5–6 weeks. The inch loss effect of the treatment usually lasts 3–5 days, depending on the client's circumstances. This effect works as an incentive to motivate the client, as well as helping circulation and improving removal of waste products and toxins. The treatment usually lasts approximately an hour.

SIGNATURE TREATMENT

S

The Spa, Sandy Lane, Barbados

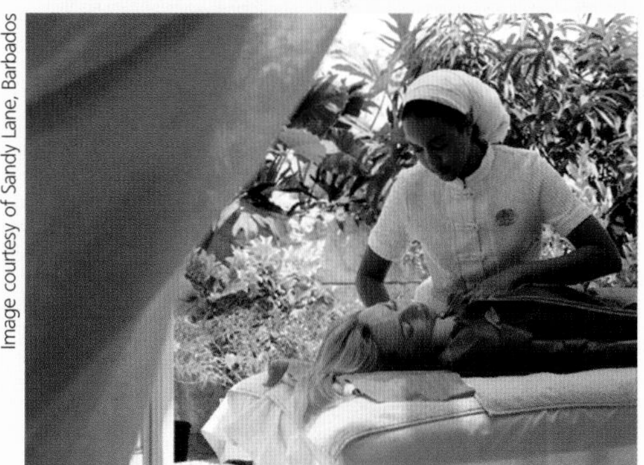

Image courtesy of Sandy Lane, Barbados

A body envelopment treatment

'Cooling Envelopment (45 mins). A soothing and cooling mixture of ingredients containing Lavender and Chamomile are applied to help ease discomfort caused by over exposure to the sun. Relax, as the whole body is gently enveloped in banana leaves, feel the heat slowly seep through your sensitised skin as you enjoy a therapeutic head massage. The treatment concludes with an application of a light, moisturising balm to calm and nourish the skin and leave the body totally relaxed.'

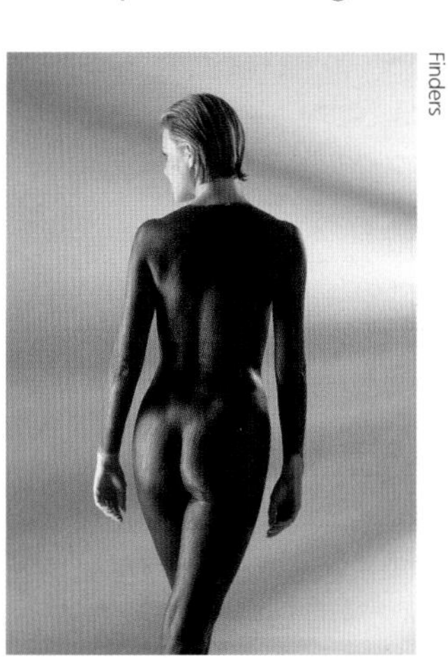

Finders

Mud envelopment treatment

EQUIPMENT LIST

- consultation/record card
- protective sheet for covering treatment couch
- 2 large towels
- 3 small towels
- 2 pieces of foil
- disposable paper briefs
- foot bootees
- cotton wool – dry and damp
- body brush
- bowl and spatula
- kettle of hot water
- active concentrate/cream
- seaweed body mask powder
- burner/candle
- duvet/blanket

Contra-indications to envelopment

Total contra-indications	*With medical approval*	*Localized*
Fever	Pregnancy	Undiagnosed lumps and bumps
Contagious or infectious diseases	Cardio vascular conditions, e.g. thrombosis, phlebitis, hypertension, hypotension, heart conditions	Varicose veins
Under the influence of drugs or alcohol	Diabetes	Cuts, bruises, abrasions
Recent operations	Any condition already being treated by another practitioner	Sunburn
Neuritis	Medical oedema	Areas of undiagnosed pain
Skin diseases	Osteoporosis	
Thyroid problems	Arthritis	
Allergies to seafood/ iodine	Epilepsy	
	Cancer	

PREPARATION OF THE CLIENT

HEALTH AND SAFETY !

Disposable paper briefs should be available to ensure a hygienic treatment. Make sure you get a variety of sizes, as nothing is more off-putting for the client than if they are too tight or, worse still, they won't fit at all.

HEALTH AND SAFETY !

Do a patch test to make sure the client isn't allergic to any of the active ingredients in the envelopment products. Apply a small amount in the crook of the elbow. If they experience redness, itching and swelling, they should not have the treatment.

- A bathing costume may be worn, or disposable briefs can be provided.
- All jewellery must be removed.
- The spa therapist must know if the body wrap contains iodine, as some clients have an allergy to it. If unsure, perform a skin test on the client using some of the product/active ingredient.
- The room must be warm, as the client soon cools down when having an envelopment treatment, even if the product is warm to begin with. The room should also smell fragrant and have soothing background music.
- Make sure you have sufficient bandages or wrapping material all ready prepared, these may need to be soaked in the active ingredient.

LINKED TREATMENTS 

A variety of treatments could be promoted to complement a seaweed envelopment/wrap, such as:

- seaweed/herbal bath (before)
- body exfoliation (before)
- dry float (when wrap is on)
- aroma-massage with pre-blended oils (after)
- facial (after).

STEP-BY-STEP: Procedure for an envelopment treatment

Treatment time: approximately 1 hour.

1 Complete a full consultation with the client, ensuring the treatment is ideally suited and safe for the individual.

2 Check contra-indications.

3 Prepare the treatment room – all equipment, towels, products, burner, soothing music, etc.

4 Prepare the couch with a sheet of foil, matt side facing upwards.

5 Client lies face up on the couch, cover with blankets for warmth and protect their hair with a towel.

6 Drape a large towel over one side of the body. Body brush the front surface of the exposed side of the body and apply the active concentrate/cream to the skin. Repeat on the opposite side of the body.

7 Cover the front of the body, turn the client over and repeat on the back surface of the body.

8 Keep the client warm whilst you mix the seaweed powder with the hot water to make a thick mud consistency. Test the temperature on the back of your hand to make sure it is an ideal temperature.

9 Adjust towel so it is draped over the buttock area. Apply the seaweed mask quickly to the back area and backs of the arms. Then continue to apply the mask to the back of each leg, covering the area from the buttock to the ankle.

10 Assist the client to turn over, placing arms close to the body. A small towel may be draped across the bust area.

11 Apply the seaweed mask to the arms, chest, abdomen and legs – working quickly so that the mask is still warm.

12 Place a large sheet of foil over the body, and tuck in carefully to seal in the heat. Bootees can cover the feet, and a duvet or blankets cover the entire body.

13 The client relaxes for 20 minutes, meanwhile the therapist stays in the room, and may apply a soothing eye mask whilst performing a light head massage.

14 Assist the client to free their feet and sit up on the bed, help them to their feet and support them in walking to the shower.

15 Hold onto the foil as the client enters the shower. Whilst the client is showering, prepare the couch.

16 Client returns to the treatment couch and lies face down, covered by a large towel.

17 Uncover one leg and massage an appropriate cream/oil into the entire area. Repeat on other leg, and then onto the back area.

18 Client turns over to face upwards, and is covered for warmth. Uncover one arm and massage the cream/oil into the area. Repeat on the other arm, chest, abdomen and both legs.

19 Allow the client to rest on the couch for at least 5 minutes before going through the recommended homecare routine.

HEALTH AND SAFETY !

Always check with your client whether they have any allergies to seafood/seaweed/iodine, and, where appropriate, carry out a patch test to ensure there will not be an allergic reaction.

SPA TIP ★

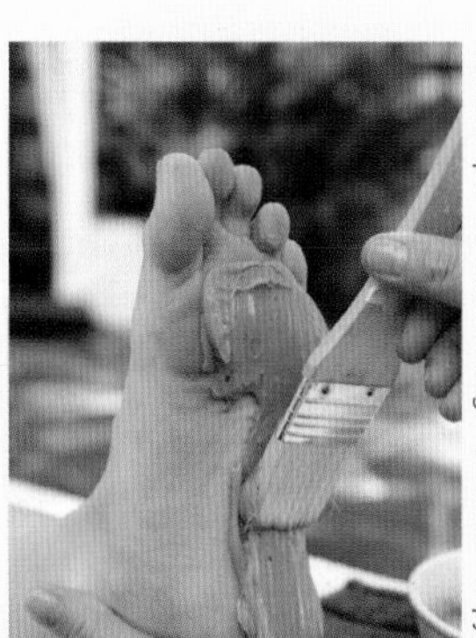

Exclusive Spas of Australia. Image Collection – Copyright

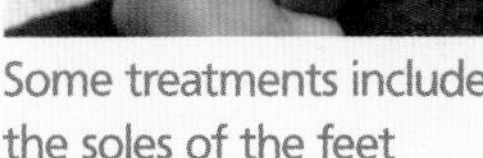

Some treatments include the soles of the feet

Some envelopment treatments keep the feet free; if appropriate then give a foot massage during the treatment.

Photos taken in Ki Day Spa

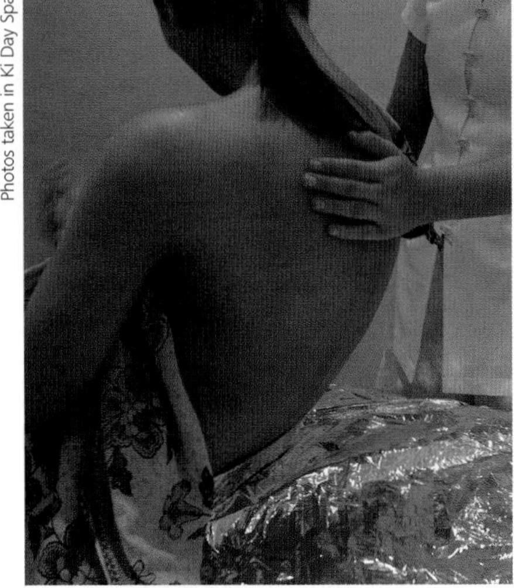
Assist the client onto the bed

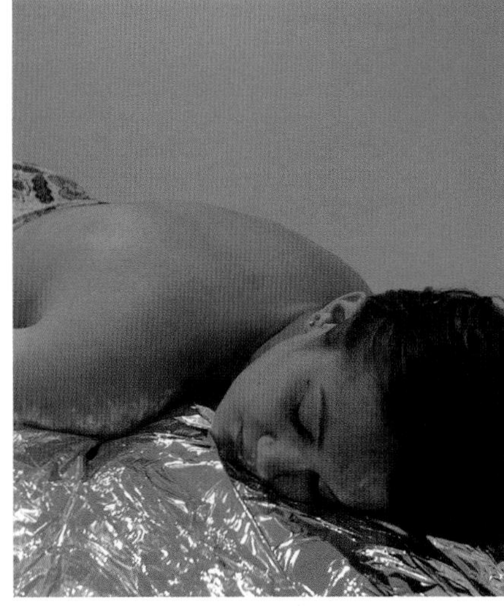
The client lies on the foil

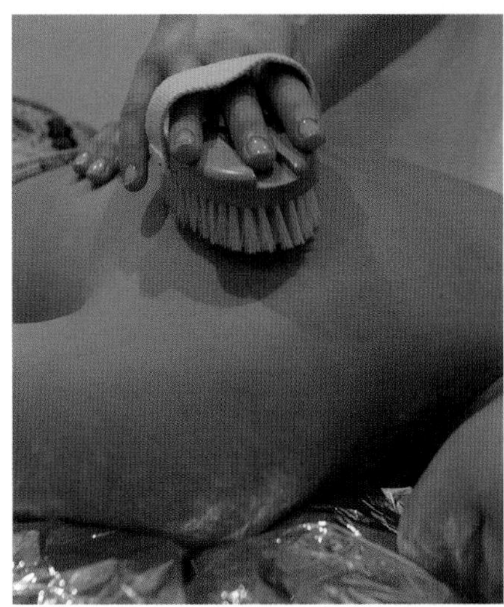
Body brush the area

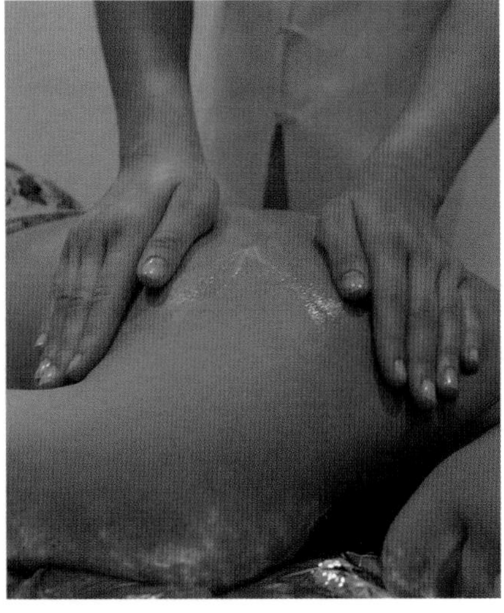
Apply the active concentrate/cream

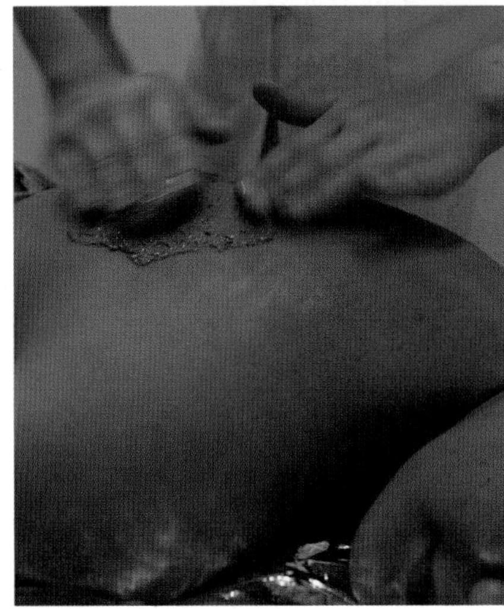
Quickly apply the warm mud

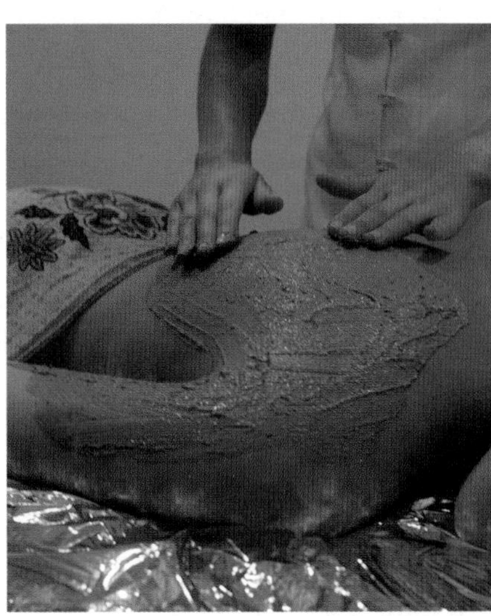
Ensure the mud is evenly applied over the entire area

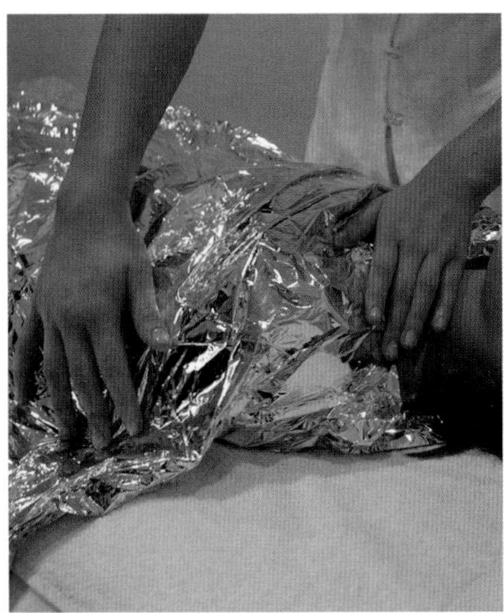
Cover the body with the foil

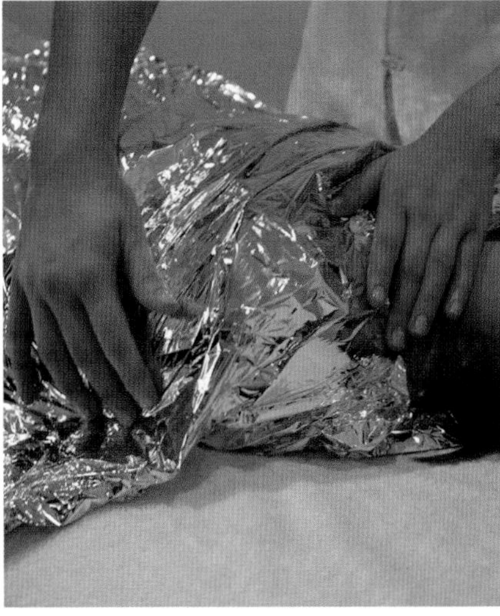
Tuck the foil in carefully to seal the heat in the 'envelope'

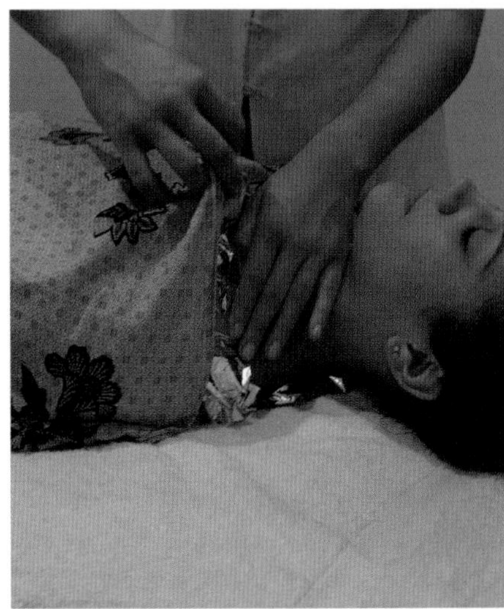
Cover with blankets or sheets to keep the client warm

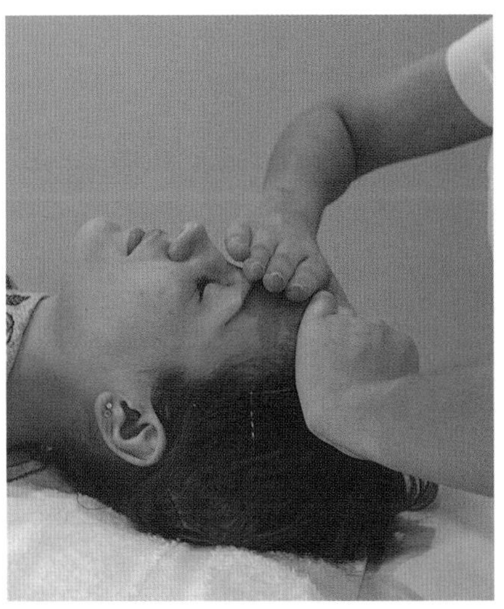
A facial massage can be carried out while the client rests

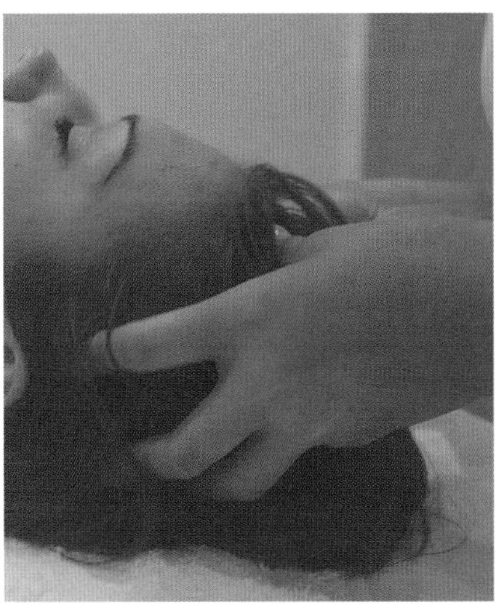
If there is time, a head massage can also be included

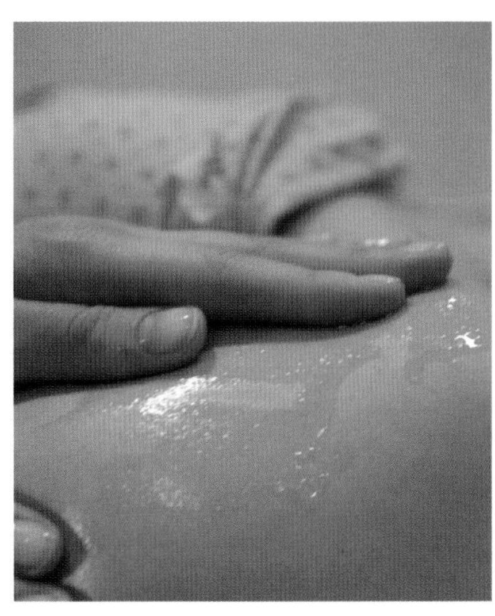
After the shower, massage the appropriate oil or cream into the skin

THAI HERBAL HEAT PACK

From as early as the fourteenth century, herbal heat packs have been used in Thailand to soothe aches, pains and bruises – today they are used in many spas to relieve pain and inflammation.

Herbs that can be used include:

- turmeric (anti-bacterial)
- camphor (cleansing)
- lemon grass (astringent)
- prai-thai herb (relieves aching muscles, sore joints).

HEALTH AND SAFETY !

Always fully prepare the shower for the client – set the water temperature, fresh towels, bath mat.

SPA TIP

In some beach spas they are using cloth bundles of sand to exfoliate the skin. In others they are packing their bundles with herbs, so that nutrients are delivered to the skin.

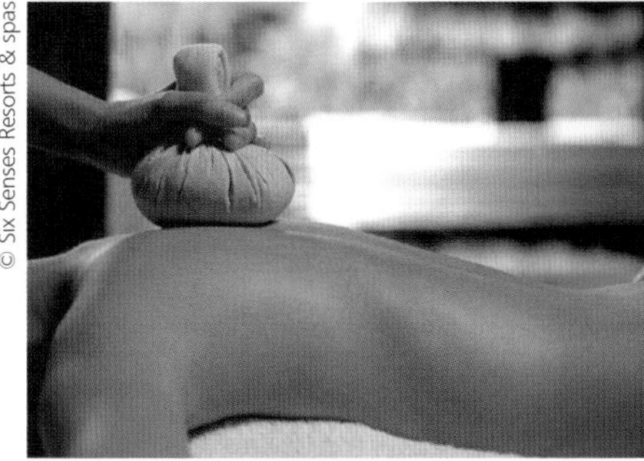

Thai herbal heat pack

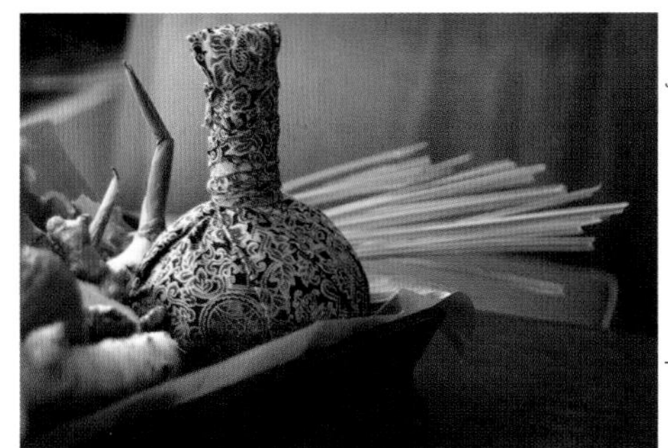

Ingredients for the heat pack

SPA PACKAGE

- spa consultation
- 'experience' shower
- algae body scrub
- seaweed envelopment/wrap treatment
- dry float treatment
- pre-blended oil massage
- relaxation room
- water/fresh fruit available

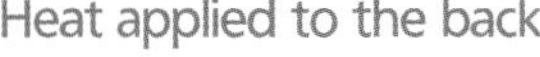

LINKED PRODUCTS

Photographs provided for use, by kind permission of the Scotsman Hotel, Edinburgh

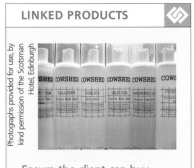

Ensure the client can buy products for home use

- body brush
- bath soak
- exfoliation cream/gel
- active oil/capsules
- toning body cream
- eye mask
- burner/candles

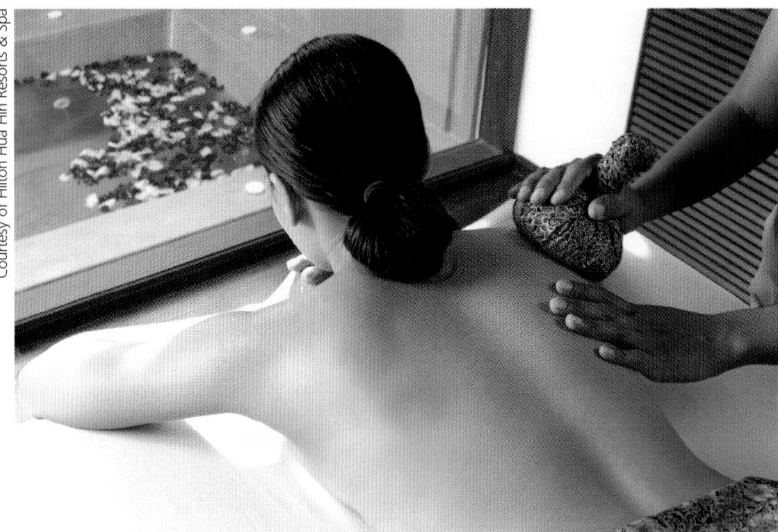

Courtesy of Hilton Hua Hin Resorts & Spa

Heat applied to the back

The herbs are packed into muslin to form a parcel roughly the size of a large grapefruit. A steamer is then used to heat the pack, and when sufficiently warm the pack is placed on the skin for a short time (30–60 seconds). The normal precautions and contra-indications to heat treatments apply, please refer to chapter 7 for details.

AFTERCARE

The client should be recommended to:

- Use retail products to continue the treatment in between visits to the spa.
- Drink plenty of water.
- Eat healthily, including unrefined, raw foods.
- Adopt a well-balanced lifestyle.

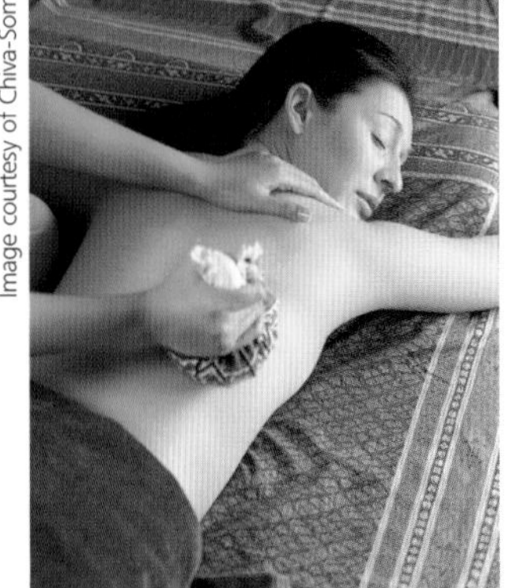

Image courtesy of Chiva-Som

Thai heat pack treatment, Chiva-Som

SIGNATURE TREATMENT

Chiva-Som, Thailand

'South Indian Body Pampering: Using three therapists, this therapy originating from Kerala in southern India is Chiva-Som's most indulgent experience. Two therapists massage warm aromatic oils into the body while a third therapist ensures the oil is kept at a comfortable temperature and spreads powdered Ayurvedic herbs over the body which results in a full body exfoliation. Steamed herb infused towels and herbal poultices are then placed over the body to encourage circulation and a profound sense of relaxation. Traditionally this treatment is used for improving skin complexion and skin problems, easing joint complaints and insomnia and improving fatigue 1 hour'.

SPA PROFILE

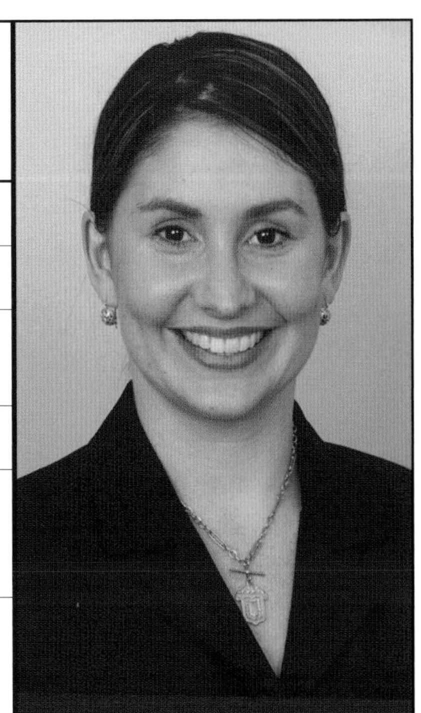

Name: Dr Angela Derks

Position: Area Spa Manager

Establishment: Six Senses Spa, The Evason Resort and Spa and Evason Hideaway, Hua Hin, Thailand

Products used: Sodashi, Decleor, Six Senses, organic ingredients from the Evason's herb garden.

Number of staff/roles: Spa Manager; Assistant Spa Manager; Spa Coordinator; 1 senior spa receptionist; 3 spa receptionists; senior spa therapist/trainer; 11 spa therapists; 3 trainee therapists; 3 spa attendants.

Training/experience: Massage diplomas/beauty therapy/paramedical aesthetician qualifications; marketing/business qualifications; naturopathy/herbalism/nutrition/ homeopathy/aromatherapy qualifications; extensive experience in Australia and Thailand.

Main responsibilities: Recruitment and selection of staff; developing new techniques and treatments; promotion and marketing; developing new 'spa suites' and treatment menus for forthcoming resort expansion.

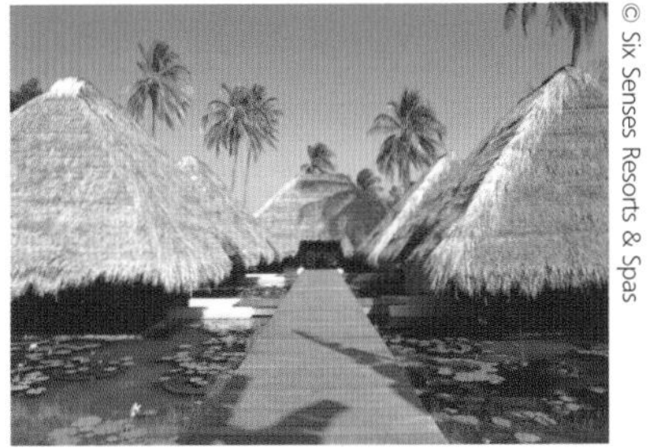

Best parts of the job: The people – my team, resort staff and our valued guests.

Developing people, on so many levels. Developing guests to be able to relax or to merely feel better. Developing spa attendants to realise they can become a spa manager if they work hard and have the right attitude and initiative.

Working in such a fantastic establishment as the Evason, with its culture of service excellence and environmental responsibility.

I love constantly developing new treatments and techniques that incorporate holistic methods.

Secrets of a successful spa therapist:

Listening.

Intuition.

Initiative and highly motivated to care and heal.

A genuine, natural, nurturing nature.

Highly skilled and confident in their techniques.

Assessment of knowledge and understanding

When you have some free time, test your understanding and knowledge by answering the following questions. Do this at regular intervals and it will reinforce your learning and help you retain the knowledge, so you are able to perform better in your assessments.

Organizational and legal requirements

1 What would you do to ensure the ambience of the spa environment is ideal for envelopment and exfoliation treatments?

Client contact and consultation

1 Why would you encourage and allow time for questions during the initial consultation?

2 Why must you never leave a client unattended during an envelopment treatment?

3 Why is it important to protect a client's modesty during an exfoliation treatment?

4 List five contra-indications that would prevent a client from having an exfoliation treatment.

Equipment and materials

1 How would you ensure the envelopment treatment is hygienic?

2 Describe how you would ensure you measured the client accurately before and after an inch-loss wrap treatment.

Exfoliation

1 Give three natural products that can be used in an exfoliation treatment.

2 What is brossage?

3 Explain what a Javanese lulur treatment is.

4 What are the benefits of body brushing the client prior to an exfoliation treatment?

5 List five contra-indications to an exfoliation treatment.

Envelopment

1 What benefits does seaweed have on the body?

2 What are the effects of an 'inch loss' wrap treatment?

3 List five precautions necessary when giving an envelopment treatment.

Aftercare advice

1 List four other treatments you could promote and 'link' with an envelopment treatment.

2 List five products you could suggest for use at home that would benefit the client after a scrub or envelopment treatment.

chapter 15

Consultation and spa etiquette

BT15

Assist with spa treatments

BT17

Provide head and body massage treatment

BT29

Provide specialist spa treatments

BT20

Provide Indian head massage treatment

BT21

Provide massage using pre-blended Gromatherapy oils

Learning objectives

This chapter covers the consultation process and how the therapist can best assess the client's needs.

It describes the skills and knowledge necessary to enable you to:

- **identify an understand the client's lifestyle and physical condition**
- **ensure the objectives of the treatment meet the client's needs**
- **recognize contra-indications and restrictions**
- **ensure client confidentiality is maintained**
- **establish a treatment plan**
- **ensure that client records are accurate and up-to-date**
- **encourage clients to ask questions and clarify any points**

When providing spa therapy services it is important to use the skills you have learnt in the following core units:

G1 Ensure your own actions reduce risks to health and safety

G6 Promote additional products or services to clients

G11 Contribute to the financial effectiveness of the business

INTRODUCTION

As the spa industry is growing so too are the numbers of new guests who are visiting a spa for the first time. These clients need to be put at ease when they schedule an appointment and arrive for their first treatment, as it will make their experience the more enjoyable. Professional spa receptionists and therapists will be aware of the trepidation some clients feel on entering a spa and the importance of putting them at ease before bombarding them with personal questions during the consultation process. Having some guidelines on spa etiquette and the use of facilities will make their spa experience more enjoyable.

SPA TIP 

A professional consultation will lead to the client being confident in the therapist and their treatment, they will be able to relax, you will get them coming back for more treatments and also recommending the spa to friends.

CONSULTATION AND RECORD CARD

When evaluating a client for spa therapies one of the most important references is the client's consultation and record card. A record card should be filled in for all spa treatments, as it is important that we retain as much information as we can about the client's lifestyle, emotional and physical state and any medical problems that may contra-indicate a treatment.

Spas can deal with gaining client information before a treatment in a number of different ways. Some spas may send out a questionnaire before the client's appointment to check that there are no medical contra-indications to treatments, and if there are any concerns a doctor's approval can be sought first. Other spas ask the client to fill out a medical history form when they arrive at reception for their first appointment, and some establishments prefer the therapist to speak to the client and fill in the record card whilst in the treatment room.

All information that is taken from the client should be stored securely in accordance with the Data Protection Act 1998 and their medical history reviewed briefly before every treatment and any changes recorded onto the card.

Questioning techniques

The client should be greeted by the therapist in a professional manner and be made to feel at ease whilst the therapist goes through the record card. When filling in the record card use open questions with a client to encourage them to give a more detailed answer than just 'yes' or 'no'. Questions which begin with 'how', 'when' or 'what' require the client to give at least a few words. This can lead the therapist into further questions and a more detailed account of the client's needs. For example: 'What spa treatments have you previously experienced?', 'Which areas of your body would you like to improve?', 'What are your expectations of the treatment?', 'How would you like to improve your skincare routine?'

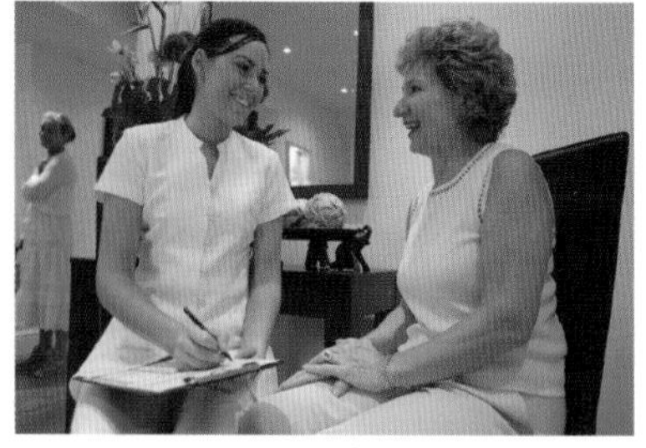

Client consultation

HEALTH AND SAFETY 

Do not risk aggravating any physical defect or interfere with a medical treatment without the doctor's consent. If in doubt always get the client to seek authorization from their doctor before giving any treatment.

SPA TIP 

Studies show that a satisfied client will tell three friends of their satisfaction, while a dissatisfied client will tell twelve people about their dissatisfaction.

ACTIVITY 

Make a list of the different types of questioning techniques that can be used in a consultation and their relevance.

A record card should contain the following information:

- Client's personal details – name, address, telephone number, email address, etc.
- Doctor's details – you may need to contact the doctor for approval prior to treatment; the client may become ill whilst having treatments.
- Client's lifestyle – stress levels, sleep patterns, exercise routine, work commitments – any problems here may be the reason they are coming for treatments.
- Diet – types of food eaten regularly, how much water, alcohol, etc., is drunk during the day, eating between meals – all of these factors will affect the client's physical wellbeing and their condition could be due to incorrect eating habits.
- Smoking – this has an effect on health and fitness levels.
- Face and body assessment – over or underweight, poor posture, muscle tone, cellulite, skin type – these will give an impression as to how healthy the client is, and again may be affecting their condition.
- Medical history – it is most important that you check for any contra-indications (as mentioned earlier) which may restrict or prevent a treatment and the products you choose.
- General health assessment – excellent, good, bad, average.
- Any additional comments – these may come from the client through your questioning or observations you have made through the consultation.
- Treatment plan – the treatment that the client is having and any recommendation for further treatments you may have made.
- Date of treatment.
- Products used – it is very important that any other therapist who treats this client knows the products used and why they were selected.
- Therapists' observations – how they felt the treatment went, any reactions/comments the client had, any retail sales that were made.
- Client's signature – it is very important that you get the client to sign the card to verify that the information they have given is accurate. If you do not do this then it leaves the client the opportunity, if anything goes wrong after a treatment, to sue the spa.

Ideally a client should follow their treatment plan, attend regularly and follow all your aftercare advice, but most clients do not fall into this category and your treatment plan will need to be adapted to suit the client's individual needs.

CONSULTATION CHECKLIST

✔ quiet private area	✔ postural check
✔ client privacy	✔ fill in record card
✔ plenty of time	✔ client signed record card
✔ client comfortable and at ease	✔ check contra-indications
✔ aims of treatment/outcome	✔ explain contra-actions
✔ treatment plan	✔ client questions

HEALTH AND SAFETY !

All record cards should be stored away in a locked box or metal filing cabinet and only be accessible by the therapists and receptionist. You must be aware of your responsibilities under the Data Protection Act 1998.

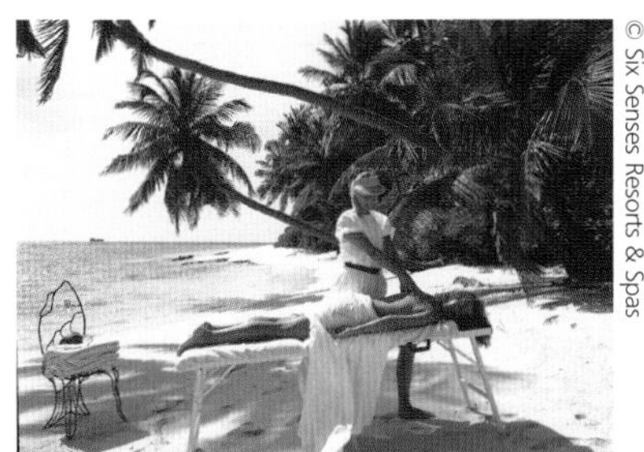

Outdoor treatment, Six Senses Spa

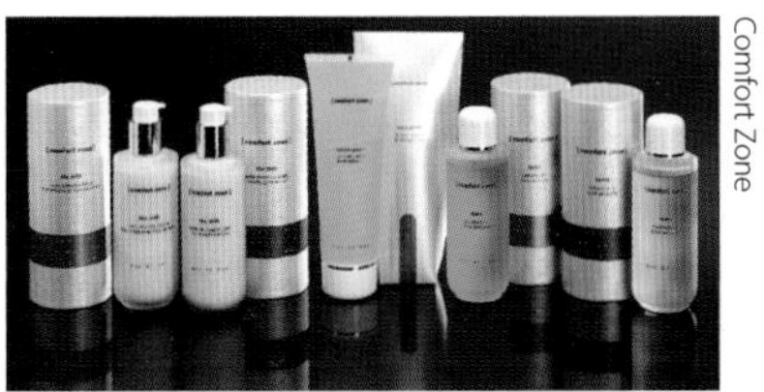

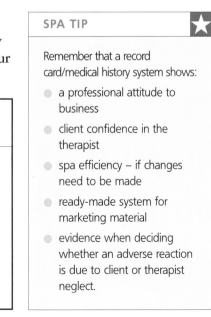

Range of treatment products

SPA TIP 

Remember that a record card/medical history system shows:

- a professional attitude to business
- client confidence in the therapist
- spa efficiency – if changes need to be made
- ready-made system for marketing material
- evidence when deciding whether an adverse reaction is due to client or therapist neglect.

SPA WORKS

Date	Spa therapist name	
Client name		Date of birth
Address		Postcode
Evening phone number	Day phone number	
Name of doctor	Doctor's address and phone number	

Related medical history (conditions that may restrict or prohibit treatment application)

Are you taking any medication (this may affect the sensitivity of the skin and reaction to the treatment)

CONTRA-INDICATIONS REQUIRING MEDICAL REFERRAL

(Prevent spa treatment application)
(Temporary CI are listed*)

- ☐ bacterial infection, e.g. impetigo*
- ☐ viral infection, e.g. verruca*
- ☐ fungal infection, e.g. tinea corporis/pedis*
- ☐ skin disorders
- ☐ skin disease, e.g. malignant melanoma
- ☐ high or low blood pressure
- ☐ heart disease/disorder ☐ recent scar tissue
- ☐ medical conditions under supervision
- ☐ history of thrombosis/embolism
- ☐ dysfunction of the nervous system
- ☐ epilepsy ☐ respiratory conditions
- ☐ liver/kidney or pancreatic conditions
- ☐ lymphatic disorders ☐ recent wax depilation/epilation
- ☐ recent alcohol consumption*
- ☐ recent heavy meal – temporary*
- ☐ recent active exercise – temporary*
- ☐ recent UV exposure – temporary*

LIFESTYLE

- ☐ dietary and fluid intake ☐ exercise habits
- ☐ smoking habits ☐ sleep patterns
- ☐ hobbies, interests, means of relaxation

EQUIPMENT/MATERIALS

- ☐ sauna
- ☐ steam room ☐ steam cabinet
- ☐ flotation bath ☐ flotation pool dry/wet
- ☐ body wrapping ☐ hydrotherapy
- ☐ relaxation room ☐ wrapping materials
- ☐ treatment products

CONTRA-INDICATIONS WHICH RESTRICT TREATMENT

(Treatment may require adaptation)

- ☐ cuts and abrasions*
- ☐ bruising and swelling*
- ☐ recent scar tissue (avoid area)
- ☐ undiagnosed lumps, bumps, swellings
- ☐ recent injuries to the treatment area*
- ☐ mild psoriasis/eczema ☐ medication
- ☐ high or low blood pressure ☐ pregnancy*
- ☐ body piercings ☐ highly anxious client
- ☐ allergies ☐ claustrophobia
- ☐ menstruation* ☐ migraine*

*temporary

TREATMENT OBJECTIVES

- ☐ improved skin and body condition
- ☐ slimming – improved contours
- ☐ lymphatic drainage ☐ relaxation

TREATMENT AREAS

- ☐ trunk – body wrap ☐ limbs – body wrap
- ☐ body – general

CLIENT PREPARATION

- ☐ exfoliation ☐ showering
- ☐ skin cleansing

PREPARATION FOR AND MONITORING OF TREATMENT ENVIRONMENT

- ☐ heat ☐ humidity
- ☐ water levels ☐ chemical concentrations
- ☐ treatment time ☐ ventilation
- ☐ consumables ☐ ambience of environment

Spa therapist signature (for reference)

Client signature (confirmation of details)

BODY ASSESSMENT

If the client is having body treatments then there may be specific conditions to look for which can benefit from different spa treatments and exercise programmes, these may be:

Stretch marks

These appear on the skin as long faint scars and are a result of fluctuating weight, e.g. pregnancy. They occur due to the skin breaking in the dermal layer and are often found on the tops of the legs, abdomen, breasts and upper arms.

SPA TIP 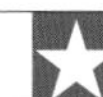

There are plenty of products and spa treatments which can improve the appearance of stretch marks and cellulite, but the client must be prepared to use the products at home to make any long-term difference.

Cellulite

Often referred to as an 'orange peel' appearance because the skin looks dimpled on the surface, it is commonly found on the bottom, thighs and knees. Quite often it is noticeable on the client when analysing the body, but it can also feel cold to the touch and if the skin is gently squeezed then lumpy nodules will be visible.

Cellulite is caused by:

- overloaded fat cells becoming compressed, which causes poor circulation to the area, resulting in poor removal of toxins and insufficient oxygen and nutrients getting to the tissues
- poor diet and a slow metabolism
- lack of exercise and a sedentary lifestyle.

This condition is not only associated with being overweight. Slim women can also suffer from cellulite, as has been recently highlighted in the media by showing pictures of celebrities appearing to be suffering with dimpled skin!

SPA TIP 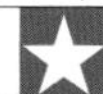

Dry skin brushing is excellent for the treatment of cellulite as it stimulates circulation and the lymphatic system to remove toxins. As homecare the client should dry brush problem areas for a few minutes before getting in the shower.

Adipose tissue

This forms the subcutaneous layer below the skin that attaches the skin to the tissues and organs beneath. It is also found among muscle fibres and around organs such as the heart. The main purpose of adipose tissue (fat) is to store fat and release it when fuel is needed by cells. It also helps to shape the body, acts as a shock absorber and helps prevent loss of body heat through the skin. On an average person, fat should account for about 10 per cent of the total body weight, but in severe obesity this may increase to 50 per cent or more. Excess fat in men tends to store around the waist area while in women it appears around the hips and thighs.

TERMINOLOGY

Manual lymphatic drainage (MLD) a type of massage where a gentle pumping action is used to help drain away pockets of water retention and toxins.

Fluid retention

Tissue fluid can accumulate due to a poor diet – one which is high in salt intake with insufficient water drunk – hormonal levels or occupational lessons if a client is standing up for long periods of time. It can be

SPA TIP 

Juniper essential oil is excellent for helping with drainage and can be used in the treatment of cellulite and fluid retention.

> **SPA TIP**
>
> Massage is very beneficial for helping to alleviate fluid retention and there are specific techniques, such as manual lymphatic drainage (MLD), which are very effective for this condition.

recognized by pressing the client's skin and checking if it remains indented and does not spring back. It is commonly found around the ankles and in the abdomen and breasts – commonly before menstruation. There is also a clinical form of oedema (swelling) which, if present, means the area must be avoided.

Poor posture

This occurs when the body is not balanced and the muscles have to work much harder to maintain an upright position. This can cause the muscles to become very tired and start to ache, and the internal organs becoming compressed can affect the digestive system and breathing.

The client's posture can be affected by:

- types of occupation
- muscular strength
- health.

Common postural faults are:

Kyphosis Round shoulders usually accompanied by the head held forward, and in old age a 'dowager's' hump can also occur. Can be caused by sitting at a desk for long periods of time or, in women, by trying to disguise a large chest or minimizing their height.

Lordosis An exaggeration of the lumbar curve which can lead to the appearance of a hollow back. The abdomen protrudes forward as does the pelvis. Can be caused by poor muscle tone of the abdomen and by carrying heavy loads with an uneven distribution of the weight.

Scoliosis A 'C' shaped curving of the spine where one shoulder is higher than the other or one hip is higher than the other. Carrying uneven loads such as shopping bags or holding children on one hip can cause this condition.

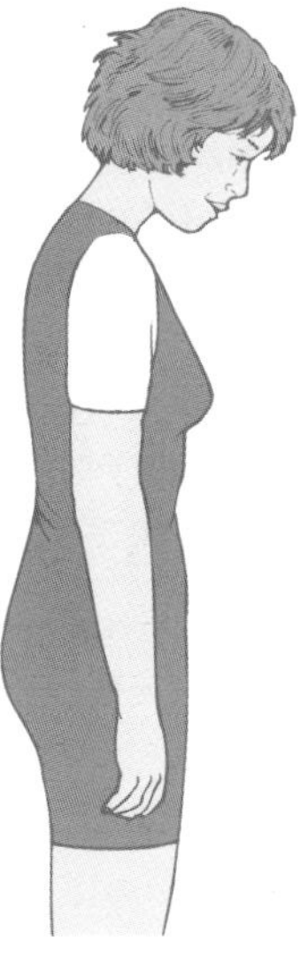

Kyphosis

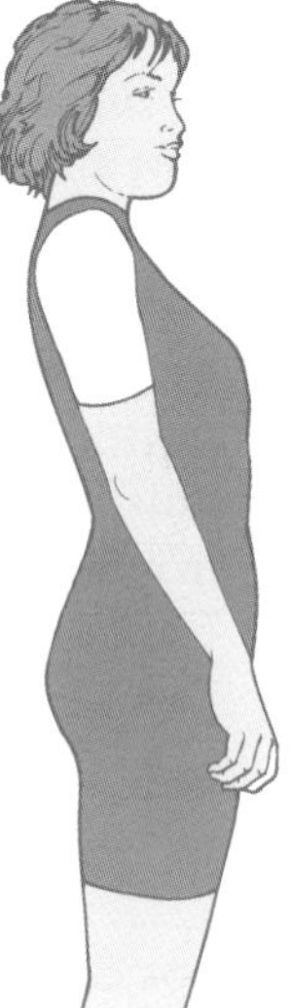

Lordosis

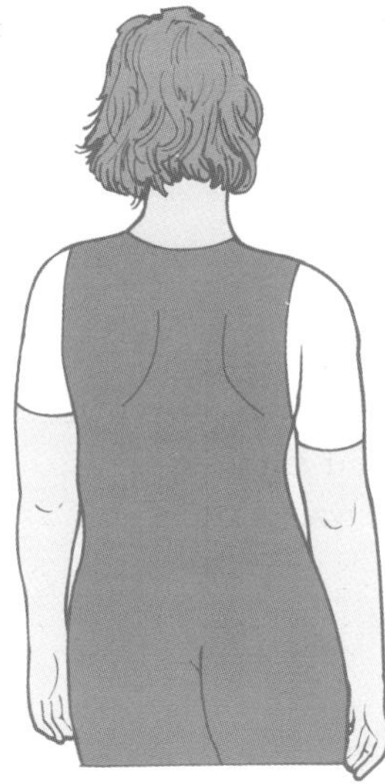

Scoliosis

Homecare advice can be given to clients, with simple exercises to try and correct the condition, but if your spa offers exercise classes such as yoga, pilates or personal training then it is important to direct the client towards the experts who will be able to devise personal correction programmes.

SPA TIP 

The **Alexander Technique** of posture alignment is taught on a one-to-one basis, where the client is re-educated to regain natural posture and use the body more efficiently. It can help with stress, breathing disorders and neck and joint pain.

SPA THERAPIST'S APPEARANCE

This must be professional at all times, no matter what the time of day or how many clients you have treated. It is essential to adhere to the following rules:

- Uniform should be clean and pressed and follow the spa's rules and regulations.
- Footwear – some spas prefer their therapists to wear flip-flops or satin slippers, or even be barefoot, to carry out treatments, as long as they are comfortable and follow the uniform guidelines for that establishment. In the UK therapists were traditionally told to wear a low white or black court shoe, but as the industry develops these ideas are changing and it is now quite often personal preference.
- Breath should be fresh, free from cigarette or strong food smells, such as garlic.
- Nails should be well manicured, short and clean with no nail varnish.
- Long hair should be tied/pinned up away from the face but still look professional.
- Make-up should be subtle as it is important for a therapist to look fresh-faced and healthy.
- Jewellery should not be worn apart from a wedding ring.

SPA TIP 

Ensure that time is set aside for getting fresh air during the day, even if it is just a quick five minute walk, as the aroma from using oils can make you a bit light-headed. Relaxation, some regular exercise and having treatments yourself are also important to ensuring that you maintain your own health and physical wellbeing.

SPA ETIQUETTE

If a client has never visited a spa before then they will appreciate guidelines and advice on what to expect, what to bring with them, and spa policies and procedures. These can be outlined in the spa brochure, website, promotional material, etc., and guidance to clients should include the following:

Appointments Always be on time for your appointments. Most spas advise guests to arrive half an hour earlier than their appointment so that they can make use of the facilities, begin to relax and familiarize themselves with their surroundings (some spas offer hydrotherapy rituals to guests such as use of the sauna and steam rooms, mineral pools, thermidarium, etc., as a pre-treatment). If you arrive late for an appointment then you may have your treatment cut short.

SPA TIP 

Ensure that you look after your own health and eat a well-balanced and nutritious diet, drink plenty of water during the day – especially after giving a massage, as you can feel quite dehydrated – and avoid drinking too much caffeine.

Making a spa appointment Try to book as far in advance as is possible to ensure that you get the date, time and therapist that you want. Always ask the receptionist if you have any queries about particular treatments or

Courtesy of the Hilton Hua Hin Resort & Spa

advice, as they will be trained and knowledgeable in all the services that the spa can offer. If you have to cancel or reschedule an appointment then most spas require at least 4 hours notice or you may be charged for the treatment.

Personal belongings Try not to bring jewellery with you on a spa visit as most spas state that they are not responsible for client's personal belongings. If staying in a destination spa or a hotel, leave all valuables in the room or hotel safe. If you have brought valuables with you make sure they are left in your locker whilst you have the treatment. Lots of clients have lost expensive jewellery by leaving them in robe pockets which end up in the laundry.

Spa attire Clients will be provided with a locker which will contain a robe and slippers for them to wear whilst in the spa and receiving treatments. If using water facilities then clients may feel comfortable bringing a bathing costume with them to use. Whilst receiving a treatment it is down to personal preference as to their attire, but some clients need reassuring that their modesty is protected at all times, and other clients feel quite comfortable being naked for a treatment! Certain spa treatments, such as Thai massage, require the client to wear loose, stretchable clothing, which is quite often provided.

Treatments for men If receiving a facial then it is advised that they have a shave at least 2 hours prior to their appointment. Some spas have communal areas and others have male and female relaxation areas, which may include sauna/steam/hydrotherapy pools, etc., for the client's comfort and privacy.

Health considerations You will have to complete a consultation card before a treatment but you may want to advise the reception when an appointment is made. These may include: high blood pressure, heart problems, allergies or pregnancy. Certain body treatments are not recommended for pregnant clients but there are specific pregnancy treatments which have been devised and are available at most spas. Always check when making an appointment.

Courtesy of Kurumba, Maldives

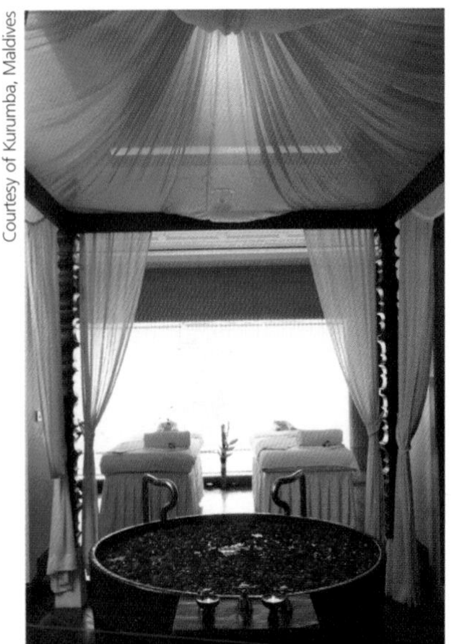

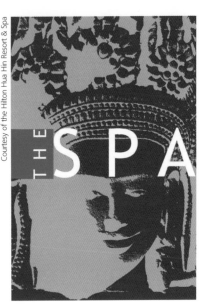

Food and drink Water and herbal/fruit teas and drinks are provided for clients during their spa visit but it is advisable that clients avoid drinking alcohol immediately before or after a treatment. If a client has just had a heavy meal then certain body treatments may need to be avoided.

Children Some spa hotels may cater for children and offer childcare facilities, but to retain a quiet, serene, relaxing environment most spas will request that children are not brought into the spa. If children under 18 are having a treatment (some spas have specific treatments designed for young girls) then the parent must sign a consent form first.

Gratuities This is usually left to the client's discretion. Most spas do not include tips on the bill, but if a client requests one can be added. Between 15 and 20 per cent is usually customary, but this may be more or less and also reflect on the quality of service that was received.

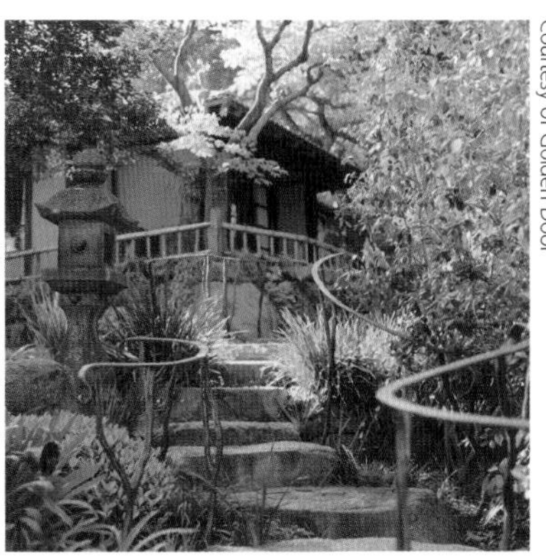
Courtesy of Golden Door

Guest room exterior, Golden Door, California

Mobile phones It is requested that clients do not bring phones or pagers into the spa. A spa visit is meant to be relaxing for the client and the idea is to switch off from the outside world and have a stress reducing experience. It is also as a courtesy to other guests.

Talking during treatments If you wish to remain silent during a treatment then the therapist will support that decision. The idea is to create a relaxing and meditative atmosphere and chattering away throughout your treatment won't allow the mind to switch off, but you may ask questions of the therapist relating to your treatment. It is the client's personal preference.

Inappropriate behaviour Therapists are part of a professional establishment and if they feel a client is behaving inappropriately then they are authorized to stop the treatment immediately.

THE CLIENT JOURNEY

A spa therapist needs to ensure the 'client journey' exceeds the client's expectations. It is important that you appreciate the importance of the five senses in each stage of the client's experience in the spa.

The five senses

Sight

The spa environment should be a total delight for the eyes. Consider every aspect; design, interior decoration, candles, soft lighting, water elements, etc. Clients can fall in love through their eyes – and you want them to return time and again to your spa.

> **TERMINOLOGY**
>
> Holistic means that you consider the complete person in the treatment of disease, often translated as the mind, body and spirit of the individual.

Smell

The 'fragrance' of a spa is very important; a smell can bring back memories and recapture experiences. Consider every fragrant step of the spa experience. Certain smells in the spa will be 'sea'-based, using algae and seaweed – these smells will invoke memories of bracing, fresh sea breezes and trips to the beach. Other smells created by aromatherapy oils, creams and candles will be more relaxing and transport the client to a peaceful, paradise-like space.

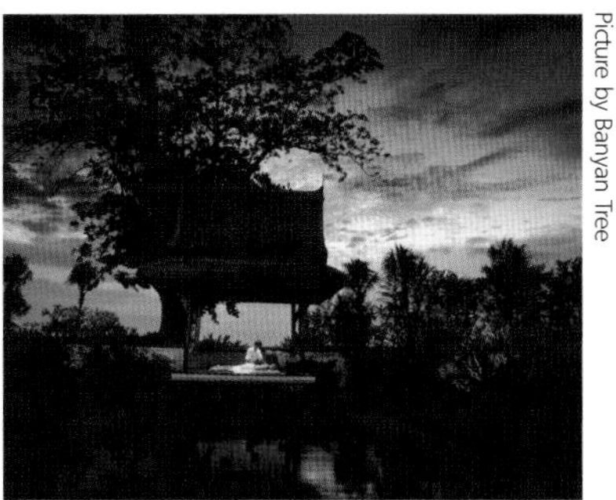
Picture by Banyan Tree

The spa environment should be a delight for the eyes

Sound

Be aware of the sounds a client will hear as this contributes to the overall sense of relaxation. Is it the sound of water, waves, bubbles or fountains? Is the music soothing and not too invasive and annoying. As part of the client's 'journey', do you consider and plan the sound used to enhance your treatments?

Picture by Banyan Tree

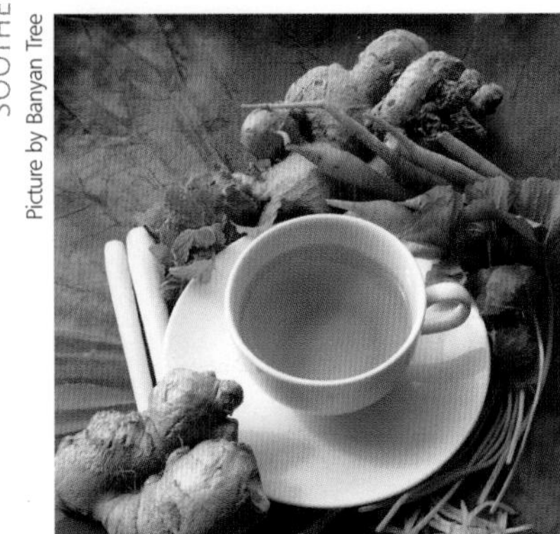

Clients need to have regular refreshment during their time at the spa

Courtesy of the Hilton Hua Hin Resort and Spa

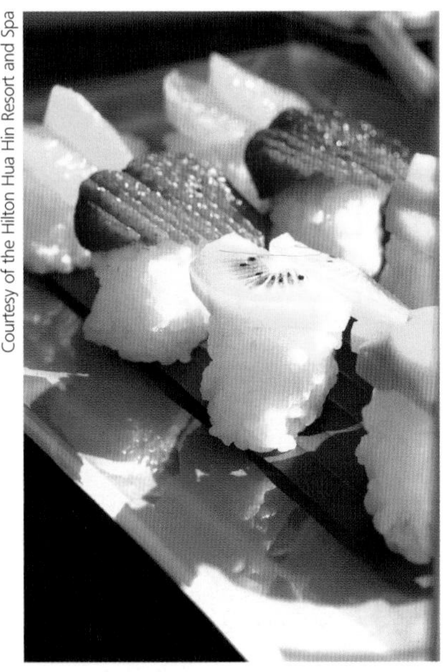

Spas encourage clients to eat and drink for health and wellness

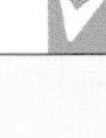

ACTIVITY

Choose a world-class spa. Conduct some research and produce a report as to how they perform against the ISPA 'Ten Elements of the Spa Experience'.

SPA TIP

Provide refreshments such as chilled water, freshly-squeezed juice, herbal teas and smoothies. Small snacks can also be provided, such as fruit platters. Some more decadent spas offer glasses of wine, chocolate brownies, etc., but many prefer to re-emphasize the healthy lifestyle by offering options such, as water and herbal teas for detoxification to accompany a de-tox treatment.

Taste

Taste can be included in the spa experience by considering the different drinks and refreshments you can offer throughout the spa experience.

Touch

Touch is one of the 'core' senses in spa therapy with treatments designed to maximize the fantastic benefits of touch on the body. Clients adore the physical feeling of 'touch' therapies – the body can feel lighter, more flexible and totally relaxed after a great body treatment. Water treatments are often extremely relaxing. The body is suspended in the water and feels 'weightless'.

THE SPA EXPERIENCE

A visit to a 'worldclass' spa should be an unforgettable experience that exceeds all expectations. The visit should be so enjoyable for the client that they can't wait to return, and they become a loyal client and an advocate for your spa.

The International Spa Association (ISPA) defines the spa experience as 'your time to relax, reflect, revitalize and rejoice'. ISPA have developed 'The Ten Elements of the Spa Experience' to help you plan and develop your spa treatments and experiences to get the best possible outcome. The ten Elements are:

- water
- nourishment
- movement
- touch
- integration
- aesthetics
- environment
- cultural expression
- social contribution
- time, space rhythms.

Integration

Some spas aim to integrate therapies and experiences that help take the client on a journey of personal fulfilment. They must then consider the relationship between mind, body, spirit and the environment. Spas may offer local cultural experiences, art, music, philosophy, as well as yoga, tai-chi and meditation.

Environment

Spas need to appreciate the environment in which they exist. Sustainability is a major influence in today's global economy so businesses have to have a strong moral compass. A spa must find a way to satisfy it's individuals and the community (locally and globally = 'glocal') by appreciating and using the earth's natural elements to enhance the health and vitality of its clients, without diminishing the health of future generations. Spas take into consideration environmental health, weather patterns, different water constitutions, cultural appreciation and the spirit of location and place.

SPA TIP 

Think how you can make your clients' spa journey as memorable and pleasurable as possible. Some spas offer a client a coin to throw into a fountain to make a wish at the beginning of the client journey. Others offer a crystal, angel card, mini-candle or small gift on leaving the spa.

SPA TIP 

Ensure you provide sufficient water in your establishment, especially in a spa with many heat and water treatments.

THE SPA JOURNEY: 'ROUTE MAP'

Stage 1. Anticipation and expectation

- Reputation.
- Website.
- Brochure/treatment menu.
- Telephone enquiry.
- Pre-information.
- Parking.
- External environment.

Stage 2: The actual journey

- Reception.
- Treatment room.
- The treatment.
- Relaxation/room.
- Reception/retail.
- Spa concierge.

SPA TIP

Freeze fruit into ice cubes, cranberries, lemon, raspberries, even mint. This looks attractive and flavours the glass of water when the ice cube melts.

Spa tip 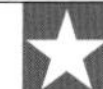

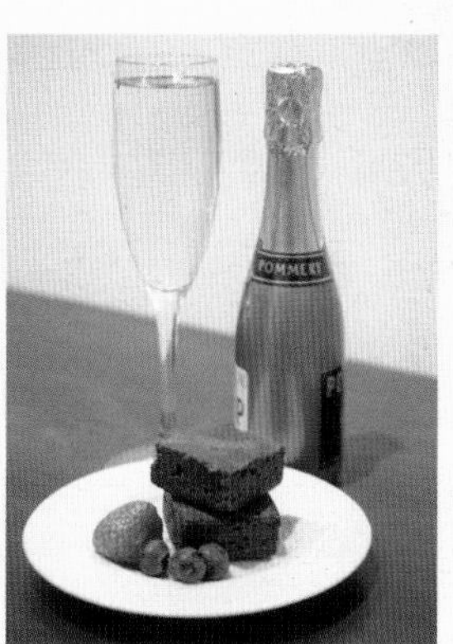

Some urban day spas offer 'indulgence packages', including champagne and chocolate brownies.

The type of spa and it's philosophy will dictate what refreshments are on offer. Chic, stylish urban day spas may want to attract a busy young 'fashionista' crowd and may offer champagne, cocktails, canapes, chocolate brownies, etc. The secret is to know your market and offer what the client wants.

Stage 3: Journey's end

- Follow-up card.
- Newsletters.
- Website – 'e-tail' opportunities.
- Promotions.

Spa cuisine

A number of spas employ nutritional specialists to work closely with the guests. They also run sessions or seminars to further educate the guests. They believe that the more the individual knows about what they are putting in their body, the healthier they will become. To ensure guests are able to continue the healthy regime at home, many spas now have their own spa cuisine books, on the spa philosophy, recipes, and menu combinations, etc.

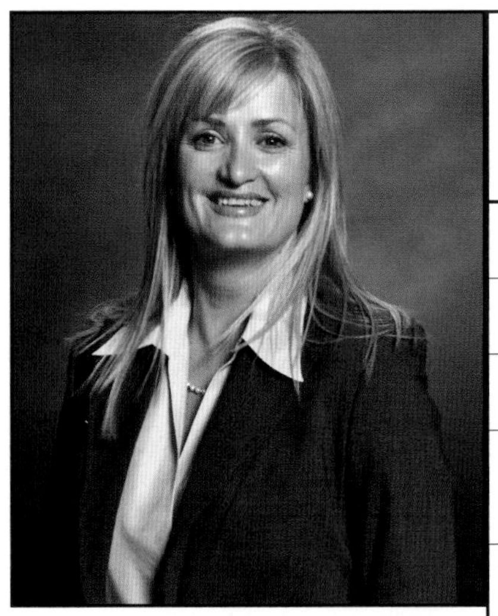

SPA PROFILE

Name: Suzanne Holbrook

Position: Executive Spa Director

Establishment: The Ritz-Carlton, Orlando, Grande Lakes, USA

Products used: Naturapathica, Carita, Acadamie, MD Skincare, Kerastase, Babor.

Number of staff/roles: 'I have 150 staff, in roles such as; spa directors, spa managers, senior spa therapists, massage therapists, fitness instructors, desk agents, spa concierges, manicure/pedicure specialists, estheticians, and retail agents.

Training/experience: 'Originally I went to college in Bury St Edmunds and did a 3-year apprenticeship in hairdressing. After years of running my own salon business I worked on cruise ships with Steiner Transocean, and quickly worked my way up in my first contract to become the spa manager. I stayed with Steiner for 6 years, and travelled all over the world. In 2000 I took a role with the Ritz-Carlton group, firstly as Spa Director in Puerto Rico, then opening a new Ritz-Carlton in Atlanta. Going on to opening a 40 000 sq ft Ritz-Carlton Spa in Orlando Florida.'

Main responsibilities: 'I head up a large department within the hotel, with 150 staff. I am a revenue manager with a high annual target. A lot of my time is spent on marketing and promotion, ensuring we maximize all business opportunities. Corporate clients, hotel guests and day guests all have individual needs, and we work hard to deliver an unsurpassed spa experience, which is consistently excellent. At the Ritz-Carlton we have a promise to the guest and a promise to the employees, and the culture of excellence runs throughout the organization.'

SPA TIP 

Luxury Spa Finder magazine found that the top five things that clients look for in spas are: weight loss, affordable, going solo, destination inclusive luxury.

SPA TIP 

At the Golden Door Spa simplicity is the key. Guests are provided with a warm-up suit, T-shirt, shorts, sandals, straw hat, rain poncho and a Japanese robe (yukata) so that the client can arrive without much luggage.

Best parts of the job: 'I love to see the spa team develop as well as the business, and focusing on achievements – I'm very target and results driven. I get huge satisfaction from making people happy, both my team and the spa guests. Fundamentally I am a revenue/income manager, and enjoy heading up a huge department with an annual revenue target in excess of $8 million.'

Secrets of a successful spa therapist: 'As an Executive Spa Director I have a passion for the business – I'm an over-achiever, and need to be careful I don't drive everybody crazy. I am very competitive and try to consistently exceed all targets. I strive to find a balance between being revenue/result driven and being caring and supportive to my staff. I believe balance is the answer to a successful business; it's a mixture of guest care, employee care and profits. The true secret to this business is the people we hire; they are the ones out there with the guests everyday, making a difference. I don't make a spa successful, my people do.'

SPA PROFILE

Name: Christine Meier

Position: Givenchy Spa Manager

Establishment: Givenchy Spa at the Health & Beauty Institute, One&Only Royal Mirage, Dubai

Products used: Givenchy

Number of staff/roles: Spa Manager, Head Therapist, Head Trainer, 7 Beauty Therapists, 3 Massage Therapists, 3 Receptionists

Training/Experience:
International School of Aesthetics, Massage School, USA – training,

School of Massage Charleston South Carolina.

Spa at Charleston Palace, Orient-Express Hotel Charleston, South Carolina, USA – Spa Director.

La Reserve, Geneva – Spa Manager.

Main responsibilities:
Meeting Income/revenue targets.

Liaison with PR/marketing.

Recruitment and selection of team members.

HR issues, appraisals, staff training and development.

Liaising with Givenchy and developing new treatments.

Best parts of the job:
'I enjoy every aspect of my role and absolutely love my job, especially: training and developing the therapists, the PR and marketing parts of the job, and meeting, greeting and talking with guests, clients and staff.'

Secrets of a successful spa therapist:
Hard work and staying focused.

Constantly trying to do the best you can – key to success in any role.

Surrounding yourself with people who have the knowledge and having a mentor who helps you develop. Never give up on knowledge. You are learning all the time, as things constantly change and as competition increases you have to stay on top. To improve you must constantly be learning.

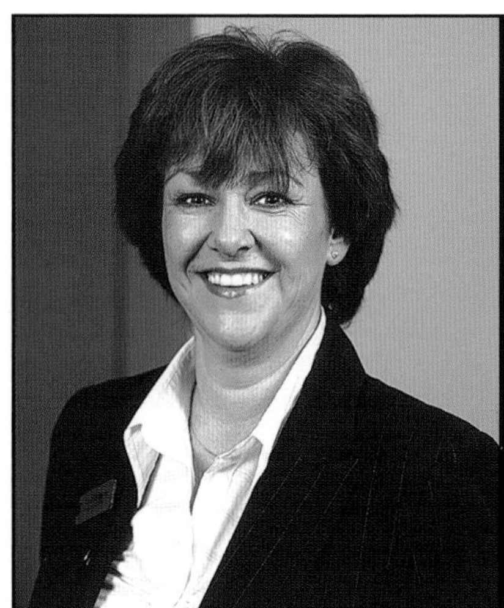

SPA PROFILE

Name: Trish Ridgway

Position: Spa Director

Establishment: Stobo Castle Health Spa, Peeblesshire, Scotland (Destination Spa)

Products used: Stobo Castle Products, Elemis, Finders, Thalgo, Phytomer, Vie, Darphin.

Number of staff/roles: 1 Spa Director, 1 Spa Manager, 1 Deputy Spa Manager, 1 Head Therapist, 10 Premier Therapists (promoted to this position), 6 Advanced Therapists (at least 2 years in the role), 8 Senior Therapists (at least a year in the role), 37 Therapists, 1 Training Manager, 1 Scheduling Manager, 1 Scheduling Assistant and 2 Spa Receptionists.

Training/experience:
Mary Reid College, Edinburgh – Beauty Therapy Qualifications

Ragdale Hall Health Spa – Therapist

Stobo Castle Health Spa – Spa Manager

Stobo Castle Health Spa – Spa Director since 2003

Main responsibilities:
Overseeing, managing and directing the spa operation.

Recruitment and selection.

Product ordering/stock checks.

Training schedule.

Appraisals and full range of HR procedures.

'Investors in People' (IiP) activity.

Managing Staff accommodation.

Ongoing liaison with the Marketing Director.

Best parts of the job:
I'm passionate about my job, Stobo castle and the spa industry generally.

I feel part of a 'family' here at Stobo. I'm very fortunate to work with such a fantastic team in a fabulous place.

I still occasionally do treatments, and love the 'hands on' part of the job.

I really enjoy developing new treatments that are unique to Stobo Castle.

Secrets of a successful spa therapist:
Commitment

Enthusiasm, a love for the industry, and that they really enjoy their job.

Great personality.

Very good personal presentation, and exceptional professional standards.

Punctual, and a good time-keeper.

Assessment of knowledge and understanding

When you have some free time, test your understanding and knowledge by answering the following questions. Do this at regular intervals and it will reinforce your learning and help you retain the knowledge, so you are able to perform better in your assessments.

1 List three types of consultation technique.

2 Where should client information be stored and in accordance with which guidelines?

3 Why is it important that records are kept accurate and up-to-date?

4 How should the therapist greet the client?

5 When should you refer a client to their doctor?

6 Why is it important to get the client's signature on the consultation record card?

7 Describe the appearance of stretch marks and cellulite.

8 List some of the causes of fluid retention.

9 List three possible causes of poor posture.

10 Describe the appearance of the postural fault lordosis.

11 Why is it important that the client and therapist are on time for appointments?

12 What is the recommended spa attire for a client's treatments?

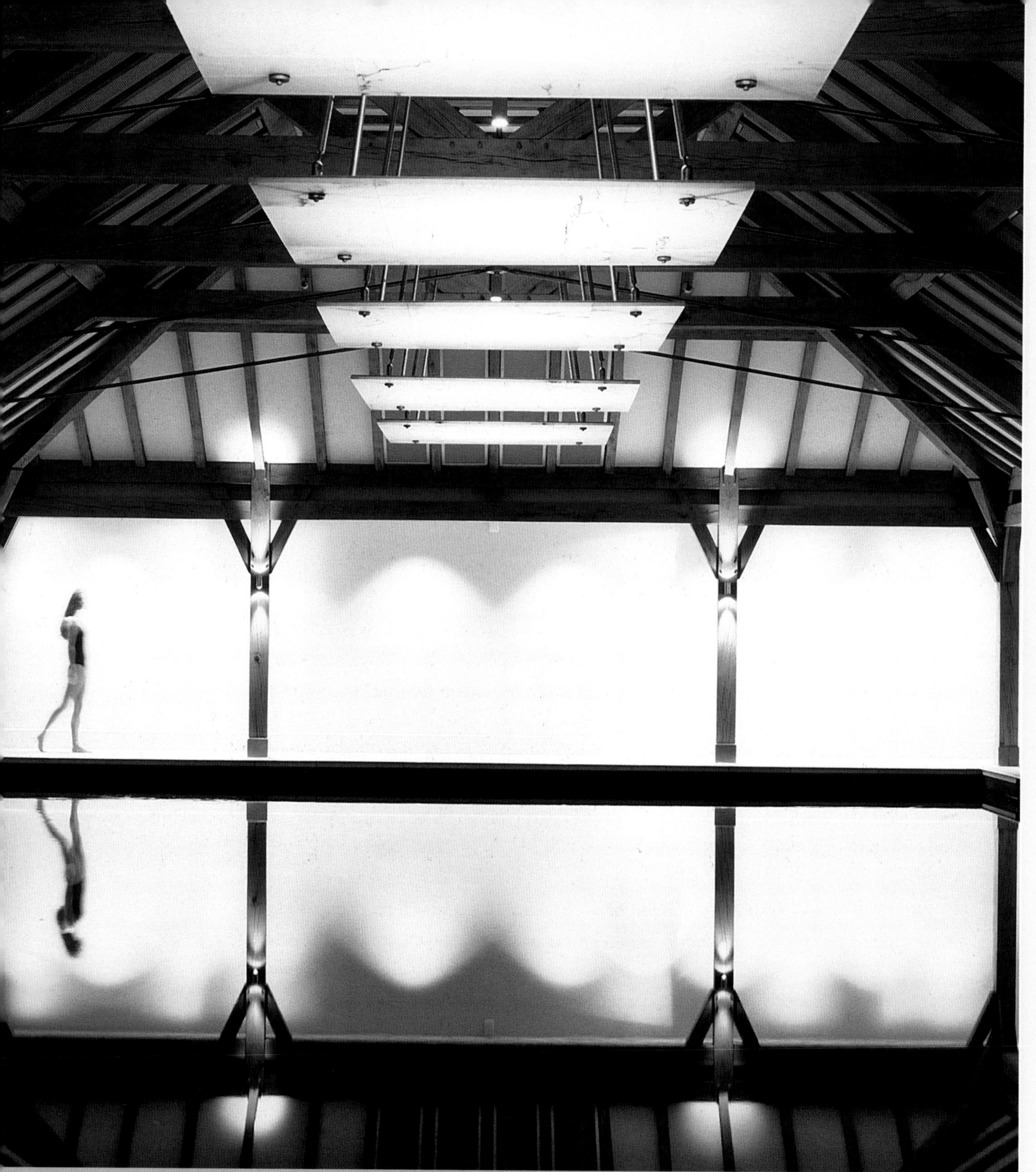

This is a **great time** to be entering the spa Industry. There is no other industry at the moment that is so open to **new talent** and which offers such **life-changing opportunities** to those who meet the demands, whether in terms of travel, personal development or career progression.

COLIN FARNDON, SPA DIRECTOR, THE GROVE, HERTFORDSHIRE

7 SEEK

The growth of the international spa industry over the past 5 years alone has been phenomenal. I'm delighted that the focus has moved toward caring for mind and spirit, not just the physical body. Mandarin Oriental were one of the first to recognize this and have made every effort to develop unique spa concepts around the world that allow our guests to find their inner balance.

HELEN NORMAN, SPA MANAGER, THE SPA AT MANDARIN ORIENTAL, LONDON

The growth of holistic awareness and therapies available is phenomenal, and has extended successfully to integrate into all types of spas. The next 10 years will be the most exciting times of the spa industry and will open doors to opportunities on a global scale. Our communities are now and will continue to obtain a deeper understanding and value concept of the health and wellness benefits that spa professionals offer to enhance their quality of lifestyle.

ANGELA DERKS ND, BHSC, MBA, AREA SPA MANAGER, SIX SENSES RESORTS AND SPA

spa directory

Clothing

Buttercups Collection
www.buttercupsuniforms.com

Cordcourt
www.cordcourt.co.uk

Daisy Chain
www.salonwear.co.uk

Dream Workwear Ltd
www.dreamworkwear.co.uk

Florence Roby
www.uniformcollection.com

Health and Beauty Wear
www.healthandbeautywear.
co.uk

Inline
www.inlinelondon.co.uk

La Beeby
www.labeeby.co.uk

Design/consultancy

Blue Spa & Leisure Consultancy
www.bluespaandleisure.com

Corporate Edge
www.corporateedge.com

HydoCo
www.hydroco.com

le spa
www.lespa.com

Spa Design Developments (SD3)
www.sd3uk.com

Spa Developments
www.spadevelopments.com

Equipment

Activewise
www.activewise.co.uk

Armadale UK
www.armadaleuk.com

Aromasteam
www.Aromasteam.co.uk

Aqua Massage
www.aquamassage.co.uk

Aquarelle Towels
www.lissadell.ie

Balnea
www.balnea.de

Barr + Wray water engineers
www.barrandwray.com

Beautelle
www.beautelle.co.uk

Beauty Express
www.beautyexpress.co.uk

Caci International
www.caci-international.co.uk

C'coon
www.transformyourtreatments.
co.uk

Cheshire Wellness
www.cheshire-spas-pools.co.uk

Comfort Zone
www.graftons.co.uk

Comfort Zone, Infrared Sauna Sales
www.comfortzoneir.co.uk

Crown Sports Lockers
www.crownlockers.co.uk

Dale Sauna
www.dalesauna.co.uk

Darley Therapy Equipment
www.darleytherapy.co.uk

Dawn Awakening Music
www.dawn-awakening-music.ltd.uk

Deckelmann Wellness
www.deckelmann-wellness.com

Ellisons
www.ellisons.co.uk

Floatworks
www.floatworks.com

Haslauer/Kurland
www.haslauer-gmbh.de

High Tech Health
www.hightechhealth.net

HoF (House of Famuir)
www.hofbeauty.co.uk

HTS (International)
www.hydrotherm.co.uk

HydroCo
www.hydroco.com

Hydro Jet Massage
www.hydrojetmassage.com

Hydro/massage
www.hydromassageuk.co.uk

Klafs
www.klafs.co.uk

LaStone Therapy
www.lastonetherapy.co.uk

Leisure Systems International Ltd
www.bodycare.co.uk

Majestic Towels
www.majestictowels.co.uk

Moor Spa International
www.moorspa.com

New World Music
www.newworldmusic.com

Nordic Saunas Ltd
www.nordic.co.uk

Oxygen Power Products
www.oxygenpower.co.uk

Salon-Relaxation
www.salonrelaxation.co.uk

Saunaland Sales
www.saunaland.com

ShouldersBack
www.shouldersback.co.uk

Solemates
www.solemates.co.uk

Sorisa
www.sorisa.co.uk

Spa Capsule
www.spacapsule.co.uk

Sterling Equipment
www.sterlingsupplies.co.uk

Stone Forest
www.stone-forest.co.uk

The (Carlton Beauty & Spa) Group
www.thecarltongroup.co.uk

The Egg, Balmoral Wellbeing Ltd
www.the-egg.co.uk

Thermarium
www.thermarium.co.uk

Totally UK
www.tuk.org.uk

Viking Saunas
www.viking-saunas.co.uk

Wave Dream, Verpo-Tech SA
www.helmuteigenmann.ch

Wellness for Health
www.wellnessforhealth.co.uk

Zen Lifestyle
www.zenlifestyles.co.uk

Products

ActiveWise
www.activewise.co.uk

Algotherm UK
www.algotherm.co.uk

Aromatherapy Associates
www.aromatherapyassociates.com

Aura-Soma
www.aura-soma.net

Babor
www.babor.de

Biodroga systems
www.beautyconcepts.co.uk

Catherine Everest (London) Ltd
www.catherineeverest.com

Clarins (UK) Ltd
www.clarins.com

Collin UK
www.collin.ltd.uk

Cosmeceuticals
www.skin-health.co.uk

Decleor
www.decleor.co.uk

Dermalogica
www.dermalogica.co.uk

Dr Sebagh
www.dr.sebagh.com

Elemis
www.elemis.com

E'Spa
www.espaonline.com

Eve Taylor Aromatherapy
www.eve-taylor.com

Finders
www.findershealth.com

Jericho Cosmetics
www.jerichocosmetics.co.uk

Karin Herzog
www.karinherzog.co.uk

Mineral Care Spa
www.mineralcare.co.uk

Natural Magic
www.naturalmagicuk.com

Nimue skin technology
www.nimueskin.com

Pevonia
www.pevonia.co.uk

Phytomer
www.phytomer.com

PLT Cosmetics & Consulting
www.plt-cosmetics.com

Premier Luxury Skin Care
www.premierskincareltd.co.uk

Repecharge
www.repechageuk.com

Sandra Day Aromatherapy Products
www.sandraday.com

Sothys
www.sothys.com

Spa Blends
www.spablends.co.uk

Thalgo
www.thalgo.co.uk

thisworks
www.thisworks.com

Tisserand
www.tisserand.com

Vitaman
www.vitaman.org.uk

Professional organizations (incl. H/S etc.)

Aromatherapy Consortium
www.aromatherapy-regulation.org.uk

Aromatherapy Trade Council
www.a-t-c.org.uk

British Association of Beauty Therapy and Cosmetology (BABTAC)
www.babtac.com

British International Spa Association (BISA)
www.spaassociation.org.uk

British Massage Therapy Council
www.bmtc.co.uk

Federation of Holistic Therapists
www.fht.org.uk

Floatation Tank Association
www.floatationtankassociation.net

Hair and Beauty Industry Authority (HABIA)
www.habia.org.uk

Health and Safety Executive
www.hse.gov.uk

Independent Professional Therapists International
www.iptiuk.com

Institute of Indian Head Massage
www.indianheadmassage.org

Institute of Optimum Nutrition
www.ion.ac.uk

International Federation of Aromatherapists
www.ifaroma.org

International Federation of Professional Aromatherapists
www.ifparoma.org

International Guild of Professional Practitioners
www.igpp.co.uk

International Spa Association (ISPA)
www.experienceispa.com

Santi Development Programmes
www.santi-santi.com

Spa Business Association
www.spabusinessassociation.co.uk

Swimming Pool and Allied Trades Association (SPATA)
www.spata.co.uk

The Prince's Trust
www.princes-trust.org.uk

Publications/books/websites

Beauty & Health Publishing
www.bhpublishing.co.uk

Great Spa Escapes (Jo Foley)
www.dakinibooks.com

Guild Press
www.beautyserve.net

Luxury Spa Finders Magazine
www.spafinder.com

Professional Spa
www.professionalbeauty.co.uk

Spa Space
www.spaspace.co.uk

Spa Style Asia
www.thamesandhudson.com

The Spirit of Yoga (Kathy Phillips)
Zen In Your Garden (Jenny Hendy)
www.tuttlepublishing.com

Recruitment

Active Connection
www.activeconnection.co.uk

Barbara Simpson-Birks (BSB)
www.idbeauty.co.uk

Beautyjobsonline.com
www.beautyjobsonline.com

Beauty Recruited.Co.Uk
www.beautyrecruited.co.uk

Beauty Recruitment Plus
www.Beautyrecruitment.com

hair and beauty jobs.com
www.hairandbeautyjobs.com

Hardings Salon & Spa
www.hardingspa.co.uk

Hardings Spa Division
www.hardingspa.co.uk

La Source Spa Recruitment
www.la-sourcejobs.com

LeisureJobs.co.uk
www.leisurejobs.co.uk

Lima Recruitment
www.limarecruitment.co.uk

Pitchblue
www.pitchblue.co.uk

Red
www.redhotcareers.co.uk

Steiner (cruiseships)
www.steinerleisure.com

Spas (UK)

Agua Bathhouse Spa, Sanderson, London
www.sandersonlondon.com

Aquarias, Wiltshire
www.whatleymanor.com

Aveda Experience, London
www.urbanretreat.co.uk

Bath House Spa
www.royalcrescent.co.uk

British Spas
www.visitbritain.com/spa

(The) Balmoral Spa, Edinburgh
www.thebalmoralhotel.com

(The) Berkeley Health Club & Spa, London
www.the-berkeley.com

Bliss Spa, London
www.blissworld.com

Calcot Spa, Wiltshire
www.calcotmanor.co.uk

Calmia, London
www.calmia.com

Cedar Falls health farm, Somerset
www.cedar-falls.co.uk

Celtic Manor, Wales
www.celtic-manor.com

Champneys Health Resorts
www.champneys.com

Chapel Spa, Cheltenham
www.chapelspa.co.uk

Chewton Glen Spa, Hampshire
www.chewtonglen.com

Cowshed Spa, Babington House, Somerset
www.babingtonhouse.co.uk

Cowshed Spa, Edinburgh
www.thescotsmanhotel.co.uk

C-Side, Cowley Manor, Gloucs.
www.cowleymanor.com

Danubius
www.danubiushotels.com

Elemis Day Spa, London
www.elemis.com

Gleneagles, Scotland
www.gleneagles.com

Ki Day Spa, Altrincham, Cheshire
www.kidayspa.co.uk

Lakeside Spa, Cumbria
www.lakesidehotel.co.uk

ONE Spa, Edinburgh
www.one-spa.com

Oyster Spa Company
www.theoysterspacompany.com

Ragdale Hall Health Hydro, Leicestershire
www.ragdalehall.co.uk

Senspa, Hampshire
www.careysmanor.com

Sequoia at The Grove, Herts.
www.thegrove.co.uk

Sienna Spa & Health Club, Manchester
www.radisson.com

St Davids Hotel and Spa, Cardiff
www.roccofortehotels.com

Stobo Castle, Scotland
www.stobocastle.co.uk

The Refinery, London
www.the-refinery.com

The Sanctuary, London
www.thesanctuary.co.uk

The Serenity Spa, Seaham Hall, Co. Durham
www.seaham-serenityspa.com

The Sodashi Spa, London
www.51-buckinghamgate.com

The Spa, Chancery Court, London
www.renaissancehotels.com

The Spa, The Lowry Hotel, Manchester
www.roccofortehotels.com

The Spa at Mandarin Oriental, London
www.mandarinoriental.com

The Spa at Pennyhill Park, Surrey
www.exclusivehotels.co.uk

Urban Retreat at Harrods
www.urbanretreat.co.uk

Spas (international)

Agua Spa at The Delano, Miami Beach
www.delanohotelmiamibeach.com

Aimia Hotel, Majorca
www.aimiahotel.com

Aman Spa, Thailand
www.amanresorts.com

Amrita Spa, Singapore
www.amritaspas.com

Ananda – in the Himalayas, India
www.anandaspa.com

Angsana Spa Bintan, Indonesia
www.angsana.com

Angsana Spa Double Bay, Australia
www.angsanaspa.com

Assawan Spa, Burj-al-Arab, Dubai
www.burj-al-arab.com

Aurora Spa retreat, Melbourne, Australia
www.theprince.com.au

Azure Spa, Lizard island, Australia
www.lizardisland.co.au

Banyan Tree Ringha, China
www.banyantree.com

Banyan Tree Spa, Bangkok, Thailand
www.banyantreespa.com

Banyan Tree Spa, Maldives
www.banyantree.com

Banyan Tree Spa, Phuket, Thailand
www.banyantree.is

Beauty Center, Positano, Italy
www.sirenuse.it

Bliss Soho, New York
www.blissworld.com

Blue Lagoon, Iceland
www.bluelagoon.is

Blue Palace, Crete
www.bluepalace.gr

Blue Spa at Carlisle Bay, Antigua
www.carlisle-bay.com

Brenners Hotel and Spa
www.brenners.com

Bulgari Hotel Spa, Italy
www.bulgarihotels.com

Canyon Ranch, California
www.canyonranch.com

Capri Palace Hotel and Spa, Italy
www.capripalace.com

Caracalla Spa, Dubai
www.leroyalmeridien-dubai.com

Chaa Creek, Belize
www.chaacreek.com

CHI, The Spa at Shangri-La, Bangkok
www.shangri-la.com/spa

Chiva-Som International Health Resort, Thailand
www.chivasom.com

Chopra Center & Spa, New York
www.dreamny.com

Chuan Spa, Melbourne, Australia
www.langhamhotels.com

Cinq Mondes Spa, Switzerland
www.brp.ch

Cleopatra's Spa, Dubai
www.waficity.com

Clinique la Prairie, Switzerland
www.laprairie.ch

Como Shambhala Retreat at Parrot Cay, Turks & Caicos
www.shambhalaretreat.com

COMO Shambhala Urban Escape, Bangkok
www.comoshambhala.bz

Daintree Eco Lodge & Spa, Australia
www.daintree-ecolodge.com.au

Danubius Hungary, Budapest
www.danubiushotels.com

Danubius Italia
www.danubiushotelsungheria.com

Delphi Spa, Ireland
www.delphiescape.com

Devarana Spa, Bangkok
www.devarana.com

ESPA at Acqualina, Florida
www.rosewoodhotels.com

Evian Roya Spa, France
www.royalparcevian.com

Givenchy Spa, One&Only Le Saint Geran, Mauritius
www.oneandonlyresorts.com

Givenchy Spa, One&Only Le Touessrok, Mauritius
www.oneandonlyresorts.com

Givenchy Spa, One&Only Royal Mirage, Dubai
www.oneandonlyroyalmirage.com

Golden Door, California
www.goldendoor.com

GSpa, Ireland
www.theghotel.ie

Habits Culti, Italy
www.habitsculti.it

Healing Waters Spa, Australia
www.silkyoakslodge.com.au

Helen Spa, Moorea
www.helenspa.com

Hotel & Spa Rosa Alpina, Italy
www.rosalpina.it

I-Spa by Algotherm, Paris
www.paris-le-grand.intercontinental.com

Kai Belte Spa, St Lucia
www.ansechastanet.com

Kalari Kovilakom, India
www.cghearth.com

Kandholhu, Maldives
www.universalresorts.com

Kurumba, Maldives
www.kurumba.com

Kuurotel Longevity Center and Spa, Brazil
www.kuurotel.com.br

La Costa Resort & Spa, California
www.lacosta.com

La Jolla Spa MD, California
www.spa-md.com

La Reserve Geneve, Switzerland
www.lareserve.ch

Las Ventanas al Paraiso, Mexico
www.lasventanas.com

Les Sources de Caudalie, France
www.sources-caudalie.com

Lilianfels Blue Mountain Resort & Spa, Australia
www.lilianfels.orient-express.com

L'Institut de Guerlain, Mauritius
www.princemaurice.com

L'Institut de Guerlain, Paris
www.guerlain.com

Mandara Spa, Bangkok
www.mandaraspa.com

Mandara Spa, Malaysia
www.ghmhotels.com

Mardavall Hotel & Spa, Mallorca
www.mardavall-hotel.com/spa

Marienbad Kur & Spa Hotels
www.marienbad.cz

Mayr health Spa, Austria
www.golfhotel.at

Mii Amo Enchantment Resort, Arizona
www.miiamo.com

Monart, Ireland
www.monart.ie

Oberoi Spa, India
www.oberoihotels.com

One&Only Maldives at Reethi Rah
www.oneandonlyresorts.com

One&Only Spa at One&Only Palmilla, Mexico
www.oneandonlyresorts.com

Oriental Spa, Bangkok
www.mandarinoriental.com

Peninsula Spa, Hong Kong
www.peninsula.com

Polynesian Spa, New Zealand
www.polynesianspa.co.nz

Rancho La Puerto
www.rancholapeurta.com

Ritz-Carlton Orlando, Florida
www.ritzcarlton.com

Samas Spa, Park Hotel Kenmare, Ireland
www.samaskenmare.com

Sanctuary Spa, South Africa
www.12apostleshotel.com

Sandy Lane, Barbados (The Spa)
www.sandylane.com

Sante Winelands Hotel & Wellness Centre, South Africa
www.santewellness.co.za

SeaSpa, Ireland
www.kellys.ie

Sereno Spa at Park Hyatt Goa Resort, India
www.goa.park.hyatt.com

Six Senses Spa, Evason Resort Hua-Hin, Thailand
www.sixsenses.com/evason-huahin

Six Senses Spa, Dubai
www.madinatjumeirah.com

Six Senses Spa, Soneva Fushi Resort, Maldives
www.six-senses.com

Six Senses Spa, Soneva Gili Resort, Maldives
www.six-senses.com

Slovak Health Spa, Piestany
www.spa-piestany.sk

Spa & Salon Bellagio, Las Vegas
www.bellagio.com

Spa Botanica, Singapore
www.thesentosa.com

Spa Chakra at W Sydney, Australia
www.whotels.com

Spa Chakra Hayman, Australia
www.hayman.com.au

Spa Village, Malaysia
www.pangkorlautresort.com

Taj Exotica Resort & Spa, Maldives
www.tajhotels.com

Terme di Saturnia Spa, Italy
www.termedisaturnia.it

Thalassa Spa, Cyprus
www.Anassa.cyprushotels.org.uk

The Bodyholiday at LeSport, St Lucia
www.lesport.com.lc

The Lyall Spa, Australia
www.thelyall.com

The Ritz-Carlton Spa, Bali
www.ritzcarlton.com

The Ritz-Carlton Spa, Miami
www.ritzcarlton.com

The Source at Begawan Giri, Bali
www.begawan.com

The Spa, Aghadoe Heights, Ireland
www.thanoshotels.com

The Spa, Hilton Hua Hin, Thailand
www.huahin.hilton.com

The Spa, Hilton Phuket, Thailand
www.hilton.com

The Spa, La Residencia, Mallorca
www.hotellaresidencia.com

The Spa, Sebel Reef House Palm Cove, Australia
www.espa.net.au

The Spa, Victoria-Jungfrau, Grand Hotel, Switzerland
www.victoria-jungfrau.ch

The Spa at Choupana Hills Resort, Portugal
www.choupanahills.com

The Spa at Four Seasons, Capsule, Australia
www.fourseasons.com

The Spa at Four Seasons Hotel George V, Paris
www.fourseasons.com

The Spa at Four Seasons Resort, Bali
www.fourseasons.com

The Spa at Four Seasons Resort, Thailand
www.fourseasons.com

The Spa at Four Seasons Resort, Whistler, Canada
www.fourseasons.com

The Spa at Mandarin Oriental, Miami
www.mandarin-oriental.com

The Spa at Mandarin Oriental, New York
www.mandarinoriental.com

The Spa at Round Hill Hotel, Jamaica
www.roundhilljamaica.com

The Spa at the Beverley Wiltshire, Los Angeles
www.fourseasons.com

The Spa at The Breakers, Florida
www.thebreakers.com

The Spa at the Lodge Torrey Pines, California
www.lodgetorreypines.com

The Spa at The Setai, Miami
www.setai.com

The Spa Retreat, Maldives
www.hilton.com

Therme Vals, Switzerland
www.therme-vals.ch

Two Bunch Palms, California
www.twobunchpalms.com

Vichy Spa at Hosteria Las Balsas, Argentina
www.lasbalsas.com

Vida Wellness Spa, Fairmont Chateau, Whistler
www.vidawellness.com

Wildflower Hall, India
www.oberoiwildflowerhall.com

Willow Steam, The Spa at the Fairmont Empress, Canada
www.willowstream.com

Willow Stream Spa, Dubai
www.fairmont.com

Spa management software

Baron Resort Manager software
www.baron.co.uk

ESP Salon/Spa software
www.esponline.info

EZ-BOOK
www.ezbook.co.uk

Gladstone MRM
www.gladstonemrm.com

Premier Software Solutions
www.premiersoftware.co.uk

Reservation Assistant
www.reservationassistant.com

Training/awarding bodies

Confederation of International Beauty Therapy and Cosmetology (CIBTAC)
www.cibtac.com

City and Guilds of London Institute (CGLI)
www.city-and-guilds.co.uk

Edexcel/BTEC
www.edexcel.org.uk

International Therapy Examinations Council (ITEC)
www.itecworld.co.uk

Vocational Training Charitable Trust (VTCT)
www.vtct.org.uk

glossary

Acupuncture tiny, fine needles are used on certain meridian points in the body to increase the flow of energy through the body and stimulate particular organs associated with these pressure points.

Acupressure a traditional Chinese form of massage which works on the same pressure points on the body as acupuncture. Instead of using needles, pressure is applied with the fingertip to release any blocked energies.

Adipose tissue the term used to describe the fatty tissue of the body. Massage cannot break down fatty tissue as this could be very dangerous.

Alexander Technique this technique of posture alignment is taught on a one-to-one basis where the client is re-educated to regain natural posture and use the body more efficiently. It can help with stress, breathing disorders and neck and joint pain.

Algotherapy marine-based products are applied to the body in order to relax and detoxify the body.

Anterior front.

Aromatherapy essential oils are applied on the body through massage, inhalation, facials, baths, treatment products, etc. The choice of essential oils and blends used will determine the therapeutic benefits.

Asanas yoga postures.

Ayurveda originally founded in India, this ancient discipline incorporates herbs, massage, diet, meditation and yoga to balance the body systems and restore health.

Bach flower remedies developed by Dr Edward Bach a simple system of 38 flower remedies to heal and balance negative thoughts, as these can lead to physical disease.

Balance sheet shows what your business has earned and spent, any assets in the bank, who owes you money and any investments you may have made such as new equipment, etc.

Balinese massage a deep tissue massage using the thumbs and palms of the hand to release tensions. Traditionally performed using coconut oil.

Balinese boreh a traditional paste made from herbs and spices is applied to the body and the client is wrapped in a blanket. The paste warms the body, which helps stimulate the circulation and relax the muscles.

Balneotherapy mineral-rich water is used for the client to bathe in, to relieve tension in the body.

Botox used to freeze muscles in the face to minimize the appearance of wrinkles and lines.

Buoyancy in water when the body is balanced and still in water due to two opposing forces: buoyancy and gravity. Buoyancy is an upward direction and gravity is a downward direction.

Bursae these are small sacs of synovial fluid that help reduce friction between a tendon and a bone. An inflammation of the sac results in bursitis.

Centre of ossification cluster of osteoblasts where bone tissue develops. There are three such centres in a long bone.

Chakras there are seven energy centres in the body, which are associated with the body's subtle energy flows.

Champissage the traditional term used in India for head massage. It originates from the Hindu word 'champi' which means head massage. In the West this term has been used to describe a hacking technique affiliated with Indian head massage.

Chill treatments Sometimes referred to as 'cold' treatments.

Chiropractic a practice of re-aligning the spine and body mechanics to alleviate backache and postural problems.

Clavicle the collarbone.

Climatotherapy treatments which use the forces of nature, including air, light, wind, sun, humidity and location.

Collagen can be injected into lines and wrinkles to plump out their appearance. Is also an ingredient of skincare and treatment products.

Colonic irrigation used to cleanse the colon and remove trapped impurities, which may have built up over years. Can be used as a form of detoxification.

Contra-action an unwanted reaction to treatment.

Contra-indication a condition of the body that prevents the treatment from being carried out.

Cranio-sacral therapy gentle manipulation of the bones of the skull which can balance the flow of the cerebrospinal fluid to stimulate the body's self-healing ability. It is very relaxing and is beneficial for migraines, dizziness and sinus problems and is suitable for use on babies.

Cryotherapy constriction of the blood vessels in the skin and muscles by applying cold or frozen products to create a lift in the skin.

Crystal therapy the use of crystals and gemstones to cleanse the body and balance energy levels.

Dead Sea therapy uses mineral-rich products from the Dead Sea, such as mud, to cleanse and relax the muscles. Products can also be used to relieve arthritis and rheumatic pains.

Desquamation the removal of dead skin cells in layers or flakes through rubbing or general friction.

Discs/menisci pads of fibro-cartilage which are attached to the bones and allow the joint to fit better, e.g. cartilage in the knee joint.

Dry skin brush a natural bristle brush that is used dry on the skin to exfoliate dead skin cells and stimulate the circulatory and lymphatic system.

Effleurage a French word meaning 'to skim over'.

Envelopment usually refers to a treatment where the body is wrapped fully – , the limbs are not wrapped individually but together with the body. This is usually carried out for detoxifying and skin conditioning purposes.

Erythaema a reddening of the skin caused by dilation of the blood vessels. It can be a result of physically increasing the blood flow, such as with massage, or because the body is hot or affected by injury or infection.

Exfoliation the removal of the top layer of dead skin cells on the body and face using scrubs, dry skin brush, peels or other techniques.

Fangotherapy mud with a high mineral content is warmed and applied on the body to help detoxify the body and warm the muscles, alleviating aches and pains.

Flotation a shallow pool or tank is filled with mineral-rich salt water where the client is allowed to float to relax and de-stress. Dry flotation takes place on a bed, which is filled with water and covered with a heavy waterproof sheet, which the client lies on before being lowered into the water.

Flexor muscles muscles which cause a 'flexion' movement, which is a bending or folding action at a joint, e.g. bending the elbow.

Four handed massage two therapists perform a massage on the body using slow, synchronized movements.

Hammam a Turkish bath which uses steam, water and oils to help cleanse the body.

Hay wrap using steamed organic alpine hay to cleanse and detoxify the body.

Hazard expose to danger.

Health spa the name given to a place where the main interest is health, and people attend for therapeutic purposes.

Herbal wrap strips of cloth are soaked in a heated herbal solution and wrapped around the body and the client is then covered with a heated blanked to maintain the temperature. Is used for relaxation and detoxifying.

Holistic the consideration of the complete person in the treatment of disease, often translated as the mind, body and spirit of the individual.

Homeopathy based on the concept that 'like cures like' for treating minor diseases using minute proportions of natural plant extracts.

Hot spring naturally occurring spring of hot mineral water, which is used in treatments for its therapeutic properties.

Humidity refers to the amount of moisture in the air. 'Relative humidity' is the measurement of moisture content as a percentage of the maximum it can hold at that temperature. The maximum capacity of moisture in the air is 100%. Dry heat treatments such as saunas have a low humidity, often as low as 10%. Whereas wet heat treatments such as steam baths have high humidity, often as high as 90%. Humidity is measured by a hygrometer.

Hydrotherapy treatments using water in jet blitzes, underwater massage, pressure showers and mineral baths.

Indian head massage a traditional Indian massage in which Ayurvedic oils are massaged into the scalp, face, neck and shoulders using acupressure massage techniques to rebalance the body's energies.

Iridology analysis of the iris in the eye, where areas are linked to specific body parts and functions. A diagnostic tool to spot any problems and recommend appropriate treatment.

Inhalation therapy using steam in treatments combined with essential oils.

Javanese lulur a traditional Balinese treatment devised for royal brides to prepare the body before the wedding. A paste of sandalwood, tumeric and powdered spices is rubbed onto the body. It is traditionally removed either with yoghurt or by bathing in a floral milk bath.

Jet blitz a jet of pressurized seawater is blasted through a hose held by a therapist onto the client's body, who is standing up against a wall. Depending on the desired effect the water can be hot or cold.

Kinesiology a diagnostic testing of muscles to diagnose and treat diseases.

Kneipp therapy hot and cold herbal baths are used by the client alternately to stimulate the circulation and create a feeling of wellbeing.

La Stone or hot stone massage using heated volcanic stones and cold marble stones in a body massage to release tension from the muscles and balance the body's energy centres.

Labour costs this is not just based on the therapist's salary but needs to include all other staffing costs involved in the spa.

Lateral outer surface.

Ligaments join bone to bone. They are made of very strong fibrous tissue, and are responsible for the stability of joints and of the body generally.

Liquid sound the use of light and music in water treatments for relaxation and visualization.

Lomi-Lomi originating from Hawaii this form of massage uses the forearms and elbows as well as the hands, to give a rhythmical, rocking massage.

Lymphatic drainage massage using a gentle pumping pressure technique to drain areas of fluid retention, stimulate lymphatic circulation and remove toxins.

Massage thought to be derived from the Arabic word 'to press softly' and the Greek word 'to knead'. Massage can be described as a 'scientific method of manipulating the body tissues'.

Medial inner surface.

Meditation can be practised in many different forms using breath techniques, a mantra, chanting and visualization to clear the mind and focus. Helps to release stress and bring about a deep sense of relaxation.

Metabolism the term used to describe how the body converts food and other substances into energy for its own use. If food is not correctly metabolized certain diseases can occur, such as obesity, gout and diabetes, while a sluggish metabolism can lead to skin problems and an overall sluggish, sallow and dull appearance.

Moor mud baths a naturally occurring mud rich in mineral and proteins, which helps ease aches and pains in the muscles. The client is coated in the mud or relaxes in a bath full of it.

Naturopathy a healthcare system that features only natural ingredients and disciplines to help the body heal itself.

Oedema means 'swelling', where the tissue fluid accumulates instead of draining away and returning to the blood system. This can be caused by poor circulation or a medical condition (contra-indicated).

Ossification the process of bone formation.

Osteoblast bone-building cells.

Osteocyte osteoblasts that have become calcified.

Overheads this may involve general overheads such as rent, rates and laundry; indirect material costs such as furniture, décor and repairs; employment costs such as staff training, uniforms and commission; and marketing costs such as brochures, price lists and posters.

Petrissage a French word, which is derived from the verb 'petrir' which means 'to knead'.

Pelotherapy mud treatments.

Phototoxic refers to some essential oils that make the skin more sensitive to sunlight.

Phytotherapy treatments using natural herbs, plants, mineral products and essential oils to heal the body.

Pilates a series of precise movements designed by Dr Joseph Pilates for dancers to help strengthen and re-align the body and improve flexibility.

Posterior back.

Prone lying lying face down.

Rasul an ancient Arabic cleansing and bathing ritual using different muds applied onto the body in a steam room where the client relaxes before a rain-like shower washes the mud off.

Reflexology a pressure point massage used on the reflex zones in the feet (and sometimes hands and ears) to promote self healing and restore energy levels in the body.

Reiki an ancient Japanese therapy which involves the laying of hands on or just above the body to balance the body's energy flow, clear blockages and promote deep relaxation.

Regression therapy healing through being taken back to previous experiences or past states.

Risk the possibility of injury or damage.

Salt glow a mixture of coarse salt and aromatic oils is massaged on the body to exfoliate and stimulate circulation.

Sauna a wooden room which is full of dry heat steam created from a thermostatically controlled heater in the room. Is used to open the pores, relax the muscles and remove toxins.

Seasonal affective disorder (SAD) a disorder in which the mood of the affected person changes according to the season of the year, typically when winter starts. They feel depressed and need to sleep a lot, and some people even feel suicidal. It is not a generally accepted illness but is believed to be caused by the lack of natural light suppressing the release of the hormone melatonin from the pineal gland, which acts as the natural 'body clock'.

Seaweed wrap freeze-dried seaweed is mixed with warm water and applied to the body and then covered with a heated blanket to detoxify and revitalize the skin.

Shiatsu a massage technique originating in Japan which uses fingertip pressure on acupressure points and meridians of the body to release blockages and improve the flow of energy in the body.

Shirodhara a traditional Ayurvedic treatment using a continuous flow of warm oil slowly poured over the client's third eye to induce deep relaxation.

Signature treatment a treatment especially created and devised by the spa or spa group and which is exclusive to their brand.

Spa thought to be derived from the Latin phrase 'solus per aqua' which means 'health from water'. 'Spa' is only used in English-speaking countries and across Europe there are a variety of names used for water related health resorts. In Germany 'kurort' may be used and means 'place of cure', and 'bad' is often used as part of a geographic location. 'Les bains' is the French name for Spa, whereas in Italy they use 'terme' and in Spain 'baños'.

Sports massage deep tissue massage which can be used before carrying out any sports activity to warm the muscles, increase the range of movement and reduce the risk of any injuries.

Sternum breastbone.

Supine lying lying face up.

Swedish massage classic massage technique using stroking, kneading and tapotement movements to stimulate circulation and relax muscles.

Swiss shower the client lies on a wet bed and powerful fine jets of water are directed on to the body from above.

T'ai chi a Chinese martial art style of movements, which are performed in a set sequence, very slowly and concentrating on the breathing whilst being carried out.

Tendon join muscles to bones. If a tendon is very flat and broad it is called an 'aponeurosis'.

Tepidarium the term given to the warm (tepidus) bathroom of the roman baths, traditionally decorated with rich marbles and mosaics.

Thai massage one of the few massages where oil is not used and the movements are performed over the client's loose clothing. Yoga-style moves are used to stretch the body, as well as kneading and exerting pressure along the meridians using the elbows, knees and palms to help release blockages.

Thai herbal heat packs a massage using a pouch of steamed herbs such as ginger, lime leaves and eucalyptus pressed against the skin to warm the tissues and relax the body.

Thalassotherapy the therapeutic use of seawater, algae and marine mud, which are rich in minerals and vitamins, as part of treatments. True thalassotherapy centres are built close to the sea.

Thermal-auricular therapy often known as hopi ear candles after the native American Indian tribe who used these herbal candles to cleanse the ears and head.

Thermodynamic using heat to reach a deeper level of massage.

Tonicite means a very bracing and toning effect.

Toxicity is what we call poisonousness. In aromatherapy this depends upon whether the oil has been taken orally or absorbed through the skin.

Tuina a traditional Chinese massage, which pummels, pulls and rolls the body to help release blocked energies and improve any muscular ailments.

Vichy shower similar to a Swiss shower, where the client lies on a wet table and a rain-like shower of varying temperature massages the body. Can be incorporated with manual massage.

Vinotherapy using grape extracts combined with essential oils in body, facial and massage treatments to hydrate, tone and relax the body.

Watsu similar to shiatsu massage but the client floats in warm water supported by a therapist who stretches and moves the limbs and uses pressure point techniques to encourage relaxation.

Wrap the client is covered in mud, seaweed, oils, creams, etc., and wrapped in either a type of foil blanket to keep in body heat or a heated waterproof blanket. The heat helps the body to absorb the products and release any toxins from the body.

Whirlpool a tub or bath of warm water in which the client bathes whilst being pummelled with jets of water, which are situated on the sides and bottom.

Yin and yang yin energy is characterized by feminine, cool, quiet, dark and wet, while yang energy is male, bright, sunny, dry and warm. The Chinese believe that to achieve a healthy body and lifestyle there should be an equal balance of the two.

Yoga an ancient Hindu practice focusing on the breath. A sequence of postures to stretch, strengthen and increase the body's flexibility whilst achieving a mental clarity.

Zen garden minimalist, simple gardens originating from Japan where they are used for meditation and relaxation.

index